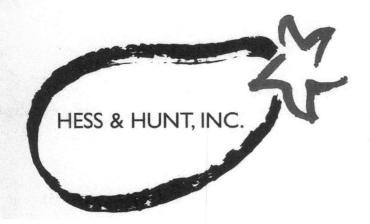

NUTRITION COMMUNICATIONS

REVIEW OF DIETETICS

Manual for the Registered Dietitian Exam

2014 – 2015 edition

Mary Abbott Hess, LHD, MS, RD, LDN, FAND, Editor

Published by Hess & Hunt, Inc.
3750 N. Lake Shore Drive, #3A
Chicago, IL 60613-4238
Phone: 773-348-2200

Printed in Eau Claire, WI by Documation, LLC.
ISBN# 978-0-9816769-6-8

For information about this book, or to order in quantity, contact:
Hess & Hunt, Inc. Nutrition Communications
E-mail: reviewdietetics@aol.com
www.reviewofdietetics.com
Phone: 847-251-6648

Individual copies are available on Amazon.com

Preface

The *Review of Dietetics: Manual for the Registered Dietitian Exam,* along with your individual study, should provide you with the skills and confidence you need to pass the registration examination and can prepare you for a successful career in dietetics. Previous editions of *Review of Dietetics* have helped thousands pass the credentialing examination.

Developing a comprehensive manual that reflects current dietetic practice is an enormous professional challenge. All of us who have worked so hard on this manual have been motivated by a desire to upgrade professional practices. We know that earlier editions of the manual have helped generations of dietetic education program graduates become registered. Over the past 30 years, the book has become a text and reference for educators, students, dietetic interns and is found in many libraries.

This manual is the most comprehensive study guide available to graduates preparing for the dietetic registration examination. In some ways, it is a "work in progress," having been constantly improved, updated, reformatted and expanded since its first edition in 1984. It is the result of thousands of hours of gathering, and updating information by dietetic educators, practitioners and content experts. There have been endless discussions of what is essential content for entry-level practice. The manual has been reviewed by many educators, RDs in practice, and by faculty who have taught review courses and we welcome suggestions from users of the book.

We realize that readers may find some inconsistencies in style and format within this manual. Please remember that this book is intended to be a set of study notes, not a perfectly edited text although we have improved formating in this edition. Comprehensive professional editing would increase the price of the book and we have not increased the selling price of the manual in 15 years to make it as affordable as possible.

The 2014-2015 edition is organized using the current *Study Guide for the Registration Examination for Dietitians* published by the Commission on Dietetic Registration (CDR) for the exams beginning in 2012. The four content domains identified by the CDR, and the outline supporting them (approved May, 2011), are the bases for the organization of this manual. This outline is indicated in the manual with bold print. We have addressed each topic that CDR includes as potential test content. Throughout the book, words printed in capital letters and bold-faced type, are followed by their definitions. The manual contains hundreds of definitions that are also referenced in the index. When a few topics were repeated in different sections of the outline, we consolidated that content into one section to avoid repetition. We are very grateful to the Commission on Dietetic Registration, especially to Executive Director Christine Reidy, for her assistance and support in helping us understand the test development process.

You may wonder why we do not provide sample questions, tests or a reading list. The reasons are quite simple:

- We believe that the outline format packs the maximum amount of information into the pages of one book. Clearly, test-takers need to know content before that information can be applied in situational questions. We assume that your undergraduate study and internship have provided considerable experience in taking problem-based tests.

- The *Study Guide for the Registration Examination for Dietitians*, published by the Commission on Dietetic Registration, provides sample questions, a test and a recommended reading list. CDR also has a practice test that can be loaded onto your computer. Exam candidates should use it to become comfortable with taking this type of exam. We also recommend practice questions available from DietitianExam.com and provide a discount certificate with each manual. Because this material is already available, we saw no reason to duplicate those efforts.

- We wanted to create a book useful before and after the registration exam. You will find the ***Review of Dietetics: Manual for the Registered Dietitian Exam*** a valuable resource for several years to come. Educators tell us that they use the book for quick updates, as a guide for preparing lectures, as well as a text for interns.

Realistically, one manual cannot summarize all of the texts, lectures and experiences that may be included in the exam. If certain areas remain unclear, or you are weak in a particular content area, consult a textbook that includes that subject in depth.

Review of Dietetics is copyrighted. Duplication of this manual is not authorized without the written permission of Hess & Hunt, Inc. The manual is for the exclusive use of individuals who purchase it.

There have been about 100 educators and practitioners who have contributed content over the years and the manual was significantly revised when the **CDR Study Guide, 9th edition, 2011,** was released. The content of Domain I was reviewed and updated by Dr. Joyce Ann Gilbert, RD, LD, former Executive Director of the Marilyn Magaram Center for Food Science, Nutrition and Dietetics at California State University, Northridge; Domain II by Susan Braverman, MS, RD, CDN, FADA, former Dietetic Internship Director at Queens College of The City University of New York, and; Domains III and IV by Rosemarie Little, MS, RD, and other staff of the Magaram Center. They did a marvelous job and I am grateful for all their work on the 2012-2013 edition. The 2014-2015 edition has many format changes and some additional information (food science, application of Dietary Guidelines, MyPlate, meats, sustainability,technology, etc.) but is not significantly different than the last edition. The CDR test format will remain the same until 2016 when we plan another full manual update.

Special thanks to Dr. Carole Zucco who manages book orders and fulfillment and Michael Dean Jones who merged all updates and corrections to create this edition and provides endless technological assistance. My most sincere thanks also go to all who have provided input, feedback and support to the ***Review of Dietetics.*** I welcome your comments that will make future editions even better.

Truly,

Mary Abbott Hess

Mary Abbott Hess, LHD, MS, LDN, RD, FAND
Editor and Publisher

Introduction

TEST-TAKING TIPS

This information on test-taking will explain the registration examination and to help you become familiar with its format. For many people, taking a "big" test creates a lot of anxiety. By using the techniques described here, you can reduce your stress level and make better decisions. Studying this manual and reviewing information from your courses/internship should give you the skills and confidence to pass the test and become a registered dietitian.. If you think you need additional help in either content review or test-taking skills, take a review course. It will help you target and plan your preparation and give you additional test-taking practice.

THE CERTIFICATION TEST

The current registration exam is practice-oriented. The majority of the questions are case study and situation-based. When you take the RD exam, you will be expected to understand the facts, apply procedures or principles and use the decision-making process to determine which facts or practices are required to solve the problem or to select the best course of action.

Only the Commission on Dietetic Registration (CDR) Examination Panel knows what questions are approved for possible use, so you will have to study broadly. Anyone who claims to possess or provide current questions is either making an error or has violated the Academy of Nutrition and Dietetics Code of Ethics in obtaining and/or sharing them. Any form of cheating, including recording or reporting test questions to others, is a breach of professional ethics.

We recommend that you order the current edition of the ***Study Guide for the Registration Examination for Dietitians***, published by the Commission on Dietetic Registration (CDR). It is available from The Commission on Dietetic Registration at www.cdrnet.org. The CDR ***Study Guide*** provides an outline of what may appear on the exam, an explanation of exam procedures, a current bibliography and a practice test with explanations of answers. Since the examination is administered only on the computer, we recommend that you use the computer practice test disk, which comes with the ***Study Guide.*** The exam is given at specified test centers by appointment.

In preparing to take the exam, you should know that all questions are the multiple-choice type, each with four potential answers. In Computer Adaptive Testing, each examinee has a custom tailored test. Test items are chosen at random from an item pool. Even though you may be taking the test on the same day as a friend, the test will not be the same. Each candidate can answer different test items and have a different number of questions. Questions are chosen to span all the content domains within in the test specifications. Regardless of the number of questions you are given, the percentage from each domain on your test will reflect the percentages as listed below. Tests will be of varying lengths and will start and stop at different times. Some of the questions are being validated for use as questions for future tests. Those do not count toward scoring and you will not know which ones they are.

The percentage of questions and general topics are as follows:

> **12% Domain I - Principles of Dietetics**
> **50% Domain II - Nutrition Care for Individuals and Groups**
> **21% Domain III - Management of Food and Nutrition Programs and Services**
> **17% Domain IV - Food Service Systems**

The type of test you will take is called **COMPUTER ADAPTIVE TESTING (CAT) FOR CLASSIFICATION**. Test items are chosen to match a decision point or performance level. Each examinee is classified into a performance category, basically "Ready for entry-level dietetics" or "Not ready for entry-level dietetics". The test will end when a candidate is classified into a performance category. Test items are presented to candidates according to their ability to distinguish between the two performance categories. A correct answer directs the computer to a preliminary status of "ready". An incorrect answer directs the computer to revise the preliminary status as "not ready". As correct answers keep coming, the preliminary status will balance in favor of "ready". When the computer has enough responses to make a clear determination of the candidate's status, it will stop the examination. You will know whether or not you have passed the exam before you leave the examination site.

PREPARING FOR THE EXAM

Long-term preparation

- Plan your review schedule.

  - Start reviewing intensively at least six to eight weeks before the exam and study several days, or most evenings, each week. The CDR **Study Guide** recommends several months of study time.
  - Schedule enough time so that you can review each section of this manual once. Then go back and review sections of content that are difficult to understand or remember.
  - Find a quiet and comfortable place to study.
  - Divide the outline into sections.
  - Assign time and dates to study each domain. Plan study sessions with stretch breaks (usually one hour of study with a 15-minute break).
  - Although you can take a test at any time, plan to take the exam as soon as you are ready. Do not put it off too long because the exam will be more difficult for you to pass if too much time elapses after you graduate.

- Use resources.

  - Thoroughly study each domain in the **Review of Dietetics**.
  - Use the CDR **Study Guide,** take the sample test and take the practice test on your computer.
  - Reread the manual for concept understanding; check additional sources, if needed, including class notes or texts. Write and analyze to increase retention; work out problems using formulas and calculations.

- Form a study group if you know others who are preparing for the exam.

  - Discuss key concepts and potential situations. Ask each other questions.
  - Consider a review course if you are not a good test-taker or have failed the exam before. Look in the *Journal of the Academy of Nutrition and Dietetics* for review courses or ask faculty or a dietetic internship director if there is a review course available in your area.

- Once you receive your test admission material from the CDR testing agency, you must schedule an appointment at one of the authorized test sites listed in the material. You will be scheduled for a 3-hour appointment. Know where you are going and how to get there.

- Stop studying and try to relax 24 hours before the exam. Eliminate stress by exercise, meditation, relaxation techniques, rest and/or enjoyable activities.

<u>**The day of the examination**</u>

- Be well rested. Organize the night before, and get a full night's sleep.
- Get started early; do not rush.
- Eat a nourishing but light meal.
- Dress comfortably.
- Bring glasses if you need them.
- Bring your notice of eligibility, admission slip and a government issued photo identification (driver's license, state photo ID or passport).
- Get to the site at least 15 minutes before the scheduled starting time. Use the restroom immediately before the exam.
- Practice a relaxation technique or think positively about all you know; visualize passing the test with ease.
- You will be given scratch paper and a simple calculator at the site. You will not be permitted to take any of these items with you at the conclusion of the exam.
- You will not be able to take any personal belongings or references into the test area.

DURING THE EXAMINATION

- Pay attention to all directions.
- The appointment time includes time to complete a tutorial designed to orient you to the computer-based testing process, the examination, and a short post-examination survey.
- Concentrate on one item at a time. Each question will require a response in order to continue the examination process. Once a question is answered and you continue on to the next question, you will not be permitted to review or change your previous answers.
- Do not dwell on questions you have already answered.
- Do not rush; take time to assess potential answers.
- Ignore distractions.

<u>**Strategies for multiple choice items**</u>

- The test panel has determined that one of the stated answers is correct, regardless of what you may think might be a better answer.
- Assume the questions and potential answers mean what they say.
  - ➢ Focus on the main idea.
  - ➢ Avoid over-interpretation and addition of variables.
  - ➢ Think of the best way to solve a problem without adding what can and cannot be done at a specific hospital because of policy, staff or tradition.
- Carefully read the stem (the question or situation part), then:
  - ➢ Formulate an answer in your mind.
  - ➢ Read all responses.
  - ➢ Look for your answer in the set of responses.
  - ➢ Eliminate obviously incorrect responses.
  - ➢ If you do not find your answer, reread the stem.
  - ➢ Choose the most inclusive of the correct responses.
  - ➢ When in doubt, make an educated guess.
  - ➢ Look for, and be wary of, irrelevant information.
  - ➢ Look for words such as *always* or *never*. Wrong responses use these words more often.

- Some questions ask for the *best* response. In this case, several are possible and you must choose the response that is most efficient, effective, reasonable or practical in the situation described. Do not "read into" the question circumstances that are particular to one institution.

TEST ANXIETY

- You can minimize test anxiety, but you cannot eliminate it. Some anxiety is normal.
  - ➢ High tension levels can cause an emotional state of mind that interferes with sound reasoning.
  - ➢ Confused thinking can be caused by fear.
  - ➢ Beverages containing alcohol or caffeine can increase tension and anxiety.

- Use anxiety-reducing techniques.
  - ➢ Avoid cramming.
  - ➢ Stop studying 24 hours before the exam.
  - ➢ Do some activity to get your mind off the test.
  - ➢ Get enough sleep.
  - ➢ Think and move calmly.
  - ➢ Do not discuss the test with anyone.
  - ➢ Use your favorite stress-reduction techniques—exercise, meditation, TV—anything you consider "play."

- Practice positive thinking. Say to yourself:
  - ➢ "I studied; I will do the best I can."
  - ➢ "I've passed plenty of tests before this one."

- Release tension.
  - ➢ When you feel tension, tense your muscles until they tremble, then relax.
  - ➢ Close your eyes and relax. Visualize yourself in the following sequence: receiving eligibility, preparing for the test, going to the test and doing well and feeling confident during the test. If at any time during the sequence you become tense, relax and try the sequence again. Practice this exercise daily. You should eventually be able to complete the sequence in a relaxed state.

- Be confident.
  - ➢ You have passed many courses and hurdles in your education. You can pass this test too.
  - ➢ Do not let preparation techniques become overwhelming; choose ones that work for you.
  - ➢ Almost all of the facts you need to pass the exam are in this book. Your study time will pay off.
  - ➢ Bring or wear something "lucky." Why not? Luck always helps.

Domain I - Principles of Dietetics

Domain I=12% of the test.

TOPIC A – FOOD SCIENCE and NUTRIENT COMPOSITION OF FOODS

1. Food science
   - Physical and chemical properties of food
     (1) Meats, fish, poultry, meat alternatives
     (2) Eggs
     (3) Milk and dairy products
     (4) Flour and cereals
     (5) Vegetables and fruits
     (6) Fats and oils
     (7) Functional foods
   - Scientific basis for preparation and storage
     (1) Function of ingredients
     (2) Effects of techniques and methods on:
         (a) Aesthetic properties
         (b) Nutrient retention
     (3) Roles of food additives

2. Composition of food
   - Sources of data, labels
   - Macro and micronutrients sources
   - Phytochemicals
   - Nutrient databases

TOPIC B – NUTRITION and SUPPORTING SCIENCES

1. Principles of normal nutrition
   a. Function of nutrients and non-nutritive substances
   b. Nutrient and energy needs throughout the life span
   c. Herbals, botanicals and supplements

2. Principles of normal human anatomy, physiology and biochemistry
   a. Gastrointestinal
         (1) Ingestion
         (2) Digestion
         (3) Absorption
         (4) Metabolism
         (5) Excretion
   b. Renal
   c. Pulmonary
   d. Cardiovascular
   e. Neurological
   f. Musculoskeletal

g. Reproductive

TOPIC C – EDUCATION and COMMUNICATION

1. Components of the educational plan
 a. Target setting/clientele
  (1) Cultural competencies and diversity
  (2) In-service education (students, health and rehabilitative service providers)
  (3) Patient/client counseling
  (4) Other (e.g., on-the-job training, telemedicine/telehealth, e-learning)
 b. Goals and objectives
 c. Needs assessment (external constraints, competing programs, illness)
  (1) Individual
  (2) Group
 d. Content: community resources, learning activities/methodology, references and handouts; audiovisual specifications
 e. Evaluation criteria
 f. Budget development
 g. Program promotion

2. Theories of educational readiness

3. Implementation
 a. Communication
  (1) Interpersonal
  (2) Group process
 b. Interviewing
  (1) Techniques of questioning: open-ended, closed, leading
 c. Counseling
  (1) Techniques: motivational, behavioral, other
 d. Methods of communication
  (1) Verbal/non-verbal
  (2) Written
  (3) Media (e.g., print, electronic, social media)
  (4) Technology (e.g., informatics)

4. Evaluation of educational outcomes
 a. Measurement of learning
  (1) Formative
  (2) Summative
 b. Evaluation of effectiveness of educational plan

5. Client information
 a. Records
 b. Confidentiality

6. Documentation

7. Orientation and training

TOPIC D - RESEARCH

1. Types of research and research design
2. Statistical evaluation, interpretation, and application
3. Evidence based research

TOPIC E - MANAGEMENT CONCEPT

Because Management is the focus of Domain III, all management content is consolidated in that Domain to avoid repetition.

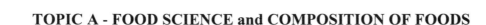

TOPIC A - FOOD SCIENCE and COMPOSITION OF FOODS

1. Food science

a. Physical and chemical properties of food

Food science of protein foods

- **PROTEINS** are large colloidal-sized molecules formed by combining basic units called amino acids with peptide bonds. Amino acids are composed of carbon, hydrogen, oxygen, nitrogen, and sometimes sulfur. Many proteins contain phosphorus; some molecules also incorporate iron, copper or manganese. The 22 amino acids in protein foods can function as acids or bases; they are soluble in dilute acid or alkali. Proteins are a source of energy providing 4 calories per gram of protein.

- Foods rich in protein include eggs, meat, poultry, seafood, milk, cheese and legumes.

- Proteins are used to make food foams (gelatin, soybean protein, cream and eggs in products like soufflés, angel food cakes and whipped cream-type products). They are also used to make gels (baked custards and pies such as pumpkin), and as thickening agents (sauces and puddings). *made from collagen*

- **DENATURATION** is the partial unfolding of the protein molecules retaining all the peptide linkages. In the later stage of protein denaturation, cross-links form and the protein molecules aggregate. Denaturation results in decreased solubility and loss of biological activity. Denaturation is not a reversible process.

- **COAGULATION** is the irreversible transformation of protein from a liquid to a solid state, either by cooking (hard-cooked egg, roast beef, Cheddar cheese curds, wheat gluten in baked bread) or by whipping (meringue). High concentrations of acid and salt can also cause protein coagulation. Over-coagulation of proteins can cause tough, rubbery or curdled products. This can occur well below boiling temperature. Coagulation, rather than denaturation, is the term used in cooking.

(1) Meats, fish, poultry, meat alternatives

MEATS

Meat composition

- Meat is composed of muscle fiber, connective tissue, bones and fat. The composition of most meat has changed over time. Many animals raised for meat are bred to have more muscle fiber and less fat. Meat is also trimmed closer so that it has less fat. Generally, the leanest cuts of meat are from the loin and the round.

- **MUSCLE FIBER** is the digestible lean tissue in meat. It should not be confused with non-digestible plant fiber that is a carbohydrate.

- **COLLAGEN** is white connective tissue in meat that can be softened or dissolved in hot water to form gelatin. Collagen sheaths coat each muscle fiber, fiber bundle and muscle. Collagen increases in meat as the animal exercises more and/or grows older. Presence of more collagen results in meat that is less tender.

- **ELASTIN** is the hard yellow elastic connective tissue in meat that is unaffected by heat or moisture. Older animals generally have a lot of elastin.

Religious Practices: ① Hindus = ∅ Beef ∅ Veal
Judaism / Islam = ∅ Pork (pig or hog)

- **FAT**, also called triglycerides, and related compounds, coat muscle tissue, cushions organs and is deposited as **MARBLING,** the fat within the lean part of muscle. Generally, the more marbling, the tenderer the meat will be. The color, texture and exact composition of fat vary with the type of animal.

Types of meat

- grass or grain based diets
~ 2 y/o

- **BEEF** comes from muscle tissue of cattle brought to market at about 2 years of age. The degree of fatness and palatability depend on the breed and feed of the cattle. Beef cattle are typically grass-fed or pasture-raised after weaning. Before slaughter, most are fed a grain-based diet if they go to feedlots. Hormones may be given to increase body weight. Some cattle are exclusively grass-fed but require more land for grazing. "Natural cattle" are grass-fed and not given antibiotics or hormones but all cattle are vaccinated shortly after birth to prevent certain diseases common to cattle. Hindus consider cows sacred and do not eat beef.

-milk based diet
~16-18 weeks old

- **VEAL** is meat from young calves raised to 16-18 weeks. Because they are taken to market early, most have had a milk-based diet or are given milk replacers if separated from their mothers shortly after birth. Guidelines from veterinary groups set standards for industry for the humane care of calves that are kept in stalls at specific temperatures. Veal is lighter in color and lower in iron than beef. Veal is generally tenderer and more expensive than beef. Hindus do not eat veal.

- **LAMB** is the meat of young sheep (4-12 months of age) and is a common entrée in the Middle East, North Africa, Central Asia and northern India. At about one year, sheep become mutton that is tougher than lamb and has a strong flavor. Lamb consumption in the U.S. is very low, less than one pound per person annually. Lamb fat is not used for food in Western cultures. It is used as tallow for candles.

Pig = < 4mo old
hog = > 4mo old

- **PORK** is the meat from pigs and hogs and is one of the most popular meats in the American diet. Animals up to 4 months are pigs and older animals are hogs. Pigs and hogs are typically raised on feed from soybean meal, fish meal, milk, meat by-products and corn. Over the years, America has been breeding hogs to be leaner. Today, many cuts of pork are leaner than beef and quite similar to poultry in levels of fat. Younger animals produce pork that is tender and mild in flavor; older, larger hogs for cured meats, bacon, ham, sausages, including hot dogs and lunch meats. Pork is a dietary staple in China and Southeast Asia. Judaism and Islam doctrine discourage consuming pork as being unclean.

- **GOAT** is the most consumed meat worldwide but not commonly eaten in the U.S. Some African and Mexican communities eat goat. On menus, it may be called cabrales, meaning young goat.

Butchering of meat

- After slaughter, the carcass is split down the backbone. Beef and veal are further divided into hindquarters and forequarters. After butchering, large **PRIMAL** or **WHOLESALE CUTS** are made. **FABRICATED CUTS,** also called **RETAIL CUTS,** sold in grocery stores for home meal preparation, are smaller cuts of meat, in menu sized or single portions.

Identification standards

- The **UNIFORM RETAIL MEAT IDENTITY STANDARDS (URMIS)** were established by the industry-wide Cooperative Meat Identification Standards Committee. They describe 314 retail cuts of beef, pork, veal and lamb. Meat package labels include the species or kind of meat, the primal or wholesale cut name and the specific retail name from the master list. Food service operators use *The Meat Buyers Guide,* a publication of the North American Meat Processors Association, which contains purchase specifications and photos of various meat cuts.

Inspection

- The **FEDERAL MEAT INSPECTION ACT OF 1906** regulates meat marketed interstate. It includes examination of the live animal, parts of the animal susceptible to disease and the packing plant. The U.S. Inspection Stamp ensuring wholesomeness is a circle with the words "*Inspected and Passed USDA.*" This stamp and the processing plant number, usually in blue ink, are placed on each quarter. This stamp does not relate to quality or tenderness, only that it is fit for human consumption.

- The **WHOLESOME MEAT ACT OF 1967** made inspection of all meat mandatory. USDA has implemented a Hazard Analysis Critical Control Point (HACCP) system in meat inspection as a result of recent food-borne illness outbreaks traced to red meat.

- USDA requires that beef, veal, pork and lamb be inspected before sale. Meats are inspected by the Food Safety and Inspection Service if meats are imported or sold interstate.

Grading

- Meat quality grading is voluntary and includes evaluation of marbling, firmness, color and texture. Grades are stamped on the outside layer of the meat of primal wholesale cuts. **USDA PRIME** grade meat is the most tender, juicy and flavorful, but also has the most fat and is the most costly. **USDA CHOICE** follows and is widely accepted and preferred by consumers. **USDA SELECT** beef is the leanest of the three common consumer quality grades. Other grades used (standard, commercial, utility, cutter and canner) are mainly for canned products, sausages and pet food. Veal and lamb have similar grading systems; however, the term "Good" is used instead of "Select" and lamb does not have a grade of "Standard." Quality grades for pork have not been established.

- Beef and lamb carcasses may also be **YIELD GRADED** by the USDA. Numbers 1-5 are used. A yield grade 1 gives the most trimmed lean meat.

- Nutritionally speaking, most nutrients in meat (protein, thiamin, niacin, iron and zinc) are similar, regardless of quality grade. The amount of fat, and therefore calories per serving, varies with quality grade.

Color

- The color of meat indicates its freshness. Color in meat is due to the pigments

MYOGLOBIN (70-80%) and HEMOGLOBIN (20-30%) that contain iron. The color changes with age, oxygen concentration, cooking and application of curing agents. Beef, exposed to air (oxygen) is typically a bright red color. Both young veal and pork are grayish pink. Older veal is a darker pink. Lamb can be light to darker pink-red, depending on what it was fed.

Meat tenderness

- Cuts from the backbone or rib area of the animal are typically the tenderest because the muscles are least exercised. Shoulders and upper legs are less tender; the least tender cuts come from the lower leg muscles, flank and neck.

Methods used to tenderize meat

- AGING is the holding of meat for a set period at a proper refrigerator temperature and humidity. Meat is aged to improve flavor and tenderness.

- MECHANICAL TENDERIZATION consists of passing meat through cutting blades or pounding it to break muscle fibers. Cross-grain cutting and thinly slicing meat can also tenderize it.

- MOIST-HEAT COOKING consists of cooking meat covered in liquid for long periods of time at low temperatures. This converts collagen to gelatin and results in more tenderness. Acids, such as vinegar, increase the water-binding capacity of fibers and thus make them more moist, but not more tender.

- ENZYMES can be used as a marinade or during cooking to tenderize muscle tissue, collagen and elastin. BROMELIN from pineapple, and PAPAIN and CHYMOPAPAIN from papaya are commonly used as meat tenderizers. Bromelin is more effective on collagen. Enzymes affect the color, flavor and texture of foods. Acids also can be used as tenderizers.

- ELECTRICAL STIMULATION is low voltage stimulation done immediately after slaughter to increase meat tenderness.

Storage and preparation of meat

- Fresh meat should be stored at 41°F or below, covered or in tightly sealed containers. The wrapping on ground meat must be air tight. Frozen meat should be wrapped in air tight packaging, labeled with the date of storage and stored at 0°F or below.

- Tender cuts generally are prepared using dry heat, while less tender cuts require moist heat and longer cooking times. DRY-HEAT COOKING, (also called HIGH-HEAT COOKING), methods for meat include broiling, roasting, pan-broiling, grilling, frying and stir-frying. MOIST-HEAT COOKING methods include stewing, braising and cooking in any liquid medium.

- Meat continues cooking after it is removed from heat. This CARRY-OVER COOKING generally increases internal temperature 5-15°F.

- Cooking at lower temperatures for a longer period of time produces less shrinkage.

- For beef steak: rare is under 145°F medium-rare 145°F; medium 160°F; well-done 170°F. Raw or rare meat may contain bacteria that cause illness. Cooking destroys these bacteria. Pregnant women, babies and those with poor immunity should not eat raw or rare meats.

- The USDA and Food Safety Inspection Service (FSIS) recommends that the temperature of cooked meats be measured by a food thermometer to assure food safety. The thermometer should be inserted in the thickest part of the lean meat, not touching fat or bone. Beef, veal, lamb and pork steaks, chops or roasts should be cooked to 145°F or above and allowed to rest 3 minutes before serving. Ground beef, lamb, veal and sausages should be cooked to 160°F; poultry to 165°F. (Prior to May 2011, for many years, the recommended safe temperature for pork was 160°F.) All meats should rest for 3 minutes after testing with a food thermometer.

- **MAILLARD REACTION** is a series of reactions between sugars and proteins caused by high heat. The browning at high temperature produces a deep brown color and caramelized crust on roasted and grilled meats.

Ground meat

- Ground meats and poultry are generally mixtures of lean meat and fat. Ground beef labeled as 95% lean usually meets the nutrient description "lean" as defined by the Nutrition Education and Labeling Act of 1990. **PERCENT LEAN** refers to the weight of the meat, not the calories it contains.

- For beef, ground round is usually the leanest, followed by ground sirloin, ground chuck and finally regular ground beef. Look for greater percentages of lean to fat. If the ground meat is cooked before adding to recipes, it should be well drained. When this process is used, less expensive, higher fat, regular ground beef can be used in recipes. Leaner ground beef carries premium prices.

- All meat, but especially ground meat, should be thawed in the refrigerator, never on the counter at room temperature.

Preserved and processed meats

- Curing meats by smoking, salting, pickling, smoking or drying them preserves meats and creates unique flavors and textures. Corned beef, ham, bacon, hot dogs and other sausages typically have added salts, sodium nitrate, sugar, and ascorbates plus seasonings. Most are high in sodium.

FISH/SEAFOOD

Types of seafood

- Seafood may be vertebrates (with fins) or shellfish. More than 500 varieties of fin-fish are sold for consumption in the U.S.

- Catfish, cod, haddock, flounder, mahi mahi, snapper, tuna and trout are a few of the finfish types. Shellfish have no bones, but have hard shells covering their bodies. Shellfish are both **CRUSTACEANS** (crab, crayfish, lobster and shrimp) with hard shells and jointed skeletons, and **MOLLUSKS** (clam, mussels, oyster, scallop, octopus, squid, abalone, conch and snail) that have no internal skeletal structure.

- Until 2002, canned tuna was the most consumed seafood in the United States. In 2002, shrimp surpassed tuna in consumption.

Seafood inspection and safety

- Fish and shellfish are very sensitive to temperature changes and microorganisms will multiply rapidly. When receiving fish and shellfish, check to ensure that internal temperature is 41°F or below.

- Lot inspection is available for shellfish. Inspection and grading of fish and fish products are voluntary services of the U.S. Department of Commerce. However, most U.S. seafood is not graded. Seafood inspection services were strengthened recently with **HACCP** requirements, and the **FDA** established a seafood telephone "hot line". Shellfish inspection receives particular emphasis because it is more likely to cause illness if not fresh or is from contaminated water.

- At peak quality, whole finfish have a fresh ocean breeze scent, are firm to the touch and have stiff fins and scales that cling tightly to the skin. Skin is shiny and "metallic." Gills are pink or bright red and free from mucous or slime. If whole, their eyes are clear, bright and protruding. Fish fillets or steaks also have a mild scent, firm and moist flesh, a translucent appearance and no browning around the edges. If wrapped, the packaging should be tightly sealed.

- Crustaceans and some mollusks are sold live. Unless frozen, canned or cooked, crab, mussels, crayfish and lobster should be alive when sold. All seafood should be kept well chilled or on self-draining ice chips to maintain temperature.

- If their shells are still on, clams, mussels and oysters must be alive; their shells should not be damaged. When these mollusks are alive, their shells are slightly open, but they close tightly when tapped. Freshly **Shucked Mollusks** (shells removed) have a mild, fresh scent. A somewhat clear liquid—not too milky or cloudy—should cover the shucked flesh.

- Scallops are almost always removed from their shells at sea. They vary in size and color ranges from creamy white to light orange, tan or somewhat pinkish. When fresh, they are not dry or darkened around the edges.

- **Surimi** is a combination of different types of fish and flavoring formed into shapes with added color. It is widely used as a substitute for lobster and crab due to lower cost.

- Vacuum-packed fish have been placed in airtight containers from which the air has been removed to prevent growth of bacteria.

- Regardless of size and color, fresh raw shrimp should have a mild odor. Shrimp is classified by count per pound and sold raw in the shell, or deveined, peeled or frozen.

- For all fish--finfish and shellfish--use your nose. A strong, "fishy" odor or ammonia smell is a sign that the fish is no longer fresh.

- Frozen seafood should be frozen solid, as a block or in individual pieces, mild in odor and free of ice crystals and freezer burn. **Freezer Burn** is indicated when drying and discoloration are present. The package should not be damaged or water stained.

- **IQF: INDIVIDUALLY QUICK FROZEN FISH OR SHELLFISH** is frozen piece by piece very quickly so that few ice crystals form. This improves quality.

- Always buy seafood from a reputable, known source. Seafood is a highly perishable food that can carry microorganisms and/or parasites. Cooking generally destroys parasites, but not the toxins that can form in some fish if the product is not properly chilled.

- Raw fish and shellfish can be contaminated with bacteria and can cause food-borne illness and other diseases. Cooking destroys the bacteria and parasites but not contamination. The FDA has issued warnings about the dangers of eating seafood from contaminated waters. Contaminants (e.g., mercury, PCBs) are stored in fish fat and build up in older (larger) fish and in mollusks, which are bottom filter feeders.

- Pregnant women and children and people with impaired immune systems are advised to avoid all raw fish and shellfish and to limit consumption of fish likely to contain mercury, including albacore tuna, King mackerel and swordfish.

Nutritional content of seafood

- Seafood is generally low in fat and high in protein and minerals. Most fat in seafood is polyunsaturated. Shrimp, squid and lobster are higher in cholesterol than clams, mussels, crab or scallops, but all are low in fat, unless additional fat is added during preparation.

- Fish that is white or light in color, such as haddock, cod, ocean perch, snapper and sole, has less fat than fish that is firm and darker in color, such as mackerel, salmon and blue fin tuna.

- Fattier fish that lived in cold water tend to have more **OMEGA-3 FATTY ACIDS** than lean fish or shellfish. Fish are the best source of omega-3 fatty acids which benefit the nervous system, brain and vascular system. *Dietary Guidelines for Americans* recommend that people eat 12 oz. of fish per week. Seafood high in omega-3's include salmon, sardines, canned tuna (especially oil-packed), mackerel, rainbow trout, herring, oysters, eel, sturgeon and Dungeness crab.

- Frozen fish is equal in nutrients to fresh fish and often less expensive.

Preparation of seafood

- Fresh fish is very perishable and should be kept well chilled and used within a day or two days, at most. Individually-portioned fish may be cooked from frozen. Finfish cooks quickly and becomes opaque when done. Fish has little connective tissue and short muscle fibers. It does not need tenderizing before cooking.

- Whole fish comes either whole (ungutted) or **DRAWN**, with entrails and gills removed. **DRESSED FISH**, in addition to being drawn, has the scales and sometimes the head removed. **FISH FILLETS** are boneless, cut lengthwise from the sides of a fish. **FISH STEAKS** are cross-section cuts from larger dressed fish usually 5/8-1-inch thick. **CUBES** are small pieces of fish used for stir-fry, soup or kebobs. **FISH STICKS** are small pieces of fish pressed together and breaded or battered and sold frozen.

- Shellfish is usually cooked by moist heat methods. Shellfish should be well cooked because it can carry bacteria. Raw oysters and raw fish as in sushi, are potentially dangerous to people with impaired immunity, pregnant women, young children and the aged.

- Lean fish cooks quickly and should be cooked just until it flakes with a fork at 145°F. Overcooking makes fish and shellfish tough.

POULTRY

- Chicken is one of the most popular protein foods in the United States. It is widely available, versatile, easy to prepare and less expensive than many other proteins. When not fried or in sauce, it is relatively low in calories and fat.

- Chicken and turkey can be purchased whole, in halves or quarters, cut into pieces or boned. Duck is purchased whole or as boneless breasts. Labor saving forms of poultry include frozen, raw cubed, sliced, frozen breaded pieces, raw or cooked rolled turkey breast, chicken patties or nuggets, turkey or chicken cold cuts, sausages and hot dogs. Many markets sell whole roasted chicken or cooked chicken in several forms.

TYPES OF POULTRY	
Broiler or Fryer:	Tender chicken, usually under 3½ lb., 9-12 weeks of age
Roaster:	Larger, older chicken (4 -8 lb.), less tender than broiler-fryer; 3- 5 months
Stewer:	Mature female, over 10 months, tough
Capon:	Castrated chicken, usually over 8 lb, under 10 months, tender
Turkey (hen):	Female turkey, usually 9 -13 lb.
Turkey (tom):	Male turkey, usually 13 -22 lb.
Cornish hen (Rock Cornish):	Small, hybrid Cornish chicken (1 -1½ lb.) that has a high proportion of bone to meat, about 5 weeks of age
Duck:	3-7 lb., several varieties (e.g., Long Island, wild, etc.)
Pheasant:	2-3 lb., with lean white meat, wild or farm raised.
Goose:	6-12 lb., under 6 months, more tender than mature goose
Quail:	Small game birds, usually about 6-8 oz. whole
Guinea:	Game bird, under 6 months, tender
Squab:	3-4 weeks, light, tender meat

Nutritional value of poultry

- Poultry is rich in protein. A 3½ oz. roasted breast of chicken with skin has about 200 calories, 30g of protein, 84g of cholesterol, and 8g of fat. Poultry has less iron than red meats, with more iron in the dark meat, leg and thigh, than in the white meat of the breast of the same bird. Chicken wings tend to be high in fat because they have a lot of skin and little lean meat.

- Fat content varies with the age, sex and species of the bird. Poultry fat is found under the skin. Much of the fat in chicken is monounsaturated. White meat is lower in fat than dark meat. Poultry skin contains fat, so skinless chicken or turkey breast is very low in fat.

Self-basting turkeys contain added fat. Much of the fat in poultry is located in the cavity directly under the skin. When poultry is cooked, the fat under the skin drains off during cooking. Removing skin before eating poultry reduces fat intake.

- **GROUND TURKEY MEAT** is ground muscle without skin, while **GROUND TURKEY** includes skin and thus is much higher in fat (5g *vs.* 13g fat/100g meat, respectively). Some ground turkey has as much fat as ground beef.

- Ducks and geese are both high-fat birds when cooked whole and eaten with skin on. Boneless, skinless duck breast is equal to chicken and turkey in fat content.

Inspection and grading

- Poultry inspection has been mandatory since 1971. A round stamp with "USDA inspected" indicates wholesomeness. Most poultry sold is Grade A.

- Currently much of the chicken sold contains salmonella or campylobacter jejuni organisms. Raw chicken should be fully cooked to destroy these organisms; surfaces and utensils that come in contact with raw poultry should be sanitized after each use. HACCP has been implemented for poultry. Some poultry is irradiated to reduce risk of bacterial contamination.

- Poultry is graded by USDA as A, B and C, with A, the highest quality. Grading of poultry for quality is voluntary, as it is for red meats. Shape, meatiness, fat distribution and general appearance determine quality. Look for meaty birds with skin that is creamy white or pale yellow and free of bruises or dry areas. The color of the fat is determined partially by the chicken feed. Tears, bruises and pinfeathers in the skin lower the grade. Young birds provide the best quality and have smooth skin, flexible joints and absence of pinfeathers.

- Kosher chicken and turkey are salted in the koshering process and are higher in sodium than regular poultry.

Storage and preparation of poultry

- Most poultry sold in this country (except stewing hens) consist of young tender birds that can be cooked by either dry or moist heat methods.

- Fresh poultry are highly perishable and should be stored chilled at 41°F or below and used within two days of purchase. Storage at temperatures between 16°F and 32°F is called **DEEP CHILL METHOD** and extends shelf life an additional 1-2 days.

- Freezing chicken at home may cause small blood vessels to expand and rupture. Pigment contained in the blood cells, once released, can have the effect of "staining" nearby bones.

- Frozen poultry can be kept up to 6 months at 0°F, tightly packaged. Defrost frozen poultry under refrigeration or in cold running water. It should not be defrosted at room temperature. Once raw poultry thaws, it should be used within 2-3 days.

- All poultry should be cooked to a minimum internal temperature of 165°F (held for 15 seconds). Overcooking makes poultry dry and tough. Cooking poultry with bones in and skin on helps to retain juiciness. Remove skin before serving or eating if fat is a concern.

Soup stocks

- The four basic types of **SOUP STOCK** are white, brown, fish, and vegetable. **WHITE STOCK** is made by covering bones (of poultry, meat or fish) and vegetables in cold water in a stock pot, simmering and skimming impurities from the surface, and straining the stock through a china cap (strainer) lined with cheesecloth. **BROWN STOCK** is made the same way, except bones are first browned.

Meat alternatives

- **MEAT ALTERNATIVES** include legumes, nuts, and seeds because these foods are storehouses of nutrients and are rich sources of protein.

- **LEGUMES** are plants that have double-seamed pods, containing a single row of seeds. Examples are lentils, peas, soybeans, peanuts and dried beans. When the seeds of a legume are dried, they are called **PULSES.** Examples are lentils and dried peas.

Nutritional value of legumes

- Legumes are a good source of protein, containing about twice as much protein per serving as cereal and about half as much protein as lean meat. Legumes have higher lysine content than grains. Legumes are low in fat, except for peanuts and soybeans. They are high in phosphorus, contain some iron, potassium, folate, zinc, are an excellent source of fiber—½ cup provides 4-10g of fiber. They also contain complex carbohydrates and are heart healthy food choices, providing no cholesterol.

- The human digestive tract lacks the enzyme necessary to digest some of the oligosaccharide found in dried beans. As a result, microorganisms in the lower intestine attack the undigested oligosaccharide ferment and produce hydrogen, which leads to flatulence in many people, when legumes are eaten.

Preparation of legumes

- Legumes must be cooked to be digestible and usually require both soaking and simmering. Dry beans will cook faster if soaked first in water. Soaking may be done overnight, or the beans may be heated in boiling water for a few minutes and then left to soak in the same water for an hour. They should be drained and cooked in fresh water. This helps to reduce flatulence.

- Add acidic foods (tomatoes, lemon juice, vinegar, wine, etc.) near the end of the cooking process because acid slows softening the legume or bean.

- The addition of a small amount (scant 1/8 tsp. per cup of beans) of baking soda may speed tenderization, but it can, in larger amounts, make the beans mushy and will destroy thiamin. It can also cause a soapy taste.

- Many canned cooked legumes (e.g., kidney beans, black beans, white beans) are available and reduce preparation time. Some legumes are available frozen.

- Legumes are economical, nutritious, have a long shelf life, and contribute flavor, color, and texture to meals. They can be used in soups, salads, as a meat substitute in vegetarian dishes, as dips, spreads and snacks.

- When purchasing, look for uniform size pieces to ensure even cooking. Legumes are graded as US 1, 2, 3, with 1 being the highest quality. Skins should be smooth and not withered. They should be stored in a cool, dark, dry place in airtight containers. Vitamin B6, found in beans, is sensitive to light. Never store dry legumes in the refrigerator. Protect legumes from moisture, which can cause mold and fungi that can produce **AFLATOXIN,** a cancer causing agent. If any evidence of mold growth is seen, discard the legumes.

Soy products

- **SOY PRODUCTS** are commonly used as meat replacements. Soybeans, which are legumes, can be processed in a variety of ways. The green soybean pod is sold fresh or frozen as **EDAMAME.**

- **TOFU** is a creamy white soy product sold in small blocks. It is made by the coagulation of the soybean protein. It is flavorless, but easily takes on the flavors and aromas of foods or seasonings with which it is cooked. The three most common forms of tofu are soft, firm or regular and extra firm. Soft has a custard like texture and a soft delicate taste. Firm or regular is the most versatile form and extra firm has a grainy coarse texture. The denser the tofu, the more calories it contains. Tofu can be used in cooking and sautéed, stir-fried or blended into a variety of products to make dips, spreads, salad dressings, cheesecakes, etc. Tofu cheeses are also available.

- **MISO** is pungent, salty seasoning paste that originated in Japan and is a combination of soybeans and a grain such rice or barley, which is fermented. It is used as a soup base or flavoring and is high in sodium.

- **TEMPEH** is a soy-based meat substitute that originated in Indonesia. For tempeh, soybeans are cooked with grains and then aged in a culture that binds the protein to form a firm product that can be sliced or formed into patties.

- **SOY MILK** is made by grinding soybeans with water. It is sold plain and in several flavors. Unlike cow's milk, it has little calcium unless it is fortified.

Nuts and seeds

- **NUTS** are the seeds or dried fruits of trees, and most have a hard outer husk to protect the softer kernel inside.

  ➢ Nuts are marketed with and without shells, and cut, sliced or ground.
  ➢ Edible seeds that we eat grow on fruit or vegetable plants and their hulls are sometimes edible.
  ➢ Peanuts are actually a legume, but are commonly considered nuts. Many peanuts in the US are sold ground as peanut butter, although nut butters can be made from other nuts.
  ➢ Nuts contain 10-25% of their calories from protein; seeds contain from 11-25% of their calories from protein but their protein is incomplete. Most seeds are low in the amino acid lysine.
  ➢ Nuts are a good source of dietary fiber.

➢ Oil-rich nuts and seeds are rich sources of Vitamin E and supply many of the B vitamins, potassium, iron, magnesium, zinc, copper and selenium.

➢ Most nuts provide over 75% of their calories from fat. TREE NUTS (almonds, cashews, Brazils, hazelnuts, macadamias, pecans, pine nuts and walnuts) are nutrient-dense foods rich in mono and polyunsaturated fatty acids. They also contain a variety of vitamins, minerals and phytochemicals.

➢ Chestnuts are the only nuts containing vitamin C. Unlike other nuts, chestnuts are mainly carbohydrate and low in fat and calories.

➢ Coconuts are a fruit seed grown on the tropical coconut palm. Unlike most nuts, the fat of coconuts and extracted coconut oil is highly saturated. Coconut oil is used in the production of some processed foods. While coconut is high in dietary fiber, it has few vitamins or minerals.

➢ Sesame seeds are a staple in many of the world's cuisines, including African, Indian and Chinese. Dark sesame oil is a common cooking ingredient in Asia. TAHINI is ground sesame seeds and has been called the butter of the Middle East. While sesame seeds are an excellent source of calcium and iron, about half of the calcium in sesame seeds is bound by oxalates and cannot be utilized.

➢ All nuts and seeds are prone to rancidity. Heat, light, and humidity will speed spoilage. Wrap nuts well and store in a cool, dry place or in the freezer.

➢ Many seeds and nuts taste better if they are toasted or roasted before they are eaten.

➢ Both tree nuts and peanuts are common allergens.

(2) Eggs

- The egg is composed of a shell, egg white (ALBUMIN) and a yolk. The albumin contains riboflavin and protein. The yolk (1/3 of weight of the egg) contains fat, protein, vitamins, iron and cholesterol. The albumin is clear and liquid when raw, and turns white and firm when cooked. The chalazae are a twisted cord-like strand of egg white that holds the yolk in the center of the egg.

- Eggs are a very economical form of protein and many nutrients, and are useful when budgets limit the quantity or quality of food. They are versatile, easily digested and a soft, easy to eat food for seniors and those with dental problems.

Grading of eggs

- Grading is done through a process called CANDLING. Eggs pass in front of a strong light and are appraised for the size of the air sac, the position of the yolk, the clearness of the white and the overall size. U.S. grades include AA, A, B and C. Grade C eggs are sold to processors but not to consumers.

  ➢ GRADE AA: The yolk of a Grade AA egg is firm and the area covered by the white is small. There is a large proportion of thick white to thin white.

  ➢ GRADE A: The yolk of a Grade A egg is round and upstanding. The thick white is large in proportion to the thin white and stands fairly well around the yolk.

  ➢ GRADE B: The yolk of a Grade B egg is flattened and there is about as much (or more) thin white as thick white.

Size of eggs

- Size is determined by weight per dozen eggs:

  ➢ Jumbo = 30 oz. per dozen
  ➢ Extra large = 27 oz. per dozen
  ➢ Large = 24 oz. per dozen (about 2 oz. per egg)
  ➢ Medium = 21 oz. per dozen
  ➢ Peewee = 15 oz. per dozen

- Standardized recipes use large eggs. Purchase large eggs when testing recipes.

Safe handling of eggs

- The **EGG PRODUCTS INSPECTION ACT OF 1970** assures egg products have been produced under inspected, sanitary conditions and are unadulterated and truthfully labeled.

- Eggs have a porous shell that allows absorption of flavor and odors. Raw eggs (in shell) should be stored at 40-45°F, up to 5 weeks, egg whites and yolks only 2-4 days.

- **SHELL EGGS** are purchased for food services by the case, containing 30 dozen eggs. Whole shell eggs may be contaminated with salmonella from the hen's body, the nest or fecal matter. To minimize contamination, care should be taken to purchase eggs that come from healthy hens and that are handled under sanitary conditions. Refrigeration retards penetration of bacteria through the shell. Shell eggs can be disinfected in water that does not exceed 130°F (higher temperature coagulates egg white); they must be dried immediately. New technology is being developed to detect salmonella-contaminated eggs and some eggs are irradiated to destroy potential salmonella. Irradiated/pasteurized eggs can safely be eaten soft cooked or raw.

- Only whole, uncracked eggs should be stored. Eggs keep well in the shell when refrigerated. Keeping eggs in the carton lessens moisture and quality loss. Hard cooked eggs are more perishable than raw eggs in the shell because the protective coating on the shell is lost during cooking.

- Raw or undercooked (cooked less than five minutes or less than 160°F) eggs are a common source of bacterial infection. For food safety, raw or undercooked eggs should not be served or eaten. Unsafe foods include Caesar salad dressing, desserts (e.g., foams like soft meringues) or beverages made with raw eggs or beaten egg whites and soft-cooked eggs. Commercial eggnog and salad dressings use pasteurized, liquid eggs and are safe, if stored properly.

- Pasteurized eggs are subject to the Egg Products Inspection Act of the U.S. (1970) that requires all liquid processed egg products to be pasteurized. Eggs for commercial food service are sold as frozen whole eggs in 30 lb. cans. A can equals 23 dozen whole eggs, 60 dozen yolks or 35 dozen whites.

- Frozen and dried eggs are available as whole eggs, whites or yolks. Because of their low bacterial count, frozen and dried eggs are used by many institutions for such items as scrambled eggs and French toast. A pound of dried whole eggs equals about 32 large eggs. Once reconstituted, they should be used immediately.

- Frozen eggs must be kept frozen until defrosted for use. Defrosting should be done under refrigeration, which may take days for bulk packages. Defrosted eggs should be used within two days.

- **EGG SUBSTITUTES** were developed for those on low cholesterol diets. Egg substitutes are subject to bacterial activity similar to liquid egg and should be handled with the same care. Two main types of egg substitute are used: (1) complete egg substitute, made from soy or milk protein, and (2) partial egg substitute, made by replacing egg yolk with egg white. The egg white substitute usually has half the fat and calories of natural eggs, a higher polyunsaturated fat/saturated fat ratio and higher sodium content. Milk-based substitutes cannot be used alone in recipes for thickening purposes, since casein does not readily coagulate; neither does soy.

- Protein coagulation, the temperature at which the egg becomes solid, varies with different parts of the egg. Whole beaten eggs coagulate at about 156°F. The egg white coagulates at a slightly lower temperature than the yolk. When making scrambled eggs with added milk, the coagulation temperature increases to 180°F. Cooked egg dishes should reach 160°F. If eggs are overcooked, the eggs protein and liquids may separate or curdle, resulting in tough, yet watery, egg dishes.

Nutritional value of eggs

- A single large egg supplies 72 calories, 10% of the daily need for protein, about 6g, along with good to excellent amounts of vitamins A, D and B-complex and some minerals. Eggs contain some iron in the yolk (which some studies suggest is poorly utilized). Eggs contain antioxidant carotenoids and are the richest source of choline, a micronutrient used to maintain cell membranes and aid in the breakdown of dietary fats.

- There is no nutritional difference between eggs with white shells and those with brown shells or fertile versus non-fertile eggs.

- Raw eggs contain the protein **AVIDIN,** which binds the B vitamin biotin, unless denatured by heat.

- Egg yolks contain sulfur that can react with the iron in the yolk to form the gray-green ring that develops when eggs are hard-cooked too long. An average large egg yolk contains 5.0g total fat, of which 1.5g is saturated (1.1g palmitic, 0.4g stearic). Egg yolks are rich in cholesterol, about 185mg per large egg yolk. New technology is being developed to centrifuge whole eggs and extract most of the cholesterol.

- Food science and the use of special chicken feeds are being used to make eggs with less cholesterol and altered fat content and some are irradiated to reduce the risk of salmonella.

Preparation of eggs

- Cooking eggs changes their form but does not alter nutritional value.

  - Eggs may be baked, boiled, poached, fried, scrambled or used as an ingredient in baked goods and sauces. To reduce fat and cholesterol, use two egg whites and one whole egg for scrambled eggs, omelets or other cooking uses.

➤ Adding vinegar or salt to cooking water may improve the shape of poached eggs since each of them speed coagulation.

➤ Hard cooked eggs are prepared by placing eggs in water, bringing to a boil, simmering for 15 minutes and cooling quickly in cold water.

➤ The texture of baked custard is improved by placing the dish in a pan of hot water. This diffuses the heat on the edges of the custard.

➤ Fat, including fat from the yolk, prevents proper whipping of egg white.

➤ Cream of tartar (an acid) is often added to egg white foams to create whiteness and to stabilize the foam.

➤ The addition of sugar slows egg coagulation.

Functions of eggs in cooking and baking

➤ Structure - the protein gives structure to baked goods and thickens custards
➤ Emulsification - natural emulsifiers help blend ingredients
➤ Aeration - beaten or whipped eggs cause baked goods to rise
➤ Flavor
➤ Color - yolks give rich yellow color and add color to crusts

Eggs as allergens

• Eggs are among the most common food allergens. The presence of eggs is listed on food labels to alert those sensitive to eggs. Plant-based egg substitutes are available for those with allergies or who must avoid whole eggs to limit cholesterol intake.

(3) Milk and dairy products

• **MILK** is the product of lactation of animals. It is a solution, a colloidal dispersion and an emulsion. The emulsion in fresh milk is weak and fat droplets will rise to the top unless homogenized. Milk is composed of water and proteins, carbohydrate (lactose), fat (mainly triglycerides), vitamins and minerals. All milk sold and processed in the U.S. is cow milk unless the label states that it comes from some other source, such as goat milk.

• According to *Dietary Guidelines for Americans,* those over the age of 9 years should drink 3 cups of low-fat milk, or the equivalent, of dairy products per day.

• Proteins in milk are curds (casein) and whey. When rennin is added to milk the curds separate out and can be used to make cheese. Often the whey is used as food for animals.

• Milk fat (cream) carries fat-soluble vitamins and essential fatty acids. It contributes to milk's texture, mouthfeel and flavor.

Processing of milk

• **HOMOGENIZATION** is a process that forces fat droplets through a small screen, reducing their size and dispersing them throughout the milk to form a stable emulsion.

➤ **PASTEURIZATION** is the process of heating milk to destroy pathogens and inactivate enzymes increasing the time milk is fresh and palatable. Major methods of pasteurization include:

> **LOW TEMPERATURE PASTEURIZATION** requires holding the product at 62°C (145°F) for 30 minutes.
> **HIGH TEMPERATURE PASTEURIZATION** holds milk at 72°C (161°F) for 15 seconds (most commonly used today).
> **FLASH PASTEURIZATION** and **ULTRA PASTEURIZATION** are newer methods using even higher temperatures for shorter periods of time to increase the shelf life of dairy products. Most cream and half and half sold have been ultra-pasteurized. This and all high and low temperature milk and cream should be kept refrigerated.
> A new form of **ULTRA HIGH TEMPERATURE (UHT) PASTEURIZATION** that kills all bacteria and makes milk shelf-stable is available. UHT is used in the United States for creamers, whipped cream and lactose-reduced milks to extend product shelf life. Many countries use UHT milk as a beverage because it requires no refrigeration until after it is opened. UHT changes milk flavor.

- Use of unpasteurized milk (**RAW MILK**) is discouraged by FDA. It can carry bacteria that cause gastroenteritis, tuberculosis, diphtheria, typhoid, undulant and scarlet fevers, salmonellosis and campylobacteriosis and other food-borne illnesses. There are specific regulations for cheeses made from raw milk including imported cheeses.

Classification of milk

- Milk is classified by the fat portion of the milk (sometimes called the "cream"):
  > **WHOLE MILK** = 3-4% fat (3.5% milk has 150 calories and 8g fat per 8 oz.)
  > **2% MILK** = 2% fat (2% milk has 121 calories and 4.7g fat per 8 oz.)
  > **1% MILK** = 1% fat (1% milk has 102 calories and 2.6g fat per 8 oz.) Also called low-fat milk.
  > **SKIM MILK** = less than 0.5% fat (skim milk has 86 calories and 0.4g fat per 8 oz.) Also called fat-free milk.
  > **LIGHT CREAM** = 18-30% fat.
  > **HALF AND HALF** = 10-12% fat. (A special variance permits "Fat-Free Half and Half" made from corn syrup and thickeners.)
  > **WHIPPING CREAM** (heavy cream) = 30-36% fat.

Nutritional value of milk and dairy products

- Milk supplies many essential nutrients including calcium, phosphorus, riboflavin, vitamins A & D, protein and water. The primary nutrients lacking in milk and other dairy products are iron and vitamin C.

- The nutrient content of low-fat milk and low-fat yogurt is often increased by the addition of dry milk solids. Vitamin D is usually added to all forms of milk; vitamin A is added to fortify lower fat milks.

- Light can destroy some of the riboflavin in milk. Riboflavin has a greenish color sometimes seen in nonfat milk. Milk is usually stored in a dark refrigerator to preserve nutrients. If milk will be exposed to light, paper or other opaque containers are preferred.

- Harder cheeses are higher in calcium than softer cheeses (cottage). The calcium in one ounce of hard cheese equals the calcium in one cup of milk.

- Greek yogurts are strained so some liquid is removed and the yogurt is thicker with more concentrated calcium and other nutrients.

- Carbohydrate content of yogurts can vary widely, ranging from 15g to 45g/serving, with fruited and sweetened yogurts containing more carbohydrate.

Milk quality

- Milk grades are based on bacterial count. Grade A has the lowest count at less than 20,000 bacteria per milliliter. Only grade A milk is sold in retail markets, and meets FDA standards.

- **BOVINE SOMATOTROPIN** (BST) is a hormone that occurs naturally in cows in small amounts. Synthetic forms can be injected to increase milk production. It is legal in the US but not in many other countries. Many people prefer non-BST milk that is often labeled as BST-free or organic milk.

Forms of milk and dairy products

- **NONFAT DRY MILK** is made from pasteurized skim milk. It contains less than 5% moisture and 1.5% milk fat by weight. Dried whole milk is also available but its fat content limits its stability in dry form.

- **BUTTERMILK** is made from low-fat milk that is treated with suitable, cultured lactic acid bacteria. Dried buttermilk is available primarily as a baking ingredient.

- **EVAPORATED MILK** has 60% of its water removed and is canned. Evaporated skimmed milk is also available.

- **CONDENSED MILK** has about 60% of the water removed and has sugar or corn syrup (44%) added and is canned. Fat-free condensed milk is also available.

- **BUTTER** is 80% or more milk fat. The fat is extracted by churning cream. It can be unsalted or salted and in sticks or whipped. European style butter is unsalted and has 82-86% fat.

- **YOGURT** is a dairy product cultured with specific enzymes. Yogurt comes in a variety of fat contents and may have fruit or flavors added. Low-fat and fat-free yogurts usually have added skim milk solids and vitamins A and D. Some yogurt contains active enzymes that aid digestion and carry a seal on the label that indicates live, active culture. Frozen yogurt has inactivated enzymes.

- **ACIDOPHILUS MILK** and other acidic milks are pasteurized and inoculated with Lactobacillus acidophilus bacterial cultures. These bacteria are normal human intestinal microbes that produce B vitamins. Acidophilus milk is often recommended for people taking antibiotics or undergoing intestinal radiation therapy to replace normal bacteria in the digestive tract and minimize gastrointestinal distress.

- **SOUR CREAM** is cultured light cream that is pasteurized and homogenized. Regular sour cream has at least 18% fat; light sour cream 40% less fat; nonfat sour cream is made from nonfat milk thickened with stabilizers.

- **Crème Fraîche** is a French version of sour cream slightly tangy in flavor. In France it is made from unpasteurized milk.

- **Cheese** is made by coagulating milk with an acid or **Rennin** (an enzyme of animal origin), and concentrating the milk casein by separating it from the whey. About 10 lbs. of milk are used to make 1 lb. of cheese. Types vary according to the treatment of cheese curds during the cheese-making process. Cheese curds may be cut or pressed differently may have molds or cultures added and may be aged for varying lengths of time. During the **Cheese Ripening** process, healthful bacteria and molds change the cheese's texture and flavor in humidity and temperature controlled environment.

- The main types of cheese are **Hard Cheese** such as asiago, pecorino romano and parmesan; **Firm Cheese** such as cheddar, Swiss, Jarlsberg, provolone and gouda; **Semi-Soft Cheese,** sliceable or sometimes veined with mold such as port salut, some mozzarella, gorgonzola, blue and Roquefort; **Soft Cheese** with creamy centers such as cottage cheese; **Fresh Soft Cheese** unripened soft cheeses such as cream cheese, ricotta, some fresh mozzarella and queso Oaxaca and feta; **Ripened Soft Cheese** such as camembert and brie.

- **Goat Cheese** may be fresh or aged. Goat cheese generally has less fat than cow milk cheeses. Read the label for fat content and type.

- **Pasteurized Processed Cheese** is a blend of one or more natural cheeses that are shredded, have an emulsifier added, and are then heated and formed. J.L. Kraft, in 1916, developed a method to make processed cheese and wrap the individual slices. Pasteurized processed cheeses melt evenly and do not separate when making sauces.

- **Cheese Spreads** and **Cheese Foods** are processed cheese-based products that have moisture added.

- Cheeses generally have a considerable amount of fat. The lowest fat cheeses in common use are pot cheese, ricotta and cottage cheese. Cheeses made with skim, part-skim or low-fat milk are generally lower in fat. High-fat cheeses include cream cheese, brie, cheddar and blue cheeses. Except for cottage-type cheeses, and those indicating they are "low fat", most natural cheeses have at least 50% calories from fat. Cheeses coagulated with acid (cottage and cream cheese) are much lower in calcium than rennin-coagulated cheeses.

- Cheeses need special care in storage and should be stored well wrapped in the refrigerator. All ripened cheeses should be served at room temperature for best flavor and should not be cut until ripe. Over-ripe cheese has an ammonia odor.

- **Ice Cream** is a churned frozen dairy-based dessert made from cream, milk, sugar and flavorings, such as chocolate or fruit. Ice cream must have at least 10% milk fat. Some premium brands have much more. Other frozen dairy desserts include gelato, frozen custard, frozen yogurt, ice milk and sherbet. They have varied amounts of milk fat and sugar. Fruit ices and sorbets are frozen desserts that are not dairy-based and do not count as servings from the dairy group.

Imitation dairy products

- For **IMITATION DAIRY PRODUCTS,** nondairy ingredients are combined and processed to produce milk-like products. Ingredients may include vegetable fat, proteins (such as sodium caseinate or soy), corn syrup solids, stabilizers, emulsifiers, water and flavorings. Nondairy creamers usually contain corn syrup and fat (sometimes coconut oil). New imitation and processed fat-free or low-fat cheeses are available and can be useful for low-fat, low-cholesterol diets, but generally have altered flavor and texture.

- Soy, almond, rice and hemp "milks" are made from plant sources. They contain no saturated fat or cholesterol and do not provide the nutrients of milk unless highly fortified. They are useful for those with milk allergy or lactose intolerance. Some can be used in cooking.

(4) Flour and cereals

- Rice, wheat and corn are the primary grains that feed the world.

- The most common seed grains from which cereals come are wheat (including bulgur), white or brown rice, corn (including hominy and grits), rye, oats and barley. Other grains include millet, quinoa, triticale, amaranth, buckwheat and wild rice. Grains and products made from them are composed largely of carbohydrates that are chemically composed of carbon, hydrogen and oxygen. Sugar molecules are the basic unit of all carbohydrates.

- There are over 100 varieties of pasta in many shapes, sizes, and flavors. Most are made from wheat flour and some liquids such as water or eggs. There are rice and pastas made from mixed grains for the gluten-free diner. Other pastas are whole wheat or protein enriched. The shape and size of pasta determines usage and ideal type of sauce. All pasta is high in carbohydrate and contains some thiamin and riboflavin. The protein content depends on the amount of semolina or grain. Pasta should be cooked in a large pot of boiling water to appropriate texture.

Composition of grain

- **BRAN** is the hull or outer coating of the grain containing cellulose, hemicellulose and vitamins (thiamin, riboflavin, niacin).

- The **ENDOSPERM** is the large central portion of the grain containing starch and protein.

- The **GERM** is a small part of the grain containing unsaturated fat, protein, iron and vitamins (thiamin, riboflavin and niacin). If the germ's fat is exposed to air, it may become rancid. Wheat germ and whole grains containing the germ are best kept refrigerated.

Processing of grain

- **MILLING** by pressure or friction breaks the grain kernel. The germ is usually removed to prevent rancidity. **WHITE FLOUR** is made from milled wheat endosperm. **WHOLE WHEAT FLOUR** is the milled whole grain, including the germ.

- Some grains are heat-treated and some are precooked. Quick-cooking oatmeal is precooked, as are some types of rice. Some grains are roasted or toasted for flavor enhancement.

Rice

- There are three basic types of rice.

  - ➤ **SHORT GRAIN RICE** has the most starch. It becomes sticky when cooked and is the most tender. A good use is for risotto.
  - ➤ **MEDIUM GRAIN RICE** is firm when it is hot, but becomes sticky when it cools.
  - ➤ **LONG GRAIN RICE** remains firm when cooked and the grains separate easily.

- All types of rice can be processed to remove the hull, the outer covering of the grain. If the grain is polished, the brown rice becomes white.

- **ENRICHED RICE** has a vitamin and mineral coating added to the grain in order to replace nutrients lost when the hull is removed.

- **CONVERTED RICE** is partially cooked with steam and removes some of the surface starch and forces some surface nutrients into the grain. Then it is polished and milled.

- Specialty rice include:

  - ➤ **ARBORIO RICE** is short grain, sticky white rice; takes 3 cups of water per 1 cup of rice to cook; best for risotto.
  - ➤ **BASMATI RICE** is extra-long grain, polished and light, sweet flavored, aged. Takes 1½ cups of water per cup of rice. Often used for pilaf.
  - ➤ **JASMINE RICE** is long grain, fragrant, and more delicate than Basmati.
  - ➤ **WILD RICE** is not a true rice, but a wild water grass; black or brown with nutty flavor; 3 grades depending on length of grain; takes 3 cups of water to 1 cup of rice.
  - ➤ **RED RICE** is also called wehani, with aromatic, earthy flavor.
  - ➤ **BROWN RICE** has the hull removed, tan color, nutty texture, takes longer to cook and needs more liquid than white rice. It contains more fiber than white rice.

- Rice should be stored in sealed containers at room temperature in a dry, dark place. Hulled rice and brown rice contain oils resulting in a shorter shelf life. White rice has hull and sprouting part removed and has a longer shelf life. Because cooked rice contains protein and has a neutral pH, it can spoil easily if left at room temperature. Refrigerate any unused, cooked rice as soon as possible.

Other grains

- **AMARANTH** is a small round herb used as a grain that is light brown. It is used in salads, baked goods, and casseroles.

- **BARLEY** is a grain available in several forms; un-milled or milled. Pearl barley is milled and polished. It has a slightly sweet flavor and chewy texture and is often added to soups to give a hearty consistency. It can also be used as poultry stuffing. Cook with 3 parts liquid and 1 part barley.

- **CORN PRODUCTS**
  - ➤ Corn can be eaten fresh, as a vegetable, or dried, as a grain.
  - ➤ As a dried grain, it is found in two main forms; **CORNMEAL** to make breads, and polenta and hominy (dried corn kernels).
  - ➤ **POLENTA** is cornmeal cooked with water or stock to a thick paste. It can also be molded and cut.
  - ➤ **HOMINY** is made by soaking dried corn in a mild lye solution until the outer layer is swollen and then removed. Hominy may be ground into grits and used for cereal.
  - ➤ **MASA HARINA** is finely ground hominy used for making tortillas and breads.

- **COUSCOUS** is a granular form of semolina that cooks quickly, sort of ground pasta. It is used for sweet and savory side dishes and salads.

- **CRACKED WHEAT** is whole wheat berries that are cracked into pieces. This unmilled grain has a brown exterior, a white interior and is high in nutrients. It is used as a hot cereal or side dish.

- **KAMUT** is a brown rice shaped grain with a nutty flavor. It is used like pasta.

- **KASHA** is hulled, roasted buckwheat groats and is often ground or cracked. It has a nutty flavor and is used for side dishes and cold salad.

- **OATS** are the berries of wheat grass. Oats can be purchased as whole grain oats or oatberries. Oatmeal is crushed, flaked oats. There are many ready-to-eat cereals containing oats. Some research shows that eating oats regularly reduces serum cholesterol and this is an approved health claim on food labels.

- **QUINOA** is small bead-like grain that is ivory colored. It has a neutral flavor and is quite high in protein. It is used for side dishes, vegetarian entrées and soups.

- **SEMOLINA** is hard grain durum wheat with bran and germ removed. Pellets are partially cooked and require brief soaking and steaming. It is used for hot cereal, dumplings and sweet puddings. Most commercial dried pastas are made from semolina flour.

- **SORGHUM** is a major food crop in Africa, Central America, China, India and Pakistan. Most sorghum in the US is used as animal feed. Some sorghum flour is used in gluten-free products.

- **SPELT** is a wheat-like product used as a whole grain or ground. It can be simmered or used in baked goods. It has a mild, nutty flavor.

- **TRITICALE** is a wheat-rye cross that has more protein and lower gluten than wheat, with a sweet, nutty flavor. It comes as berries, flour, flakes, and is used in side dishes, casseroles and as hot cereal.

Nutritional value of grain

- Grains and cereals are sources of carbohydrate, protein, fiber, vitamins and minerals. Protein, in most cereal grains, is deficient in two amino acids; lysine and tryptophan. Altering the genes of a plant augments the deficient amino acids, as in high lysine corn or Triticale, which is also higher in lysine.

- Grains are usually dried for storage and cooked with liquid to make them edible.

- **ENRICHMENT** restores some nutrients lost during processing (iron, riboflavin, niacin, thiamin and folate). The FDA sets standard levels for enrichment. Most flour sold in the United States is enriched.

- **FORTIFICATION** adds nutrients, such as folic acid, to grain products over and above levels normally found in the product. As of January 1998, folic acid is being added to most enriched breads, flours, corn meals, pastas, rice and other grain products, to reduce the risk of neural tube defects in newborns. The level added is 0.43-1.4mg/lb of product. Many breakfast cereals are highly fortified with vitamins and minerals.

- Whole grain products naturally contain **PHYTIC ACID**, which binds some calcium and iron, thus reducing absorption of these minerals.

Gluten

- **GLUTEN** is formed when hydrated particles of flour are manipulated (e.g., kneaded) in a flour-water paste. The elastic character of gluten allows it to trap CO_2 as it forms during leavening, and gives volume and structure to baked goods. Sugar and fat inhibit gluten development. Sugar draws water away from gluten and fat coats flour and prevents water from making contact.

- Individuals with **CELIAC DISEASE (CELIAC SPRUE)** have an immune reaction to the gliadin part of gluten. They must avoid all products containing gluten or damage to the digestive tract and other severe symptoms may occur. About 1% of the population has celiac disease; another 5-10% may have some degree of gluten intolerance. Others choose a gluten-free diet believing it has health benefits or will promote weight loss.

- Gluten-free products are now widely available in most food categories and there are standards required for a food to carry a gluten-free label.

- Gluten-free flours include rice, potato, corn, teff, buckwheat, soy, chickpea and pure oat flours. These flours must be processed on equipment that has not been used for milling any grains containing gluten.

- Flours can be produced from a mixture of grains, excluding sources of gluten, to make products usually made with wheat flour.

Wheat flour mixtures

- Classification of wheat flour may be according to color (red, white), season of planting, (winter, spring) or texture (hard, soft).
  - ➤ **DURUM WHEAT** is a very hard variety of wheat with high-protein (gluten) content and is used for pasta.
  - ➤ **HARD WINTER WHEAT** forms strong gluten and is used mainly for bread flour.
  - ➤ **SOFT SUMMER WHEAT** forms weak gluten and is used for cake flour.

- The functions of ingredients in flour mixtures, as in bread baking, are:
  - ➤ Flour provides the basic structure.
  - ➤ Liquid moistens the flour protein, gelatinizes starch, dissolves sugar and salt, releases CO_2 from baking powder and activates yeast.

- ➢ Fat tenderizes the dough, improves texture and aids leavening by creaming, which mixes air into solid fat.
- ➢ Sugar adds flavor, browns crusts and tenderizes. Sugar also softens the gluten and raises the coagulation point of eggs.
- ➢ Eggs add flavor, color, structure and nutritive value to baked products. Eggs act as an emulsifying agent and a leavening agent by trapping air when beaten.
- ➢ **LEAVENING** is a process that adds ingredients or uses techniques to incorporate air, CO_2 and steam. Air for leavening is incorporated into products by beating, whipping and sifting.
- ➢ Microorganisms or chemical reactions produce CO_2. Adding baking soda (sodium bicarbonate) to an acid chemically produces CO_2. Cream of tartar, vinegar, lemon juice, buttermilk or yogurt may provide the acid. With baking powder, the soda and acid are not activated until a liquid is added. For double-acting baking powder, heat is required for the second reaction.
- ➢ Products leavened by steam have high water content and use high heat in the beginning of the baking process to produce steam.
- ➢ Eggs are used in steam-leavened products to strengthen the batter.
- ➢ Yeast growth also produces CO_2 gas, allowing bread to rise.

Proportions of ingredients

- Structural ingredients, i.e., flour and eggs, are balanced against tenderizing ingredients, such as fat and sugar. Liquids (milk, egg and fat) are balanced against dry ingredients (mainly flour). General proportions for baked goods are as follows:

  - ➢ Weight of shortening = weight of whole eggs
  - ➢ Weight of eggs + milk = weight of flour
  - ➢ 1½ teaspoons double-acting baking powder to each cup of flour

- Batter proportions for quick breads leavened with air, steam or chemicals are:

  - ➢ Pour batter = 1 part liquid: 1 part flour (popovers, pancakes)
  - ➢ Drop batter = 1 part liquid: 2 parts flour (muffins, some cookies)
  - ➢ Soft dough = 1 part liquid: 3 parts flour (biscuits, yeast bread)
  - ➢ Stiff dough = 1 part liquid: 4 parts flour (pie crust, rolled cookies, noodles)

Mixing dough

- **CONVENTIONAL MIXING** creams fat with the sugar, and then alternately adds liquid and flour (e.g., cakes).

- **QUICK/SPEED METHOD** adds fat and milk to the dry ingredients and mix, then adds eggs and mixes again (e.g., cakes, quick breads).

- **MUFFIN METHOD** mixes the liquid (often oil) and dry ingredients separately, then combine them just until the dry ingredients are moistened (e.g., popovers, pancakes, muffins).

- **PASTRY METHOD** cuts semi-solid fat such as butter, lard or shortening into dry ingredients, then adds liquid while stirring (e.g., pastry, biscuits).

Manipulating dough

- **STIRRING** is a rotary motion that distributes ingredients.

- **BEATING** is a rotating motion more vigorous than stirring that provides a smooth distribution of ingredients.

- **CREAMING** is beating together fat and sugar to incorporate air, causing the batter to become light and fluffy.

- **KNEADING** is manipulation by pressure, alternating folding and stretching. It develops a smooth, elastic product and may be done by machine or hand.

- **CUTTING-IN** is a technique to incorporate solid fat into flour mixture, with blades or chopper, to divide fat into flour.

- **FOLDING-IN** is a method of gently combining beaten egg whites (a source of air leavening) with a mixture of other ingredients.

Yeast breads

- Yeast breads are leavened by CO_2 produced by the cells of the microorganism Saccharomyces cerevisiae. The yeast ferments the sugars in the bread dough (sucrose, glucose, fructose, and maltose). Yeast is available in compressed cakes of fresh yeast, or as dry yeast granules called **ACTIVE DRY YEAST** or **QUICK RISING YEAST**. It is perishable and an expiration date is provided. Fresh yeast must be refrigerated or frozen.

Quality

- The quality of baked products depends on proper proportions of ingredients, freshness and quality of ingredients, proper mixing techniques, and appropriate baking times and temperatures.

High altitude baking

- Baking at altitudes greater than 3,000 ft above sea level requires adjustments to recipes. Lower atmospheric pressures cause excessive expansion of leavening gases, which stretch and weaken the cell structure being formed in the oven. The resulting product may have a coarse, irregular grain, or it may collapse. Recipes should be adjusted to contain less baking powder, harder flour, more water, higher baking temperature or less shortening or sugar.

COMMON BAKING PROBLEMS

Product	Problem	Cause
Muffin	Tunnels, peaked top pale slick crust	Over mixing
Cake	Low volume, flat top, brown specks	Under mixing (undissolved soda)
	Tough crust	Too little fat or sugar
	Hump in the middle	Oven too hot
	Uneven texture	Incomplete mixing or too short baking time
	Bitter flavor	Too much baking powder

STARCHES

- **STARCHES** are digestible complex carbohydrates used to thicken sauces, gravies, cream soups and puddings. Starches are not sweet and are not readily absorbed in cold liquids. Starches are composed of **AMYLOSE**, straight chains of glucose units and **AMYLOPECTIN**, branched chains of glucose units. Amylose produces organic gels, while amylopectin produces clear thickening. Amylopectin is more stable and less likely to break down.

- Starch can be processed from corn, wheat, tapioca, potato, arrowroot, etc. The thickening power of starches varies. Cornstarch is an excellent thickener. Modified (cross-bonded) starch is used to thicken and improve the texture of frozen foods, many processed foods and baby foods.

- When starch granules are watered and heated, they swell or **GELATINIZE**, increasing the viscosity of the suspension as they form a paste. As the mixture cools, the paste forms a gel. Stirring a starch mixture after it thickens may break the swollen starch grains and cause a loss of thickening or stickiness. Adding sugar keeps the starch paste thick. Both sugar and fat have a tenderizing effect.

- **DEXTRINIZATION** or partial starch hydrolysis is caused by acid, heat and enzymes. Dextrins thicken less than most starches. A starch and liquid mixture should be cooked before an acid is added.

- Lumps usually occur when a dry starch is mixed with warm or hot water. The exterior of the granules becomes sticky, causing clumping. To decrease lumping, mix starch with cold water first forming a **SLURRY**, then add it to the hot liquid with continuous stirring. Other methods of preventing lumps are mixing the dry starch with sugar or fat before adding to warm water. Melted fat cooked with flour is called a **ROUX**. A roux can be cooked to caramelize, creating the dark roux typical in Cajun cooking.

- **SAUCES** are flavored, thickened liquids, usually formed by adding seasonings and a thickening agent to stock, juice or other liquids.

- There are five basic sauces, called **MOTHER SAUCES** or **LEADING SAUCES:** Béchamel,

Tomato, Espagnola, Velouté and Hollandaise. Other sauces are made from them by adding other ingredients. Additional sauces are made from chopped or pureed fruits or vegetables, such as salsas and fruit sauces. Thickening agents, such as flour or cornstarch, are used to thicken sauces. Sauces are changed by the addition of seasoning, herbs and flavoring.

BASIC SAUCE PROPORTIONS

Consistency	Proportion of Flour: Liquid	Typical Use
Very thin	2 tsp: 1 cup	soup with starchy veg.
Thin	1 Tbsp: 1 cup	soup, nonstarchy veg.
Medium	2 Tbsp: 1 cup	gravy, sauce
Thick, very thick	3-4 Tbsp: 1 cup	soufflé, croquettes

---

(5) Vegetables and fruits

VEGETABLES

- **VEGETABLES** are edible plants. Different parts of the plant, including flowers, seeds, stems, roots, leaves and underground stems (tubers) can be eaten. Some fruits that are not sweet are also commonly considered vegetables because they are prepared and served like vegetables (i.e., tomatoes).

- At meals, half the plate should be fruits and vegetables. *MyPlate* recommends 2 ½ cups of vegetables per day, on a 2,000 calorie diet, to provide the vitamins, minerals, fiber, water, phytochemicals and carbohydrates needed for health.

TYPES OF VEGETABLES

Category	Examples	Desirable Characteristics
Cabbage Family	Cauliflower, broccoli, cabbage, Brussels sprouts, bok choy	Heavy for size, good color, unblemished
Fruit-Vegetables	Tomatoes, eggplant, avocados	Firm flesh, smooth skin, good color, unblemished
Leafy Greens	Spinach, kale, lettuces, beet and collard greens	Crisp, bright leaves without brown spots
Onion Family	Onions, garlic, shallots, leeks	Firm flesh, good color, dry, clean surface
Seeds and Pods	Green beans, corn, lima beans, sugar snaps, peas	Firm, well shaped, without blemishes or dried spots
Squashes	Hard shell and summer squashes, cucumbers, zucchini, pumpkin	Firm, free of blemishes, heavy for size, no mold
Stems, Stalks, Shoots	Celery, asparagus, sprouts, pea shoots	Firm, unblemished, no burning of leaves
Tubers and Roots	Carrots, radishes, turnips, parsnips, potatoes, yams	Firm, unwrinkled, good color, smooth surfaces, no soft spots

Storage and use of vegetables

- Although most vegetables are ripe when purchased, most continue to ripen depending on storage conditions. All vegetables are freshest and best quality when picked and eaten in season. Small vegetables are usually more tender.

- Potatoes, winter squash and onion family vegetables should be stored at 60-70°F in a dark, dry place. If refrigerated, they lose flavor and texture, and the starch in potatoes turns to sugar. Tomatoes should be stored at room temperature. Most other vegetables should be refrigerated at 40-45°F, with high humidity. Fresh vegetables and fruits should be stored in bags or loosely wrapped in the refrigerator. Do not wash fruit or vegetables before storing as they will stay fresher longer if not washed until use.

- Fresh vegetables should be carefully washed immediately before cooking to remove sand, grit, chemicals and insects. Root vegetables should be scrubbed with a brush. Cabbage family vegetables should be soaked in salted water for a few minutes to draw out insects. Wash leafy green vegetables in a water bath or under running water. Store all cut vegetables in the refrigerator.

- Frozen vegetables are a convenient alternative when fresh vegetables are out of season or not readily available. Nutrients and colors are maintained.

- All frozen vegetables should be stored at 0°F and used when thawed. Do not refreeze thawed vegetables.

- Discard potatoes with green skin or green spots on skin. These contain **SOLANINE**, a toxin caused by prolonged exposure to light. Solanine is not destroyed by heat and does not dissolve in water. This toxin can cause gastrointestinal and central nervous system problems.

- Canning preserves flavor and texture of some vegetables; such as tomatoes, corn and beans. But canning softens some vegetables and some nutrients go into the liquid in the can. The net weight of canned vegetables is the weight of the entire contents of the can including packing liquids.

- The high heat used in canning destroys microorganisms. If cans are not properly sealed, processed or handled and have any dents or swelling they should be discarded, as should cans that contain discolored food.

Vegetable preparation

- When cut, some vegetables, like potatoes, turn brown as cells oxidize. Enzymatic browning of vegetables and fruits can be reduced by immersing them in cold water or by adding a small amount of antioxidants, such as lemon juice.

- Many vegetables can be cooked with dry or high heat to preserve flavor and nutrients. Methods include grilling, roasting, broiling, baking, sautéing or stir-frying.

- Moist-heat cooking methods include blanching, poaching, braising, simmering. Green vegetables should be cooked without a cover; red vegetables should be cooked covered to preserve color.

- Sulfur compounds in strong-flavored vegetables of the onion family are water-soluble and lost in steam when the vegetables are cooked without a lid. Sulfur compounds in the cabbage family are released and become apparent upon over-cooking or in the presence of acid.

- Most vegetables should be cooked in minimum amounts of water for short periods to preserve nutrients, flavor and color. Addition of baking soda to cooking water prevents color changes in vegetables by neutralizing acid, but also reduces nutrient value and is not recommended.

- Excess water and heat may lead to loss of vitamins. Vitamin C is leached into cooking water and oxidized. Small amounts of some B vitamins are destroyed by heat. Vitamin A can be oxidized by heat.

- Microwave cooking or steaming of vegetables preserves nutrients, color and texture.

- Long cooking of green vegetables causes undesirable color changes. Low-acid vegetables can cook longer without experiencing color changes. Adding some acid retains the best color of red cabbage and beets.

STANDARD VEGETABLE CUTS

Baton
1/4 x 1/4 x 2 inches (small stick)

Brunoise
1/8 x 1/8 x 1/8 inch (extra small dice)

Chiffonade
Thin ribbons

Chips
1/8 inch thick slice

Diagonal
Bias-cut slices

French Fry
1/2 x 1/2 x 3 inches

Fine Julienne
1/16 x 1/16 x 2 inches

Mirepoix
1/2 inch average rough cut

Julienne
1/8 x 1/8 x 2 inches (short matchstick)

Tourne
7 sided; 2 inch long barrel

Small Dice
1/4 x 1/4 inch squares

Waffle
1/8 inch thick slice, perforated

Round
Round disks of varying thickness

Medium Dice
1/2 x 1/2 inch squares

Stick
3/8 x 3/8 x 2 inches

Large Dice
3/4 x 3/4 inch squares

FRUITS

- *MyPlate* recommends 2 cups of fruit per day for a 2000 calorie diet. Fruits are rich sources of carbohydrate, fiber, water and many vitamins, minerals and phytochemicals.

- Fresh fruit adds color, flavor and nutrients to any meal.

- Using local fruits in season reduces cost and generally increases quality but, due to quick shipping, many fruits are available year round.

- USDA has voluntary grading for fresh fruits. Most fresh fruit is US Fancy. Premium quality and lesser grades are typically made into jams, jellies and sauces.

TYPES OF FRUIT

Category	Examples	Desirable Characteristics
Berries	Strawberries, blueberries, raspberries, blackberries, gooseberries	Juicy, thin-skinned fruit with tiny seeds, picked when ripe. Sweet, plump, even color. No mold or spots.
Citrus	Oranges, grapefruits, lemons, limes, tangerines, tangelos	Smooth, clear, bright colored skin. No soft spots.
Drupes	Peaches, nectarines, plums, apricots, cherries, mango	Thin skin, slightly soft flesh, firm plump without bruises, smooth skin.
Exotics	Persimmon, pomegranate, prickly pear, lychee	Semi-soft skin, slightly heavy, good color, bright skin.
Grapes	Seeded and seedless red, green, black grapes	Plump and juicy, rich color, firmly attached to stems.
Melons	Cantaloupe, honeydew, watermelon, canary melon	Netted or smooth rind. Heavy for size. Firm, with good aroma and no soft spots.
Pommes	Pears, apples	Firm, thin skinned with no blemishes, bruises, soft spots.
Tropicals	Papaya, mango, banana, kiwi, pineapple	Firm, plump, good color, unblemished.

Storage and use of fruit

- There are color, flavor, and texture changes as fruits ripen. The flesh becomes soft, juicier, and less tart and flavor and aroma intensify. Some fruits are shipped unripe (like bananas) and continue to ripen after shipping. Others (like pineapples) must be picked when fully ripe.

- Ripe fruits, except bananas, should be refrigerated.

- When fruits ripen, they release **ETHYLENE GAS**, a colorless, odorless gas emitted from fruits. This gas triggers enzymes, causing other fruits to ripen. To ripen firm pears, peaches and other fruit, put them in a paper bag and seal the top, hold at room temperature, checking daily to determine when they ripe. To stop fruits from ripening further, chill and isolate them from fruits that need more ripening. Melons, apples, and bananas emit more of this gas than other fruits.

- Canned fruit, in heavy or light syrup, water or fruit juice is available. Canned fruit softens in texture, but nutrient content of the fruit is not diminished. The syrup can be drained or eaten depending on caloric needs. Canned fruit includes cooked fruit products, like applesauce. For food safety reasons and for ease in chewing, canned fruits are preferred options for individuals with immunity problems who cannot eat fresh produce, and for some who have difficulty eating fresh fruit. Canned fruit has a long shelf life. Discard any bent or bulging cans as contents are not safe to eat.

- Frozen fruit, especially **INDIVIDUALLY QUICK FROZEN (IQF) FRUIT**, can be very good quality, although freezing often breaks down the cell structure of fruit. Frozen fruit must be kept at a constant temperature of 0°F or lower.

- Dried fruits should be stored in airtight containers in a cool, dark place. Avoid sunlight and moisture.

- **COMPOTES** are fresh or dried fruits cooked in sugar syrups.

- **CHUTNEY** is a condiment of fruit, vinegar, sugar, and spices. It can be hot or mild and served cold, warm, or hot, often with poultry or meats.

- Treating fresh produce with sulfur dioxide (**SULFITES**) to avoid browning has been banned because some people are allergic to it. Dried fruits (such as golden raisins and apricots) that are processed with sulfites must note on the package that they contain sulfites.

- The cut surfaces of some fruits (e.g., apples, pears) are susceptible to **ENZYMATIC BROWNING**. Phenolic substances act as a substrate for enzymes released when fruit is cut or damaged. Lowering the pH of the fruit, with an acid juice dip (typically pineapple or lemon juice) can control the reaction that inactivates the enzyme. Immersing fruit in sugar syrup or chilling it also helps prevent browning.

Preparation of fruit

- When heated in water without sugar, fruit releases its sugar and flavor, creating a fruit sauce.

- Cooking fruit in sugar syrup preserves its shape and firmness.

- Cooking destroys microorganisms on fruits and vegetables.

- Fruits may be poached by submerging in liquid (juice or syrup) and cooking at low temperature to retain texture and shape.

- Fruit, such as pineapple slices, peaches, nectarines and pears may also be grilled as an accompaniment to an entrée or as part of a salad.

Structure of vegetables and fruits

- The cell walls of plant products contain **LIGNIN**, **CELLULOSE** and **HEMICELLULOSE** fibers that support the contents of the cell. Lignin, a non-carbohydrate polysaccharide found in cell walls, is indigestible to humans and is not softened by cooking. PECTIC SUBSTANCES (PECTIN) act as the intercellular cement in fruits. Used with acid and sugar, they form gels and are used in the preparation of jellies and jams.

Color of vegetables and fruits

- Pigments in vegetables and fruits include two fat-soluble pigment groups found in cell plastids that are in the cytoplasm. Green pigments (primarily CHLOROPHYLL) play a vital role in photosynthesis. Magnesium in chlorophyll is the center of the porphyrin ring. It is replaced with hydrogen, dulling the color in the presence of heat and acid.

- CAROTENOIDS are also fat-soluble substances ranging in color from yellow to orange-red and are of two types: (1) carotenes, containing carbon and + hydrogen, and (2) xanthophylls, containing carbon + hydrogen + oxygen. Carotenoids are the most stable pigments, but heating and oxidation decrease the intensity of the color slightly. Carotenoids are biologic antioxidants.

- FLAVONOIDS are water-soluble phenolic pigments found in cell sap. These include anthocyanins (blue-red, purple), anthoxanthins (colorless, pale yellow) and phenolic compounds or tannins (clear, white, brown). These produce more intense food color in presence of acid. Adding a tiny bit of lemon juice, cream of tartar or vinegar to the water reduces color change. Apples, pears, peaches, bananas and avocados are subject to enzymatic browning. Adding a small amount of orange or lemon juice prevents browning.

Quality

- High-quality vegetables and fruits are young, succulent, tender, crisp, unbruised and have nonfibrous tissue. TURGIDITY is the degree of crispness caused by water pressure in plant material. Sugar or salt added to fruits or vegetables causes the cells to lose interior fluid and become limp (e.g., salt on cucumbers).

Grading

- Grading of vegetables and fruits is voluntary. Standards define the color, shape, size, maturity and number and degree of defects. Some products also have standards for flavor and tenderness.

- Vegetables and fruits are graded in two groups:
  - 1. Fresh: U.S. Fancy, U.S. No. 1, U.S. No. 2
  - 2. Processed: U.S. Grade A (Fancy), U.S. Grade B (Choice for fruits and Extra Standard for vegetables) and U.S. Grade C (Standard)

Labeling

- The top-twenty selling vegetables and fruits currently have nutrition labeling provided at point-of-purchase, but not on each package. This is "voluntary" but may become mandatory if the voluntary system is not widely implemented.

(6) Fats and oils

- Some fats and oils contain only carbon, hydrogen and oxygen; others also contain phosphorus, nitrogen or sulfur.

Fatty acids

- **FATTY ACIDS** are important structural components of lipids. Most naturally occurring fatty acids have straight carbon chains, even numbers of carbon and hydrogen atoms attached to the carbons, except at the carboxyl carbon. Most dietary fats and oils are **TRIGLYCERIDES** containing three fatty acids and a molecule of glycerol. Some fatty acids have branched chains, odd numbers of carbons or a hydroxyl group in place of a hydrogen, which occur in trace amounts in some foods.

- Fatty acids differ in carbon chain length (usually 4-24 carbons in food) and in degree of saturation (0 double bonds = **SATURATED**, 1 double bond = **MONOUNSATURATED**, 2 or more durable bonds = **POLYUNSATURATED**). Saturated fats are more chemically stable.

- **CIS-FATTY ACIDS** and **TRANS-FATTY ACIDS** are terms to describe the positioning of the hydrogen atoms attached to the double bonds in the fatty-acid molecule. A cis configuration occurs when the hydrogen attached to carbons that have a double bond is on the same side of the carbon-carbon double bond. Cis is the typical natural configuration of hydrogen atoms in fatty acids. A trans configuration occurs when the hydrogen attached to carbons, forming a double bond, is on opposite sides. Trans-fatty acids are similar to saturates in raising plasma cholesterol levels. Trans-fatty acids are a result of partial hydrogenation of cis bonds. Trans-fatty acids are made because they are more stable to heat and more resistant to rancidity. Vegetable oil is virtually all cis bonds. Stick margarine from vegetable oil typically has 25-30% trans-fatty acids versus 13-20% trans-fatty acids in soft tub margarine. Since 2006 when the FDA required that the amount of trans-fatty acids be listed on the Nutrition Facts label, many products that contained trans-fatty acids have been reconfigured either to lower the amount of trans fatty acids or to remove them entirely. The *2010 Dietary Guidelines for Americans* recommend avoiding trans fats and the FDA banned the addition of trans fats in processed foods in 2013.

Fat crystallization

- Solid fats consist of crystals suspended in oil. The higher the proportion of crystals, the more solid the fat is at room temperature. Crystalline forms of fat include alpha (small, unstable), beta (large, stable) and beta prime (smaller than beta, stable). Lipids with a cis double bond are difficult to arrange in a crystal because the molecule tends to bend. **PLASTICITY** of fat is determined by the volume of crystals to oil and the melting point of the fat in the crystals.

COMMON FATTY ACIDS IN FOODS

Common Name	International Union of Chemistry (IUC) Name	Abbreviation	Source
Saturated			
	No double bonds		
Butyric	Butanoic	4:0	Butter
Caproic	Hexanoic	6:0	Butter, coconut and palm nut oils
Caprylic	Octanoic	8:0	Butter, coconut and palm nut oils
Capric	Decanoic	10:0	Butter, coconut and palm nut oils
Lauric	Dodecanoic	12:0	Laurel oil, coconut oil, spermaceti
Myristic	Tetradecanoic	14:0	Coconut oil, nutmeg oil, animal fats
Palmitic	Hexadecanoic	16:0	Plant and animal fats
Stearic	Octadecanoic	18:0	Plant and animal fats
Archidic	Eicosanoic	20:0	Peanut & rapeseed oils, butter lard
Behenic	Docosanoic	22:0	Peanut oil
Lignoceric	Tetracosanoic	24:0	Peanut oil, glycolipids, phospholipids
Monounsaturated			
	One double bond		
Myristoleic	Cis-9-tetradecenoic	14:1	Butter, sperm oil, fish liver oils
Palmitoleic	Cis-9- hexadecenic	16:1	Butter, fish oils, animal fats
Oleic	Cis-9-octadecenoic	18:1	Plant and animal fats
Vaccenic	Cis- and trans-11- octadecenoic	18:1	Butter
Gadoleic	Cis-9-eicosenoic	20:1	Brain phospholipids, fish liver oils
Erucic	Cis-13-docosenoic	22:1	Rapeseed oil, various seed oils
Polyunsaturated			
	Two double bonds		
Linoleic	Cis-9, cis-12- octadecadienoic	18:2	Plant and animal fats
	Three double bonds		
Linolenic	Octadecatrienoic cis-9, cis-12, cis-15	18:3	Linseed oil, mammal fats, fish liver oil
Eleostearic	9, 11, 13-octadecatrienoic	18:3	Chinese wood oil, seeds, fats
γ-Linolenic	6, 9, 12- octadecatrienoic	18:3	Primrose seed oil
	Four double bonds		
Moroctic	4, 8, 12, 15- octadecatetraenoic	18:4	Fish oils
Arachidonic	5, 8, 11, 14- eicostaetraenoic	20:4	Animal phospholipids, fats
	Five double bonds		
Timnodonic	4, 8, 12, 15, 18-eicosapentaenoic	20:5	Sardine oil
Clupanodonic	4, 8, 12, 15, 19- docosapentaenoic	22:5	Brain and liver phospholipids
	Six double bonds		
Nisinic	4, 8, 12, 15, 18, 21- tetracosahexaenoic	20:6	Sardine oil

Melting point

- The **MELTING POINT** is the temperature at which a solid changes to a liquid.

- Factors that affect the melting point of fat include:

  - **CARBON CHAIN LENGTH:** The melting point decreases with an increase in the number of double bonds from -4°C for a 4-carbon, to 80°C for a 22-carbon fatty acid.
  - **DEGREE OF SATURATION:** Melting point will increase according to the degree of saturation. Saturated fats have higher melting points. Double bonds make crystallization more difficult and require less energy for melting after crystallization occurs.
  - **CONFIGURATION:** The trans form of fatty acid has a higher melting point than the cis form. The bend in a chain with a cis configuration inhibits crystal formation.
  - **CRYSTALLINE FORMATION:** Alpha crystals melt faster than beta prime and beta prime crystals melt faster than beta crystals.
  - **COMPONENT FATTY ACIDS:** The melting point of a triglyceride is determined by the melting point of the component fatty acids. Monoglycerides have higher melting points than triglycerides.

Processing of fats

- **HYDROGENATION** is a process that saturates or hardens oils or soft fats by the addition of hydrogen in the presence of a catalyst (usually nickel) and pressure. The process is used to make shortening or margarine; hard margarine sticks are more hydrogenated than soft, tub margarine. Many stick margarines are made from polyunsaturated oils and become monounsaturated (partially in the trans form) as a result of hydrogenation.

- Trans bonds (even in fats that are monounsaturated) act in the body similar to saturated fats and may be hypercholesterolemic. Tiny amounts of trans fatty acids are in a few foods but most trans bonds are in processed foods.

- **INTERESTERIFICATION** changes the arrangement of fatty acids on triglycerides to produce a more random distribution. The fat molecules become heterogeneous; the fat is less coarse and grainy and more plastic over a wide range of temperatures. Lard processed this way forms smaller crystals and creams more easily.

- **WINTERIZATION** is a process in which oil is chilled until more saturated molecules begin to crystallize. Then the solid material is removed by filtration. The process produces oils that will stay clear in the refrigerator.

- **ANTIOXIDANTS** may be added to prevent fat from becoming rancid when it is oxidized or when the fatty acids are liberated from glycerol by enzymes.

  - The primary FDA approved antioxidants are **BHA** (butylated hydroxyanisole), **BHT** (butylated hydroxytoluene) and **PROPYL GALLATE.**
  - Tocopherols, such as vitamin E, are naturally-occurring antioxidants.
  - Metal contaminants may catalyze oxidation. Their activity can be curtailed by chelating substances, such as citrate, ascorbate, phosphate and ethylenediaminetetraacetate acid (**EDTA**).

Use of fat in food preparation

- Fats contribute to characteristic flavors, richness, textures and aromas of foods. They also contribute to a feeling of satiety, carry fat-soluble vitamins and are the source of essential fatty acids.

Fats and oils in cooking

- The most healthful oils for cooking are canola and olive oil because of their high unsaturated fat content and versatility.

- **CANOLA OIL** is a bland oil made from the pressing of rapeseed or field mustard plants. It contains both Omega-3 and Omega-6 fatty acids.

- **OLIVE OIL** and **EXTRA VIRGIN OLIVE OIL (EVO)**, that come from the first pressing of the olives has a more intense flavor and is used in dressings and drizzles. Olive oils come in varied colors depending on the amount of chlorophyll and carotenoid pigments. There are also different flavors based on the olive-growing region. Regular olive oil can be used for most cooking uses. Extra virgin is reserved for dressings. Extra virgin is much more expensive than regular olive oil. When extra virgin is heated, there is little difference in flavor compared to regular. The nutrient values of both types of oil are the same.

- **SOYBEAN OIL** is an inexpensive oil that has a high smoke point and is good for frying. It is high in monounsaturated fatty acids unless it is hydrogenated.

- **SUNFLOWER OIL** is rich in Vitamin E protecting it from rancidity. It is used in some trans-fat-free shortenings.

- **COTTONSEED OIL** has more saturated fatty acids than most other oils.

- **GRAPESEED OIL** has the highest smoke point, is rich in linoleic and oleic acid and has a slightly grapy flavor. It is an expensive oil used by some chefs for very hot searing of foods.

- **NUT OILS**, hazelnut, walnut and other nut oils are intensely flavored. They are expensive and used primarily for drizzles and finishing foods rather than in cooked foods.

- **TROPICAL OILS** (coconut, palm and palm kernel oils) are highly saturated. All are used widely in Africa and parts of Asia where they add needed calories to the diet. Some recent research shows some health benefits of coconut oil.

Uses of fats

- Fats are good conductors of heat and can be heated to temperatures substantially above the boiling point of water. Heated fats can brown the surface of foods. The highest temperature for cooking fat is 390°F.

- At very high temperatures, fats begin to smoke (**SMOKE POINT**), then they flash (**FLASH POINT**) and then the fat will burn (**FIRE POINT**).

- Fat with a high initial smoke point (at least 420°F) is good for frying. Free fatty acids in fat lower the smoke point. Cooking oils and hydrogenated fats decompose at higher temperatures than lard, butter and mixtures of animal and vegetable fats.

- Smoke point is lowered by repeated or prolonged use of the fat, by salt, water, food particles or emulsifiers in the fat and by increased exposed surface area. Thus, the smoking point of fats heated in shallow, wide pans with slightly sloping sides is lower than that of fats heated in narrow deep pans with vertical sides.

- Fat should be filtered and refrigerated after each use. To restore flavor, fresh fat should be added whenever fat is reused. Fat used to fry fish or other strong-flavored food should only be reused to fry similar items.

- Fats expand and foam when heated, so pans should not be filled more than half way when frying. A cup of melted fat weighs more than a cup of solid fat.

- Shortening (firm fats, such as hydrogenated oils, butter, lard, and margarine) is used as shortening in pastry products. It interlaces between protein and starch structures making the gluten strands shorter. For example, flaky pie pastry results when small flakes of gluten are separated by fat and then leavened by steam. Fat also creates tenderness in baked goods by preventing water and flour interactions to form gluten. Shortening traps air that increases volume and tenderness of baked goods.

- Fat forms emulsions with water and air. Fat globules may be suspended in a large amount of water (e.g., milk, cream, salad dressing). Water droplets may be suspended in a large amount of fat (e.g., diet margarine). Air may be trapped as an emulsion in fat (e.g., butter cream icing, whipped butter).

Rancidity

- **RANCIDITY** is spoilage of fat caused by the reaction of triglycerides with water molecules breaking them down to volatile compounds with off flavors. Rancidity can also be caused by oxidation when heat or light cause lipids to break down and cause free radicals with altered taste and aroma. Adding antioxidants and storing in containers that block light and air can delay rancidity of oils.

Fat replacers

- **FAT REPLACERS** can be made from a variety of compounds that mimic the desirable flavor, texture or cooking properties of fats.

- Carbohydrate-based fat replacers are non-sweet carbohydrates; some are **GRAS** (generally recognized as safe) and others have FDA approval. Carbohydrate-based fat replacers have 0-4 calories per gram, depending on type.

CARBOHYDRATE-BASED FAT REPLACERS

Ingredient	Description	Example/Name	Use
Cellulose (GRAS) 0 – 4 calories/g	Microparticles to create mouthfeel of fat and retain moisture in food	Cellulose gel Avicel®, Methocel® Solka-Floc®	Dairy products, salad dressing, frozen dessert
Dextrin (GRAS) 4 calories/g	Derived from tapioca, corn or other starches. Gels thickens, stabilizes	N-Oit®, Amylum	Salad dressing, puddings, spreads, frozen desserts
Fiber (GRAS) 4 calories/g	Structural functions, volume, and shelf stability	Opta™, Oat Fiber, Snowite Z-Trim, Uttracel™	Baked goods, meat spreads, extruded products
Gums (GRAS) 0 calories/g	Thickening, gelling, creamy texture	Xanthen gum, Keltrol®, Kelcogel®, Slendid™	Baked goods, dairy, frozen desserts, soups, processed meats, sauces
Inulin (GRAS) 1 calorie/g	Fiber and bulking agent extracted from chicory root	Raftiline®, Fruitafit®, Fibruline®	Yogurt, cheese, frozen desserts, filling, whipped cream, processed meats
Maltodextrin (GRAS) 4 calories/g	Hydrolyzed food starch, texture modifier, and bulking agent. Not for frying	Maltrin®, Paselli®, Star-Dri®, Lycadex®, Lorelite, CrystalLean®	Baked goods, filling, and frostings, frozen desserts, dairy, salad dressing
Nu-Trim	Beta-glucan rich fat replacer made from oat and barley		Baked goods, milk, cheese, ice cream
Oatrim (GRAS) 1-4 calories/g	Enzyme treated oat starch, used for texture, adds fiber	Beta Trim™, Trim Choice, Replace	Baked goods, fillings, dairy, cheese, salad dressing, candy
Polydextrose (FDA approved additive)	Water-soluble polymer of dextrose, with small amounts of sorbitol and citric acid	Litesse™, Sta-Lite™	
Polyols (GRAS) 1.6-3 calories/g	Hydrolyzed, hydrogenated starches to replace bulk in fat reduced and fat-free products	Xylitol, Mannitol, Isomalt, Sorbitol	Frozen dairy desserts, baked goods, fillings, frosting
Modified food starch	Fat replacer from potato, corn, oat, rice, wheat or	Amalean® I & II,	Processed meats, salad dressing, baked

FAT-BASED FAT REPLACERS

Ingredient	Description	Example/Name	Use
Caprenin (FDA petition pending)	Reduced calorie triglyceride with melting characteristics of cocoa butter.	Caprenin	Candy, chocolate
Esterified Propoxylated Glycerol (EPG)	Reduced calorie. May partially or fully replace fats and oils in many products and in baking and frying.		
Mono & di-glyceride emulsifiers (GRAS) 9 calories/gram, but less is used compared to fat; therefore calories are reduced.	Glycerines react with specific fatty acids. Allow fat and water to mix.	Dur-Lo® EC™	Cake mixes, cookies, icing, dairy products
Olestra—calorie free (FDA approved)	Sucrose polyester; non-absorbable from sucrose and oils but may cause diarrhea in some people. Inhibits fat-soluble vitamin absorption, but is supplemented to prevent effect. Stable under high heat, such as frying.	Olean®	Potato, corn tortilla chips, crackers, cheese puffs
Salatrim (FDA petition pending) 5 calories/gram	Reduced calorie fat from glycerol and short chain fatty acids and stearic acid. Not for frying.	Benefat™	Chocolate, cookies, crackers, sour cream, cheese, margarine, snacks
Sorbestrin approximately 1.5 calories/gram	Low calorie, heat stable liquid fat substitute made of fatty acid including esters of sorbitol.		Vegetable oil
Fantesk	Mixture of starch, water and oily substance using pressurized steam.		Frostings and bakery products.

- Trans fats are to be avoided when possible according to *Dietary Guidelines for Americans*. Food labels now require declaration of content of trans fats. Ingredients with trans fats were used to increase shelf life of many processed foods. Manufacturers now try to limit use of trans fats from hydrogenated by using various technologies including fat blends, fat replacers and substitutes and pectin gels. The *2010 Dietary Guidelines for Americans* recommend avoiding trans fats and the FDA banned the addition of trans fats in processed foods in 2013.

I. PRINCIPLES OF DIETETICS (12%)

- Protein-based fat replacers cannot be used in baking or fried foods because heat changes the proteins. The body digests these as proteins.
  - Simplesse®, (GRAS) micro-encapsulated spheres of egg white or whey protein, mimics fat-like texture and creaminess, is used in frozen desserts, sour cream, and salad dressing, margarine, coffee creamer, etc. It provides 1-2 calories per gram. It is digested as a protein.
  - Dairy-Lo® is a modified whey protein concentrate. Controlled thermal denaturation results in a functional protein with fat-like properties. It is used in cheese, yogurt, sour cream, ice cream and salad dressing.

(7) Functional Foods

- **FUNCTIONAL FOODS** have been defined by The Institute of Medicine (IOM), a branch of the National Academy of Sciences, as those that include "any modified food or food ingredient that may provide a health benefit beyond the traditional nutrients it contains."

- Functional foods used to be known as **NUTRACEUTICALS** or **DESIGNER FOODS**. Surveys show that consumers are interested in products that provide health benefits so food manufacturers are designing and offering them. Examples include margarine with substances that reduce blood cholesterol, cereals with added fibers that promote cholesterol reduction, soy added to reduce risk of cardiovascular disease and various foods with live cultures.

- Quality, flavor, cost and safety are concerns when using engineered foods. Each must be evaluated individually to determine if it meets consumer needs and uses technology and ingredients that are safe.

- A variety of engineered foods have been developed as a result of advances in food technology. Some engineered foods are nutritionally equal or superior to whole foods in that fats or other components have been reduced. Some engineered foods (i.e., surimi, fortified fruit drinks) are more economical than the foods they replace.

- **BIOENGINEERING** produces foods **GENETICALLY-MODIFIED ORGANISMS (GMO)** that have been genetically altered to change their properties. Examples are vegetables resistant to crop diseases, varieties with increased yields and tomatoes that are red and ripe for a longer time without rotting. Many individuals, organizations, and nations oppose GMOs and are concerned about allergens and unknown effects of bioengineered foods especially those that put genes from animals into vegetables and other foods.

b. Scientific basis for preparation and storage

(1) Function of ingredients

SUGARS

- **SUGARS** are the basic, simple chemical units of carbohydrates. Sugars generally provide 4 calories per gram. Sugars, regardless of the form eaten, are converted to glucose for use in the body.

- The term **SUGAR** generally refers to refined sucrose derived from sugar beets or sugar cane. These two sugars are the same and are 99.5% pure sucrose. Sugar in recipes refers to granulated beet or cane sugar.

Functions

- Sugars are an active agent in non-enzymatic browning reactions. Sugars **CARAMELIZE** when cooked, causing browning and flavor changes.

- Sugars modify the properties of egg, starch and gelatin gels. Sugars dehydrate pectin micelles to permit pectin gels to form. They stabilize egg white foams and tenderize starch gels and gelatins.

- Sugars provide food for yeast in breads, help foods retain moisture, tenderize baked products by widening the gluten strands, and are a base for making icing.

- Sugars provide sweetness to many foods and form the crystalline structure of candies. A **CRYSTAL** is a closely-packed molecule arranged in a pattern and closely bound by plane surfaces or faces. Sucrose, for example, has 18 faces.

  - ➤ **CRYSTALLIZATION** occurs when a solution is supersaturated. If only one or two nuclei are formed, the crystal size will be large. If nucleus formation is rapid, many small crystals will form. Small crystal formation is desirable for food products.
  - ➤ Factors affecting crystal formation are the nature of the substance, the concentration of the solution, the temperature, the agitation (stirring) and the presence of impurities.
  - ➤ Stirring a mixture of sugars and acid (cream of tartar) enhances small crystal formation.
  - ➤ In candy making, sugar is crystallized and the sugar to moisture ratio is controlled to make a sweet confection.
  - ➤ The state of crystallinity and the percentage of moisture in confections are determined by the nature of its ingredients, the heat used, the concentration of sugar syrups, the way syrups are cooled and the degree of agitation (stirring).

- Sucrose is the main sweetener and crystal former in candy making. At room temperature, two parts of sucrose dissolve in one part of water. At higher temperatures, more sucrose is dissolved, which produces a higher concentration of syrup. High-fructose corn syrup is produced in this way.

Types of sugar

- **GRANULATED SUGAR (TABLE SUGAR)** may be labeled "granulated," "fine granulated" or "extra fine granulated." These designations do not indicate definite particle size, but preference in manufacturer terminology. It is the most commonly-used sugar and is extracted from sugar cane or sugar beets. One teaspoon provides 16 calories.

- **INVERT SUGAR** is made from hydrolysis of sucrose to form a mixture of dextrose and levulose. The confectionery trade refers to glucose as dextrose and fructose as levulose. An invert sugar/sucrose combination is sweeter than sucrose alone.

- **SUPERFINE GRANULATED SUGAR** is a specially screened, uniformly fine-grained sugar, designed for use in cakes, meringues, mixed drinks and other products that require quick creaming or rapid dissolving.

- **POWDERED** or **CONFECTIONER'S SUGAR** is granulated sugar that has been crushed or screened to the desired fineness. It usually contains a small amount of cornstarch to prevent caking.

- **BROWN SUGAR** contains varying amounts of molasses, non-sugars (ash) and moisture. Designations of "light brown," "dark" or "old-fashioned brown" indicates the color characteristics and the intensity of the molasses flavor, which increases with the color.

- **MAPLE SUGAR** is the solid product resulting from evaporation of maple syrup or maple sap. It consists of sucrose, invert sugar and ash.

- **MAPLE SYRUP** is made by evaporating maple sap or a solution of maple sugar. It contains not more than 35% water and weighs not less than 11 pounds per gallon. Imitation maple syrup (maple flavored corn syrup) is popular because real maple syrup is expensive.

- **CORN SUGAR** is crystallized dextrose (glucose) obtained by hydrolyzing cornstarch with acid.

- **CORN SYRUP** is obtained by partial hydrolysis of cornstarch by acid, alkaline or enzymatic catalysts. The liquid is neutralized, clarified and concentrated to syrup consistency. Corn syrup retards crystallization, increases the viscosity of confections, is less fragile than sucrose and contributes to the confection chewiness.

- **RAW SUGAR** is processed from cane sugar and retains some of the cane sugar molasses. It can contain contaminants, such as molds, fibers and waxes. Raw sugar should not be given to infants.

- **HONEY** is produced by honeybees from the nectar of plants. Its principal ingredients are **FRUCTOSE (LEVULOSE)** and **GLUCOSE (DEXTROSE)**. Honey should not be given to infants or individuals with impaired immune responses because it contains spores that may cause botulism in vulnerable individuals.

- **ORGANIC SUGAR** is from sugar cane that has been cultivated without chemical pesticides or herbicides meeting USDA standards for organic foods. It is used as an ingredient in other foods labeled organic because they must have all organic ingredients. It performs identically to refined sugar.

- **MOLASSES** is the thick, dark liquid from sugar cane juice. Premium grades have a lighter color and milder flavor.

- **TURBINADO SUGAR** is raw sugar from sugar cane that has been cleaned by steam to make beige-colored coarse crystals with delicate molasses flavor.

ZERO CALORIE SUGAR SUBSTITUTES

Scientific Name	Trade Name	Sweetness Index**	Discovery	FDA status	Safety	Assets/Uses/ Limitations	ADI*
Saccharin	Sweet 'n Low, Sugar Twin, Sweet 10, Necta Sweet	300-600	1879	1910-approved; safety: 1977 required to carry a warning label; 2001 warning label lifted	Actual risk, if any, appear slight	Heat and shelf stable; bitter & metallic aftertaste	5mg/kg/body weight/day
Cyclamate	Sucaryl liquid	30-60	1937	1950 approved; 1970 banned in U.S.; 50 countries allow use including Canada	NAS -"no proof of mutagenicity, or carcino-genicity"	Stable, soluble, low sweetening power	N/A
Aspartame	Equal, Nutrasweet, Insta Sweet	160-220	1965	1981 approved	FDA—"one of the most tested substances ever approved"	No aftertaste, sweet, clean taste; heat labile; shelf stable for 10 months; those with PKU should not use	50mg/kg/body weight/day
Acesulfame-K	Sunette; Sweet One	200	1967	1988 approved	Not digested or absorbed	Highly soluble, shelf stable; some say bitter aftertaste	15mg/kg/body weight/day
Neotame-a derivative of dipeptide composed of aspartic acid and phenylalanine	Neotame (is ingredient)	7,000 – 13,000	~1980	2002 approved	Not digested or absorbed	Good stability	18mg/kg/body weight/day
Stevia	Reb-A, Truvia, PureVia			Centuries of use, natural GRAS		Slow onset, may have licorice like aftertaste	4mg/kg
Sucralose	Splenda	400-800	1976	1998-99 approved	Tested for more than 20 years with no reported problems	Heat stable, no aftertaste; can be used in baking; also sold blended with sugar	5mg/kg/body weight/day
Xylitol, mannitol, sorbitol, sugar alcohols		1.0 or less		Approved	Long shelf life; acts like sugar, non-carcinogenic	Probably OK.; metabolized independently of insulin In "diabetic foods." Some diarrhea if excess; used in sugar free gums; partially absorbed.	
Erythritol	Nectress (from monk fruit)	150	1848	Approved		Can be used in baking	

*ADI: (Acceptable Daily Intake) "The amount of a food additive that can be safely consumed on a daily basis over a person's lifetime without any adverse effects.
**In relation to sucrose.

(2) Effects of techniques and methods on:

(a) Aesthetic properties

- Meals need variety, including contrasting flavors, colors and textures to be interesting, but the combinations should be acceptable. Balance spicy and bland, sweet and sour. Avoid serving foods of similar taste; vary preparation methods, and size and shape of the food on the plate.

FOOD ACCEPTABILITY

Qualitative (subjective) evaluation

- Observing plate waste and conducting consumer surveys will provide information about food acceptance. Foods offered but not chosen and foods yielding high-plate waste should be reevaluated for quality and acceptability.

Sensory aspects of meals

- **APPEARANCE** refers to the size, shape, wholeness, gloss, transparency, color, attractiveness and consistency of individual foods and of the total meal.

- **FLAVOR** is determined by tastes perceived by taste buds (sweet, salty, sour, bitter and umami), aroma, texture and temperature and by the strength of flavoring materials. Herbs, spices and flavoring extracts affect flavors and food acceptability to individuals. Method of preparation, such as grilling or frying, imparts specific mouthfeel that contribute to flavor.

- **AROMA**, the odor or fragrance of food, is closely associated with flavor and anticipation of flavor and can stimulate salivation and appetite. Heat intensifies aroma (i.e., baking bread, burning coffee). Aroma is a major factor in what most people consider as the taste of food.

- **TEXTURE** refers to the hand and mouthfeel of firmness, softness, juiciness, crispness, chewiness and the fibrous and crystalline qualities of the food.

Qualitative (sensory) tests

- Discrimination tests:
  - ➤ **PAIRED COMPARISON** compares only two samples at one time. A judge is given the samples and asked to indicate how they differ. This testing is valuable for controlling and maintaining the quality of a product.
  - ➤ **TRIANGLE TESTS** present judges with three samples, two of which are identical. The judge must decide which two are alike. This method is useful when only small differences exist between samples.
  - ➤ **DUO-TRIO TESTS** present judges with one identified sample first (control). The judge then receives two coded samples (one is the same as the identified sample) and must determine which of the two coded samples is like the control sample. There is a 50% chance of guessing the correct answer with this method, so the paired comparison and triangle tests may be more valuable.

- Descriptive tests:

  - In **RANKING,** judges rank samples according to the intensity of the characteristic being evaluated. This is useful for evaluating samples on a single quality characteristic (i.e., saltiness, crispness).
  - **SCORING** involves giving a product a score on a scale, such as 1-5 or 1-10, for a given characteristic. Much information about the product can be accumulated because both qualitative and quantitative data can be collected. This type of testing requires trained judges and well-established standards.
  - **FLAVOR PROFILES** involve a specially-trained panel working together to produce a written record of the aroma and flavor of the product. Aroma and flavor are examined separately and tabulated according to individually detected components or character, intensity of each, order of appearance and aftertaste.

Quantitative (objective) evaluation

- Quantitative measures use instruments and test procedures to measure food qualities. **IMITATIVE TESTS** measure food properties the way humans perceive them. **NON-IMITATIVE TESTS** measure the chemicals of the physical properties of food.

(b) Nutrient retention

- The degree of nutrient loss during cooking must be considered in relation to the amount of the nutrient present in the food. For example, vitamin C lost from pasteurizing milk is insignificant since milk is not a major source of that vitamin.

- Heat processing increases bioavailability of protein, CHO, and niacin and increases palatability, resulting in increased nutrient consumption. Water-soluble vitamins are sensitive to heat, especially thiamin, riboflavin, vitamin B_6 and vitamin C. The percentage of vitamins retained after cooking varies by food and length of cooking time. Refrigeration preserves the nutrient quality of fresh foods. Most cooked vegetables retain about 95% of minerals after cooking and about 95% of most B vitamins. Cooked vegetables retain at least 75% of vitamin C except for fried potatoes, which retain 50% of the vitamin and cooked green, leafy vegetables that retain 60% of their vitamin C value.

- When foods are cooked in water, some water-soluble vitamins and minerals may be lost through leaching and blanching if the liquid is not consumed. For example, some nutrients from vegetables are released into the added liquid when soup is cooked.

- Due to oxidation, fat-soluble vitamins (A, D, E, K) are subject to losses if exposed to air, as are some water-soluble vitamins like vitamin C. Cut fruit and juices should be covered when refrigerated.

- Drying and fermentation cause only small nutrient losses, especially if antioxidants are added.

- Microwaving retains nutrients equivalent to that of foods cooked in a moderate amount of water. A short cooking time increases vitamin retention. Foods prepared in advance and reheated in a microwave have less nutrient loss than foods held on a steam table.

- Irradiation retains nutrients comparable to that of heat-processed food. Irradiation destroys pathogens without changing the nutrient profile.

- Canning and freezing of commercially processed food cause fewer nutrient losses than fresh unprocessed foods that are held for several days.

- Properly storing covered food at safe temperatures preserves nutrients and food quality.

- Vegetables typically lose 10-20% of their vitamins during cooking. However, cooking softens fibers so that nutrients within cell walls are more available, i.e., cooked carrots have more available Vitamin A than raw carrots.

- When greens, such as spinach, are cooked, the cell walls break and water is released. This causes condensing of the spinach; thus, a serving of cooked spinach has far more nutrient value than a serving of raw spinach, as in a salad.

- Cooking vegetables in the skin avoids some nutrient losses. Cutting them in large pieces, as opposed to small pieces with extra surface area, also preserves nutrients.

- Cooking has little effect on carotenoids, but long exposure to oxygen destroys them.

- Cooking destroys some naturally-occurring toxins in foods, such as in the small amounts of cyanide in lima beans.

- Cooking converts some nutrients from unusable forms to forms the body can absorb. For example, the form of lysine in corn is only bioavailable when cooked.

- Processing can affect nutritional value of food. Brown rice has more fiber and nutrients than white rice; whole grain breads have more fiber and micronutrients.

(3) Roles of food additives

- **FOOD ADDITIVES** are substances, or mixtures of substances, added to basic foodstuffs as a result of any aspect of production, processing, storage or packaging. The Food and Drug Administration, in accordance with the Federal Food, Drug and Cosmetic Act, regulates the use of food additives.

- About 3,000 additives are used in foods sold in the United States with sugar, salt, corn syrup and dextrose used in the largest quantity -- over 90% by weight of all additives ingested.

- Over 600 substances appear on the **GENERALLY RECOGNIZED AS SAFE (GRAS)** list because experts agree that they are safe under the conditions of intended use.

- Additives provide a number of common functions. Those functions include:

  - Acidity or alkalinity control. The acidity or alkalinity of a food affects its flavor, texture and cooking qualities. Acetic acid, adiptic acid, citric acid, lactic acid, malic acid, phosphoric acid, potassium acid tartrate, sodium citrate and tartaric acid are used for acidity and alkalinity control.
  - **ANTI-CAKING AGENTS** prevent caking or lumping of finely powdered or crystalline substances such as salt (e.g., calcium silicate, iron ammonium citrate, silicon dioxide, sorbitol, etc.)

- **ANTIMICROBIALS** are substances that prevent food spoilage by molds, fungi, bacteria or yeast. Calcium propionate, caprylic acid, potassium propionate, potassium sorbate, sodium benzoate, sodium nitrate, sodium nitrite, sodium propionate and sulfur dioxide are used as antimicrobials.
- **ANTIOXIDANTS** reduce undesirable color and flavor changes caused by oxygen in the air. They retard food spoilage and lengthen shelf life by delaying the rancidity of fats or the browning of fruits. Ascorbic acid (Vitamin C), BHA (butylated hydroxyanisole), BHT (butylated hydroxytoluene), citric acid, EDTA (ethylenediaminetetraacetate acid), erythorbic acid, sodium erythorbate, sulfur dioxide, tartaric acid and vitamin E (tocopherol) are commonly used antioxidants.
- **BLEACHING** and **MATURING AGENTS** remove the yellowish color caused by natural pigments especially in flour. The maturing and bleaching agents also modify the gluten in the flour to give improved baking results (e.g., acetone peroxide, hydrogen peroxide).
- **EMULSIFIERS** permit the dispersion of particles of one liquid in another liquid. Emulsifiers allow liquids, such as salad dressings, to stay mixed and not separate into oil and other liquids in the dressing. Emulsifiers are also used to improve the uniformity and fineness of grain of bakery goods and ice cream. Lecithin, mono and diglycerides, polysorbates and propylene glycol monostearate are used as emulsifiers.
- **FLAVORS** and **FLAVOR ENHANCERS** are the largest and most diverse group of food additives. Extracts, herbs, hydrolyzed vegetable protein, monosodium glutamate (MSG), natural flavors, spices, synthetic flavors, vanilla and vanillin are flavors and flavor enhancers.
- Food colors give foods appetizing and characteristic colors. Examples of food colorings are annatto extract in cheese, caramel, citrus red no. 2 in soft drinks, dehydrated beets, F. D. and C. colors: Blue No. 1, Red No. 3, Red No. 40, Yellow No. 5, paprika, tumeric and saffron in grain dishes and sauces.
- **GELLING AGENTS,** such as gelatin and pectin are used in baked desserts, fillings, sherbets, preserves, and glazes.
- **HUMECTANTS** keep the moisture in foods. Glycerine, glycerol monostearate, propylene glycol and sorbitol are humectants used in cereals, baked goods and candy.
- **LEAVENING AGENTS** are substances that make foods lighter in texture and increased in volume. Yeast produces carbon dioxide as its leavening agent. Air and steam are physical leavening agents. Chemical leavening agents include baking powder (e.g., calcium phosphate, monocalcium phosphate, sodium aluminum sulfate and baking soda/sodium bicarbonate).
- Vitamins and minerals are commonly added to foods to restore nutrients lost in processing or to improve the nutritional value of the food. Ascorbic acid, carotene, iron (ferrous sulfate, ferrous fuminate), niacinamide, potassium iodide, riboflavin, thiamin, tocopherol (Vitamin E), Vitamin A and Vitamin D are common additions.
- **SEQUESTRANTS** bind trace minerals and prevent them from causing undesirable changes in the product (e.g., EDTA, calcium disodium EDTA.)
- **STABILIZERS** and thickeners are used to maintain smooth, uniform flavors and textures. These keep foods such as jams, puddings, and pie fillings at the desired consistency. Calcium alginate, cellulose, gelatin, guar gum, gum arabic, carrageenans, cornstarch, modified food starch, pectin, sodium alginate, vegetable gums and xanthan gum are used as stabilizers.

> ➢ Sweeteners improve the flavor characteristics of food. Examples of sweeteners include corn syrup, dextrose, fructose, glucose, honey, invert sugar, mannitol, non-nutritive sweetener, saccharin, sucrose and xylitol.

- **SULFITES,** including sulfur dioxide, sodium sulfite and sodium and potassium bisulfite, are listed as GRAS. Common uses of sulfites include as antimicrobials against gram-negative and gram-positive bacteria, molds and yeast. Sulfites are used widely in the wine industry to control the fermentation of wines by promoting the growth of fermentative yeasts while preventing bacterial growth; as anti-browning agents to control the discoloration of dried fruits, white raisins, apricots, apples, potatoes and mushrooms; and on shrimp and lobster to prevent enzymatic action that causes black spots on fresh shellfish. Because some people (particularly those with asthma) are sensitive to sulfites, current labeling laws require that foods containing sulfites indicate that on the label.

- **TARTRAZINE** (FD & C Yellow #5) is another substance that has been shown to cause severe adverse reactions, particularly in those sensitive to aspirin. Tartrazine, if present, is also labeled.

- **MONOSODIUM GLUTAMATE (MSG)** is a flavor-enhancer used worldwide, particularly in Asia. In the United States, it is used primarily in processed foods. The active ingredient is glutamate. Natural glutamate is found in larger amounts in ripe tomatoes and parmesan cheese than in most foods with added MSG. Most scientific and medical organizations report that MSG is safe food additive and that true MSG sensitivity is very rare. (Note: The editor/ publisher acknowledges that she has been a consultant to Ajinomoto, USA)

2. Composition of food

a. Sources of data, labels

- The Food and Drug Administration (FDA) has requirements for providing nutrition information for standard menu items in certain chain restaurants and similar retail food establishments. The Affordable Care Act, in part, amended the Federal Food, Drug, and Cosmetic Act. Among other things, ACA requires restaurants, similar retail food establishments that are part of a chain with 20 or more outlets and vending machine operators with 20 or more machines offering for sale the same menu items, to provide calorie and other nutrition information for standard menu items, including food on display and self-service food. Restaurants and similar retail food establishments not covered by the law may choose to become subject to the Federal requirements by registering every other year with the FDA.

Food labeling

- The **NUTRITION LABELING AND EDUCATION ACT (NLEA)** of 1990 mandates that most processed and packaged foods carry a nutrition label that includes a Nutrition Facts panel to identify the nutrient value of food. Revisions of the label format to make it easier to understand are being considered but new nutrition labeling has not been released at the time of this publication.

- NLEA requires that almost all food products under FDA jurisdiction (domestic or imported) carry labels that include the following information in a box titled **NUTRITION FACTS:**

  - ➤ Standardized serving sizes in standard household and metric measure (grams) for 139 food categories (sometimes a count, e.g., 2 cookies.) This is not necessarily the same as the suggested serving size on MyPlate or *Food Exchanges* and can cause confusion.
  - ➤ Number of servings per container is rounded to nearest whole portion for foods that are packaged and sold separately.
  - ➤ Calories per serving and calories from fat.
  - ➤ Grams of total fat and saturated fat, plus a percentage of daily value for each (based on 2,000 calorie diet with 30% of calories from fat, no more than 10% of calories from saturated fat).
    - o Trans fats must be listed
    - o Milligrams of cholesterol and percentage of daily value.
  - ➤ Milligrams of sodium and percentage of daily value.
  - ➤ Grams of total carbohydrate and grams of sugars.
  - ➤ Grams of dietary fiber and percentage of daily value.
  - ➤ Grams of total protein.
  - ➤ Percentages of daily value of vitamin A, vitamin C, calcium and iron.
  - ➤ Percentage of fruit or vegetable juice in beverages (if applicable).
  - ➤ Single-serving packages that contain 50-200% of the reference amount will be labeled as one serving, for example, a soft drink in a 12-oz. can with reference amount of 8 oz. will include nutrients in the whole can.
  - ➤ Listing of calories or other nutrients from saturated fat, polyunsaturated fat, monounsaturated fat, potassium, soluble fiber, insoluble fiber, sugar, alcohol and additional non-required but essential vitamins and minerals will be allowed on a voluntary basis.
  - ➤ The bottom of the label shows the total (g or mg) values for 2,000 and 2,500 calorie diets; the top part shows the percentage of daily value based on the 2,000 calorie level.

% Daily Value

- **DAILY VALUE** (DV) is a percentage on a food label that shows how a food fits into the total daily diet. DVs for energy producing nutrients are based on the number of calories consumed per day. Few consumers understand the % DV information. For labeling purposes, 2,000 calories, (intentionally set as a rounded number to make calculations easier), is the established reference for this calculation. DV for cholesterol, sodium and potassium are not based on caloric intake. They are recommended levels for all adults. Each nutrient listed has, in addition to the DV and %DV, dietary advice or a goal. Total fat might have the term "*less than*" listed, while total CHO might have "at least" listed. All nutrients must be declared as percentages of the DV, in addition to the actual amount of the nutrient contained in the package. This may be omitted when labeling laws change.

Ingredient listing

- The label must list what is in the food, beginning with the ingredient that is present in the largest amount by weight. (Foods with only one ingredient are exempt.) Other ingredients are listed in descending order, according to weight. In the labeling law, all ingredients must be listed even in standardized foods. Foods with **STANDARDS OF IDENTITY** (meaning that in order to use the name of that food, only specific ingredients may be used) are not exempt. The ingredient list includes identification of FDA certified food additives, sources of protein hydrolysates used as flavors or enhancers, a declaration that casein is a milk derivative, the total percentage of juice in juice beverages, and presence of common allergens.

- Ingredients likely to be of concern to consumers (based on specific health concerns) include the following:

  - **Vegetable sources of saturated fat:** Coconut oil, palm kernel oil, palm oil, coconut oil, some hydrogenated oils, vegetable shortenings, sources of trans-fatty acids.
  - **Animal sources of saturated fat:** Lard, beef fat, bacon fat, salt pork, butterfat, milk-fat, cream cheese, dried or frozen liquid whole eggs, egg yolks (not egg whites).
  - **Primary sources of sweeteners:** Glucose (glucose, dextrose, corn syrup); fructose (fructose, fruit sugar, fructose corn syrup, levulose); honey (honey, raw honey, unpasteurized honey, invert sugar, invert sugar syrup, tupelo honey); maltose (maltose, malted syrup, maltodextrin, dextrins); sorghum (sorghum molasses, grain sorghum syrup); lactose (milk sugar, whey); sugar alcohols (sorbitol, mannitol, xylitol). All sweeteners are grouped together and listed within parentheses in order of weight.
  - **Primary sources of sodium:** Sodium chloride (salt), monosodium glutamate (MSG), seasoned salts, calcium disodium phosphate, EDTA, whey, dried buttermilk powder, cheeses, Dutch-processed cocoa, soy sauce, baking powder, baking soda, Worcestershire sauce, barbecue sauce, fish sauce.
  - **Potential allergens:** Tartrazine and other artificial colors, monosodium glutamate, sulfites, nitrites, milk, eggs, fish, crustaceans, shellfish, peanuts, tree nuts, wheat and soy.

Simplified format

- A simplified format can be used when a food contains insignificant amounts of seven or more of the mandatory nutrients and total calories. Foods with a small label area may also use a simplified format. Baby foods have a simplified format because there are no DVs for infants.

Labeling exemptions

- The following foods are exempt from label requirements:

  - Packages with less than 12 square inches for labeling (must have address or phone number, but not full labeling).
  - Foods produced by small businesses for example, businesses with food sales of less than $50,000/yr, businesses with fewer than 100 FTE employees that have sales of fewer than 100,00 units annually.

- ➤ Restaurant food unless a health claim is made. Health claims trigger disclosure of label information.
- ➤ Food served for immediate consumption (vending machines, hospital cafeterias, airplanes, shopping malls, sidewalk vendors.)
- ➤ Ready-to-eat food that is not for immediate consumption, but is prepared primarily on-site (bakery, deli, candy store items.)
- ➤ Foods shipped in bulk, not for sale in that form to consumers.
- ➤ Medical foods.
- ➤ Plain tea, coffee, spices and foods with no significant amount of any nutrient.
- ➤ Nutrient supplements, herbs and related products.

Voluntary labeling

- The 20 most frequently consumed fresh fruits, vegetables and fresh fish, and 45 major cuts of fresh meat and poultry, must have nutrition information at point of purchase. If voluntary compliance standards are not met, labeling will become mandatory.

Nutrient content descriptors

- Claims that wrongly imply that a food does or does not contain a nutrient are prohibited. Thus, "made with oat bran" cannot be used unless the food is a "good source" of fiber.

- FREE means no amount, or only trivial or "physiologically inconsequential" amounts, of one or more of these components—fat, saturated fat, cholesterol, sodium, sugars and calories.

- CALORIE-FREE means fewer than 5 calories per serving and SUGAR-FREE and FAT-FREE both mean less than 0.5g per serving. Synonyms for "free" include "without," "no," and "zero."

- LOW means foods that could be eaten frequently without exceeding *Dietary Guidelines for Americans* for one or more of these components. Synonyms for "low" include "little," "few" and "low source of."

- LOW FAT means 3g or less per serving.

- LOW SATURATED FAT means 1g or less saturated fat per serving.

- LOW SODIUM means 140mg or less sodium per serving.

- VERY LOW SODIUM means 35mg or less sodium per serving.

- LOW CHOLESTEROL means 20mg or less cholesterol and 2g or less saturated fat per serving.

- LOW CALORIES means 40 calories or less per serving.

- LEAN and EXTRA LEAN can be used to describe the fat content of meat, poultry, seafood and game meats.

  - ➤ LEAN means less than 10g of fat, less than 4.5g or less of saturated fat and less than 95mg of cholesterol per serving and per 100g.
  - ➤ EXTRA LEAN means less than 5g of fat, less than 2g of saturated fat and less than 95mg of cholesterol per serving and per 100g.

- **HIGH** means the food contains 20% or more of the DV for a particular nutrient in a serving.

- **GOOD SOURCE** means one serving of a food contains 10-19% of the DV for a particular nutrient.

- **NO SUGAR ADDED** means no sugar is added during processing or packaging of a food that normally contains added sugar.

- **REDUCED** means a nutritionally-altered product that contains 25% less of a nutrient or of calories than the regular, or reference, product. This claim cannot be made if reference product is "low."

- **LESS** means a food, whether altered or not, that contains 25% less of a nutrient or of calories than the reference food. "Fewer" is also acceptable.

- **LIGHT** means an altered product that contains one-third fewer calories or half the fat of the reference food. If the food derives 50% or more of its calories from fat, the reduction must be 50% of the fat, In addition, " light" may be used on food in which the sodium content of a low calorie, low fat food has been reduced by at least 50%. "Light in sodium" may be used on a food in which the sodium content has been reduced by at least 50 %. "Light" still can be used to describe such properties as texture and color, as long as the label explains the intent; for example, "light brown sugar" and "light and fluffy."

- **MORE** means the product contains a nutrient that is at least 10% of the DV more than the reference food. The 10% of DV also would apply to "fortified," "enriched" and "added" claims.

- **PERCENT FAT-FREE** is used only on low-fat or fat-free products. It is based on amount of fat present in 100g of the food. Thus, if a food contains 2.5g of fat per 50g, the claim must be "95% fat-free."

- **HEALTHY** describes a food that is low in fat and saturated fat and contains limited amounts of cholesterol and sodium per serving. In addition, it must have at least 10% DV of one or more of 6 key nutrients, vitamins A, C, iron, calcium, protein or fiber, if it is a single item food. Raw meat, poultry and fish can be labeled "healthy" if a serving contains no more than 5g of fat, 2g saturated fat and 96mg cholesterol.

- **FRESH** is a food that is raw, has never been frozen or heated and contains no preservatives. (Irradiation at low levels is allowed.) "Fresh frozen," "frozen fresh" and "freshly frozen" can be used for foods that are quickly frozen while still fresh. Blanching (brief scalding before freezing to prevent nutrient breakdown) is allowed. Uses like "fresh bread" are still allowed.

- For meals and main dishes:
  - **LOW CALORIE** means the meal or main dish contains 120 calories or less per 100g.
  - **LOW SODIUM** means the food has 140mg or less per 100g.
  - **LOW CHOLESTEROL** means the food contains 20mg cholesterol or less per 100g and no more than 2g saturated fat.
  - **LIGHT** means the meal or main dish is low fat or low calorie.
  - Claims that a meal or main dish is "free" of a nutrient, such as sodium or cholesterol, must meet the same requirements as those for individual foods.

- Processed meats have mandatory labeling, but fresh meat and poultry are not required to have labels on each package. Information about game meats (e.g., deer and quail) may be available at point of purchase.

- **HEALTH CLAIMS** are statements on a package label or advertisement that attribute a specific medical benefit from consumption of a food or nutrient. FDA must approve the terminology and use on the label. Claims must be supported by significant scientific evidence and must undergo a lengthy approval process.

- The FDA is currently permitting **QUALIFIED HEALTH CLAIMS** to be added to a food label. Each of the "qualified claims" is considered on an individual basis, but there is currently no rule for their use. These claims do not meet the "significant scientific" standard, but there is emerging evidence for a relationship between a food, food component, or dietary supplement and reduced risk of disease or health related condition, but not conclusive. This claim requires a disclaimer, such as "scientific evidence suggests but does not prove that…" (See **www.fda.gov** for specific claims.)

- **STRUCTURE FUNCTION CLAIMS** may be used without FDA permission. Claims such as "fiber maintains bowel regularity" or "calcium builds strong bones" are examples of this type of claim.

- **HEALTH CLAIMS BASED ON AUTHORITATIVE STATEMENTS** allow certain health claims to be used on foods based on an "authoritative statement" from a scientific body of the U.S. Government or the National Academy of Sciences. This claim is not allowed on dietary supplements. Each claim must meet specific guidelines for amount of the specific nutrient mentioned. Examples include:

  - **Calcium** and **Osteoporosis:** A calcium-rich diet may help prevent osteoporosis, a condition in which bones become thin and brittle. The claim must indicate the disease depends on many factors by listing risk factors or the disease, such as gender, race and age. Must also include additional factors necessary to reduce risk such as eating healthful meals and regular exercise. Foods or supplements containing more than 400mg of calcium must state that total intakes of more than 2,000mg of calcium provide no added benefits to bone health.
  - **Dietary Fat** and **Cancer:** Limiting the amount of total fat you eat may help reduce your risk for some cancers. The product must be low in fat.
  - **Dietary Saturated Fat** and **Cholesterol** and **Risk of Coronary Heart Disease:** Limiting the amount of saturated fat and cholesterol you eat may help prevent the risk of heart disease. The food must be low in total fat and must include the terms Coronary heart disease or Heart disease. Must also include physician advisory statement.
  - **Fruits, Vegetables and Grain Products that contain Fiber (particularly soluble fiber) and Risk of Coronary Heart Disease:** Diets low in saturated fats and cholesterol and rich in fruits, vegetables and grain products that contain some types of fiber, especially soluble fiber (at least 0.6g without fortification), may help prevent coronary heart disease.
  - **Sodium** and **Hypertension:** Limiting the amount of sodium you eat may help prevent hypertension, or high blood pressure. Hypertension is a risk factor for heart attacks and strokes. Individuals with high blood pressure should consult their physicians.

> **Fruits** and **Vegetables** and **Cancer:** Eating fruits and vegetables that are low in fat and are good sources of dietary fiber, vitamin A or vitamin C may help prevent some cancers.

> **Dietary Non-carcinogenic Carbohydrate Sweeteners and Dental Caries:** The sugar alcohols must be those that may be used are specified, such as xylitol, sorbitol, mannitol, maltitol, isomalt, lactitol, hydrogenated starch hydrolysates, hydrogenated glucose syrups, erythritol or a combination of these. The claim must imply that the specific sugar alcohol does not promote or may reduce the risk of tooth decay and must name the sugar alcohol. A statement that frequent between-meal consumption of foods high in sugars and starches can promote tooth decay. Small packages may use a shortened claim.

> **Plant Sterol/stanol Esters and the Risk of Coronary Heart Disease:** The claim must specify these are part of a diet low in saturated fat and cholesterol and the daily amount of the plant sterol or stanol ester necessary to reduce CHD risk and that it should be consumed with 2 different meals daily. Spread and salad dressings that exceed 13g of fat per 50g must bear the statement "see nutrition information for fat content." It also must say "may" or "might" reduce the CHD risk.

> **Potassium and the Risk of High Blood Pressure and Stroke:** The food must be a good source of potassium, be low in sodium, total fat, saturated fat, and cholesterol. Required wording on the label is "Diets containing foods that are a good source of potassium and that are low in sodium may reduce the risk of high blood pressure and stroke."

- The term **ORGANIC** can be used on a food label if foods meet certain criteria. Organic products must contain at least 95% organic ingredients, excluding water.

b. Macro and micro-nutrient sources

- Nutrients are presented in the following section in a format that includes sources with nutrient functions along with other information about each nutrient.

- **MACRONUTRIENTS** are nutrients needed by the body in larger amounts. They include carbohydrates, protein, lipids and water. Their requirements are measured in grams or grams needed per kilogram of body weight.

- **MICRONUTRIENTS** are nutrients needed by the body in very small amounts. Vitamins and minerals are micronutrients. The amounts required are measured in milligrams or micrograms. While they help regulate the production of energy from macronutrients, they are not energy yielding.

c. Phytochemicals

- **PHYTOCHEMICALS** are naturally occurring plant chemicals that protect against diseases or have health-enhancing benefits. Many are antioxidants, protect against cellular changes that lead to cardiovascular damage, neurodegenerative diseases or various forms of cancer. Phytochemicals are sometimes called phytonutrients, although they are not truly nutrients.

- When foods are cooked or processed, phytochemical content may be increased or decreased. For example, tomato sauce has more lycopene than fresh tomatoes while apple juice has fewer phenols than fresh apples. Processing grain removes almost all of the phytochemicals in whole grains because those are found in the bran and germ of the grain.

PROTECTIVE PHYTOCHEMICALS

Phytochemical	Food Source
Allyl sulfides/other organosulfurs	Garlic, onions, leeks, scallions
Anthocyanosins	Red, purple and blue pigments in plants such as Eggplant, cherries, red grapes and blueberries
Capsaicin	Chili peppers
Carotenoids (i.e., Lycopene)	Orange, red and yellow fruits and vegetables
Catechins	Tea, especially green tea
Dithiolthiones	Cruciferous vegetables, broccoli, cabbage, kale
Ellagic acid	Walnuts, strawberries, raspberries, grapes, apples, cranberries
Flavonols (i.e., Quercitin)	Cocoa, chocolate, apples, grapes, wine, tea
Flavenones	Citrus fruits
Indoles	Cruciferous vegetables, broccoli, cabbage, kale
Isoflavones (i.e., Genestein)	Soybeans, other legumes, licorice
Lutein, zeaxanthin	Kale, greens, spinach, corn, citrus
Sulphorophane	Cruciferous vegetables
Lignans	Flaxseed, berries, whole grains, licorice
Limonene	Citrus peel
Monoterpenes	Oranges, lemons, grapefruits
Phenolic acids	All plants
Phytosterols	Nuts, seeds, whole wheat, corn, soybeans, legumes, vegetable oils
Protease inhibitors	All plants, especially soy foods, seeds, legumes
Resveratrol	Grapes and wine
Saponins	Garlic, onions, licorice, legumes
Silymarin	Artichokes
Triterpenoids	Citrus fruit, mushrooms, licorice
Flavenones	Citrus fruits

d. Nutrient databases

- The nutrient content of food is best determined by laboratory analysis. The free on-line USDA database **www.ars.usda.gov/ba/bhnrc/ndl** is constantly being updated, but still contains some data from samples analyzed many years ago. Much information from other sources is drawn from this database.

- Nutrient composition figures are also available from current books, computer analysis programs, journal reports, food labels and food manufacturers. Food manufacturers are required to substantiate nutrient composition by food analysis of multiple samples before nutrition labeling. By comparing and keeping track of the nutrient content of foods, individuals can determine the relative value of individual foods and calculate their daily intake of specific nutrients.

TOPIC B - NUTRITION and SUPPORTING SCIENCES
1. Principles of normal nutrition

a. Functions of nutrients

- **NUTRIENTS** are essential chemicals to be supplied by or derived from food and are required by the body for growth, maintenance and reproduction. They provide energy, contribute to structure and regulate body processes. The six classes of nutrients are: 1) carbohydrates; 2) fats; 3) proteins; 4) vitamins; 5) minerals; and, 6) water. About 45 nutrients are considered essential to human life.

- Essential nutrients are not manufactured by the body, or cannot be produced in sufficient quantity to meet physiological need; examples are the essential amino acids, minerals, vitamins, linoleic and linolenic fatty acids and water.

CARBOHYDRATES

- **CARBOHYDRATES (CHO)** provide energy for the body and are the main source of fuel for energy in the cells and for the nervous system. They provide 4 calories per g. They spare protein from being used for energy and aid in the oxidation of fat for energy. In fibrous forms, carbohydrate promotes peristalsis and aids normal elimination of waste. Dietary fiber, because it is not digested or absorbed, does not supply calories. The Dietary Reference Intake report on macronutrients states to meet the body's daily energy and nutritional needs, while minimizing the risk for chronic disease, adults should consume 45% to 65% of their calories from CHO, with at least 130 grams per day for adults and children and no more than 25% of energy from added sugars. The Adequate Intake (AI) for total fiber is set at 38 and 25g per day for men and women ages 19 to 50 years, respectively.

- Carbohydrates consist of carbon, hydrogen and oxygen combined into simple sugar units ($C_6H_{12}O_6$), with either an aldehyde or ketone group. These simple sugar units form the basic structure of monosaccharides, disaccharides and polysaccharides, starch and fiber.

- **MONOSACCHARIDES** are single sugar units. The only monosaccharides that can be absorbed by humans are glucose, fructose and galactose. All are hexoses, 6 carbon sugar units. They differ in taste, degree of sweetness, chemical behavior and dietary source because of differences in their chemical structure. Fructose has a ketone on the second carbon, whereas glucose and galactose have an aldehyde group on the first carbon. All monosaccharides are converted to glucose for use in the body.

  - **GLUCOSE** is found in fruits, vegetables and honey and is also derived from maltose, lactose and sucrose digestion. It is the most widely distributed sugar in nature.
  - **DEXTROSE** is glucose produced from the hydrolysis of cornstarch.
  - **FRUCTOSE,** also called **LEVULOSE** or **FRUIT SUGAR**, is found in fruits and honey and is also derived from sucrose digestion. It is the sweetest of all monosaccharides.
  - **GALACTOSE** is derived from lactose digestion.

- **DISACCHARIDES** are two monosaccharides linked together between the aldehyde or ketone and a hydroxyl on another sugar. Important disaccharides are sucrose, lactose and maltose.

- ➤ **SUCROSE** is table sugar. It is found in sugar beets, sugar cane, maple syrup and molasses. It breaks down into glucose and fructose.
- ➤ **LACTOSE** is milk sugar. Lactose breaks down into glucose and galactose and is less sweet than other sugars.
- ➤ **MALTOSE,** also known as malt sugar, is produced from the digestion of starch.
- ➤ **LACTULOSE,** a synthetic disaccharide, is not metabolized and is used in laxatives.
- ➤ **TREHALOSE** is found in mushrooms and yeast. It breaks down into two alpha-glucose units.

- ● **POLYSACCHARIDES** (glycogen, starch, dextrins and fiber) have more than two simple sugar units linked together. They are sometimes referred to as complex carbohydrates. Some polysaccharides are digestible; others are not.

  - ➤ **GLYCOGEN** is the storage form of carbohydrate in animals and humans, where it is stored in the liver and muscle tissues. It is found in liver, fresh oysters and in small amounts in most cuts of meat. Glycogen is a branched glucose polymer.
  - ➤ **STARCH** occurs in two forms; amylose and amylopectin. It is found in plants and plant-derived foods, such as cereals, breads, pasta, rice, dried beans, potato and starchy vegetables (e.g., corn). **AMYLOPECTIN** has many branches, has a very high molecular weight, and is more abundant in the food supply. Most of the starch in grains and starchy tubers is amylopectin. **AMYLOSE** is a smaller molecule with few branches.
  - ➤ **DEXTRINS** are intermediate products in the hydrolysis of starch. They are found in toast or parched (browned) flour.
  - ➤ **FIBER** is a carbohydrate structure with bonds that cannot be broken down by the digestive enzymes of humans. All components of dietary fiber, except for lignin, are made up of polysaccharide chains. Fibers include insoluble cellulose, hemicellulose, lignin and soluble gums and pectins.
  - ➤ **CELLULOSE** is a simple polymer of glucose, the most abundant organic compound in nature. This long molecule provides structure. It cannot be digested by the human digestive tract but can be digested by many animals. Best sources are bran, whole grains and vegetables.
  - ➤ **TOTAL FIBER (TF)** is the total amount of dietary fiber and functional fiber.
  - ➤ **DIETARY FIBER** is the edible, non-digestible part of carbohydrates and lignin that are naturally found in plants; such as cereal bran, sweet potatoes, legumes, corn cereal and onions.
  - ➤ **FUNCTIONAL FIBER** is extracted from natural sources or is synthetic with similar health benefits as dietary fiber. Pectin is an example.
  - ➤ **SOLUBLE** and **INSOLUBLE FIBER:** Fiber can be classified as water-soluble or insoluble. While human enzymes cannot break down these fibers, soluble fiber may be absorbed after breakdown by bacteria in the digestive tract. Soluble fibers swell in water, bind cholesterol secreted in bile and may help lower blood cholesterol.
  - ➤ **SYNTHETIC NON-NUTRITIVE FIBER** is a food ingredient made from plant material not usually consumed, such as the highly-refined cellulose from wood pulp that is added to some reduced-calorie breads, or used as a thickener in some low-calorie salad dressings.
  - ➤ **RESIDUE** is the total solid feces produced from undigested, unabsorbed food and metabolic and bacterial products. Milk, after digestion, yields residue but contains no fiber.

FIBER: TYPES, SOURCES AND PHYSIOLOGICAL EFFECTS

Types	Food Sources	Physiological Effects
Soluble Forms Soluble pectin, gums, mucilages, soluble hemicelluloses	Oat bran, barley, beans and legumes, fruits and vegetables, (especially seaweed), citrus fruit peel, sugar beet pulp, apples, guar gum, locust bean gum, carob bean gum, psyllium (cillium), Fiberall®, Metamucil®, some bran cereals)	Accelerate intestinal transit and fecal weight; slow starch hydrolysis; delay glucose absorption; decrease serum cholesterol; may reduce serum triglycerides; fill the stomach, creating a sense of fullness (useful in weight reduction); increase viscosity of the food mass
Insoluble Forms Cellulose, insoluble hemicelluloses and insoluble pectins	Primarily cereals, wheat grains, bran, rice; cabbage, Brussels sprouts, root vegetables, nuts, seeds	Prevent and relieve constipation by adding fluid and bulk to stool; decrease intestinal transit time; may protect against colon cancer, diverticulosis and hemorrhoids because of faster transit time through the colon

HIGH FIBER FOODS

Foods With Over 2g Dietary Fiber Per Standard Portion

Cereals	Legumes	Vegetables	Fruits
All-Bran	All canned peas and beans	Asparagus	Fresh apple
40% Bran	Lentils	Canned beets	Fresh pear
Corn bran	Navy, kidney and pinto	Broccoli	Canned plums
Fiber 1	beans have over 5g	Brussels sprouts	Dried fruits
Grape-Nuts	per ½ cup cooked portion	Kale (frozen)	Banana
Oat Bran		Potato w/skin	Fresh orange
Rolled oats		Spinach	
Wheaties			
Whole wheat flour (2 ½ tbsp)			

Foods With Over 1g Soluble Fiber Per Standard Portion

Cereals	Legumes	Vegetables	Fruits
Oat Bran	Black-eyed peas	Brussels sprouts	Fresh citrus
Rolled oats	Kidney beans	Carrots	Fresh apple
Barley	Navy beans		Canned plums
	Pinto beans		
	Split peas		

PROTEINS

- **PROTEINS** are complex nitrogenous compounds made up of amino acids with peptide linkages.

Functions of protein

- Dietary protein furnishes the body with amino acids for making body protein. Proteins are needed to provide structure, regulate body functions and, in some cases, provide energy. They provide 4 calories per g. Structural functions include proteins in all body cells, membranes, cytoplasm and organelles; including muscle, skin and bone structure.

- Protein regulates body processes by providing components of enzymes, transport molecules in blood and cells, immune system molecules, hormones and molecules that aid in muscle contractions, fluid balance, acid-base balance and nerve transmissions.

- Protein can be used as an energy source. If the diet provides insufficient energy, protein of the body is broken down and used as fuel.

- For healthy adults, protein intake is suggested as 10-15% of calories, or about 0.8g of protein per kg of body weight per day (0.8g/kg/day). This is equivalent to about 50g of protein for a 138-pound person. The 2002 Dietary Reference Intake Report on macronutrients states that adults should get 10% to 35% of their calories from protein.

Composition and structure of proteins

- Proteins are made of carbon, hydrogen, oxygen and nitrogen and are the most diverse and complex molecules in the human body. All enzymes, antibodies, hormones and tissues of the body are proteins. Proteins are synthesized from basic units called amino acids. **AMINO ACIDS** are composed of a carbon atom attached to a carboxyl group (COOH), a hydrogen atom (H), an amino group (NH_2) and an amino acid radical. A protein is a chain of amino acids linked together by peptide bonds to form a molecule. The **PEPTIDE BOND** connects the amino group of one amino acid to the carboxyl group of the adjacent amino acid. All amino acids have a similar structure but each has a different side chain.

- **INDISPENSABLE AMINO ACIDS,** also called **ESSENTIAL AMINO ACIDS,** cannot be formed in the body in sufficient amounts to support life and growth, so they must be supplied by the diet. There are nine essential amino acids: 1) Histidine; 2) Isoleucine; 3) Leucine; 4) Lysine; 5) Methionine; 6) Phenylalanine; 7) Threonine; 8) Tryptophan; and, 9) Valine.

- The **DISPENSABLE AMINO ACIDS,** also called **NON-ESSENTIAL AMINO ACIDS,** (Alanine, Aspartic acid, Asparagine, Glutamic acid, Serine) can be formed from other compounds (amino acids) in the body in sufficient amounts, so the body is not dependent on dietary sources of these amino acids.

- **CONDITIONALLY ESSENTIAL AMINO ACIDS -** Currently, there are also six amino acids that are considered, conditionally indispensable. These are : 1) Arginine; 2) Cysteine; 3) Glutamine; 4) Glycine; 5) Proline; and, 6) Tyrosine. Under most conditions, the body can synthesize these from precursors to meet metabolic needs, but there may be certain physiological conditions or pathological states when that is not possible.

- The instructions for making each protein are transmitted by way of the genetic information contained in **DNA** (deoxyribonucleic acid). A section of DNA serves as a template for making a strand of **RNA** (ribonucleic acid). Known as messenger RNA, this molecule escapes through the nuclear membrane and attaches itself to one of the ribosomes. Transfer RNA collects amino acids from the cell fluid and brings them to the messenger. Each of the 20 amino acids has its own transfer RNA. The amino acids are lined up in the appropriate sequence and enzymes bind them together. Finally, the completed protein is released.

- **TRANSAMINATION** is the transfer of an amino group from one compound to another. This reaction is used to produce nonessential amino acids and the process requires Vitamin B_6.

- **DEAMINATION** is the removal of an amino group from an amino acid. In this way, the liver converts amino acids into non-nitrogen compounds that can be used for energy.

- Each protein molecule contains approximately 16% nitrogen. Nitrogen excreted from the body in urine, feces and sweat must be replaced by dietary nitrogen. The weight of nitrogen lost is multiplied by a factor of 6.25 to determine the grams of protein needed to replace the loss.

- A few amino acids have specific medical applications. Lysine, in supplemental form, is known to relieve herpes infections and cold sore symptoms. Glucosamine sulfate, in some studies, has been shown to promote cartilage repair and to revitalize bones at joints to relieve osteoarthritis pain.

Sources of protein

- Dietary protein, with all essential amino acids present in appropriate ratios for utilizing and building body proteins, is called **HIGH BIOLOGICAL VALUE PROTEIN.** Proteins from animal sources (except gelatin) are of high biological value. Plant sources of protein are considered **INCOMPLETE PROTEIN (LOW BIOLOGICAL VALUE)** because they do not contain all essential amino acids or do not contain the essential amino acids in the correct proportion to create body proteins.

- Those who eat few complete proteins or those consuming only plant-proteins, need to choose **COMPLEMENTARY PROTEINS**, especially during growth periods. Complementary proteins are two or more foods that together provide all essential amino acids. (For example, combining legumes with rice, corn or wheat, or mushrooms with broccoli.) If protein intake is varied and caloric intake is sufficient, amino acids may complement one another when eaten within the same day.

- **NET PROTEIN UTILIZATION (NPU)** is another method of measuring protein quality. It measures protein actually used by comparing the amount of dietary protein in the diet against nitrogen losses, using the formula [N (g) x 6.25 = protein (g)]. The amount of nitrogen retained in the body is compared with the amount eaten to calculate the NPU, which ranges from about 40-94. Protein from animal sources has higher NPU than that from vegetable sources.

- Another method of measuring protein quality is the corrected **PROTEIN DIGESTIBILITY CORRECTED AMINO ACID SCORES (PDCAAS),** which has been adopted by both the

FDA and the World Health Organization (WHO). This measurement, based on amino acid requirements for children ages 2-5 years old, corrects for digestibility of proteins. Scores that are equal or greater than requirements have a PDCAAS of 1.0.

- The **PROTEIN EFFICIENCY RATIO** also measures protein quality. This method determines how well a specific protein supports weight gain in rats. It is used to evaluate the protein quality in infant formulas and baby foods.

PROTEIN IN FOOD		
Food	**Portion**	**Grams of Protein**
Cottage cheese, low fat	1 cup	30
Chicken, broiled, skinless, some bone	3 ½ oz.	29
Turkey, roasted breast, skinless	3 oz.	25
Tuna, water packed	3 oz.	25
Beef, lean sirloin, broiled	3 oz.	25
Hamburger, broiled	1 med. (4 oz.)	20
Fish, halibut, broiled	3 oz.	23
Pork chop, pan fried	1 med. (4 oz.)	18
Chili, beef and beans	1 cup	15
Ravioli, meat, canned	1 cup	11
Taco, beef	1 med.	11
Tofu (bean curd)	½ cup	10
Split pea with ham soup	1 cup	10
Garbanzo beans, canned	1 cup	12
Peanuts, dry roasted	¼ cup	9
Peanut butter	2 Tbsp	8
Milk, skim, 1%, 2%, whole	1 cup	8
Pumpkin seeds, roasted	1 oz.	7
Bologna, beef	2 oz.	6
Egg, boiled	1 large	6
Oatmeal, quick cooked	2/3 cup	5
Almonds, roasted	1 oz.	5
Broccoli, cooked	1 cup	5
Spaghetti, cooked, no sauce	1 cup	5
Potato, baked	1 med.	5
Peas	½ cup	4
Rice	1 cup	4
Chicken noodle soup	1 cup	3
Tomato soup	1 cup	2
Ice cream, vanilla	½ cup	2
Cornflakes	1 cup	2
Bread, white	1 slice	2

FATS

- Fats supply energy. They are a concentrated source of calories, providing 9 calories per gram. They provide the **ESSENTIAL FATTY ACIDS (EFA)** linoleic and linolenic acids. Fats are important components of all membranes particularly of the brain and nervous system. Fats aid in the absorption and transport of fat-soluble vitamins and other nutrients. Fat is stored in adipose tissue and cushions organs protecting them from shock. Adults should get 20% to 35% of their calories from fat. Infants and younger children need 25% to 40% of their calories from fat. There is no RDA, EAR or AI for total fat.

Composition of fats

- **FATS,** also called **LIPIDS,** like carbohydrates, are composed of carbon, hydrogen and oxygen. Fats are classified according to their chemical structure.

- **SIMPLE LIPIDS** are esters of fatty acids with an alcohol. Monoglycerides, diglycerides and triglycerides are simple lipids, as are some sterol esters. **COMPOUND LIPIDS** are esters of fatty acids with glycerol, plus other compounds (e.g., lipoproteins, phospholipids, and lecithin). **DERIVED LIPIDS,** such as mono and diglycerides, are substances resulting from digestion that have characteristics of lipids.

- The basic units of a lipid compound are **FATTY ACIDS** composed of a long hydrogen chain attached to a carboxyl group. Fatty acids have an even numbered carbon chain and differ in length and degree of saturation.

- **GLYCEROL** forms the backbone to which fatty acids attach. About 95% of lipids in food are **TRIGLYCERIDES.** They have a backbone of glycerol to which three fatty acids are attached. The remaining 5% of lipids are **PHOSPHOLIPIDS** (e.g., lecithin) and sterols (e.g., cholesterol). Phospholipids contain both glycerol and fatty acids. They are major components of cell membranes. They have both hydrophilic and hydrophobic properties and are therefore ideal emulsifiers (e.g., bile).

- **SATURATED-FATTY ACIDS** are those in which every available bond in the hydrocarbon chain is attached to a molecule of hydrogen. Foods containing primarily saturated-fatty acids are generally solid at room temperature and come primarily from animal sources (butter, beef, etc.) Vegetable sources of saturated-fatty acids include tropical oils (palm oil, palm kernel oil and coconut oil) and cocoa butter.

- **MONOUNSATURATED-FATTY ACIDS** have one double bond in the hydrocarbon chain that is not fully saturated with hydrogen. Foods rich in monounsaturated- fatty acids are usually liquid at room temperature. Monounsaturated-**OLEIC ACID** is the predominant fatty acid in olive oil, sesame oil and canola (rapeseed) oil. Chicken fat and partially-hydrogenated margarines also contain monounsaturates.

- **POLYUNSATURATED-FATTY ACIDS** have two or more double bonds in the hydrocarbon chain. Polyunsaturated fats are liquid at room temperature and are mainly from plant sources. The location of the double bond closest to the omega (methyl) end of the fatty-acid chain defines a fatty-acid's family.

  - ➤ **OMEGA-3 FATTY ACIDS** are polyunsaturated, with the first double bond starting from the methyl end located at carbon 3. Alpha linolenic, is an 18 carbon essential fatty acid and has three double bonds. The body can use it to synthesize new compounds, such as eicosanoids, that have an influence on inflammatory processes, blood clotting, and blood vessel constriction and dilation. The AI for alpha linolenic acid is 1.6 and 1.1g per day for men and women over age 14, respectively.

➤ **OMEGA-6 FATTY ACIDS** are polyunsaturated, with the first double bond starting from the methyl end located at carbon 6. The essential fatty acid, linoleic acid, has two double bonds and 18 carbons. The body can convert it to arachidonic acid, a 20 carbon-fatty acid with 4 double bonds from which eicosanoids can be formed, as well. The AI for linoleic acid is 17 and 12g per day for men and women between the ages of 19 and 50, respectively. Eicosanoids can have different physiological effects, depending on from which fatty-acid family they are derived.

➤ **OMEGA-9 FATTY ACIDS** are monounsaturated, with the double bond at the methyl end located at carbon 9.

- **TRANS-FATTY ACIDS** can be formed during the hydrogenation process to solidify liquid fats. One hydrogen is added on each side of the double bond, as opposed to **CIS-FATTY ACIDS**, where two hydrogens are on the same side of the double bond. Research suggests that trans-fatty acids promote development of atherosclerosis and several other disorders. Since January 1, 2006, food labeling regulations require manufacturers to declare the content of trans-fatty acids. Some localities have passed legislation to ban trans-fatty acids in all restaurant foods. The *2010 Dietary Guidelines for Americans* recommend avoiding trans fats and the FDA has banned the addition of trans fats in processed foods..

- Actually, most fats contain a mixture of the three basic types of fatty acids. When a food is considered a monounsaturated fat, for example, it has more monounsaturated acids than poly or saturate- fatty acids.

- **CHOLESTEROL** is a major structural component of all cell membranes, especially brain and nerve tissue. Cholesterol is the precursor of sterol hormones, estrogens, progestins, glucocorticoids, androgens, estrogens and vitamin D.

  ➤ Cholesterol is an example of a **STEROL,** a complex ring structure that is a monohydric alcohol. Food cholesterol is esterified and must be hydrolyzed by pancreatic esterase. Cholesterol is present in animal (not plant) foods, but is also manufactured in the human body. All of the carbons in cholesterol come from acetyl CoA. Serum cholesterol can be derived from different compounds in the body, such as glucose or fatty acids. Serum cholesterol in the body is transformed into a related compound (bile), excreted, or deposited in body tissues, where it may accumulate in the arteries, causing atherosclerosis. It is the principal constituent of gallstones.

  ➤ Humans produce more cholesterol in the skin, liver and intestines than the average diet supplies. There is a genetic component for degree of cholesterol synthesis. Serum cholesterol synthesis seems to be promoted by high intakes of saturated fats. Reducing total dietary fat and saturated fat intake may help reduce serum cholesterol. Substituting monounsaturated and polyunsaturated-fatty acids for saturated fats may help lower serum cholesterol, as well.

  ➤ Cholesterol is present in all animal fats. Egg yolks contain the highest cholesterol level of any commonly consumed food (186mg per large egg yolk). Organ meats (331mg/3oz. cooked beef liver) and fish roe are also cholesterol-rich.

COMPARISON OF DIETARY FATS

Dietary Fat	Cholesterol (mg/Tbsp)	Saturated	Polyunsaturated Linoleic	α--Linolenic	Monounsaturated
Canola oil	0	7%	21%	11%	61%
Safflower oil	0	10%	76%	trace	14%
Sunflower oil	0	12%	71%	1%	16%
Corn oil	0	13%	57%	1%	29%
Olive oil	0	15%	9%	1%	75%
Soybean oil	0	15%	54%	8%	23%
Peanut oil	0	19%	33%	trace	48%
Cottonseed oil	0	27%	54%	trace	19%
Lard	12	43%	9%	1%	47%
Beef tallow	14	48%	2%	1%	49%
Palm oil	0	51%	10%	trace	39%
Butterfat	33	68%	3%	1%	28%
Coconut oil	0	91%	2%	0%	7%z

Nutrient recommendations

- The standards used in the United States and Canada are called **DIETARY REFERENCE INTAKES (DRI)**. Values have been set for all vitamins, minerals, carbohydrates, fiber, lipids, protein, water and energy. The DRI is comprised of a set of four lists that are used to assess and plan the diets of healthy people.

- The **RECOMMENDED DIETARY ALLOWANCES (RDA)** and **ADEQUATE INTAKES (AI)** specify nutrient intake goals for individuals in specific life stages and gender groups. The RDAs are based on research evidence. The AI are based on available scientific evidence and observation and where the scientific data are not sufficient to establish an RDA. The RDA and AI are meant to be used as nutrient goals for individuals and both are used for meal planning and assessment.

- **TOLERABLE UPPER INTAKE LEVELS (UL)** are defined as "the highest average daily nutrient intake level that is likely to pose no risk of toxicity to almost all healthy individuals of a particular life stage and gender group." Intakes above the specified levels may place a person at risk of nutrient toxicity.

- **ESTIMATED AVERAGE REQUIREMENTS (EAR)** are defined as "the average daily nutrient intake estimated to meet the requirement of half of the healthy individuals in a particular life stage and gender group." These are used for setting policies and in research. RDA values are set based on these estimates.

- Another group of standards set by the DRI committee is **ACCEPTABLE MACRONUTRIENT DISTRIBUTION RANGES (AMDR).** These are described as "values for carbohydrate, fat and protein expressed as percentages of total daily caloric intake." This was established to assure the provision of an adequate amount of total energy and nutrients and an attempt to reduce the risk of chronic illnesses.

- The **DAILY VALUE (DV)** is a United States standard that is meant to reflect the needs of an average person. They should be used mainly to compare the nutrients in different foods.

VITAMINS

- **VITAMINS** are organic compounds needed in very small amounts in the diet for normal growth, development and maintenance of the body. They do not provide energy but are necessary for metabolic reactions within cells. The deficiency of each vitamin causes a specific disease or metabolic disorder. Vitamins are classified as water-soluble or fat-soluble.

Water-soluble vitamins

- **ASCORBIC ACID** (Vitamin C) is a highly unstable, water-soluble vitamin. Heat, alkali and light can destroy vitamin C. It is oxidized on exposure to air. Ascorbic acid is stable in dry form, but it may be destroyed during storage and processing. Ascorbic acid is almost completely absorbed, but the body has limited storage capacity for this vitamin, so excess intake is excreted in urine.

  - ➢ **Functions:** Ascorbic acid aids the body in enhancing nonheme iron absorption from foods eaten in the same meal by keeping it in the reduced-ferrous form. It also improves stability of folic acid, and helps recycle oxidized vitamin E for reuse in the cells. Vitamin C aids in the hydroxylation of proline and lysine during formation of collagen, essential for cell function, resistance to infection, capillary integrity and wound healing. It is necessary for the metabolism of proteins, synthesis of neurotransmitters and hormones. It is a biological antioxidant, required for carnitine and norepinephrine synthesis, and is required for hydroxylation of cholesterol for bile-acid synthesis. Vitamin C also helps lymphocytes and other cells of the immune system to function properly.
  - ➢ **Sources: ACEROLA** (Puerto Rican cherry), oranges and other citrus, broccoli, Brussels sprouts, kiwi fruit, tomatoes, strawberries, cabbage, red and green peppers and other sweet peppers, melons, guava, baked potatoes, papaya and mango.
  - ➢ **Dietary Reference Intakes:** The adult RDA for vitamin C is

    > Men: 19+ years 90mg/day
    > Women: 19+ years 75mg/day;
    >   85mg/day during pregnancy for those over age 19;
    >   120mg /day during lactation
    > +35mg/day for smokers

    For smokers and those who live or work with smokers, the intake is 125mg/day for men and 110mg/day for women. Tolerable Upper Intake Levels (UL) for adults have been established at 2000mg/day and at 1800g/day for pregnant and lactating women over age 19.

- **BIOTIN** is soluble in water and alcohol. It is stable to heat and light. Strong acid, alkali or oxidizing agents can inactivate it. It is present in animal products as a water-insoluble protein complex and in plant products in a water-soluble form.

  - ➢ **Functions:** Biotin is involved in carbohydrate and lipid metabolism and in deaminating residues of some amino acids. Each of the biotin-dependent carboxylases catalyzes a carbon-dioxide fixation reaction, and biotin functions as carrier of carbon dioxide on the enzyme. This results in elongation of carbon chains in carbohydrate and fat metabolism.

> **Sources:** Egg yolk, liver, dried beans, cauliflower, mushrooms and brewer's yeast; some biotin is synthesized by intestinal bacteria.
> **Dietary Reference Intakes:** AIs have been established for biotin. No RDAs or EARs have been established.

Adults: 25-30mcg/day
30mcg/day during pregnancy
35mcg/day while breastfeeding

- **COBALAMIN (VITAMIN B₁₂)** is a dark red crystalline compound containing cobalt. It is slightly soluble in water, soluble in ethanol and insoluble in organic solvents. The vitamin is destroyed by oxidizing and reducing agents and by sunlight. Large amounts are stored in the liver. There are at least five different coenzyme forms.

  > **Functions**: Cobalamin is required, along with folate, in the synthesis of DNA and RNA. It is necessary for the synthesis of the myelin sheath of nerves, for fat and carbohydrate metabolism, for normal red blood-cell maturation and to maintain folic acid in its active form. Pernicious anemia results when **INTRINSIC FACTOR**, that is produced in the stomach and is necessary for the absorption of B_{12}, is absent.
  > **Sources:** Organ meats, meat, poultry, fish, clams, oysters and milk. Vegetarians often require supplements.
  > **Dietary Reference Intake:** RDAs have been established for vitamin B_{12} for most individual life cycle categories and AIs for infants. The Food and Nutrition Board of the Institute of Medicine advises "because 10 to 30% of older people may malabsorb food- bound B_{12}, it is advisable for those older than 50 years to meet their RDA mainly by consuming foods fortified by B_{12} or a supplement containing B_{12}."
  Men: 14+ years 2.4mcg/day
  Women: 14+ years 2.4mcg/day
  2.6mcg/day during pregnancy
  2.8mcg/day during lactation

- **FOLATE (FOLIC ACID, FOLACIN, PTEROYLGLUTAMIC ACID)** is a yellow-orange crystal slightly soluble in water and sensitive to light and heat in acidic solutions. Appreciable losses occur during storage and cooking. Folate is stored primarily in the liver. The form of folate used in fortified foods is highly bioavailable and folate is now required to be a part of fortification of flour, cornmeal, rice and other grains.

  > **Functions:** Folate is a critical nutrient for the formation of RNA and DNA and is especially important wherever rapid cell production and turnover occurs in the body (e.g., blood cell production, maintenance of the GI tract). Folate is necessary for the transfer of single carbon units in amino acid metabolism and nucleic acid synthesis. It is required for the synthesis and catabolism of amino acids. Needs are particularly high in pregnancy because of the rapid rate of cell division in the fetus. Recent research recommends supplementing the diets of all premenopausal women because inadequate folate very early in pregnancy increases the rate of birth defects. It is also

protective against heart disease and colon cancer. High levels of homocysteine and low levels of folic acid increase one's risk of fatal heart disease. An important function of folate in the body is to break down homocysteine, which will accumulate in the body, enhancing arterial wall deterioration and blood clot formation.

> **Sources:** Legumes, soybeans, peanuts, sunflower seeds, green leafy vegetables, asparagus, oranges, tofu, folate enriched grain, breads, pasta, and cereals. Some folate is synthesized in the intestinal tract.

> **Dietary Reference Intakes:** RDAs have been established for folate. RDAs, which are almost twice the 1989 amounts, have been established for children and adults. AIs have been established for infants.

    Men: 19+ years 400mcg Dietary Folate Equivalent (DFE)/day
    Women: 19+ years 400mcg DFE/day
        600mcg   DFE/day during pregnancy
        500mcg   DFE/day during lactation

    The UL, which applies to synthetic forms obtained from supplements and/or fortified foods (including pregnant and lactating women) is 1,000mcg DFE/day for adults.

- **NIACIN (NICOTINIC ACID)** is the most stable of all vitamins. It is resistant to heat, light, air, acid and alkali, but it is soluble in hot water and ethanol. It occurs as nicotinic acid in plants, and as nicotinamide in animals. Niacin is stored to a limited extent.

  > **Functions:** The coenzymes nicotinamide adenine dinucleotide (NAD) and nicotinamide adenine dinucleotide phosphate (NADP) or their reduced forms, are required for oxidation of carbohydrate, synthesis of fatty acids, and functioning of the Krebs cycle in all energy- production reactions and electron transport. Large doses of niacin (3g) have been used to reduce serum cholesterol, but there are some side effects. Niacin can be synthesized from tryptophan in humans, with 60mg tryptophan equivalent to 1mg nicotinic acid. Niacin values are expressed in **NIACIN EQUIVALENTS (NE),** the total of preformed niacin and tryptophan that can be converted to niacin.

  > **Sources:** Liver, meats, poultry, fish and shellfish, peanuts, mushrooms, whole and enriched grains and breads.

  > **Dietary Reference Intakes**: RDAs have been established for niacin. AIs have been established for infants and ULs. Values are expressed in mgNE, except for recommendations for infants less than six months of age, which are expressed as preformed niacin.

      Men: 14+ years 16mgNE/day
      Women: 14+ years 14mgNE/da
          18mg NE/day during pregnancy
          17mg NE/day while breastfeeding

      The UL for all adults (including pregnant and lactating women) is 35mgNE/day.

- **PANTOTHENIC ACID** is a water-soluble vitamin that is fairly stable during ordinary processing and storage, but it is sensitive to high temperatures and is easily hydrolyzed in hot acid or base solutions. Pantothenic acid is widely distributed in plants and animals in bound form. It occurs in body tissues in a bound form that is liberated by proteolytic enzymes. Small amounts are stored in the liver and kidneys.

- ➢ **Functions:** Pantothenic acid is a constituent of **COENZYME A (CoA),** that is required for the oxidation of carbohydrate, protein and fat for energy. It acts in the synthesis of sterol, steroid hormones, porphyrins, acetylcholine, cholesterol and ketones. CoA is required in the synthesis of fatty acids. Utilization depends on the presence of folate and biotin.
- ➢ **Sources:** Beef, poultry, whole grain cereals, potatoes, tomatoes, broccoli.
- ➢ **Dietary Reference Intakes**: AIs have been established for pantothenic acid. No RDAs or EARs have been established.
  Men: 14+ years 5mg/day
  Women: 14+ years 5mg/day
       6mg/day during pregnancy
       7mg/day during lactation

- • **RIBOFLAVIN (VITAMIN B₂),** is slightly soluble in water, readily destroyed by exposure to light, and unstable in an alkaline medium. Riboflavin has a yellowish pigment with a green fluorescence (sometimes seen is in skim milk and meats.) It is stable to dry heat, acids and oxidizing agents. Riboflavin's absorption is increased when food is in the GI tract. There is little body storage of riboflavin.

  - ➢ **Functions:** Riboflavin is necessary for conversion of B₆, folate, niacin and vitamin K to their active forms; coenzyme form FMN (flavin adenine mononucleotide) and FAD (flavin-adenine dinucleotide); is involved in cellular oxidation-reduction reactions and other metabolic reactions including biosynthesis of niacin from tryptophan. Riboflavin also maintains body tissue, helps form red blood cells and protects against common skin and eye disorders.
  - ➢ **Sources**: Milk, liver, dark green leafy vegetables, cheese, fortified cereals, enriched grains, brewer's yeast, lean meats, eggs and mushrooms.
  - ➢ **Dietary Reference Intakes:** RDAs have been established for riboflavin and AIs for infants. The RDAs are based on the vitamin's function and excretion in the body. Pregnant and lactating women have increased needs.
    Men: 14+ years 1.3mg/day
    Women: 19+ years 1.1mg/day
         1.4mg/day during pregnancy
         1.6mg/day during lactation

- • **THIAMIN (VITAMIN B₁)** is a water-soluble vitamin that is stable in dry form and in a slightly acidic medium, but is readily destroyed in a neutral or alkaline medium and by high temperatures.

  - ➢ **Functions:** Thiamin regulates muscle tone of the gastrointestinal tract. It is necessary for the normal functioning of nerves, maintains muscle tone for heart function and acts as a coenzyme in carbohydrate metabolism. When combined with phosphorus (as the coenzyme thiamin pyrophosphate), it plays a key role in carbohydrate metabolism, in decarboxylation of keto acids such as pyruvate and ketoglutarate and the transketolase reaction in the pentose-phosphate pathway.
  - ➢ **Sources:** The largest concentrations of thiamin are found in brewers yeast, lean pork and ham, Brazil nuts, pistachios and pecans. Other sources are lentils, wheat germ, whole grains, dried beans, nuts, seeds, enriched flours, breads and cereals.
  - ➢ **Dietary Reference Intakes:** RDAs have been established for thiamin and AIs for

infants. The RDAs are based on levels of energy intake because of thiamin's role in energy metabolism. The AIs for infants are based on levels of thiamin generally found in human milk.

Men: 14+ years 1.2mg/day
Women: 19+ years 1.1mg/day
        1.4mg/day during pregnancy
        1.4mg/day during lactation

- **VITAMIN B$_6$** is very water-soluble. It is stable in acid and alkaline solution and in the presence of heat, but it is rapidly destroyed by light in a neutral or alkaline solution. Vitamin B$_6$ is the class name given to include three compounds with Vitamin B$_6$ activity; **PYRIDOXINE, PYRIDOXAL** and **PYRIDOXAMINE**. Body storage is limited. All three compounds can be converted to the coenzyme form, pyridoxal phosphate.

  ➤ **Functions**: B$_6$ coenzymes are required in amino acid metabolism, conversion of tryptophan to niacin, formation of nonessential-amino acids and formation of neurotransmitters in the brain from amino acids. They are also necessary for glycogen, fatty-acid metabolism, immune function and reduced risk for atherosclerosis.

  ➤ **Sources**: Liver, meats, poultry, brewer's yeast, mango, potatoes, beans, nuts and seeds (especially filberts, sunflower seeds, peanuts and peanut butter). Vitamin B$_6$ is available in a large variety of unprocessed foods. Food processing can result in losses of 50-70%.

  ➤ **Dietary Reference Intakes**: RDAs have been established for vitamin B$_6$, AIs for infants and ULs for both children and adults. The need for vitamin B$_6$ increases as intake of protein increases.

  Men: 14-50 years 1.3mg/day; 51+ years 1.7mg/day
  Women: 14-18 years 1.2mg/day; 19-50 years 1.3mg/day; 51+ years 1.5mg/day
          1.9mg/day during pregnancy
          2.0mg/day during lactation

  The UL for vitamin B$_6$ is: 14-18 years 80mg/day 19+ years 100mg/day, including pregnant and lactating women.

Fat-soluble vitamins

- **CALCIFEROL (VITAMIN D)** is insoluble in water and stable to heat, acid, alkali and oxidation. It can be acquired preformed in food or by exposure of the skin to sunlight. A natural prohormone found in the skin, **7-DIHYDROXY VITAMIN D**, becomes **CHOLECALCIFEROL (D$_3$)** on exposure to sunlight. It is stored in the liver, spleen, lungs and brain. **ERGOCALCIFEROL (D$_3$)** is a plant form of vitamin D.

  ➤ **Functions:** Vitamin D promotes mineralization of bone by enhancing absorption of calcium, increases reabsorption of calcium by the kidneys and helps maintain normal blood levels of calcium and phosphorus. D$_3$ appears to be more biologically available that D$_2$.

  ➤ **Sources:** Fortified milks (400 IU per quart), fish oils, fortified margarine and cereal, liver, fatty fish (sardines, herring, mackerel and salmon), butter.

  ➤ **Dietary Reference Intake:** AIs have been established for vitamin D. They are expressed as cholecalciferol and assume an absence of adequate exposure to sunlight.

People who wear clothing that covers the entire body, especially those who live in cold climates, should be advised to take a supplement. One mcg of cholecalciferol is equal to 40 IU of Vitamin D. EAR for Vitamin D is now 10mcg/day.

Men and women: 14-70 years 15mcg/day

               70+ 15mcg/day

               20mcg/day during pregnancy and lactation

The UL for all age groups except infants is now 1000mcg/day.

- **RETINOL (VITAMIN A)** is insoluble in water and unstable in air, but it can be stabilized by the addition of antioxidants. Vitamin A is stable at high temperatures in the absence of oxygen and it is stable to acid, alkali and normal cooking temperature. Provitamin A exists in yellow and green plants in several isomeric forms; alpha-carotene, beta-carotene and cryptoxanthin. **BETA-CAROTENE** is the most potent, but only 50% of carotene can convert to active vitamin A. Excess accumulations of pigment can turn skin yellow or orange. Vitamin A is stored in the liver as an ester, primarily as vitamin A acetate, transported as retinol (alcohol form) and active as retinaldehyde. Vitamin A is measured in **RETINOL ACTIVITY EQUIVALENTS (RAE)**. The RAE is a measure of vitamin A activity of beta-carotene and other vitamin A precursors that shows the amount of retinol the body will get from a food containing the precursors. Vitamins A and D were formerly measured in International Units (IU).

       1 RAE = 1mcg retinol

       1 RAE = 12mcg beta-carotene

       1 RAE = 24mcg other carotenoids

  - **Functions:** Vitamin A maintains the integrity of skin and epithelial tissue, is required for night vision and growth, regulates structure and functions of cellular and subcellular membranes, helps bone and tooth formation and also plays a role in the body's immune reactions. Some carotenoids are antioxidants that may have the ability to protect cells from carcinogenic changes. The American Cancer Society promotes consumption of fruits and vegetables rich in carotenoids.
  - **Sources:** Liver, fish (and fish liver oils), egg yolk, whole or fortified milk, cheese, butter and margarine; carotenoids such as beta-carotene are precursors of vitamin A and are found in dark yellow, green and orange fruits and vegetables (carrots, pumpkins, sweet potatoes, mango, spinach, broccoli, dark leafy greens and cantaloupe).

  Dietary Reference Intakes: The RDAs for vitamin A, expressed as RAE are:

  Men: 14+ years 900mcg/day

  Women: 14+ years 700mcg/day

              770mcg/day during pregnancy (over age 19)

              1300mcg/day during lactation (over age 19)

  The UL for vitamin A applies to the preformed vitamin only and is 3000mcg/day for all adults, including pregnant and lactating women. Those who take supplements, use fortified foods, and eat diets high in animal protein, are in danger of vitamin A toxicity (hypervitaminosis A).

- **TOCOPHEROL (VITAMIN E)** is stable at high temperature and in acid, but readily oxidizes in the presence of lead, iron salts and rancid fat. It is destroyed by high heat processing, such as deep-fat frying. It decomposes in ultraviolet light. Eight tocopherols have been isolated, but only four are considered biologically active. **ALPHA-TOCOPHEROL** is the most potent. Vitamin E content of food is expressed in milligrams. Small amounts of vitamin E are stored in fatty tissue and in the liver.

> **Functions:** Vitamin E protects cell membranes and red blood cells from oxidative damage or breakdown by inactivating free radicals. It has a sparing effect on vitamin A, carotene and polyunsaturated-fatty acids because it prevents their oxidation. Vitamin E also protects red and white blood cells and improves immune response.
> **Sources:** Seeds and vegetable oils (particularly corn, soy and sunflower), nuts, green and leafy green vegetables, wheat germ, whole wheat, margarine and salad dressings, and mangos.
> **Conversion factors:** To estimate the alpha tocopherol content of foods shown as tocopherol equivalents multiply by 0.8.
> **Dietary Reference Intakes:** RDAs for vitamin E are:
> Men: 15mg /day
> Women: 15mg /day, including pregnancy
> Lactation: 19mg/day
> The UL for all adults (including pregnant and lactating women) for vitamin E is 1000mg/day and applies to any form of supplemental D tocopherol, fortified foods or a combination of the two.

- **VITAMIN K** has at least three forms all belonging to a group of chemical compounds known as **QUINONES**. **PHYLLOQUINONE (K_1)** is found in green plants; **MENAQUINONE (K_2)** is formed by bacterial action in the intestinal tract. **MENADIONE (K_3),** the synthetic form, is the most biologically reactive. Vitamin K is stable to heat, oxygen and moisture, but it is unstable to alkali and ultraviolet light. Vitamin K is synthesized in the gut of adults and children, but infants do not have the intestinal flora necessary for synthesis.

> **Functions**: Vitamin K is required for the synthesis of blood clotting factors such as prothrombin, and other proteins (e.g., bone, plasma, kidney).
> **Sources**: Green leafy vegetables, liver, cabbage family, milk, eggs.
> **Dietary Reference Intakes:** AIs have been established for vitamin K
> Men: 120mcg/day
> Women: 90mcg/day
> 90mcg/day during pregnancy and while breastfeeding

Vitamins as antioxidants

- Vitamin C, vitamin E and beta-carotene function in the body as effective antioxidants. **ANTIOXIDANTS** inhibit oxidation and the resulting free radical damage in many body tissues, thus preventing the onset of degenerative diseases that are often associated with age, such as cancers (lung, gastrointestinal and breast), heart disease and stroke, immune system dysfunction, cataracts and certain neurological disorders such as Parkinson's disease.

- Since the early 1980s, there have been reports in the scientific literature that biologic antioxidants can protect against diseases. Studies to determine the optimal levels of vitamin intake to promote health are testing the effectiveness of supplements at levels that are generally beyond normal dietary intakes.

- The *Dietary Guidelines for Americans* encourage increased intakes of fruits and vegetables. Diets rich in fruits and vegetables have been correlated with decreased cancer risk in many studies. The protection is thought to be not only from antioxidants, but also from fiber and other carotenoids. Other carotenoids (alpha-cryptoxanthin, lutein, lycopene and zeaxanthin) have antioxidant properties, but have not been as widely studied.

- In addition to vitamins C, E and beta-carotene, there are other biological antioxidants. Antioxidant enzymes include superoxide dismutase, catalase and glutathione peroxidase. Zinc, copper, manganese and selenium are nutritional precursors needed to form these antioxidant enzymes. Non-enzymatic oxygen scavengers include uric acid, glutathione, thiols in protein, bioflavonoids in citrus fruits, transferrin, ubiquinone (coenzyme Q_{10}) and ceruloplasmin, a copper-binding substance in plasma. Many phytochemicals are antioxidants.

MINERALS

- **MINERALS** are inorganic materials that cannot be synthesized by the body. Major minerals, are required in larger amounts by the body than are the trace minerals. Caution must be taken not to exceed the ULs, especially because there are some vitamin:vitamin; vitamin: mineral; and mineral: mineral interactions that cause medical problems.

- **CALCIUM (CA)** makes up from 1.5% to 2% of adult body weight. About 99% is found in bones and teeth. The remainder is found in body fluids, soft tissue and blood, where it is used for regulatory functions. It is the most abundant mineral in the body. The calcium ion has a positive charge.

  - ➤ **Functions:** Calcium is necessary for the structure of bones and teeth, blood coagulation, muscle function, transmission of nerve impulses, production and activity of numerous enzymes and hormones and regulation of cell wall permeability. Recent research suggests that it may play a role in prevention of certain diseases. One of the most important functions of the body is calcium homeostasis. An imbalance of blood calcium is regulated by the intestines, bones, and kidneys along with Vitamin D, and the 2 hormones, **PARATHROMONE** and **CALCITONIN** that regulate calcium.
  - ➤ **Sources:** Dairy products (hard cheese, milk, yogurt, etc.), sardines, nuts (almonds, filberts, brazil nuts) blackstrap molasses, shellfish, green leafy vegetables and soy products; such as green soybeans, soy nuts and tofu (from calcium added in processing).
  - ➤ **Dietary Reference Intakes:** AIs and ULs have been established for calcium. EAR is now 800-1,000mg/day.
    Men and women, RDA: 1,000-1,300mg/day depending on age
    The ULs for calcium are 2,000-3,000mg/day for all groups over age 1

- **CHLORIDE (CL)** is the principal anion in extracellular fluid. Normal concentrations in plasma are about 103mEq/liter.

  - ➤ **Functions**: Chloride works with sodium and potassium to maintain normal fluid balance, acid-base balances and cell-membrane transfer. It is also important for the digestion of food.
  - ➤ **Sources:** Chloride is abundant in food, particularly salt. Sources include table salt,

seafood, milk, meat, eggs and many processed foods.

> **Dietary Reference Intakes**: AIs have been established for chloride.
> Men and women: 1,800-2,300mg/day
> Pregnancy and lactation: 2,300mg/day

- **CHROMIUM (CR)** is present in the body in very small amounts and is found mainly in glandular organs. Chromium assumes different charges, but the positively charged form is more stable and the one most commonly found in foods.

  > **Functions:** Chromium makes insulin action more effective and maintains glucose homeostasis. Chromium has a role in carbohydrate and fat metabolism. However, current research suggests that chromium supplementation does not improve glucose or insulin response in diabetics.
  > **Sources:** Brewer's yeast, oysters, liver, wheat germ, beer and unprocessed, unrefined foods.
  > **Dietary Reference Intakes**: AIs have been established for chromium.
  > Males: 30-35mcg/day
  > Females: 20-25mcg/day
  > Pregnancy 19+: 30mcg/day
  > Lactation 19+: 45mcg/day

- **COPPER (CU)** is concentrated mainly in the liver, kidney, spleen and heart. An adult body has about 100mg of copper that is stored in the liver.

  > **Functions**: Copper is a part of many enzymes, including those necessary for red blood cell synthesis, nerve tissue maintenance and connective tissue formation. Copper is required for the absorption of iron in the formation of hemoglobin. While all copper containing enzymes have differing metabolic roles, they are all involved with reactions that consume oxygen or oxygen radicals.
  > **Sources:** Liver, other organ meats, oysters and clams meat, shellfish, green leafy vegetables, whole grains, legumes, nuts, seeds, molasses, chocolate, and brewer's yeast.
  > **Dietary Reference Intakes:** RDAs and ULs have been established for copper. The RDAs are:
  > Adults 19+: 900mcg/day
  > Pregnancy: 1,000mcg/day
  > Lactation: 1,300mcg/day
  > The ULs for all adults (including pregnant and lactating women) is 10,000mcg/day.

- **FLUORIDE (F)** is found in very small amounts in the body, but is a vital component of bones and teeth.

  > **Functions:** Fluoride functions in the mineralization of teeth and bones. It inhibits dental caries by increasing the integrity of tooth enamel.
  > **Sources:** Fluoridated water, fish and foods prepared with fluoridated water and fluoride added to toothpaste and mouthwashes.
  > **Dietary Reference Intakes:** AIs and ULs have been established for fluoride. The AIs are: Men: 3-4mg/day
  > Women14+ years: 3mg/day, including pregnancy and lactation
  > The UL for all adults including pregnant and lactating women is 10mg/day.

- **IODINE (I)** is found mainly in the thyroid gland (about 80% of total iodine).

  - **Functions:** Iodine is necessary for the synthesis of thyroxin, the thyroid hormone that regulates cellular oxidation and basal metabolism.
  - **Sources:** Iodized salt, saltwater fish and shellfish, vegetables grown in areas with high levels of iodine in the soil, milk from cows that graze on plants from soil containing iodine.
  - **Dietary Reference Intakes:** The RDAs established are:

Adults:	150mcg/day
Pregnancy:	220mcg/day
Lactation:	290mcg/day

    The ULs are 1100mcg/day for all adults including pregnant and lactating women.

- **IRON (FE)** is a trace mineral vital for life but needed in only small amounts. An adult has about 3-5g of body iron: 70% in hemoglobin and 10-20% in myoglobin. The remainder is stored mainly in the liver, bone marrow, and spleen. In food, iron is found mainly in its ferric form. About 1 to 1.5g of iron are normally stored as hemosiderin ferritin in the body. Iron is transported as transferrin.

  - **Functions:** It acts as a component of heme, enables tissues to utilize oxygen and eliminate carbon dioxide, is necessary for red blood cell synthesis, is a component of enzymes required for cellular oxidation and it strengthens the immune system.

  - **Sources:** Organ meats, red meat, poultry, fish, shellfish, legumes, enriched grains, fortified cereals, most dried fruits and green leafy vegetables. Absorbability of iron varies widely; heme forms from meat are absorbed more readily than the non-heme forms from all vegetable and some animal sources.
  - **Dietary Reference Intakes:** RDAs and ULs have been established for iron.
    The RDAs are:

Men: 19+ years:	8mg/day
Women: 19-50 years:	18mg/day
51+ years:	8mg/day
Pregnancy:	27mg/day
Lactation:	9mg/day

    The ULs are 45mg/day for all adults including pregnant and lactating women.

- **MAGNESIUM (MG)** totals about 21-28g in an adult, with 60% of that in bones and teeth and the remainder in muscle (26%), soft tissue and body fluids.

  - **Functions:** Magnesium is required to stabilize the structure of ATP in certain enzyme reactions; is a cofactor for many enzymes that are involved in metabolism of food components, helps maintain muscle contractibility and nerve irritability. Magnesium is required for fatty acid, nucleic acid and protein synthesis
  - **Sources:** Nuts, seeds, legumes, dark green leafy vegetables, whole grains, meats, milk.
  - **Dietary Reference Intakes:** RDAs and ULs have been established for magnesium.
    The RDAs are:

Men:	400-420mg/day
Women:	310-320mg/day (and during lactation)
Pregnancy:	350-360mg/day (ages 19-30)

- **MANGANESE (MN)** is present in an adult body at a level of about 20mg and is concentrated in the bones, the liver, kidneys and pancreas.

  - **Functions:** Manganese is necessary for many enzymes involved in the metabolism of carbohydrates, fats and amino acids. Manganese has a role in the formation of connective tissue and skeletal tissue, in addition to growth and reproduction.
  - **Sources:** Wheat germ, whole grains, legumes, nuts, beet greens, blackstrap molasses, pineapples and blueberries.
  - **Dietary Reference Intakes:** AIs and ULs have been established for manganese. The AIs are:
    Men: 2.3mg/day
    Women: 1.8mg/day
      Pregnancy: 2.0mg/day
      Lactation: 2.6mg/day
    The UL for all adults (including pregnant and lactating women) is 11mg/day.

- **MOLYBDENUM (MO)**

  - **Functions:** is required in the enzyme xanthine oxidase, which aids in formation of uric acid. It is also a component of several enzymes necessary for the conversion of food to energy and mobilization of iron from storage. It is known to be especially important for people who are on long term TPN feedings.
  - **Sources:** Legumes, dried beans, nuts, whole grain cereals, dairy products and dark green leafy vegetables. It is widely distributed in foods that are commonly eaten.
  - **Dietary Reference Intakes:** RDAs and ULs have been established for molybdenum. The RDAs are:
    Adults 19-70+:   45mcg/day
      Pregnancy and lactation: 50mcg/day
    The UL for all adults 19-70+ years (including pregnant and lactating women) is 2000 mcg/day.

- **PHOSPHORUS (P)** Adult tissues contain about 700 grams of phosphorus, with 85% of that in bones and teeth. The remainder is in extra-cellular fluid and in soft tissue, especially striated muscle. Phosphorus is a component of ATP, DNA, RNA, B vitamin coenzymes, lipoproteins and buffers. The ion has a negative charge.

  - **Functions:** Phosphorus aids in the transport of fatty acids and the absorption of glucose and glycerol through phosphorylation. Phosphates (phosphorus salts) are found in all cells of the body. They are part of a major buffer system important in intracellular fluid and the kidney tubules, where phosphate aids in the excretion of hydrogen ions.
  - **Sources:** Pumpkin seeds, sunflower seeds, soy nuts, nuts (almonds, Brazil nuts, cashews and pistachios), sardines, fish, brewer's yeast, milk, meats and poultry.
  - **Dietary Reference Intakes:** RDAs and ULs have been established for phosphorus. The RDAs are:
    Adults 19-70+ years, including pregnant and lactating women: 700mg/day
    The UL for adults 19-70 years (including lactating women): 4000mg/day and for pregnant women, it is 3500mg/day, for adults over age 70: 3000mg/day.

- **POTASSIUM (K)** is the major cation of intracellular fluid. A small amount of potassium is present in extracellular fluid.

  - **Functions:** Potassium works with sodium to maintain fluid balance and cell integrity. It works with calcium to regulate neuromuscular activity. Potassium helps maintain acid-base balance and cell-membrane transfer.
  - **Sources:** Fruits, vegetables, juices, milk, cooked dried beans and peas, whole grains, fresh meats, poultry, fish and shellfish. Most Americans do not get enough potassium in their diets.
  - **Dietary Reference Intakes:** AIs have been established for potassium. ULs have not been established because potassium from food is usually safe and unless it is taken in supplemental form, it does not usually pose a problem. When taken in supplemental form, potassium can cause fatal cardiac arrhythmias, unless the dosage is carefully controlled. When some diuretics are prescribed, potassium is also prescribed, because these medications can deplete the body's potassium.
    The AIs for adults are:
    Ages 19-70+ (including pregnant women): 4700mg/day
       All lactating women: 5100mg/day

- **SELENIUM (SE)** is deposited in highest concentrations in the liver, kidneys, heart and spleen. It acts as an antioxidant.

  - **Functions:** Selenium is an active cofactor in glutathione peroxidase, that removes hydrogen peroxide and other hydroperoxides from the cell. It works with vitamin E in prevention of free-radical formation, which some research suggests has a role in cancer prevention.
  - **Sources:** Selenium content of food is dependent upon the amount of selenium in the water and soil where food is grown. Major sources are Brazil nuts, organ meats, shellfish, meats and poultry; and grains grown in selenium-rich soil.
  - **Dietary Reference Intakes:** RDAs and ULs have been established for selenium. If a person's diet is very high in saturated fatty acids, selenium intake may need to be increased, because of its antioxidant activity.
    The RDAs are:
    Adults: 55mcg/day
                 60mcg/day during pregnancy
                 70mcg/day during lactation
    The UL for all adults, including pregnant and breastfeeding women is 400mcg/day.

- **SODIUM (NA)** is the principal cation of extracellular fluid. About half of the body's sodium is in extracellular fluid, 10% is in intracellular fluid and the remaining 35-40% is in the skeleton.

  - **Functions:** Sodium works with chloride to maintain osmotic pressure in the extracellular fluid compartment, including plasma volume. Sodium also works to maintain fluid balance. It aids in conducting nerve impulses and muscular contraction. Its ion has a positive charge.
  - **Sources:** Table salt (NaCl), of which 40% is sodium, dairy products, meat, fish, poultry, eggs, some vegetables, soy sauce, seasonings and many pickled and processed foods. Fruit is generally low in sodium.
  - **Dietary Reference Intakes:** Diets are not usually low in sodium and because the

body can adapt to lower intakes, deficiencies are not usually seen. Most Americans eat too much sodium. AIs and ULs have been established for sodium. Recommendations are set at low levels to protect against hypertension, but they are high enough for people to eat a diet adequate in other nutrients. The AIs for sodium are:

Adults aged 19-50: 1,500mg/day, including pregnancy and lactation
Adults aged 51-70: 1,300mg/day
Adults aged 70+: 1,200mg/day
The UL for all adults, including pregnant and lactating women is 2300mg/day.

- **SULFUR (S)** is present in every cell, especially cells in hair, nails and cartilage. The body uses sulfur as a component of other compounds; but it does not use sulfur itself, as a nutrient. It is found in insulin, melanin and in the amino acids cysteine and methionine. It is also a component of thiamin, biotin and pantothenic acid. Sulfur is an essential constituent of cell proteins, activates enzymes and provides structure for proteins. Its ion has a negative charge. All protein foods are sources. There is no DRI for sulfur because no deficiencies are known.

- **ZINC (ZN)** is widely distributed in the body. Adults have about 2g concentrated in skin, hair, nails, testes, liver, muscles and bones.

  - **Functions:** Zinc is required for the synthesis of DNA and RNA and for carbohydrate, protein and alcohol metabolism by enzymes. It is also needed for energy metabolism, growth, healing wounds, immune response and reproduction. Zinc is a constituent of enzymes and insulin.
  - **Sources:** Oysters, red meats, soybeans, nuts and wheat germ.
  - **Dietary Reference Intakes:** RDAs and ULs have been established for zinc.
    The RDAs are:
    Men 14-70+ years: 11mg/day
    Women 14-18 years: 9mg/day; 19-70+ years; 8mg/day
           11mg/day during pregnancy: 12mg/day during lactation.
    The UL for all adults including pregnant and lactating women is 40mg/day.

WATER

Functions

FLUID BALANCE			
Average Fluid Intake		**Average Fluid Output**	
Beverages	1,250ml	Urine	1400ml
Water in Foods	900ml	Feces	100ml
Water (food oxidation)	350ml	Skin (perspiration)	700ml
	2,500ml	Lungs (expiration)	300ml
			2,500ml

- A large portion of the body weight is water. Intracellular fluid (within cells) is about 45% of body weight. Extracellular fluid (blood, lymph, spinal fluid and secretions) and interstitial fluid (around and between cells) comprise about 20% of body weight. Water is a medium for all metabolic processes and transports nutrients to cells and waste or toxic substances from cells. Water is a solvent for body compounds, lubricates the joints and water plays a principal role in the regulation of body temperature.

Fluid balance

- Water needs vary and depend on many factors, such as the foods one eats, the environmental temperature and humidity, activity levels and state of health. The body seeks to maintain electrolyte concentrations in intracellular and extracellular fluid. This is accomplished by small shifts of fluid from one body compartment to another. Sodium and potassium are the primary minerals controlling this movement.

Intake and output

- Dietary sources of water include beverages and foods. Water is also available to the body as a result of the oxidation of food. Fluid is lost through urine, feces, skin (perspiration) and the lungs (expiration). Intake and environment influence total output. Water intake is regulated by thirst, which is controlled by the hypothalamus. The following chart illustrates typical fluid intake and output.

  > **Dietary Reference Intakes:** AIs have been established as goals for individual intake.

  For infants 0-6 months: 0.7L/day
  For infants 7-12 months: 0.8L/day
  For children ages 1-3: 1.3L/day
  For children ages 4-8: 1.7L/day
  For males ages 9-13: 2.4L/day
  For males ages 14-18: 3.3L/day
  For males ages 19-70+: 3.7L/day
  For females ages 9-13: 2.1L/day
  For females ages 14-18: 2.3L/day
  For females ages 19-70+: 2.7L/day
  For pregnancy: 3.0L/day
  For lactation: 3.8L/day
  Total water intake includes all water contained in food, beverages and drinking water.

Water in foods

- Water is the most abundant nutrient in most foods. Each molecule of water contains 2 molecules of hydrogen and one molecule of oxygen. Water changes forms depending on temperature:

  > Water freezes at 32° F (0° C) by forming a crystalline network holding the molecules. When water freezes, the volume expands.
  > Pure water boils at 212° F (100° C) when the vapor pressure equals the atmospheric pressure. The molecules vaporize and become steam. Atmospheric pressure is lower at higher altitudes requiring longer cooking times.

➢ Pressure cookers allow boiling to occur at higher temperatures so foods cook in shorter periods of time

- Fresh foods have high water activity making them susceptible to microbial spoilage. Food preservation methods that reduce water activity or delay spoilage include dehydration, freezing, salting and the addition of sugars in jams.

- Mineral salts, such as bicarbonates and/or sulfates of calcium and magnesium, determine the "hardness" of water. Hard water can cause cloudiness in tea, mineral deposits on cooking vessels and increase cooking times of legumes. Hard water can have minerals removed by ion-exchange processes but the resulting "soft water" contains far   more sodium.

- Water in foods is useful as a method for heat transfer, as a solvent to form solutions and for chemical reactions necessary for cooking and freezing foods.

b. Nutrient and energy needs throughout the life span

Growth charts

- Growth charts are used as clinical and research tools to assess the nutritional status of infants, children and adolescents.

  ➢ Growth charts include BMI for age charts, in addition to development of additional percentiles.
  ➢ There are now both Spanish and French versions, in addition to the English version.
  ➢ BMI calculators for children aged 2-20 are also available:
    http://apps.nccd.cdc.gov/dnpabmi/
  ➢ The charts and other information are available on the Center for Disease Control web site: **www.cdc.gov/growthcharts**

Infancy

- Infants have the highest calorie and protein needs per body weight of any time in the life cycle because of rapid growth and development and high activity rates. Based on the 2002 National Academy of Sciences report on Dietary Reference Intakes (DRI) for Macronutrients, the ESTIMATED ENERGY REQUIREMENTS (EER) for infants, which are based on human milk consumption, should be derived by the following formulas:

  EER = TEE (total energy expenditure) + Energy Deposition
  0-3 months   (89 x weight of infant [kg] – 100 + 175 (kcal for Energy Deposition)
  4-6 months   (89 x weight of infant [kg] – 100 + 56 (kcal for Energy Deposition)
  7-12 months (89 x weight of infant [kg] – 100 + 22 (kcal for Energy Deposition)

- **Protein requirements for infants are:**
  0-6 months 1.5g/kg/day (AI) (~9.1g/d).
      This recommendation is based on the observed average intake of infants who are fed mostly human milk. Infants who are fed only human milk for the first 6 months of life receive adequate amounts of protein.
  7-12 months 1.5g/kg/day (RDA) (~11.0g/d)

- **Carbohydrate requirements are:**
  0-6 months 60g/day (AI)
  7-12 months 95g/day (AI)

- **Fat requirements are:**
  0-6 months 31g/day (AI)
  7-12 months 30g/day (AI)

- **Linoleic acid requirements are:**
  0-6 months: 4.4g/day (AI)
  7-12 months 4.6g/day (AI)

- **α-Linolenic acid requirements are:**
  0-6 months 0.5 (AI)
  7-12 months 0.5 (AI)

- Full term infants are born with a fetal iron reserve sufficient for three to six months. Although human milk may meet an infant's need for iron, iron supplementation is recommended beginning at four months. Iron-fortified infant formula and fortified infant cereals are recommended for the first year of life. Supplementation with vitamin D and fluoride is recommended for breast-fed babies. Fluoride can be provided through formula prepared with fluoridated water or fluoride supplements. It is recommended that babies fed infant formula receive ascorbic acid supplementation until fruits and vegetables are introduced, at about four to six months. Breast-fed babies rely on their mothers' intake of ascorbic acid.

- Breastfeeding is the preferred method of feeding, because breast milk is tailored to meet infant needs. It provides the baby with some degree of immunity and facilitates bonding between mother and child. The American Academy of Pediatrics recommends breastfeeding through the first year, if possible. Nutrient requirements of an infant can be met with formula for the first year of life.

- Breastfeeding should be an individual decision. Women who choose to bottle-feed because of personal values, lifestyle, inadequate milk supply, work demands or other reasons should not be made to feel guilty for this choice. Many, many babies have thrived on bottle feeding and there are many excellent baby formulas available.

- The American Academy of Pediatrics advises that whole cow's milk should not be used during the first year. Whole milk should be used during the second year because it contains essential fatty acids, which are necessary for healthy development particularly of the brain and nervous system.

- The FDA regulates the minimum level of nutrients required in commercial infant formula in the United States. Standard formulas differ somewhat, but most are formulated to be as similar to human milk as possible. Human milk protein is 60% whey (mainly lactalbumin) and 40% casein. Most of the popular commercial infant formulas have modified the protein to reflect this ratio. The carbohydrate source in the majority of cow's milk based formulas is lactose, although maltodextrin is combined with lactose in one formulation. All fat in commercial milk based formula comes from vegetable oil, but each product has a different blend. All contain linoleic and linolenic acids and some companies have begun to add DHA because it is considered to be essential for brain development. Some recent research has suggested that formula fed babies do not have the high levels of DHA that breast fed babies have. This is thought to be caused by the fact that while the precursors of DHA (linoleic and linolenic acids) are present, the precursors in breast milk are more biochemically active.

- Specialty formulas are available for infants who are unable to tolerate standard formulas. Protein and/or carbohydrate change is most common. These include soy and/or lactose-free products. Hypoallergenic formulas may contain "partially hydrolyzed protein." In these formulas lactose, is removed, and another carbohydrate is added (usually corn syrup but sometimes sucrose, cornstarch or tapioca.) If fat malabsorption is a problem, MCT oil is often used. MCT oils contain no essential fatty acids, so these should be supplemented.

- **COLOSTRUM,** the first fluid secreted by the breast, has higher concentrations of carotene, protein and minerals than mature human milk. It contains immunological factors that protect an infant. Concentrations of fat and lactose increase in milk as colostrum diminishes (usually within a day or two.)

- Breast milk contains a lipase that aids rapid digestion and absorption of milk fat. Water-miscible vitamin D in breast milk is well utilized by infants. The GI tract and kidneys are too immature to process solid foods until four to five months. Some babies have trouble digesting regular cow's milk before age one. The American Academy of Pediatrics recommends iron-fortified formula until age one for bottle-fed infants.

- Infant tolerance of solid foods varies, but introduction of solids is not recommended before four months because solids are poorly digested as the GI tract is immature and doesn't handle solids well. Some children are ready to have solid foods earlier than others, but by six months of age, children should be ready to have some solid food to fulfill certain nutrient needs and to handle foods of varying textures and flavors. Other foods are generally introduced in the following order: fortified infant cereals (usually rice cereal first), vegetables, fruit and fruit juices, teething biscuits, meat, fish and poultry and finally eggs, cheese and food mixtures. Many physicians suggest avoiding or limiting baby desserts and giving primarily basic foods to avoid preference for sweets.

- Introduce single foods to infants one at a time, rather than in mixtures, to detect intolerances. Introduce a variety of soft table foods by age one. One year olds should receive over 50% of calories from table food. Also at one year, babies may be given whole milk. Children under two years of age should not be given skim milk. (For further information, see: *Position of the Academy of Nutrition and Dietetics: Nutrition Guidance for Healthy Children Ages 2 to 11 years, J Am Diet Assoc. 2008:108:1038-1047.)*

- Generally, healthy full-term babies double their birth weight by approximately five months and triple their birth weight by a year. The length increases an average of 10 inches. The first six months are critical for brain growth. The rate of growth in the first four months is faster than at any other time. From four to eight months, growth rate slows and assessment of physical growth is the way to assess nutritional status.

- Height, weight and head circumference charts for children provide standards for "normal" values. For children, height and weight are recorded as percentiles, according to sex to determine the growth curve. Children under 24 or 36 months (depending on reference) should be measured recumbent (lying flat); those over three years are measured standing up to determine height. Actual measurements are plotted at various stages of development and the growth rate is evaluated and compared to percentages of other children of the same age and sex.

- The American Society of Pediatrics states that newborns should be fed whenever they show signs of hunger. Formula-fed newborns usually take 2-3 ounces at a feeding.

- Avoid giving foods that can cause choking (e.g., raisins, small pieces of hot dog, grapes, nuts or hard candy). Do not give honey, which can carry botulism spores. Use care in heating baby foods by microwave. Microwave ovens heat food unevenly and some babies have been severely burned.

Young children (toddler and preschool)

- Feeding problems can be avoided by offering a variety of acceptable, healthful foods and letting the child decide what to eat and how much to eat. Eating patterns of young children fluctuate greatly from day to day. Growth, over a period of time, is the best indicator of nutritional well-being. **FOOD "JAGS"** are common among younger children who want the same food repeatedly. Parents may give the preferred food, but should continue to offer a choice. Jags are not generally considered a nutritional threat. Overweight children should not be put on very low-calorie, weight reduction diets. Some behavior modification techniques including increased activity may begin; activities may be increased until the height/weight ratio is in an acceptable range.

- The protein and calorie needs of young children are as follows:

  ➢ Age 1-3 years: The RDA for protein for males and females is 1.1g/kg/day (~13g/day)
  ➢ Age 4-8 years: Caloric needs increase to 90kcal/kg. The RDA for protein for males and females is 0.95g/kg/day. (~19g/day)

- Based on the 2002 National Academy of Sciences report on Dietary Reference Intakes (DRI) for Macronutrients, the Estimated Energy Requirements (EER) should be derived by the following formulas:

  EER for males and females ages 13 – 35 months: (89 x weight of child [kg] – 100 + 20 (kcal for Energy Deposition) EER for boys 3 – 8 years:
  88.5 – 61.9 x Age [y] + PA (physical activity) x (26.7 x Weight [kg] + 903 x height [m]) + 20 (kcal for Energy Deposition) EER for girls 3 – 8years:
  135.3 – 30.8 x Age [y] + PA x (10.0 x Weight [kg] + 934 x Height [m] + 20 (kcal for Energy Deposition)

- **Carbohydrate needs are:**
  ➢ Age 1-3 years: 130g/day (RDA)
  ➢ Age 4-8 years: 130g/day (RDA)

- **Total fiber needs are:**
  - ➢ Age 1-3 years: 19g/day (AI)
  - ➢ Age 4-8 years: 25g/day (AI)

- **There is no recommendation for fat.**
- **Linoleic acid needs are:**
  - ➢ Age 1-3 years: 7g/day (AI)
  - ➢ Age 4-8 years: 10g/day (AI)

- **α-Linolenic acid requirements are:**
  - ➢ Age 1-3 years: 0.7g/day (AI)
  - ➢ Age 4-8 years: 0.9g/day (AI)

- The rapid rate of growth during infancy is followed by deceleration in the preschool and school years. Weight gain approximates 4-6 lbs/year. Length increases about 3 inches per year to age 7 and then 2 inches per year until the puberty growth spurt.

- Brain growth is about 75% complete by the end of the second year. By 6-10 years, brain growth is complete. Progressive growth is influenced by genetics, nutritional and health status, as well as foods consumed.

- During preschool years there is a decrease in the intake of calcium, phosphorous, riboflavin, iron and vitamin A because of discontinuation of iron-fortified infant cereals, a reduction of milk intake and a disinterest in vegetables. Between ages 3 and 8 there is usually an increase in intake of all nutrients.

- To support a child's efforts at self-feeding, offer simple, unmixed dishes, foods at room temperature, finger foods, colorful foods and small portions.

- Recent studies show a dramatic rise in the incidence of childhood obesity. Children should be monitored carefully for adequate nutrient intake and normal weight gain before adolescence, if possible. Many parents who fear obesity for their children restrict the diet severely, eliminating too many calories and fat. Because diet restriction can hinder growth, it is best to reduce the rate of weight gain or to maintain weight as the child continues to gain in height and to stress physical exercise. (For further information, see *Position of the Academy of Nutrition and Dietetics: Nutrition Guidance for Healthy Children Ages 2 to 11 years, J Am Diet Assoc. 2008; 108:1038-1047.*)

School-age children

- In children, 9-13 years, there is a decline in the food requirement per unit of body weight. Protein requirements are 0.95g/kg body weight for both males and females—about 34 grams/day (RDA)

  - ➢ Based on the 2002 National Academy of Sciences report on Dietary Reference Intakes (DRI) for Macronutrients, the Estimated Energy Requirements (EER) should be derived by the following formulas:
  EER for boys 9 – 18 years:
  88.5 – 61.9 x Age [y] + PA x (26.7 x Weight [kg] + 903 x Height [m]) + 25 (kcal/day for Energy Deposition)

EER for girls 9 – 18 years:
135.3 – 30.8 x Age [y] + PA x (10.0 x Weight [kg] +934 x Height [m]) +25 (kcal for Energy Deposition)

- **Carbohydrate needs are:**
  - Males and females aged 9-13 years 130g/day (RDA)

- **Total fiber needs for ages 9-13 are:**
  - Males-31g/day (AI); Females - 26g/Day (AI)

- **Linoleic acid needs for ages 9-13 are:**
  - Males-12g/day (AI); Females - 10g/day (AI)

- **α Linolenic acid for ages 9-13 are:**
  - Males - 1.2g/day (AI);
  - Females: 1.0g/day (AI)

- There is no recommendation for total fat for this age group.

- School-age children generally have a rather consistent but slow growth rate. They are gaining in fine and gross motor skills and developing social skills.

- Peers increasingly affect food choices and feeding programs at school contribute to food intake. This is the time to support active daily physical activity patterns.

- Snacks provide about 1/3 of average daily energy. Breakfast should be encouraged because those who eat breakfast have better school records than those children who skip breakfast do.

- The extent to which food, particularly artificial color, flavor additives and sugar, affects behavior remains controversial. Research has found that relatively few children respond negatively to additives when double-blind tests are used. Definite evidence that sugar causes behavioral problems in children has not been found. However, the 2002 Dietary Reference Intake Report recommends that "added sugars should comprise no more than 25% of total calories consumed."

- Children with family history of hyperlipidemia or heart attacks should be tested for serum cholesterol. Children's total cholesterol should be less than 170mg/dL or dietary interventions should be initiated.

Adolescence

- Adolescence is a period of rapid growth and physiological development, but individuals grow and mature at different rates. Calcium, iron and vitamin A are the nutrients most lacking in this age group, especially in girls. Menstrual iron losses for girls and increase of muscle mass in boys account for the increase in iron needs. Dieting is contraindicated during periods of growth.

- Caloric needs during adolescence are described previously in Domain I. The RDA for protein for males 14-18 years is: 52g/day and for females age 14-18 years is 46g/day.

- Carbohydrate needs for all males from age 14 through 70 and non-pregnant, non-lactating females age 14 through 70 is 130g/day. (RDA) Needs for pregnant women are 175g/day and for lactating women 210g/day.

- Total fiber needs for males age 14-50 are 38g/day (AI) and females age 14-18 are 26g/day. For pregnant females, the AI is 28g/day and for lactating women age 14-50 the AI is 29g/day.

- Eating habits are influenced by peer pressure, body image and a desire for independence from parents. Common problems include crash diets, unusual food habits, missed meals and eating disorders. Diets affect growth, physical performance and future risks for chronic diseases.

- All mineral intake requirements increase during adolescence, especially during the adolescent growth spurt. During this time, needs for calcium, iron, zinc, magnesium and protein are high. Low intakes are often due to food choices, overuse of convenience and fast foods and sugar-containing snacks. Soft-drink consumption contributes to low-calcium intakes and the caffeine in many soft drinks further increases calcium excretion.

- Iron requirements increase significantly for adolescents of both sexes and teens of all races and socioeconomic levels. Iron needs increase for females as soon as they begin to menstruate, regardless of their age. Requirements increase for males when lean body mass develops. In early adulthood, requirements decrease for males, but remain high for females until they stop menstruating.

- Teenagers are vulnerable to nutrition misinformation and unsafe practices and are greatly influenced by media and friends. Many take ergonomic aids, try very restricted diets, take supplements inappropriately, have excessive alcohol intakes, or other harmful practices.

- **ANOREXIA NERVOSA** and **BULIMIA NERVOSA** are eating disorders common among teen and college-aged females.

Adults

- The primary goals of adult nutrition are the promotion of good health and the prevention of disease. A healthy lifestyle will delay development of chronic disease in adults. Components of a healthy diet include attention to risk factors of excess fat, cholesterol, sodium and body fat; regular physical exercise; stress management; smoking cessation and avoidance of alcohol abuse.

- The **BASAL METABOLIC RATE (BMR)** declines 2% each decade after early adulthood. Body composition changes account for some decline in the BMR, because the percentage of lean body tissue decreases.

- Most nutrient needs, other than energy, remain the same. Iron needs for women decrease after menopause.

- Exercise and activity level are key for weight maintenance throughout life. New weight charts reflect that some weight gain after the age of 35 may be normal and without medical risk.

- During middle and older adulthood, there is gradual cell loss and a reduced rate of cell metabolism, reducing organ performance (e.g., nephrons lost from kidneys), diminishing secretion of digestive juices, decreasing motility of the GI tract, decreasing absorption and utilization of nutrients and decreasing senses of smell and taste.

- Coronary heart disease, diabetes mellitus, hypertension and other diseases common in adults are described in Domain II.

- For adult women, breast cancer and osteoporosis are health concerns with nutritional influences. There is a strong genetic role in the development of both breast cancer and osteoporosis. One in 10 American women will get breast cancer. Prevention of breast cancer may be aided by a low-fat, high-fiber diet. Maintenance of a diet adequate in calcium throughout life reduces risk of osteoporosis, especially when combined with physical activity and control of hormone status.

Pregnancy and lactation

Weight gain

- Adequate weight gain during pregnancy promotes healthy infants. Mothers who gain inadequate weight (generally less than 15 pounds) have a greater incidence of **LOW BIRTH WEIGHT BABIES (LBW)**, babies that weigh less than 5.5 pounds. LBW babies have higher rates of infant mortality and are more likely to have physical handicaps, lower IQs, visual and hearing problems and behavioral disorders.

- Maternal age and pre-pregnancy weight is an important factor. Desired weight gain for most normal-weight healthy women is 25-35 pounds (11-16kg). Underweight women should gain more than normal-weight women should gain (28-40 pounds). Overweight women should attempt to gain 15-25 pounds. Young teens should aim for the higher end of each weight range. Even obese women should gain a minimum of 15 pounds. The target weight gain for a woman carrying twins is 35-45 pounds, and for triplets 50-60 pounds.

- Generally, a pregnant woman should follow these guidelines from the Institute of Medicine (2009), for weight gain:

RECOMMENDED WEIGHT GAIN FOR PREGNANT WOMEN

BMI	Recommended gain	Gain/week after 12 weeks
BMI < 18.5	12.7 – 18.2kg (28 -40 lb)	0.5kg (~ 1 lb)
BMI 18.5 – 24.90	11.4 – 15.9kg (25 – 35 lb)	0.4kg
BMI > 25.0 – 29.9	6.8 – 11.4kg (15 – 25 lb)	0.3kg
BMI > 30.0	5.0 -6.8kg (11-15 lb)	
Other		
Twin pregnancy	15.9 – 20.4kg (35 – 45 lb)	0.7kg
Triplet pregnancy	Overall gain of 22.7kg (50 lb)	

- Weight gain should be gradual and progressive throughout pregnancy. Sudden weight gains are caused by excess fluid retention and require treatment, but mild, generalized edema is clinically normal.

- The blood sugar of pregnant women is usually tested for diabetes in the 22-24 week of pregnancy. Women with gestational diabetes require careful monitoring to reduce maternal and fetal complications and excessive weight gain.

Nutrient needs

- The percentage of absorption of some nutrients, especially calcium and iron, is increased during pregnancy. The digestive process is slowed to allow for increased absorption of nutrients. Excess vitamin and mineral intake during pregnancy can harm the fetus. All supplements should be medically prescribed. There are two RDA levels for lactation, reflecting differences in the amount of milk produced in the first and second six months of lactation.

- Energy: The Estimated Energy Requirements (EER) for pregnancy should be derived by the following formulas:

  14 – 18 years:
  1st trimester = Adolescent EER + 0
  2nd trimester = Adolescent EER + 160kcal (8kcal/wk x 20 weeks) + 180kcal
  3rd trimester = Adolescent EER + 272kcal (8kcal/wk x 34 weeks) + 180kcal

  19 – 50 years:
  1st trimester = Adult EER + 0
  2nd trimester = Adult EER + 160kcal (8cal/wk x 20 weeks) + 180kcal
  3rd trimester = Adult EER + 272kcal (8cal/wk x 34 weeks) + 180kcal

  The EER for lactation: 14-18 years:
  1st six months = Adolescent EER + 500-170
  2nd six months = Adolescent EER + 400 – 0

  19 – 50 years:
  1st six months = Adult EER + 500 -170
  2nd six months = Adult EER + 400 – 0

- Protein: The RDA for pregnancy is 1.1g/kg/day or ~71g/day for all age groups. The RDA for lactation is the same as for pregnancy for all age groups. Extra energy-dense foods will help conserve protein for pregnant vegetarian women.

- Vitamins: The RDA for vitamin A during pregnancy is 750mcg/day for women under age 19 and 770mcg/day for women over age 19, with a UL of 2,800 and 3,000 respectively. The RDA for Vitamin A during lactation is 1,200mcg/day for women under age 19 and 1,300mcg/day for women over age 19. This is recommended to maintain maternal liver reserves, to account for variations in milk volume and to provide a margin of safety. The UL is the same as for pregnancy. Need for folate increases to 600mcg. in pregnancy and 500mcg during lactation. The UL for pregnancy and lactation is 800mcg/day for women under age 19 and 1,000mcg/day for women over age 19. Folate is essential for cell division and is included in prenatal supplements. Increasing fruits, vegetables and enriched grain products in the diet can also help meet needs.

- Minerals: AIs for calcium during pregnancy and lactation, call for 1000mg/day for women over age 19 and 1300mg/day for those under age 19. The UL is 2500mg/day for all age groups. Most fetal calcium is deposited during the third trimester when the baby's bone and teeth structures calcify. Pregnant women need iron to replace the usual iron turnover, to allow expansion of red blood cells in increased blood volume, to provide iron to the fetus and placenta and to replace blood lost during delivery. There is little need during the first trimester, because cessation of menstruation compensates for increased need; this is also true for non-menstruating lactating women. The RDA for iron for pregnant women of all ages is 27mg/day and cannot be met by diet. Therefore, the National Academy of Sciences and the American College of Obstetrics and Gynecology recommends a daily supplement of iron. To maintain fluid balance and increased blood volume, sodium should not be restricted during pregnancy unless there is a specific medical reason to do so. Diuretics upset fluid balance and sodium levels and may be harmful.

- Food avoidance, cravings and aversions are common in pregnancy. Data are limited and mostly anecdotal. **PICA** is a compulsive food behavior that is potentially dangerous. It is the persistent ingestion of non-food substances such as consumption of dirt, clay (**GEOPHAGIA**) or laundry starch (**AMYLOPHAGIA**). Consuming other food substances such as stones, cigarette ashes, mothballs, baking soda, coffee grounds and wall plaster have been reported. The practice of pica is not related to geographic area, race, culture or status within a culture. Some pica substances interfere with absorption of nutrients, others can cause lead poisoning, obstruction, anemia or infection.

- **FETAL ALCOHOL SYNDROME (FAS)** occurs when a woman consumes excessive alcohol during pregnancy (3 or more drinks/day or excessive binge-drinking.) The result is abnormal fetal development. Infants are born with anomalies of the eyes, nose, heart and central nervous system. Physical growth and mental development may be retarded. These anomalies become permanent disabilities and there is high postnatal mortality among infants with FAS. **FETAL ALCOHOL EFFECTS (FAE)** is a result of moderate intake of alcohol during pregnancy leading to the birth of a baby with more subtle features of FAS. Children are born with cognitive and behavioral problems that continue throughout life. There is no evidence that one drink, or an occasional alcoholic beverage causes FAS or FAE.

Aging adults

- Chronological age is a poor measure of physical health and mental alertness.

- The United States Census reports older people as:
  - Those aged 65-74 as the young-old; those aged 75-84 as the aged; and those aged 85 and older as the oldest-old.
  - All groups are quite diverse, but those who are the oldest are most likely to have serious health problems and require assistance with tasks in their daily living.

- Leading causes of death in the United State are heart disease, cancer and stroke. All are related to degenerative changes associated with aging and personal lifestyle.

- Maintaining adequate calcium throughout life builds bone strength and minimizes chances of broken hip or other bones from falls that are common among the aged.

Physical changes in aging adults

- In most individuals, aging causes a gradual decrease in physiologic functions including:

  - Decreased tolerance to fats, decreased sensory acuity, and/or depressed appetite may occur.
  - Dental problems or poorly fitting dentures require correction to eliminate reliance on soft foods.
  - Changes in cardiovascular function reduce cardiac output and a decline of kidney function.
  - Lactose intolerance may develop. Small amounts of milk or cooked or fermented milk may be tolerated. Lactase (or Lactaid®) may be added to fluid milk. Lactose-reduced milk is also available.
  - Decreased carbohydrate tolerance raises the risk of diabetes. Regular exercise may improve cell response to insulin and offset this.
  - Slowed peristalsis, decreased HCl production in the stomach, loss of digestive enzymes and atrophic gastritis may interfere with absorption of iron, calcium and vitamin B_{12} and cause gastrointestinal upsets.
  - Immobility may cause constipation and contribute to the development of decubitus ulcers (skin ulcers), obesity and osteoporosis.
  - There is an increased need for modified diets for high blood pressure and other problems prevalent in aging.
  - Use of multiple medications can cause nutrition problems.
  - Nutrients of concern include vitamins D and C and calcium. Intakes of folate, pyridoxine, zinc and vitamin B_{12}, are typically low. There is some evidence that the elderly have altered nutrient requirements (in part because of impaired absorption), but there is little evidence that intake above the RDA is necessary or will prevent changes associated with aging. DRIs have been established for males and females in age categories 51-70 and above 70.

Mental changes

- Brain cells are lost with advancing age and there may be decreased blood flow to the brain from atherosclerotic change. There are likely to be fewer neurotransmitters. Parkinson's disease and Alzheimer's disease become more common.

- Memory loss and decreased attention span may make diet instruction or obtaining a diet history difficult. Short, frequent counseling sessions, supplemented with handouts, should be scheduled.

Social changes

- Economic limitations and isolation may decrease food intake. Participation in community programs (e.g. Supplemental Nutrition Assistance Program, Meals-on-Wheels and congregate feeding programs) should be encouraged to maintain social contacts and support systems. Most elders prefer to remain in their homes and every attempt should be made to foster and encourage independent living with support appropriate to meet individual needs.

c. Herbals, botanicals and supplements

Herbals

- **HERBAL THERAPY (**also known as **HERBALISM**), **HERBAL MEDICINE** or **PHYTOTHERAPY** is folk and traditional medicine, based on the use of plants and plant extracts.

  - ➢ Thousands of plants have been used as healing agents since earliest recorded history. The use of herbs and other plants to treat disease is almost universal in non-industrialized societies and plants yield useful medicinal compounds.
  - ➢ Chinese herbal medicine and Ayurvedic medicine from India use primarily herbal therapies.
  - ➢ Many commonly used pharmaceuticals used in Western medicine (opiates, aspirin, digitalis, quinine, etc.) are derived from plants and the phytochemicals derived from them are being evaluated for the treatment of diseases.
  - ➢ In Europe, botanicals have long been considered complements to conventional drugs.
  - ➢ **GERMAN COMMISSION E** has been evaluating herbal medicine for years and has published 400 monographs containing information on actions, side effects, dosage and cautions of various botanicals.
- As of 2004 the National Center for Complementary and Alternative Medicine began funding clinical trials into the effectiveness of herbal medicine because use of natural products is the most common use of complementary and alternative medicine. About 600 botanicals are sold in the U.S., but few have been carefully tested. For further information, refer to **http://nccam.nih.gov**

- Andrew Weil, MD and other physicians and medical facilities who advocate complementary care, promote and prescribe herbal remedies. Most Americans use herbal therapy including coffee, tea, ginger, garlic, herbs and other foods that contain biologically active compounds that have medicinal effects. More and more Americans are using complementary medications and seeking foods and botanical products to promote health.

Botanicals

- A **BOTANICAL** is a plant or plant part valued for its medicinal or therapeutic properties, flavor, and/or scent. Botanicals are sold in many forms such as fresh or dried products; liquids or solid extracts and tablets; capsules, powders and tea bags. Herbs are a subset of botanicals. Products made from botanicals that are used to maintain or improve health may be called herbal products, botanical products, or **PHYTOMEDICINES.**

- The safety of a botanical depends on its chemical makeup, how it works in the body, how it is prepared, and the dosage used. Preparation methods include infusions, such as tea, which is made by steeping fresh or dried botanicals in boiling water. Some roots, barks, or berries may need to be steeped in boiling water for longer periods of time to extract the desired ingredients. Tinctures, made by soaking the botanical in a solution of alcohol and water, are sold as liquids and are used to concentrate and preserve the botanical. For further information, see **http://ods.od.nih.gov**

- The actions of botanicals range from mild to potent. A botanical with mild action may have subtle effects.
  - Chamomile and peppermint, both mild botanicals, are usually taken as teas to aid digestion and are generally considered safe for self-administration.
  - Ginger relieves nausea and motion sickness.
  - Some mild botanicals may have to be taken for weeks or months before their full effects are achieved.
  - For example, valerian may be effective as a sleep aid after 14 days of use but it is rarely effective after a single dose. However, there is no information available about the long-term safety of valerian.
  - In contrast a powerful botanical produces a fast result. Kava, as an example, can have an immediate and powerful action affecting anxiety and muscle relaxation. However, in recent years, several countries have restricted the sale of kava-containing products based on hepatic adverse events and some documented hepatic toxicity.

- The dose and form of a botanical preparation also play important roles in its safety.
  - Teas, tinctures, oils and extracts have different strengths. The same amount of a botanical may be contained in a cup of tea, a few teaspoons of tincture, or an even smaller quantity of an extract.

- Also, different preparations vary in the relative amounts and concentrations of chemical removed from the whole botanical.
  - For example, peppermint tea is generally considered safe to drink but peppermint oil is much more concentrated and can be toxic if used incorrectly.
  - It is always important to follow the manufacturer's suggested directions for using a botanical and never exceed the recommended dose without the advice of a healthcare provider.

Health roles for herbs and plants

- **ALOE VERA** (Aloe ferox, A. barbadensis) - Taken internally, concentrated Aloe ferox resin is used as a strong laxative. Externally, the clear gel from the A. barbadensis leaf, is used to treat burns, abrasions, skin injuries and in cosmetic products. Early studies show that the topical aloe may help heal burns and abrasions, but does not prevent burns from radiation therapy. Diarrhea that is caused by the laxative effect of oral aloe vera can decrease the absorption of many drugs, including glucose-lowering medications and may also lower blood glucose levels. A juice made from the gel can be used as a drink. The green part of the leaf surrounding the gel can be used to produce a juice or a dried substance called latex that is taken by mouth. The strong laxative properties come from the latex. The FDA has approved aloe vera as a natural food flavoring.

- **ASTRAGALUS** (Astragalus membranaceous) - Used in traditional Chinese and East Indian medicine for its immune-enhancing and tonic properties. The root of the astragalus plant is typically used in soups, teas, extracts or capsules. Evidence for its use is limited. Results from small or preliminary studies suggest that it may benefit heart function and help the immune system fight infection. Possible side effects are not well known because it is usually used in combination with other herbs, such as ginseng, angelica and licorice. It may interact with medications that suppress the immune system, such as cyclophosphamide, which is taken by cancer patients and similar drugs taken by organ transplant recipients.

- **BILBERRY** (Vaccinium myrtillus) - A European version of blueberry. Historically, bilberry fruit was used to treat diarrhea, scurvy and other conditions. Bilberry leaf is used for entirely different conditions, including diabetes. Bilberry extract, rich in purple/blue pigments may be of benefit for some eye and other circulatory problems, diarrhea, menstrual cramps, varicose veins and venous insufficiency. The extract is also used to help increase microcirculation by stimulating new capillary formation, strengthening capillary walls. There is not enough scientific evidence to support the use of Bilberry fruit or leaf for any health conditions. High doses may be toxic.

- **CASCARA SAGRAND** (Rhamnus purshiana) - The bark is used as a stimulant laxative, especially in cases of chronic constipation. As an approved safe and effective laxative, cascara is found in some over-the-counter laxative preparations. It should not be used within two hours before or after taking other medicines.

- **CAPSICUM** (Cayenne, hot pepper, capsicum species) - Internally, cayenne acts as a circulatory stimulant, induces perspiration and is used to stimulate digestion. It should be used with caution if a person has an upset stomach, stomach ulcers, irritable bowel problems, kidney disease or if one is taking medication for high blood pressure, blood thinning seizures, migraine headaches, sedation or muscle relaxation. Several products for external use in arthritic and rheumatoid conditions contain capsaicin as the active pain-relieving ingredient. Topical capsaicin preparations are also used for the relief of pain associated with herpes zoster ("shingles").

- **CHAMOMILE** (Matricaria recutita) - There are two types of chamomile used for health conditions, Roman chamomile and German chamomile. The two are thought to have similar effects on the body and the German variety is more commonly used in the U.S. Chamomile flowers are antispasmodic and are used to make teas, liquid extracts, capsules or tablets. A popular remedy for indigestion, flatulence, gastrointestinal spasms and inflammation of the gastrointestinal tract, it is often used as a bedtime beverage, because of its mild sedative effects. However, it has not been well studied in people and there is, at this time, little evidence to support its use for any condition. Externally, chamomile creams or ointment are used for inflammation of skin and extracts are used as a mouth rinse. There are reports of rare allergic reactions in people who have eaten or come in contact with chamomile products.

- **CRANBERRY** (Vaccinium macrocarpon) - Recently, cranberry products have been used to prevent or treat urinary tract infections or *H pylori* infections that can lead to stomach ulcers, or to prevent dental plaque. It has also been thought to have antioxidant and anticancer activity. Some studies testing cranberries for their ability to prevent urinary tract infection have shown promise, but the results are not yet considered to be conclusive. Studies for other uses are being funded, but no conclusions may be drawn at this time.

- **DANDELION** (Taraxacum officina/e) - Dandelion greens are edible and are a rich source of Vitamin A. The leaves and roots are used fresh or dried in teas, capsules or extracts. Dandelion leaves are used in salads or as cooked greens and the flowers are used to make wine. It is used by some people as a liver or kidney "tonic", as a diuretic and for minor digestive problems. At this time, there is no compelling evidence for its use for any medical condition. There are rare reports of upset stomach and diarrhea and some allergic reactions. Persons with inflamed or infected gallbladder or blocked bile ducts should not use dandelion.

- **DONG QUAI** also spelled Tang kwei or Danggui (Angelica sinensis) - One of the most widely used herbs in traditional Chinese medicine, it is primarily used in herbal formulas as a "female tonic" to treat muscle cramps and pain associated with difficult menstrual periods. Dong quai should not be used with warfarin, aspirin, and during pregnancy and lactation.

- **ECHINACEA** (Echinacea purpurea and related species) - Also called purple coneflower and native to the U. S., this plant was the most widely used medicinal plant of the Central Plains Indians, being used for a variety of conditions. For upper respiratory infections, many trials on humans have found Echinacea to reduce duration and severity, especially when treatment was initiated early. Research conducted in the US is inconclusive and more studies have been funded.

- **ELEUTHERO** (Siberian ginseng) (Eleutherococcus senticosus) - This distant relative of true ginsengs grows in Siberia, Manchuria, China and Northern Japan and is not considered true ginseng. Used as a general tonic and to reduce physical and mental stress. In Germany, Siberian Ginseng is approved as a tonic to invigorate and fortify the body during fatigue or weakness and to increase work and concentration as well as for patient rehabilitation.

- **EPHEDRA** is a naturally occurring substance that comes from botanicals. The principal active ingredient ephedrine is an amphetamine-like compound that can powerfully stimulate the nervous system and heart. Ephedrine alkaloids are found naturally in a number of plants, including the Ephedra species (also known as ma huang, Chinese Ephedra or epitonin). Ephedra products were marketed as dietary supplements to promote weight loss, increase energy and enhance athletic performance. The FDA, in 2004, banned the sale of dietary supplements containing ephedrine alkaloids because they found that these supplements present an unreasonable risk of illness or injury to consumers. They confirmed that Ephedra was effective for short-term weight loss but that since it raises blood pressure and stresses the heart, there is an increased risk of heart problems and stroke, which negates any benefits of the weight loss and that there is no evidence that these products enhance athletic performance. The rule does not apply to traditional Chinese herbal remedies or herbal teas that are regulated as conventional foods. It also does not apply to products regulated as drugs containing chemically synthesized ephedrine, used for asthma, bronchitis and allergic reactions.

- **EVENING PRIMROSE OIL** (Oenothera biennis) - Evening primrose oil (EPO) is a relatively recent herbal remedy, having been marketed since the 1930s for eczema and other conditions involving inflammation, such as rheumatoid arthritis. More recently, it has been used for conditions affecting women's health, such as breast pain associated with the menstrual cycle, menopausal symptoms and premenstrual syndrome. Some recommend its use for diabetes and cancer. Evening primrose oil may have modest benefits for eczema and may be useful for rheumatoid arthritis and breast pain, but study results are not definitive at this time.

- **FEVERFEW** (Tanacetum parthenium) - Feverfew has been used as a folk medicine for menstrual cramps since Greco-Roman times. At least three published clinical studies in England in the 1980s confirm the efficacy of feverfew leaves for prevention and moderation of the severity of migraine headaches. The dried leaves and sometimes the flowers and stems are used to make supplements in the form of capsules, tablets and liquid extracts. It appears to be safe for short-term use. Long term safety is not known. Feverfew can cause allergic reactions in people who are allergic to the daisy family. Other side effects include diarrhea and other stomach upsets, may cause mouth irritation and sores in those who chew fresh leaves of the plant. It may also interact with some medications. Some research suggests that feverfew may help to prevent migraine headaches, but results are mixed. There have been few published studies regarding its ability to reduce rheumatoid arthritis symptoms.

- **GARLIC** (Allium sativum) - Garlic may mildly display a host of benefits but current research in the U.S. is inconclusive. Research in the U. S. has been focused on its effect on certain types of cancer prevention and decrease in total cholesterol and blood pressure. Garlic is used in Europe as an approved remedy for cardiovascular conditions, especially high cholesterol and triglyceride levels associated with risk of atherosclerosis. Some believe it is a preventative measure for colds, flu and other infectious diseases. It should not be taken in large amounts by those on anticoagulant therapy and specific HIV medications.

- **GINGER** (Zingiber officina/e) - Ginger is a plant used as a food, beverage, spice or medicine. It has been used to treat nausea, motion sickness and vomiting. Ginger has a long history of use for all types of digestive upset and can be helpful to increase appetite.

- **GINKGO** (Ginkgo biloba) - A standardized extract of ginkgo leaf increases circulation and has shown antioxidant activity. Many European studies have confirmed the use of standardized ginkgo leaf extract for a wide variety of conditions associated with aging, including memory loss and poor circulation. Ginkgo extract is also used clinically in Europe for tinnitus (ringing in the ears), vertigo and cold extremities. A recent study found it to be ineffective in lowering the overall incidence of cognitive decline, dementia and Alzheimer's disease in the elderly. Research is still being conducted in the United States with Ginkgo and other symptoms and diseases. There are some data suggesting that there may be some serious side effects such as increased bleeding risk, so people who take anticoagulant drugs, have bleeding disorders or have scheduled surgery or dental procedures should use caution. Uncooked ginkgo seeds may cause seizures and, if consumed in large quantities, may cause death. Gingko leaf and leaf extracts do not seem to have the same effect.

- **ASIAN GINSENG** (Panax ginseng) - One of the world's most famous herbs. Ginseng is classed as an "adaptogen", a relatively recent term coined by Russian researchers to describe ginseng's general tonic properties. **ADAPTOGENS** are herbs that increase the overall resistance to all types of stress. Other herbal adaptogens include astragalus, Siberian ginseng and schizandra. Asian ginseng (Chinese and Korean) is thought to increase energy and endurance. Some studies have shown that Asian Ginseng may lower blood glucose. Other studies have indicated possible beneficial effects on immune function. At this time, all studies are inconclusive. People with diabetes should use caution in taking this because Asian ginseng may lower blood sugar levels and if medicines are used to lower blood sugar, there may be a large drop in blood sugar levels.

- **GOLDENSEAL** (Hydrastis canadensis) - Goldenseal root is a Native American herb used by Indians and early settlers for its antiseptic wound healing properties. It is also used for its soothing action on inflamed mucous membranes. It is a popular remedy for colds and flu, often used in combination with echinachea. At this time, few studies have been published regarding goldenseal's safety and effectiveness and there is little scientific evidence to support its use for any health problems.

- **HAWTHORN** (Crataegus oxyacantha) - Hawthorn has a long reputation in both folk medicine and clinical medicine as a heart tonic. In Europe, hawthorn berry preparations are widely used by physicians in treating heart conditions, such as mild forms of angina. It has also been used for digestive and kidney problems. More recently Hawthorn leaf and flower have been used for heart failure, for which there is scientific evidence of safety and efficacy. There is insufficient evidence of efficacy for other heart problems. The leaf and flower are also used to make extracts, usually with water and alcohol and dry extracts are put into capsules and tablets.

- **LICORICE (**Glycyrrhila glabra and G. uralensis) - Licorice is one of the most widely used medicinal plants in the world, in several traditional medicine systems. It is soothing to inflamed mucous membranes; often in gastric and duodenal ulcers and cough and asthma remedies. Licorice extract displays a stimulating action on adrenal glands. Licorice and its extracts are safe for normal use in moderate amounts. However, long-term use or ingestion of excessive amounts can produce headache, lethargy, sodium and water retention, excessive loss of potassium and high blood pressure.

- **MILK THISTLE** (Silybum marianum) - Milk thistle is used in European folk medicine as a liver tonic. Silymarin from milk thistle is believed to have a protective effect on the liver and to improve its function. It is typically used to treat liver cirrhosis, chronic hepatitis and gallbladder disorders. Other claims for effectiveness include lowering cholesterol levels, reducing insulin resistance in people with type 2 diabetes who also have cirrhosis and reducing the growth of cancer cells in breast, cervical and prostate cancers. At this time, research in the U.S. is ongoing for the use of the role of milk thistle for chronic hepatitis C and other types of liver disorders. It is also being studied for cancer prevention and to treat complications in HIV.

- **PASSION FLOWER** (Passif/ora incarnata) - Contrary to the implications of its name, it has mild sedative and calmative properties. Taken internally, passion flower is usually combined with other sedative herbs for various types of nervous conditions, including insomnia and related disorders.

- **PEPPERMINT** (Mentha piperita) - Internally, peppermint is an antispasmodic, with a calming effect on the stomach and intestinal tract. As a tea, extract or in a capsule, peppermint is useful for indigestion, cramp-like discomfort of the upper gastrointestinal and bile duct, irritable bowel syndrome and gum inflammation or irritation.

- **PSYLLIUM** (Plantago ovata and P. major) - Psyllium is a major source of fiber. The primary use of psyllium seed and/or psyllium seed husks is as a bulk laxative, especially for cases of chronic constipation. The tiny seeds contain a coating of gelatinous material, which swells upon contact with moisture. This increases the movement (motility) within the colon thus producing a bowel movement. Psyllium husk is an approved over-the-counter laxative.

- **SAW PALMETTO** (Sabal, Serenoa repens, Sabal serrulata) - Saw palmetto extract is a popular remedy for enlarged prostate (benign prostatic hypertrophy-BPH), a condition common in men over 50 years of age. Saw palmetto should be taken only after a physician properly diagnoses disease. Some clinical studies indicate that the extract can increase urine flow and reduce frequency of nighttime urination.

- **SENNA** (Cassia senna) - Both senna leaves and pods (fruits) were used in ancient Arab medicine as safe and effective laxative. Today, senna is one of the most popular, safe and reliable stimulant laxatives. As with all stimulant laxatives, long-term dependence may develop, so only short-term use is recommended.

- **VALERIAN** (Valeriana officinalis) - Valerian has long been used for sleep disorders and anxiety. The roots and rhizomes of the plant are usually used to make the supplements including capsules, tablets, liquid extracts and tea. Research suggests it may be helpful for insomnia, but research has not yet confirmed it. There is not enough scientific evidence at this time to determine if valerian is effective for anxiety, depression or headaches. Valerian is generally safe to use for short periods of time. No information is available about long-term safety.

- **VITEX** (Chaste Tree) (Vitex agnus-castus) - The small fruits of the Mediterranean tree have been used by women, for menstrual disorders since Greco-Roman times. Extract of vitex is a plant preparation, which adjusts the monthly menstruation cycle on a natural basis and causes premenstrual discomforts to subside. An extract of vitex is approved in Germany for menstrual disorders, PMS and painful breasts.

- **WITCH HAZEL** (Hamamelis virginiana) - The astringency of the leaves and bark makes witch hazel a popular ingredient for various skin conditions as well as for bruises and varicose veins. It is approved for use in hemorrhoid products. For additional information see **http://nccam.nih.gov.**

Dietary supplements

- **DIETARY SUPPLEMENTS** are products intended to supplement the diet. They contain a vitamin, mineral, herb, botanical or amino acid. They may also contain a concentrate, metabolite, constituent or extract of these ingredients. They must be labeled as dietary supplements and cannot be represented as a conventional food or as a sole item of a meal or diet.

- Dietary supplements come in many forms such as tablets, capsules, gel caps, powders and liquids. While multivitamin and multimineral supplements are generally safe, high-potency supplements have much more than the daily need and may be harmful to the kidney, liver, nerves, etc. Current laws do not limit potency except for folacin.

- In 1994 federal legislation, the **DIETARY SUPPLEMENT HEALTH AND EDUCATION ACT (DSHEA)**, passed removing "dietary supplements" from FDA control. Manufacturers can now suggest benefits on their packages and in ads, without any proof of safety or efficacy, but cannot make direct medical claims. FDA cannot require testing of supplements prior to marketing. FDA can only take action if a product is unsafe or mislabeled.

- Supplements are labeled as to potency, although testing shows that many labels do not accurately reflect contents. DSHEA requires that manufacturers provide information that is factual and not misleading. The **UNITED STATES PHARMACOPEIA (USP) www.usp.org** is an independent nongovernmental organization that sets standards and monitors for quality and integrity. Products that meet those standards have a USP mark on their labels. They are also dated with an expiration date.

- In 2000, FDA published a rule that dietary supplements could carry structure/function claims but could not relate the claim to a disease state. Separate rules related to disease claims now apply.

- The **OFFICE OF DIETARY SUPPLEMENTS (ODS)** is responsible for coordinating research on dietary supplements at the National Institutes of Health. Get current information on supplements at their website: **www.ods.od.nih.gov**.

- Hundreds of supplements are available. The following are among the most commonly used.

COMMONLY USED SUPPLEMENTS		
Supplement	**Claims, Benefits**	**What to Know**
Bee pollen	Improves physical performance	Can cause severe allergic reactions. To be avoided by those with kidney disease or gout.
Beta carotene	Prevents cancer and heart disease and boosts immunity	Don't take if you're a smoker: studies suggest an increase in lung cancer risk for smokers taking these pills. Beta carotene is plentiful in vegetables and some fruits and is beneficial in this form. The 600 other carotenoids are also important for health and are found in yellow, red and deep green vegetables and fruits.
Blue green algae (spirulina)	"Purifies" blood; "cures" most diseases	Not a medicine or good source of nutrients. Benefits unproven.
Brewer's Yeast	Decrease constipation, cure diabetes, lower blood pressure, improve athletic performance	No evidence to support claims. Can cause diarrhea and nausea.
Calcium	Prevents or slows osteoporosis	Women over 50 (postmenopausal) and men over 65 may need supplements if they don't get 1,500 milligrams a day from food. Safe and effective. Should be taken at meals, and be combined with an exercise program. Calcium should also come from dietary sources, such as low-fat or fat-free milk and many leafy greens.
Chaparral	Anti-cancer activity; "purifies" blood; arthritis remedy	Unsafe for human consumption. No proven medical value. Linked to liver disease and acute poisoning.
Chromium picolinate	Builds muscle, prevents and cures diabetes, promotes weight loss	Chromium is an essential mineral, but deficiency is rare in the US. No evidence that chromium picolinate supplements perform as claimed, promote weight loss, or benefit healthy people. Some evidence that they may harm cells. Diabetics should take only on medical advice.
Coenzyme Q-10	Cure-all; prevents heart disease; increases immune response	An interesting antioxidant; may be effective against heart failure. Animal studies show it helps immune system. Expensive. Benefits for healthy people unproven.
Creatine (and other amino acids)	Improves athletic performance	Amino acid manufactured in the body. Some studies show short-term boost for muscle strength for young, highly trained subjects. Meaningless for casual exercisers.
DHEA	Slows aging, prevents chronic diseases, cures some cancers	Human hormone. May have powerful positive or negative effects-research ongoing. What is sold in the health-food stores may not be DHEA.

COMMONLY USED SUPPLEMENTS, cont.

Folic acid	Reduces plasma homocysteine levels. Prevents certain birth defects, heart disease, possibly some cancers	Solid evidence for these claims. All women capable of becoming pregnant should get 400 micrograms of folic acid a day from a supplement, in addition to what they get from food. Other people not eating a good diet (fruits, vegetables, fortified grains and cereals) should also consider taking a multivitamin containing folic acid.
Garlic pills	Lower blood pressure and blood cholesterol, prevent stomach cancer	No clear evidence that garlic pills are beneficial. No one knows which element in garlic is beneficial. Eat garlic, it can't hurt, might help. Pills should not be taken with blood pressure medication.
Ginseng	Improves athletic performance, fights fatigue, cures cancer and heart disease, lowers blood sugar, aphrodisiac	Little solid evidence that ginseng does anything, though it has been used for thousands of years as a cure-all and energizer. Ginseng plant contains many pharmacologically active elements, but they vary from one type to another. Can cause headaches, sleep and gastrointestinal disorders. Many products on the market contain no ginseng at all.
Glucosamine & chondroitin sulfate	Halt, reverse or cure arthritis	Probably harmless, but does not reverse arthritis. Test show it reduces joint pain for some people. Don't substitute for conventional treatment.
Lysine	Cures cold sores (herpes)	Some evidence that 1,000 to 3,000 milligrams daily might head off recurrences, but such high doses may be dangerous. Should not be taken over long periods. Prescription drugs are available and effective, but very expensive.
Melatonin	Promotes sleep, counters jet lag, improves sex life, etc.	A human hormone. Shows promise as sleeping pill. May have serious side effects. Research in progress.
Minerals, chelated	Better absorbed than other mineral supplements	These minerals are bonded to certain amino acids. They may be less well absorbed than others.
Minerals, colloidal	Cure-all, claim that is better absorbed	Probably no advantage. Get minerals from food instead or a standard multivitamin/mineral supplement.
Multivitamins /minerals	Compensate for a poor diet	No supplement can make up for a poor diet. But a daily multivitamin/mineral pill that does not exceed the daily need for any nutrient, is a good idea for the elderly, those with restricted diets or others who may have nutritional shortfalls. Also multivitamins tailored for women, elderly, children, etc.
Pycnogenol	Cure-all	Pine bark extract. No evidence of effectiveness against diseases.

COMMONLY USED SUPPLEMENTS, cont.		
Rose hips	More "natural" vitamin C source	Expensive source of vitamin C.
Sassafras	Performance booster, "blood purifier"	Contains safrole, an aromatic oil known to cause cancer in animals. Banned by FDA, as unsafe and ineffective.
St. John's wort	Alleviates depression	Preliminary evidence shows efficacy against mild forms of depression. Should not be taken as a diet drug or with prescription antidepressants.
Selenium	Prevents some cancers, possibly heart disease	Evidence is preliminary; food is best source (fish, grains). Very high doses are toxic.
Vitamin C	Prevents or cures colds; may help prevent cancer, heart disease, cataracts	This powerful antioxidant may protect against chronic diseases. Not a cold cure but can reduce symptoms. Get as much as possible from produce, which contains other beneficial substances. Take 250 to 500 milligrams daily as a supplement. Great excess may cause kidney stones. Abrupt discontinuance at high doses may cause rebound scurvy.
Vitamin E	May help prevent cancer, heart disease, cataracts	Another powerful antioxidant, but not plentiful in foods, except vegetable oils, nuts, and seeds. Take 200 to 800 IU daily as a supplement.
Zinc	Cures/shortens colds; relieves prostate symptoms; slows/prevents macular degeneration (eye condition that can cause blindness)	Not recommended for prostate problems. Evidence of effects against macular degeneration is weak.

2. Principles of physiology and biochemistry

a. Gastrointestinal

- **INGESTION** is the act of taking food into the body and swallowing it.

Physiology of ingestion

- In the mouth, food is broken into small particles through **MASTICATION**, the process of biting and chewing with teeth and jaws. Incisor teeth cut, while molars grind. Mastication breaks food into small particles that are then exposed to enzymes. Fine particles ease swallowing and passage through the GI tract. The soft mass of chewed food swallowed at one time is call the **BOLUS**.

- The bolus is swallowed and passed down the esophagus through rhythmic **PERISTALTIC WAVES** controlled by nerve impulses. Eating in a sitting position facilitates this process because gravity helps move the food downward. At the entrance to the stomach, the **GASTROESOPHAGEAL-CONSTRICTOR MUSCLE** relaxes to allow food to enter. This muscle then constricts to keep the food from being regurgitated.

Pathophysiology of ingestion

- Conditions that interfere with mastication or swallowing include a broken jaw, missing teeth, periodontal disease, ulcers in the mouth, poorly fitted dentures, dental caries, surgery or radiation therapy to head or neck and sensitivity to hot or cold.

- **DYSPHAGIA** is difficulty in swallowing. It may be physical or psychological.

- **ACHALASIA** is a dysfunction of the esophagus. There are two clinical conditions: **CARDIO SPASM,** caused by a malfunctioning cardiac-sphincter muscle and **HIATAL HERNIA,** a protrusion of the upper stomach into the thorax. Achalasia is dangerous because the person may aspirate food in the esophagus into the lung, leading to serious infection. Persons with achalasia can tolerate only small servings of liquids or semi-liquids. Tube feedings or parenteral feeding may be required to prevent malnutrition.

- **REFLUX ESOPHAGITIS** is an irritation in the lower esophagus caused by stomach acids that come up to the esophagus when the cardiac sphincter does not close tightly.

b. Digestion

- **DIGESTION** is the process by which complex foods are broken down chemically into their simpler parts in the gastrointestinal tract.

Physiology

- The digestive system consists of the **GASTROINTESTINAL TRACT (GI TRACT)** or **ALIMENTARY CANAL.** The GI tract is a flexible, muscular tube about 26 feet long that goes from the mouth past the epiglottis to the esophagus, through the cardiac sphincter to the stomach, through the pylorus to the small intestine (the duodenum, with entrance from the gallbladder and pancreas, then the jejunum; then the ileum), through the ileocecal valve to the large intestine, past the appendix to the rectum and ending at the anus.

Biochemistry

- As the bolus passes along the tract, glands and organs secrete materials (enzymes, hydrochloric acid and buffer ions) into the tract that promote the breakdown of the food. Water and electrolytes produce the necessary chemical medium and circulate organic substances. Throughout digestion, chemical processes occur at different pH levels. The stomach normally remains at pH 1.5-1.7 and hormones start and stop the production of hydrochloric acid (HCl). **CHYME** is the semifluid, gruel-like material produced by gastric digestion of food. Intestinal contents are slightly alkaline because the pancreas adds bicarbonate. Fat digestion takes longer than carbohydrate digestion and therefore fat provides satiety for a longer period of time, but carbohydrate is used more quickly for energy.

Pathophysiology

- **DYSPEPSIA,** also called **INDIGESTION,** is a vague abdominal discomfort in the GI tract, primarily the stomach. Indigestion is a symptom, not a disease, and is aggravated by tension, eating too much or eating too fast.

- **NAUSEA** is the queasy feeling before vomiting and can be triggered by odors, sights or motions. It often accompanies pregnancy and also can be a side effect of medications. If vomiting is prolonged, fluids and electrolytes must be replaced.

- An inflammation of the stomach, **GASTRITIS,** is characterized by anorexia, nausea, vomiting, belching, feeling of fullness and pain just above the stomach. Aspirin or other drugs, alcohol abuse, food irritants, allergies, food poisoning, stress, infections and radiation can cause gastritis. Eliminating the irritant and/or instituting a liquid or bland diet treat gastritis.

- **FLATULENCE** is an expulsion of gas through the mouth and rectum, usually after eating certain foods. Bacteria in the gut can produce **METHANE** gas. Poor carbohydrate digestion (e.g., lactose intolerance) may cause flatulence. Some foods that may cause gas include legumes, apples, beans, Brussels sprouts, cabbage, flax seeds, citrus fruits, melon, milk products, onions, potatoes, prune juice, raisins, wheat germ and uncooked starches.

OVERVIEW OF DIGESTION AND ABSORPTION

MOUTH AND ESOPHAGUS

Carbohydrate The salivary glands secrete a watery fluid into the mouth to moisten the food. The salivary amylase enzyme begins digestion:

Salivary amylase (ptyalin)
Starch ✂ Smaller amylase polysaccharides and/or starch maltose

This action continues in the esophagus.

Fiber The mechanical action of the mouth crushes and tears fiber in food and mixes it with saliva to moisten it for swallowing. There are no changes in the esophagus.

Fat Glands in the base of the tongue secrete a lipase known as *lingual lipase*. Some hard fats begin to melt as they reach body temperature. There are no changes in the esophagus.

Vitamins No action on vitamins occurs in the mouth or the esophagus.

Minerals/Water The salivary glands add water to disperse and carry food. There are no changes in the esophagus.

STOMACH

Carbohydrate Gastric secretions (hydrochloric acid, gastric lipase, mucus, intrinsic factor, and gastrin) are mixed with food and fluid and most of the food turns into a semi-liquid state (chyme.) To a small extent, stomach acid hydrolyzes maltose and sucrose:

HCl
Maltose ✂ Glucose + Glucose

HCl
Sucrose ✂ Glucose + Fructose

Fiber There are no changes in the stomach.

Protein Stomach acid uncoils protein strands and activates pepsin:

pepsin and HCl
Protein ✂ Small polypeptides

Fat The gastric lipase hydrolyzes single-bond triglycerides to produce diglycerides and fatty acids. Small degree of hydrolysis by lingual lipase occurs for most fats, but it may be more for milk fats.

Vitamins Intrinsic factor attaches to vitamin B_{12}.

Minerals/Water Stomach acid acts on iron to reduce it, making it more absorbable. The stomach secretes enough watery fluid to turn moist, chewed mass of solid food into liquid CHYME.

OVERVIEW OF DIGESTION AND ABSORPTION (cont.)

SMALL INTESTINE

Carbohydrate   The pancreas produces amylases and releases them through the pancreatic duct into the small intestine:

pancreatic amylase
Polysaccharides ✂ Maltose

Then enzymes on the surfaces of the small intestinal cells break these into monosaccharides, and the cells absorb them:

maltase
Maltose ✂ Glucose+Glucose

sucrase
Sucrose ✂ Glucose+Fructose

lactase
Lactose ✂ Glucose+Galactose

Fiber   Unchanged.

Protein   Pancreatic and small intestinal enzymes split polypeptides further:

pancreatic and intestinal proteases
Polypeptides ✂ Di- and tri-peptides and amino acids

The enzymes on the surface of the small intestinal cells hydrolyze these peptides and the cells absorb them as amino acids:

intestinal di- and tri-peptidases
Peptides ✂ Amino acids

OVERVIEW OF DIGESTION AND ABSORPTION (cont.)	
Fat	The stomach's churning action mixes fat with water and acid. A gastric lipase continues to hydrolyze a little fat. BILE (an important emulsifier of fats) flows in from the liver (via the common bile duct.)
	Bile Fat ✂ Emulsified fat
	Pancreatic lipase flows in from the pancreas:
	Pancreatic lipase Emulsified fat ✂ Monoglycerides, glycerol and fatty acids
Vitamins	Bile emulsifies fat-soluble vitamins and aids in their absorption fats. Water-soluble vitamins are absorbed here.
Minerals/Water	The small intestine, pancreas and gallbladder add enough fluid so the total secreted into the intestine in a day approximates two gallons. Many minerals are absorbed. Vitamin D, through hormonal action, indirectly aids in the absorption of calcium.
LARGE INTESTINE **Carbohydrate**	Carbohydrate is already absorbed.
Fiber	Most fiber passes intact through the digestive tract to the large intestine. Here bacterial enzymes digest some fiber:
	bacterial enzymes Some fiber ✂ Glucose
	Fiber holds water, regulates bowel activity and binds cholesterol, some minerals, carrying them out of the body.
Protein	Protein is already absorbed as amino acids.
Fat	Some fat and cholesterol, trapped in fiber, is excreted in feces.
Vitamins	Intestinal bacteria produce vitamin K, which is absorbed here.
Minerals/Water	Additional minerals and most of the water are absorbed here.

c. **Absorption**

- **ABSORPTION** is the process by which digested food material passes through the epithelial cells of the GI tract (mainly the small intestine) into the blood or lymph.

- **BIOAVAILABILITY** is the degree to which an ingested nutrient gets absorbed and is available to the body. Some forms of vitamins and minerals are more bioavailable than other forms. Medications can influence bioavailability by either blocking or enhancing absorption. Bioavailability of other nutrients is influenced by the acidity or alkalinity within portions of the digestive tract. Bioavailability is also influenced by substances in food (phytates and oxylates), drugs (antibiotics) and body stores (iron, calcium and zinc).

- The small intestine has an enormous absorptive surface. Folds of the mucosa are covered with finger-like projections called **VILLI**. They encapsulate tiny capillaries and lymph vessels that lead to the larger circulatory systems. Each villus is covered with microvilli that make up the brush border. Nutrients are absorbed through villi to enter the bloodstream.

Mechanisms

- Some nutrients require energy and protein carriers to move from the intestinal lumen into the mucosal cell. When the concentration within the cell is greater than the concentration in the lumen, these nutrients move by **ACTIVE TRANSPORT**. Glucose and amino acids are pumped across membranes this way.

- **DIFFUSION** is the process of free transfer of substances across a membrane resulting in equalization on both sides of the membrane. Sodium follows water passively.

- Movement of nutrients across a semi-permeable membrane from a higher to a lower concentration is **FACILITATED DIFFUSION**. A carrier may shuttle nutrients across the membranes. This is also called **CARRIER-MEDIATED DIFFUSION.**

- **PINOCYTOSIS** occurs when a large area of the membrane engulfs particles and "swallows" nutrients into cells. Sometimes a whole protein enters the body in this way. Pinocytosis can allow allergens to enter the body.

- The small intestine is the primary site for nutrient absorption.

Pathophysiology

- **MALABSORPTION** is an abnormal condition where products of digestion are not properly absorbed. Most often fat absorption is not normal and there is usually a decreased absorption of fat-soluble vitamins and some minerals.

- **DIARRHEA** is characterized by loose stools and frequent bowel movements, which causes decreased absorption of nutrients. It is caused by GI disease and may be a symptom of infection (e.g., cholera), food-borne illness (e.g., salmonellosis), tuberculosis, renal failure or enteritis (inflammation of intestine).

- Fatty diarrhea (**STEATORRHEA**) occurs when fat is poorly absorbed. Other diseases that can cause steatorrhea are Crohn's disease, celiac disease, dumping syndrome and ulcerative colitis. Malnutrition may occur as a result of malabsorption. Fluids and electrolytes must be replaced to avoid dehydration when prolonged or serious diarrhea occurs. Effective nutritional management depends on the cause and the needs of the individual.

- **LACTOSE INTOLERANCE** is a disorder resulting from a deficiency of **LACTASE,** a brush-border enzyme that splits the disaccharide lactose into glucose and galactose. Undigested lactose in the bowel increases the osmotic load and causes a pull of fluid into the intestine. This results in diarrhea, bloating and cramping. Bacterial action on the lactose further contributes to the symptoms by producing organic acids and gas. Symptoms can be very mild or quite severe, depending on the degree of enzyme deficiency. Some infants are intolerant of lactose (milk sugar) and require a soy-based or lactose-free formula. After infancy and early childhood, less lactase is secreted and lactose intolerance is common, especially in Blacks, Asians, Native Americans and certain ethnic groups; including Jews. Lactase tablets (Lactaid®), special milk with added lactase, or smaller portions of milk may reduce symptoms of intolerance. Yogurt or buttermilk may be tolerated when milk is not, because the enzymes used to culture them aid digestion and reduce the need for lactase.

VITAMIN ABSORPTION

Ascorbic Acid	Almost completely absorbed from small intestine by active mechanism and diffusion. Excess is excreted and some is oxidized and exhaled as carbon dioxide.
Biotin	Not readily absorbed. Absorption is prevented by **AVIDIN,** a protein in raw egg white that is inactivated by heat.
Calciferol (vitamin D)	Absorbed as either preformed vitamin D from foods or exposure of skin to sunlight. Absorbed from the intestine by the lymphatic system with the aid of fat and bile. Metabolized to 25-hydroxycholecalciferol (the most active biological form.)
Cobalamin (vitamin B_{12})	Needs **INTRINSIC FACTOR** (mucoprotein enzyme from stomach) to be absorbed in the ileum. Some B12 is recycled from bile.
Folate	Readily absorbed from both the upper and lower GI tract by active transport. The physiologically active form of the vitamin is tetrahydrofolic acid.
Niacin	Absorbed in the intestine. Cereal forms of niacin are poorly absorbed.
Pantothenic acid	Readily absorbed from the small intestine and excreted in the urine.
Retinol (vitamin A)	Aided by bile, retinol is absorbed from the intestines and transported via the lymphatic system. Mineral oil interferes with absorption. The conversion of provitamin A (carotene) to vitamin A occurs mainly in the intestinal cell wall, although some conversion takes place in the liver and the kidneys.
Riboflavin	Absorption occurs through intestinal wall and then it is transported by protein or linked to a phosphate molecule such as flavin adenine dinucleotide (FAD) or flavin mononucleotide (FMN). Absorbed better when food is in GI tract.
Thiamin	Absorbed primarily in the duodenum through active transport.
Tocopherol (vitamin E)	Absorbed through the lymphatic system. Requires fat and bile salts for optimal absorption.
Vitamin B_6	Completely absorbed in the upper small intestine and found as pyridoxine which circulates in blood as pyridoxal phosphate, the coenzyme form. Lower pH boosts absorption rate.
Vitamin K	Absorbed from the intestine through the lymphatic system. Requires bile and pancreatic juice for optimal absorption. Some vitamin K is synthesized in the intestines.

MINERAL ABSORPTION

Calcium	Usually 20-30% of ingested calcium is absorbed through the duodenum with rate dependent on need. Vitamin D, an acid medium, ascorbic acid, lactose and protein enhance absorption. Excess absorbed through the colon, with kidneys regulating amount retained. Fat, laxatives, fiber, binding agents (phytates, phosphates and oxalates), lack of exercise, antacids and any condition increasing GI motility can interfere with calcium absorption. Metabolism is regulated by 1,25 dihydroxy-cholecalciferol (vitamin D), parathyroid hormone, estrogen, testosterone and calcitonin.
Chloride	Absorbed through the colon, with kidneys regulating amount retained.
Chromium	Readily absorbed through GI tract.
Copper	Absorbed with amino acids from small intestine and transported in the form of ceruloplasm through the portal circulatory system for storage in the liver. Zinc can interfere with copper absorption. Copper absorption can be blocked by phytates.
Fluorine	Absorbed in small intestine.
Iodine	Absorbed in the small intestine in the form of iodide and transported to the thyroid.
Iron	Absorbed from the upper part of the small intestine. Absorption controlled by body levels and need. Normally, little iron is absorbed. Iron in the body is recycled many times. Iron from animal sources (**HEME IRON**) is absorbed better (30%) than that from plant sources (**NON-HEME IRON**) of which only 2-10% is absorbed. Absorption of non-heme iron is enhanced by ascorbic acid, gastric hydrochloric acid and "meat factor." Factors interfering with iron absorption include tea and coffee (regular and decaffeinated), whole grains, bran and legumes (beans) and living at a low altitude. Iron is lost through the GI tract, urine, sloughed off skin, menstrual flow, nails, hair and sweat. Bleeding or blood donation also causes significant iron loss.
Magnesium	Absorption through the upper intestine is enhanced by parathyroid hormone and hindered by excess fat, phosphate, calcium and binding agents like phytates and oxalates.
Manganese	Poorly absorbed, with only 3-5% entering the bloodstream.
Molybdenum	Readily absorbed from the GI tract.
Phosphorus	Teens and adults absorb 50-70%; infants absorb 85% from human milk. Absorbed from the intestines aided indirectly by hormonal action of vitamin D. Absorption is hindered by excess aluminum, iron and other binding agents. Prolonged therapy with some antacids may interfere with absorption.
Potassium	Absorbed in small intestine, but about 90% is lost in urine and feces.
Sodium	Absorption through large intestine, but 90% is normally excreted in urine. Levels controlled by the kidney's renin-angiotensin-aldosterone system.

MINERAL ABSORPTION (cont.)	
Sulfur	Absorbed in its free form. Excreted in relation to protein intake and catabolism.
Zinc	Absorbed from the small intestine, transported across mucosal cells and stored in the liver. Absorption affected by body size, the level of zinc in the diet and the presence of interfering or competing substances: fiber, phytates, copper, iron and GI diseases.

d. Metabolism

- **METABOLISM** is the sum of reactions and processes that convert nutrients into energy, functional units or parts of body tissues.

- **ANABOLISM** refers to the synthesis of cellular materials for growth, maintenance and repair of tissue. Anabolic processes use energy.

- **CATABOLISM** refers to reactions that break down cellular materials into less complex compounds for energy production or excretion. Catabolic reactions release energy.

- **GLYCOLYSIS** is an anaerobic stage of glucose metabolism. The changes in glycolysis take place in the cell cytoplasm and involve breaking glucose, which has six carbons, into two three-carbon compounds of pyruvic acid. Two molecules of **ADENOSINE TRIPHOSPHATE (ATP)** are required for glycolysis, but four molecules of ATP are produced, thus resulting in a net gain of two molecules of ATP available for immediate energy. Pyruvic acid is further reduced to lactate, which goes out of the cells into the bloodstream.

- **OXIDATIVE DECARBOXYLATION** is the second stage of carbohydrate metabolism. It is known by several names: **KREBS CYCLE, TRICARBOXYLIC ACID CYCLE (TCA)** or the **CITRIC ACID CYCLE**. This process takes place in the mitochondria and as a result, six molecules of carbon dioxide and 20 atoms of hydrogen are released from every molecule of glucose or every two molecules of pyruvic acid. The coenzyme involved is coenzyme A, with acetyl-CoA the active molecule. The reaction also requires niacin, riboflavin and thiamin.

- The electron transport system is responsible for a process known as **OXIDATIVE PHOSPHORYLATION**. The TCA cycle involves dehydrogenation that cannot occur without oxidation of hydrogen to water. The electrons from the hydrogen carriers pass from one series of electron carriers to another, losing some energy and heat at each stage, as adenosine diphosphate (ADP) is converted to adenosine triphosphate and heat is released.

- The **UREA CYCLE** is the process of synthesizing urea from the deamination of amino acids. Carbon dioxide and NH_3 (ammonia) combine with ornithine to form arginine. This reaction uses energy from ATP.

Energy metabolism

- The energy value of food is expressed in terms of units of heat. A **KILOCALORIE (KCAL)** is the amount of heat required to raise the temperature of one kg of water from 14.5 to 15.5 **CELSIUS** (also called **CENTIGRADE)**. A kcal is different from the calorie (c), which equals 0.001kcal. The kcal, or Calorie (C), equals 1,000 calories. However, the term "calorie" is commonly used to describe the kcal or Calorie when describing food value.

- The **ENERGY VALUE** of food is the number of kcal a food will yield when oxidized by the body or a calorimetry device.

- A **JOULE** is a measure of mechanical energy more precise than the kcal measure of thermal energy. One **KILOJOULE (KJ)** is the energy involved in moving a one kg weight one meter by one Newton (a unit of force).

4.18 kilojoules = 1 kilocalorie = 1 Calorie

- **OXIDATION** is any chemical reaction involving addition of oxygen, removal of hydrogen or a loss of electrons and an increase in valence. Oxidation in biological systems requires energy. During cellular respiration, cellular oxidation reactions take place, yielding energy. Oxidation-reduction reactions occur simultaneously in cellular respiration. Oxidation involves the loss of electrons and reduction results in a gain of electrons. The electron donor or receptor is itself oxidized or reduced during the process. The reactions are reversibly catalyzed by oxidoreductase.

- **CELLULAR OXIDATION** of carbohydrate (CHO) and fat yield energy, heat, water and carbon dioxide. Protein (PRO) oxidation yields energy, heat, water, carbon dioxide and urea. Water, carbon dioxide and urea are removed from the body as waste.

- In the body, food is not completely digested and absorbed. Normally about 98% of CHO, 92% of PRO and 95% of fat is absorbed, so values of CHO = 4kcal/g; PRO = 4kcal/g; fat = 9kcal/g; and alcohol = 7kcal/g are used to estimate energy values for an average, mixed American diet. This is sometimes referred to as the **COEFFICIENT OF DIGESTIBILITY.** For most purposes, the 4:4:9:7 values are used as the net energy to humans after food is digested and metabolized.

- During fasting, starvation or intense physical exercise, the body draws energy from its own stores. The initial source is stored adenosine triphosphate (ATP) and creatinine phosphate in cells, but this source is depleted in a few minutes. Oxidative phosphorylation of body nutrients, the primary source of energy during starvation or fasting, results in the breakdown of glycogen, protein and fat. Glycogen has a 12 to 24 hour energy reserve in the liver and muscle tissue. There is a limited energy reserve of protein in the muscle mass, but larger than in glycogen stores. The glycogen can be broken down into glucose units if the blood sugar gets low and the brain needs glucose as fuel. The capacity for energy storage in adipose (fat) tissue is unlimited. The supply of available energy varies from one person to another, depending on the size of the individual's fat stores.

- **CALORIMETRY** is the measurement of heat released when foodstuffs are burned for energy. **DIRECT CALORIMETRY** measures heat loss from the body by placing a subject in an insulated, box-like chamber. The rise in temperature of the water circulating in the tubes surrounding the chamber is noted. The **ATWATER CALORIMETER** and **BENNIGER'S APPARATUS** are two examples of equipment used for direct calorimetry in humans. The **BOMB CALORIMETER** is used to measure heat released when food is burned in the chamber of the calorimeter. The subsequent heat release is measured.

- **INDIRECT CALORIMETRY** determines the heat produced by an individual by calculating oxygen consumed and/or carbon dioxide expelled over a given period of time. A specific amount of heat is liberated per liter of oxygen used in oxidizing carbohydrate, protein and fat. A ratio exists between the oxygen and CO_2 used to oxidize each nutrient. This ratio is known as the **RESPIRATORY QUOTIENT (RQ):**

$$RQ = \frac{\text{moles } CO_2 \text{ expired}}{\text{moles } O_2 \text{ consumed}}$$

- Under basal conditions, the caloric value of one liter of oxygen is 4.82kcal and the average RQ is 0.82. The normal range of RQ is 0.7-1.0.

- In the laboratory and in clinical settings open-circuit indirect calorimetry is very widely used. Indirect calorimetry is thought to be more accurate than the use of predictive equations to determine REE.

- Indirect calorimetry is a non-invasive technique and is reasonably easy to use. Most systems in use today are computerized, portable and are relatively inexpensive.

- To improve the accuracy of the outcomes, the test should be done before daily activities begin to assure that the individual is in a rested state. If the person has traveled to the site, he or she should lie down and rest for a minimum of 20 minutes before starting the test.

- Individuals who will undergo this testing should avoid strenuous physical activity for at least 14 hours before the test and moderate physical activity for at least 2 hours.

- The person should be instructed to fast for at least six hours and avoid caffeine consumption and medication usage, where possible overnight, and nicotine for at least two hours before the test. Ideally, women should be tested between the 15 – 23 day of their menstrual cycle.

ENERGY VALUE OF NUTRIENTS IN FOOD		
Food item	Actual Energy Value (In a calorimeter)	Estimated (net) Energy Values (In the human body)
Carbohydrate	4.10kcal/g	4kcal/g
Protein	5.65kcal/g	4kcal/g
Fat	9.45kcal/g	9kcal/g
Alcohol	7.0kcal/g	7kcal/g

Hormones that affect energy metabolism

- Secreted by beta cells of the pancreas, **INSULIN** lowers blood glucose levels, increases liver and muscle glycogen formation, inhibits gluconeogenesis in the liver and increases the rate of glucose utilization by body tissues. Insulin is required for the entrance of glucose, protein and fats into cells.

- Produced by the alpha cells of the islets of Langerhans of the pancreas, **GLUCAGON** is a hyperglycemic-glycogenolytic factor of the pancreas, which increases the blood glucose level by stimulating the breakdown of glycogen to glucose in the liver. Glucagon is secreted in response to hypoglycemia and exercise. Insulin and glucagon are antagonistic. In other words, insulin moves glucose out of the bloodstream and into the cell, thus reducing blood glucose levels. Glucagon initiates the breakdown of glycogen from the liver to increase blood glucose.

- **EPINEPHRINE (ADRENALIN)** is secreted by the adrenal medulla in response to fear or stress. It raises the blood glucose level by stimulating the breakdown of liver and muscle glycogen to produce glucose. Epinephrine causes a quick release of readily available glucose from stored glycogen for immediate use. Epinephrine constricts blood vessels, increases blood pressure and accelerates heartbeat to prepare for the "fight or flight" syndrome.

- **THYROXINE** is the principal hormone secreted by the thyroid gland. It raises the blood glucose level because it influences the rate of insulin destruction, glucose absorption from the intestine, and the release of epinephrine. Thyroxine is the principal hormone regulating BMR and oxygen consumption.

- **GROWTH HORMONE(GH)** and **ADRENOCORTICOTROPIC HORMONE (ACTH)** are secreted by the anterior pituitary; GH and ACTH raise the blood glucose level by acting as insulin antagonists, by increasing amino acid uptake and by increasing the rate of protein conversion to glucose. These hormones influence protein and fat metabolism.

Factors affecting energy intake

- **HUNGER** is a physiological phenomenon, whereas **APPETITE** is a learned response. Food intake is regulated by two phases of appetite control: short-term regulation (daily food consumption) and long-term regulation (homeostatic mechanisms for maintenance of body weight). The hypothalamus sends a hormonal message from the central nervous center to the digestive system to trigger hunger and satiety. The ventromedial hypothalamus, the **SATIETY CENTER,** within the brain, produces **SEROTONIN** in response to increases in circulating glucose, amino acids, cholecystokinin and insulin. Serotonin produces the satiety effect. The lateral hypothalamus is the feeding center. It responds to opiates and monoamines, which produce a feeling of hunger.

- Inappropriate caloric consumption, impaired digestion and/or inefficient absorption are physiologic influences on energy intake.

- Psychological influences include emotions that trigger hormonal responses and increase or decrease appetite. Some people eat for comfort; others are primarily motivated by external cues and habits.

- **ENERGY BALANCE** is equilibrium between energy intake and energy expenditure. **POSITIVE ENERGY BALANCE** (weight gain) occurs when energy intake exceeds expenditure. Extra energy is stored by the body, results in weight gain. When energy intake is less than energy needs, **NEGATIVE ENERGY BALANCE** and weight loss occur.

- The interrelationships of metabolism of carbohydrate, protein and fat ultimately determine the final use of nutrients. Carbohydrate and fat can spare protein from being used as an energy source. Excess protein and carbohydrate can be stored for use as energy later. Some excess protein can enter muscle. Glucose can be synthesized from glycerol and amino acids to maintain blood glucose levels. Limited amounts of glucose can be converted to glycogen for storage in the liver. Excesses of carbohydrate, protein, fat and alcohol can be converted to fat for storage, if there is an excess of calories over current needs.
- **KETONURIA** is a condition that occurs if there is a high concentration of **KETONES** in the blood from incomplete oxidation of fatty acids and the excess ketones are excreted in the urine. Ketones are produced during fasting or when diabetes is poorly controlled. High ketone levels in the blood can cause neurological damage.

e. Excretion

- **EXCRETION** is the separation and elimination of waste matter and water from the blood, tissues or organs. Major excretion wastes include urine, feces and perspiration.

Physiology

- Within a 24 hour period (usually about 4 hours after a meal has been consumed), most of the chyme leaves the **ILEUM**, the last part of the small intestine, and enters the large intestine. The **LARGE INTESTINE** is divided into four parts: **CECUM, COLON, RECTUM** and **ANAL CANAL**. A valve controls the passage of the semi-liquid mass. Normally the valve remains closed, but peristaltic waves relax the valve, allowing small amounts of chyme to enter the cecum. Peristaltic waves move the mass slowly along the large intestine, aided by mucus secreted from glands in the colon. Chyme moves from cecum to colon in about 10 hours. Mass movements propel fecal contents into the colon, where they are stored until defecation. **GASTROCOLIC REFLEX** eventually pushes fecal matter into the rectum. Desire to defecate is triggered by stretch receptors in the rectum. Elimination is accomplished by strong contractions of the rectal wall and relaxation of anal sphincters.

- **UREA** is the principal nitrogen-excretion product of metabolism. It contains ammonia, a strong smelling, potent substance produced by the liver during the degrading of amino acids to energy or fat. Urea circulates in the blood, then passes through the kidneys where it is removed and excreted as **URINE**. Water is required to keep urea diluted and in solution, which is why individuals on high protein diets should drink more water than usual.

- **FECES** is composed of small amounts of food residue, especially indigestible fiber, microflora, wastes from desquamated cells, bile pigments, cholesterol and unabsorbed minerals, such as calcium and iron. Bile pigments impart the characteristic color to feces. Typical daily excretion is about 100-200grams.

Biochemistry

- As the chyme reaches the large intestine, almost all nutrients and water have been absorbed. The large intestine secretes alkaline juices with a large amount of mucus but no hydrolytic enzymes. There is very little absorption of nutrients at this point.

- Vitamin K synthesis takes place in the colon.

- Microflora in the large intestine are resistant to dietary change. Predominant bacteria are **ESCHERICHIA COLI.** Bacteria in the large intestine release gases, including ammonia, methane, carbon dioxide and hydrogen, lactic and acetic acid and substances that have toxic properties such as indole and phenol.

Fiber and physiologic conditions

- **CONSTIPATION** involves infrequent or difficult bowel movements. Prunes contain **ISATIN,** a natural laxative. Dietary fiber increases stool bulk and volume, decreases transit time and reduces colonic pressure. Coarsely ground bran, often consumed as bran cereal, seems to be more effective in relieving constipation than fruits and vegetables.

- **DIVERTICULI** are sacs or pouches on the walls of the colon. **DIVERTICULITIS** is an inflammation of the diverticuli. Symptoms may include nausea, vomiting, fever, abdominal tenderness, distension, pain and intestinal spasms. A high-fiber diet may relieve symptoms over time, but is contraindicated during periods of inflammation, perforation or abscess. Nuts or seeds should not be used because they may get caught in the sacs causing irritation and pain.

- **WATER-SOLUBLE FIBERS** (gums and pectin) can lower serum cholesterol. Suggested mechanisms for this effect include decreased intake of fat and kcal, reduced cholesterol and fat absorption and binding of bile cholesterol so that it is not reabsorbed.

- A **HIGH-FIBER DIET** contains increased amounts of cellulose, hemicellulose, lignin and pectin and provides approximately 12 or more g of crude fiber (25-35g of dietary fiber). Emphasis is placed on increasing the intake of whole grain breads and cereals, fresh fruits and vegetables and legumes that are high in fiber content. Fiber supplements in the form of tablets, powders or wafers may be included. The intake of refined carbohydrate is reduced because it is displaced by unrefined foods. The caloric content is not substantially different from a normal diet. Liquid is generally increased in a high fiber diet.

- Reliance on large quantities of foods high in phytate content (wheat bran) to increase fiber intake may interfere with vitamin and mineral absorption by binding them. A mixed high fiber diet is a better choice.

c. **Renal**

- The primary functions of the kidneys are maintenance of homeostasis through control of fluid, pH and electrolyte balance.

Anatomy

- The paired kidneys are reddish organs shaped like kidney beans. An average adult kidney measures about 10-12cm long, 5 – 7.5cm wide, and 2.5cm thick. Near the center of the medial concave border, the ureter exits the kidney through the hilus. The hilus is the entrance to the renal sinus. Three tissue layers surround the kidney. The renal capsule is the inner layer, the adipose capsule is the middle layer and the outer layer is called the renal fascia.

- There are two internal sections of the kidney, the cortex and the medulla. Within the medulla are the renal pyramids whose apexes are termed renal papillae. Together the cortex and the renal pyramids make up the parenchyma, the functional portion of the kidney. The functional unit of the kidney is the **NEPHRON**.

- Nephrons consist of two portions, a renal corpuscle and a venal tubule. The renal corpuscle has two components, the glomerulus and Bowman's capsule. The renal tubule has three sections, proximal convoluted tubule, loop of Henle and the distal convoluted tubule. The distal convoluted tubules of several nephrons are linked to a single collecting duct. The loop of Henle connects the proximal and distal convoluted tubules. The descending limb of the loop of Henle dips into the medulla and the ascending loop of Henle returns to the cortex.

Physiology

- The nephrons are the working unit of the kidney. In this capacity, the nephrons carry out three functions: 1) they control blood concentration and volume; 2) regulate blood pH; and, 3) remove waste.

  - The initial step in the formation of urine is glomerular filtration. This process uses blood pressure to force fluid and solutes through the glomerulus capillaries. There are three main pressures involved in blood filtering: 1) glomerular blood hydrostatic pressure (GBHP); 2) capsular hydrostatic pressure (CHP), the pressure opposing pressure exerted by filtrate in the glomerular that is being pushed back into the capillaries; and, 3) blood colloid osmotic pressure (BCOP) and another force opposing filtration due to the presence of protein in the blood. The net filtration pressure (NFP) is GBHP-(CHP+BCOP). The amount of filtration formed by the kidneys is termed the **GLOMERULAR FILTRATION RATE (GFR)**. In normal adults this is about 125ml/minute.

  - Tubular secretion removes solutes from the blood and returns them to the filtrate for elimination in urine. As with reabsorption, secretion occurs all along the length of the renal tubule.

  - About 99% of filtrate passing through the tubules is reabsorbed into the blood, leaving only 1% to be excreted as urine. The movement of water and solutes back into the blood is termed tubular reabsorption. Solutes that are reabsorbed by both active and passive diffusion include glucose, amino acids, urea and several charged ions. Water reabsorption occurs by osmosis. Other small molecules are generally reabsorbed by pinocytosis. The proximal convoluted tubules (PCT) make the largest contribution to reabsorption with the more distal portions responsible for homeostatic balances.

Biochemistry

- There are three principal mechanisms used to control the glomerular filtration rate and blood pressure: 1) renal autoregulation of GFR; 2) hormonal regulation of GFR; and 3) neural regulation.

  - Renal autoregulation of GFR is a negative feedback regulation of GFR by the juxtaglomerular apparatus (JGA). The process begins with a stimulus that disrupts the

NFP and GFR. Receptors in the JGA detect the decrease in flow of fluid and sodium and chloride ions and inhibit secretion of vasoconstrictors while the arterioles dilate, allowing more blood to flow into the glomerular capillaries, thus increasing the NFP and GFR and a return to homeostasis.

➢ Hormonal regulation of GFR is controlled by two hormones, angiotensin II and atrial natriuretic peptide (ANP) as a part of the renin-angiotensin system. The process begins with the release of renin from juxtaglomerular cells in response to a stimulus such as decreased delivery of fluid and NaCl to the macula densa and increased frequency of nerve impulses in renal sympathetic nerves. Once in the blood, renin acts on angiotensinogen, a plasma protein produced in the liver, converting it to angiotensin I. As angiotensin I passes through the lungs it is converted to the active hormone angiotensin II by angiotensin converting enzyme (ACE). Angiotensin II acts on: 1) arterioles to constrict, increasing glomerular hydrostatic pressure; 2) adrenal cortex to secrete aldosterone increasing sodium and water reabsorption increasing blood volume; 3) hypothalamus to signal increased thirst further increasing blood volume; and 4) posterior pituitary gland stimulating the release of antidiuretic hormone increasing water retention that also increases blood volume. The process returns homeostasis. The second hormone, ANP, promotes diuresis and natruresis when released (secondary to stretching of the heart) in response to increased blood volume. This hormone also increases GFR while suppressing secretion of ADH, aldosterone and rennin. This lowers blood pressure and reduces edema.

➢ Through neural regulation, the blood vessels of the kidneys are supplied by vasoconstrictor fibers of the sympathetic portion of the autonomic nervous system. At rest, there is minimal sympathetic stimulation and the renal blood vessels are maximally dilated. When there is sympathetic stimulation (exercise, flight or fight), vasoconstriction of the arterioles occurs, decreasing GFR.

Reabsorption

- A major mechanism for sodium reabsorption in the tubules and collecting ducts is by an electrochemical gradient where sodium ions passively diffuse from filtered fluid in the tubule lumen through leakage channels in the brush boarder into the tubule cell. Concurrently, sodium pumps expel sodium and import potassium, which can diffuse back out through leakage channels. The active transport of sodium promotes reabsorption of water by osmosis. As water leaves the filtrate, the concentration of other solutes is increased, thus creating concentration gradient for substances such as K^+, $Cl-$, HCO_3- and urea and promoting their reabsorption by passive diffusion.

- Glucose, amino acids and other useful metabolites are reabsorbed by Na^+ symporters PCT. Substances brought into PCT by symporters leave by facilitated diffusion through the basolateral membrane. The reabsorption of these metabolites also results in the re-absorption of water by osmosis. Although the majority of solutes are reabsorbed in the PCT, some are also reabsorbed in the loop of Henle by symporters. Most reabsorption of water occurs together with reabsorption of solutes in PCT, in the descending loop of Henle and DCT.

Secretion

- Tubular secretion removes materials from the blood adding them to the filtrate having two principal effects; it rids the body of waste materials and helps control blood pH to maintain K homeostasis in body fluids. The cells in the collecting ducts secrete K^+ in exchange for reabsorbed Na^+. Secretion of K^+ is controlled by aldosterone, K^+ concentration in plasma and Na^+ concentration in OCT. The secretion of H^+ takes place in the PCT. Most of the H^+ secreted into tubular fluid combines with filtered HCO3- to form H_2CO_3, which then disassociates into CO_2 and H_2O. The CO_2 diffuses into tubule cells joining with water to form H^+ and HCO3-. As the H^+ is secreted into the tubular fluid by Na^+/H^+ antiporters the HCO_3 is re-absorbed into the blood along with Na^+. Ammonia production in the PCT depends on blood pH. It is secreted into the filtrate by Na^+/NH_4^+ antiporters.

d. Pulmonary

Anatomy

- External anatomy - The lungs are paired cone-shaped organs housed in the thoracic cavity. The pleural membrane encloses and protects each lung and consists of an outer layer, the parietal pleura and an inner layer, the visceral pleura. Between these two layers is a small space, the pleural cavity, containing a lubricating fluid secreted by the membranes to reduce friction between the membranes during breathing. The base of the lung is concave and fits over the convex area of the diaphragm. The superior portion of the lung is termed the apex. The costal surface is rounded to match the curvature of the ribs. The medial surface contains the hilus, through which bronchi, pulmonary blood vessels, lymphatic vessels and nerves enter and exit. The right lung is thicker and a bit shorter than the left lung due to the diaphragm and higher on the right side due to the liver. The left lung contains the concave cardiac notch, where the heart lies. Each lung is divided into lobes. Both lungs have a superior and inferior lobe and the right lung also has a middle lobe. Each lobe receives its own secondary lobar bronchus. These secondary bronchi give rise to tertiary bronchi which supply the bronchopulmonary segments.

- Internal anatomy - Each bronchopulmonary segment of the lungs contains many lobules wrapped in connective tissue and containing a lymphatic vessel and arteriole, a venule and a branch from a terminal bronchiole. The terminal bronchioles divide into respiratory bronchioles which subdivide into alveolar ducts.

- Alveolar anatomy - Around the alveolar ducts are alveoli and alveolar sacs. The alveoli walls contain cells that secrete alveolar fluid which contains a surfactant, which reduces the surface tension of alveolar fluid. Around the alveoli, the arteriole and venule of the lobule form a capillary network.

Physiology

- Inspiration: For air to flow into the lungs, the pressure inside the lungs must become lower than the pressure in the atmosphere. This is achieved by expanding the lungs through contraction of the diaphragm and intercostal muscles. When the volume of the lungs increases the alveolar pressure inside the lungs decreases and air enters from the atmosphere into the lungs due to a gas pressure difference. Air continues to move into the lungs until the gas pressure difference no longer exists. The atmospheric air entering the alveoli of the lungs contains oxygen. The exchange of oxygen and carbon dioxide between alveoli and pulmonary blood capillaries results in the conversion of deoxygenated blood coming from the heart to oxygenated blood returning to the heart. The fully oxygenated blood is pumped into the aorta, through the systemic arteries and then to the capillaries of the tissue cells.

- Expiration: For air to flow out of the lungs, the pressure inside the lungs must become higher than the pressure in the atmosphere. Normal expiration is passive process involving no muscle contraction. As the diaphragm relaxes, the lungs recoil inward and the alveolar pressure increases. Air then flows from the area of higher pressure in the alveoli to the area of lower pressure in the atmosphere.

- **PULMONARY VOLUME** - During normal breathing, about 500ml of air moves into and out of the lungs, this volume of air is called the tidal volume. Only about 35ml of the tidal volume reach the alveoli; the residual 150ml remain in airspaces known as anatomic dead space. The total air breathed in one minute is termed the minute volume of respiration (MVR). The inspiratory reserve volume is the additional inhaled air following a very deep breath and averages 3000ml above tidal volume. If one inhales normally but exhales forcibly, the additional exhaled air is called the expiratory reserve volume. The residual volume is the air remaining in the lungs even after the expiratory reserve volume is expelled.

- **PULMONARY CAPACITY** - Inspiratory capacity is the sum of **TIDAL VOLUME** plus inspiratory reserve volume (about 3600ml) and represents the total inspiratory ability of the lungs. The sum of residual volume plus expiratory reserve volume (about 2400ml) is the functional residual capacity. **VITAL CAPACITY** is the sum of inspiratory reserve volume, tidal volume and expiratory reserve volume (about 4800ml). Lastly, total lung capacity is the sum of all volumes (about 6000ml).

Biochemistry

- Transport of O_2 and O_2-. Since oxygen does not dissolve easily in watery blood plasma, a majority of it (98.5%) is carried in combination with hemoglobin inside red blood cells. Each hemoglobin unit has four heme groups and each heme group can carry one molecule of oxygen. The most important factor determining how much oxygen combines with hemoglobin is pO_2. When the pO_2 is high, hemoglobin is saturated. When pO_2 is low, hemoglobin is only partially saturated and oxygen is released from hemoglobin. In pulmonary capillaries where the pO_2 is high, a lot of oxygen binds to hemoglobin. However, in tissue capillaries where pO_2 is lower, oxygen is less bound to hemoglobin and is released for diffusion into tissue cells.

- Under normal conditions about five percent of deoxygenated blood contains carbon dioxide (CO_2). The CO_2 is carried in the blood as dissolved CO_2, carbaminohemoglobin and bicarbonate ions. The smallest percentage (7%) is dissolved in plasma and diffuses in the alveoli of the lungs. The formation of carbaminohemoglobin is dependent on pCO_2. The higher the pCO_2, the greater the affinity of CO_2 for hemoglobin. A relatively low pCO_2 is found in pulmonary capillaries, which allows CO_2 to split from globin and diffuse into the alveoli. Most CO_2 (70%) is transported in blood as bicarbonate ions. As CO_2 diffuses into tissue capillaries into red blood cells (RBC), it combines with water to form carbonic acid which dissociates into hydrogen ions and bicarbonate ions. The accumulation of bicarbonate ions inside the RBC causes some to diffuse into plasma. The ionic balance between the RBC and the plasma is maintained by shifts of chloride.

- Gasses exchange in lungs and tissues. As CO_2 leaves tissue cells and enters blood cells, it causes more oxygen to disassociate from hemoglobin allowing more CO_2 to combine with hemoglobin and more bicarbonate ions are produced. As oxygen diffuses from the alveoli into blood cells, hemoglobin becomes saturated with oxygen. Hemoglobin saturated with oxygen is a stronger acid than when combined with CO_2. As a result, the more acidic hemoglobin releases more hydrogen ions, which bind to bicarbonate ions to form carbonic acid. The carbonic acid disassociates into water and CO_2, with the CO_2 diffusing from the blood in the alveoli.

d. Cardiovascular

Anatomy

- Heart - The heart is about 12cm long, 9cm at its widest point, and 6cm thick. The apex is formed by the tip of the left ventricle. Opposite the apex is the base, the upper posterior portion of the heart, formed by the atria. The pericardium is a triple-layered membrane consisting of two principal portions, the fibrous pericardium and the serous pericardium. The fibrous pericardium anchors the heart to the mediastinum. The serous pericardium is a double-layered membrane consisting of the outer parietal later and the inner epicardium which adheres tightly to the heart. Between these layers is the pericardial cavity containing the pericardial fluid which reduces friction between the layers as the heart beats. The heart wall consists of three layers: the epicardium (outer layer), myocardium (middle layer), and the endocardium (inner layer). The interior of the heart contains four chambers that receive the circulating blood. The right and left atrium are the two superior chambers and each contain an auricle that increases the volume of the atria. The inferior chambers are the right and left ventricle. Coronary sulcus separate atria from ventricles. Interatrial and interventricular septums separate the atria and ventricles respectively.

- Arteries - Blood flows from the right atrium into the right ventricle and into the lungs via the pulmonary trunk. The pulmonary trunk divides into a right and left pulmonary artery each carrying blood to one lung. The blood returns to the heart through the pulmonary vein and into the ascending aorta. Next the blood flows into the coronary arteries which carry blood to the arch of the aorta, thoracic aorta and the abdominal aorta which, along with their branches, carry blood throughout the circulatory system.

- Veins - The right atrium receives deoxygenated blood from the body through three veins. The superior and inferior vena cava bring blood from areas of the body superior and inferior to the heart respectively. The coronary sinus drains blood from vessels supplying the wall of the heart. Two veins, the great cardiac and middle cardiac, are the vessels that carry blood to the cardiac sinus.

- Valves - The heart has valves to prevent the backflow of blood. These valves open and close in response to changes in pressure as the heart contracts and relaxes. Atrioventricular (AV) valves are located between the atria and ventricles. Between the right atrium and the right ventricle is the tricuspid valve; between the left atrium and left ventricle is the mitral valve. The two arteries exiting the heart also have valves. The pulmonary semilunar valve is located in the opening where the pulmonary trunk leaves the right ventricle. At the opening between the left ventricle and the aorta is the aortic semilunar valve.

- Auto rhythmic cells - A small portion of cardiac muscle fibers become auto rhythmic, which enable them to rhythmically generate impulses. They set the rhythm of the heart and ensure the heart contracts in a coordinated manner. The components of this conduction system include: sinoatrial and atrioventricular nodes; the left and right bundle branches and the Purkinje fibers.

Physiology

- Muscle contraction - An impulse is initiated by the sinoatrial node and spreads to the contractile fibers thus opening Na^+ ions channels increasing membrane permeability (allowing inflow Na^+ producing depolarization), opening Ca^{2+} channels allowing Ca^{2+} to enter the cytosol. Ca^{2+} maintains the depolarization. Next, Ca^{2+} binds to troponin allowing actin and myosin filaments to slide past one another to build tension. Repolarization occurs when the Na^+ and Ca^{2+} channels close and K^+ channels open. As the K^+ ions diffuse out along their concentration gradient and few Na^+ and Ca^{2+} enter the fiber, the negative resting membrane potential is restored and the muscle fiber relaxes.

- The **CARDIAC CYCLE** are all the events associated with one heartbeat. As the atria and ventricles alternately contract and relax, pressure changes occur causing blood to flow from areas of higher pressure to ones of lower pressure. In a normal cardiac cycle, the two atria contract while the two ventricles relax. Then the two ventricles contract while the atria relax. The phase of contraction is termed **SYSTOLE**. The phase of relaxation is called **DIASTOLE**. A cardiac cycle consists of systole and diastole of the atria and a systole and diastole of the ventricles.

- **CARDIAC OUTPUT** is the amount of blood flow from the ventricle into the aorta each minute. The variables include the stroke volume and the number of heart beats per minute. Cardiac reserve refers to the ratio between the maximum cardiac output one can achieve and the cardiac output at rest.

Biochemistry

- Two substances in the body, hormones and ions, have major effects on the heart. The adrenal medulla releases two hormones (epinephrine and norepinephrine) that increase both heart rate and contractility. Thyroid hormone has a similar effect on heart rate and heart muscle contractility. The relative concentration of three cations (Na^+, K^+ and Ca^2) impact cardiac functionality. Elevated levels of K^+ or Na^+ in blood decreases heart rate and contractility. Whereas a moderate increase in Ca^{2+} speeds and strengthens heart rate, excess K^+ can also block impulse generation.

e. Neurological

Anatomy

- In spite of the complexity of the nervous system, it consists of only two main cell types: neuroglia and neurons.

- **NEUROGLIA CELLS** support, protect and nurture neurons by maintaining homeostasis of the fluid surrounding neurons. There are four types of neuroglia in the central nervous system (CNS): astrocytes; oligodendrocyte; microglia; and ependymal. Two neuroglia are found in the peripheral nervous system (PNS), Schwann cells which produce myelin sheaths around the PNS, and neurons and satellite cells which support neurons in ganglia. In the CNS, the star-shaped astrocytes participate in metabolism of neurotransmitters, generation of impulses, brain development and help form the blood brain barrier. Oligodendrocyte are smaller than astrocytes and form the myelin sheath around neurons. Microgalia are derived from monocytes and protect the CNS from invading microbes. Lastly, ependymal are generally ciliated squamous and columnar shaped cells that line brain ventricles and the central canal of the spinal cord.

- **NEURONS** are nerve cells consisting of a cell body, dendrites and an axon. The cell body contains a nucleus surrounded by cytoplasma with typical cell organelles along with neurofibrils. Dendrites are short highly branched and usually not myelinated. Axons are long thin, cylindrical projections that tend to be myelinated. The synaptic end bulb of the axon contain vesicles that store neurotransmitters. A nerve fiber is the term for a dendrite or axon. A **NERVE** is a bundle of nerve fibers that course along the same path in the peripheral nervous system.

Physiology

- Resting membrane potential (RMP) - For neurons to communicate, their plasma membranes have electrical voltage and specific ion channels open and close to allow the ions to move across the cell membrane. The RMP exists because there are negative charges on the inside of the cell and positive charges on the outside of the cell. The phospholipid layer of the plasma membrane is a good insulator allowing current to flow across the membrane only through ion channels. The membrane potential changes when ion channels open or close. Therefore, the factors contributing to RMP are the distribution of membranes and the relative permeability of the plasma membrane to Na^+ and K^+. Extracellular fluid has a higher concentration of Na^+ and Cl- ions. The intracellular fluid has a higher concentration of K^+, organic phosphates and amino acids in proteins. Also, the permeability of the plasma membrane to K^+ is 50 to 100 times greater than that of Na^+ in a resting neuron.

- The two basic types of ion channels are leakage and gated. Leakage channels are always open whereas gated channels open and close in response to four types of stimuli: voltage, chemicals, mechanical pressure and light. The voltage-gated ion channel gives the plasma membrane the ability to respond to stimuli by producing impulses. The chemically-gated ion channels open and close in response to chemical stimuli such as neurotransmitters, hormones and some ions by either direct or indirect changes of the membrane permeability. Mechanically-gated ion channels respond to mechanical vibration or pressure, whereas light-gated channels open and close in response to light.

- Action potential - In a typical neuron, during an action potential, both the Na^+ and K^+ voltage-gated ion channels open then close. Depolarization is brought on by the rapid opening of Na^+ voltage-gated ion channels. Repolarization occurs with the slower opening of the voltage-gated K^+ channels and the closing of the open Na^+ channels. Together, the depolarization phase along with the repolarization phase, comprise an action potential.

- **SYNAPSES** are the functional junctions between a neuron and an effector, such as muscle or a gland. They may be either electrical or chemical in nature. An electrical synapse allows an electrical current to spread between cells through gap junctions. Electrical synapses allow faster communication than chemical synapses and they are able to synchronize a group of neurons or muscle fibers. In chemical synapses, the pre and post-synaptic neurons are separated by the synaptic cleft. The presynaptic neuron releases a neurotransmitter that diffuses across the synaptic cleft and acts on receptors in the plasma membrane of the postsynaptic neuron to produce a graded potential. The depolarization opens voltage-gated Ca^+ and Na^+ channels. Ca^{2+} is more concentrated in extracellular fluid so Ca^{2+} flows inwards. The increase intracellular Ca^{2+} triggers exocytosis of synaptic vesicles releasing neurotransmitter molecules into the synaptic cleft. A chemical synapse is only a one-way information transfer from presynaptic neuron to postsynaptic neuron, muscle fiber or gland cell.

Biochemistry

- Excitatory and inhibitory neurotransmitters are located in both the PNS and CNS. A neurotransmitter may show either an excitatory or inhibitory response depending on the nature of the receptor. Acetylcholine (ACh) is a neurotransmitter that is excitatory at the neuromuscular junction acting to open chemically-gated cation channels and an inhibitory neurotransmitter at other synapses, indirectly opening ion channels via protein receptors on the plasma membrane. Two amino acids, glutamate and aspartate, are excitatory neurotransmitters. Two others, gamma amino butyric acid (GABA) and glycine, are inhibitory neurotransmitters. Catecholamine neurotransmitters (epinephrine, norepinephrine, and dopamine) are synthesized from tyrosine and can be either excitatory or inhibitory. Neurotransmitters, once released into the synaptic cleft, must be removed for normal synaptic function. The neurotransmitter may be removed through diffusion out of the cleft, enzymatic degradation by neurotransmitter specific enzymes or by reuptake of the neurotransmitter into the neuron that secreted it.

f. Musculoskeletal

Anatomy

- The **MUSCULOSKELETAL SYSTEM** in humans is an organ system that provides stability, support and movement using the muscular and skeletal systems. The musculoskeletal system consists of the skeleton, muscles, cartilage, tendons, ligaments and joints. The system determines how skeletal bones are connected to one another and to muscle fibers via tendons and ligaments. The skeleton provides stability, is the main storage area for calcium and phosphorus and protects organs. Muscles keep the bones in place and provide movement of the skeleton. Joints connect different bones and allow movement. Cartilage surrounds the ends of bone to prevent bones from directly rubbing against each other.

- The average human has about 206 bones. There are five general classifications of bones: long, short, flat, irregular and sesamoid. There are two divisions of the skeleton, the axial and appendicular. The regions of bone may be categorized as compact or spongy. Structurally, the skeletal system consists of cartilage, bone tissue, bone marrow and the periosteum.

- A typical long bone consists of the following parts:
  - ➤ Epiphysis: Ends of the bone.
  - ➤ Metaphysis: The region where the diaphysis joins the epiphysis.
  - ➤ Articular cartilage: A layer of hyaline cartilage covering the epiphysis where the bone forms a joint with another bone.
  - ➤ Periosteum: The membrane around the surface of the bone. It has two layers, fibrous and osteogenic.
  - ➤ Medullary: The space within the diaphysis containing the bone marrow.
  - ➤ Endosteum: The lining of the medullary. It is a membrane containing osteoprogenitor cells.

- There are four types of cells in bone tissue:
  - ➤ Osteoprogenitor: These cells are unspecified cells derived from mesenchyme.
  - ➤ Osteoblast: The cells that form bone.
  - ➤ Osteocytes: Mature bone cells derived from osteoblasts.
  - ➤ Osteoclasts: The cells engaged in bone resorption.

- Muscle - There are three types of muscles; cardiac, skeletal and smooth. Only skeletal and smooth are part of the musculoskeletal system and only skeletal muscle is responsible for movement.
  - ➤ **SKELETAL MUSCLE** - The neurons that stimulate muscle contraction are called motor neurons. Deep fascia is connective tissue that holds muscle together. Three layers of connective tissue extend from the deep fascia to further protect and strengthen skeletal muscle. The epimysium encircles the whole muscle and is the outer most layer. The perimysium surrounds bundles of fibers and the endomysium surrounds individual muscle fibers. The sarcolemma is the plasma membrane of the muscle

fiber. It surrounds the sarcoplasm of the muscle fiber. The sarcoplasm contains myofibrils, the contractile units of skeletal muscle. The myofibrils contain myofilamets which are arranged in compartments call sarcomers. The two contractile proteins that form the myofilaments are actin and myosin.

> **SMOOTH MUSCLE** - Myofilaments are also in smooth muscle. There are two types of smooth muscle tissue: visceral and multiunit. The fibers in visceral muscle tissue form large networks and contain gap junctions. Multiunit smooth muscle tissue consists of individual fibers with their own motor neuron.

Physiology

- Skeletal - The process by which bone forms is called **OSSIFICATION**. The formation of bone is either intramembranous ossification or endochondral ossification. Intramembranous ossification is the formation of bone on or within the fibrous connective-tissue membrane. Formation of bone in the hyaline cartilage is referred to as endochondral ossification. Both mechanisms replace pre-existing connective tissue with bone. The process begins with migration of mesenchymal cells to an area where bone formation is starting. The mesenchymal cells become osteoprogenitor cells which then become osteoblasts. In the absence of capillaries the osteoprogenitor cells become chondroblasts which are responsible for the formation of cartilage.

- Bone growth - The epiphseal plate allows the bone to grow in length and it also shapes the articular surfaces. The region between the diaphysis and the epiphysis of a bone, where the calcified matrix is replaced by bone, is termed the metaphysis. The rate of growth is controlled by hormones. As growth ensues, the cartilage cells, produced on the epiphyseal side of the plate, are destroyed and replaced by bone on the diaphyseal side of the plate. Eventually the epiphyseal cartilage cells stop dividing and bone replaces cartilage. The epiphyseal line, a remnant of the epiphyseal plate, is formed and bone stops growing in length. Osteoclasts destroy the bone lining the medullary cavity and osteroblasts add new bone tissue to the area.

- Muscle - Muscle contraction and relaxation is initiated when a nerve impulse arrives at the axon terminal of the motor neuron, triggering the release of acetylcholine (ACh). The ACh diffuses across the synaptic cleft, binding to its receptors and triggers an action potential. The action potential causes the release of Ca^{2+} from the sarcoplasmic reticulum into the sarcoplasm. Ca^{2+} binds to troponin on the myofilament exposing the binding site for myosin and it binds ATP. The shape change that occurs when myosin binds to actin produces the power stroke of contraction. The myosin swivels to the center of the sarcomere. Drawing the thin myofilaments past the thick myofilaments, myosin releases ADP. Once the power stroke is complete, ATP again binds with myosin causing myosin to detach from actin ATP site further along the thin myofilament. Relaxation occurs when acetylcholine esterase destroys ACh in the synaptic cleft, disallowing another muscle action potential and closing the Ca^{2+} releasing channels. Ca^{2+} active transport pumps remove Ca^{2+} from the sarcoplasm into the sarcoplasmic reticulum. As the Ca^{2+} levels in the sarcoplasm drop the tropomyosin-troponin complex slides back over the myosin binding sites on actin, preventing further binding of myosin to actin and the myofilaments go back to their relaxed state.

Biochemistry

- Calcium homeostasis - The role of bone in Ca^{2+} homeostasis is as a regulator of blood Ca^{2+} levels. When Ca^{2+} blood level decreases, Ca^{2+} is released from the bone; when the blood level increases, Ca^{2+} goes back into the bone. If some stimulus causes blood Ca^{2+} levels to fall, receptors on the parathyroid gland detect the change and release parathyroid hormone (PTH) into the blood. PTH increases the number and activity of osteoclasts, increasing bone resorption resulting in the release of Ca^{2+} (and phosphate) into the blood. PTH also affects the kidneys and intestines. The kidneys are stimulated to reabsorb more Ca^{2+}, eliminate phosphate and produce the active form of vitamin D, calcitrol. The calcitrol acts on the intestines by stimulating Ca^{2+}receptors which causes increase absorption of Ca^{2+}. Ca^{2+} levels become elevated the thyroid gland speeds Ca^{2+} uptake by bone from the blood and increases Ca^{2+} deposit into bones. The net result of these two hormones maintains calcium homeostasis.

- Muscle metabolism during contraction is dependent on the phosphagen system. This system consists of creatine phosphate and ATP and provides enough energy for muscles to contract maximally for 15 seconds. Creatine phosphate is formed while the muscle is at rest. The creatine phosphate transfers a high-energy phosphate group to ADP, forming ATP and creatine. When muscle activity continues and the supply of creatine phosphate is depleted, muscle glycogen is broken down into glucose. The metabolism of glucose via glycolysis splits the glucose molecule into two molecules of pyruvic acid and two ATP. Since glycolysis does not require oxygen, it is an anaerobic process. Without sufficient oxygen, the pyruvic acid will be converted lactic acid. If sufficient oxygen is available, enzymes in the mitochondria can completely oxidize pyruvic acid to CO_2, water, ATP and heat. Through the process of cellular respiration, muscle tissue can obtain oxygen by diffusion of oxygen into muscle fibers from the blood and oxygen is released by myoglobin inside muscle fibers.

g. Reproductive

Anatomy

- Males - Sperm are produced in the testes, located in the scrotum, and transferred to the epididymis for maturation and storage. Upon ejaculation, sperm travels from the epididymis to the vas deferens, which have ejaculatory ducts at the ends. The seminal vesicles empty into the ejaculatory ducts which then empty into the urethra. The top portion of the urethra is surrounded by the prostate gland. Along the urethra, and below the prostate, are the Cowper's glands that produce fluid that is a lubricant. The urethra goes through the penis which contains three layers of spongy erectile tissue.

- Females - The organs of female reproduction include the ovaries, which produce oocytes that, when fertilized, become mature ova. Within the ovary, each oocyte is surrounded by a follicle. Following puberty, one ova is released during ovulation. The two Fallopian tubes transport ova to the uterus. The lining of the uterus is the endometrium. The bottom end of the uterus is termed the cervix. The vagina serves as a birth canal and a repository for sperm. The opening to the vagina is covered by an inner skin layer, the labia minora, and an outer skin layer, the labia majora. At the end of the labia is the clitoris, the female equivalent of the male penis.

Physiology

- **OOGENESIS** is the process by which an oogonium becomes an ovum through meiosis. It begins soon after fertilization when germ cells travel to the gonads. They become oocytes once they enter the stages of meiosis. They are made up of oogenic cells and surrounded by follicle cells. At puberty the follicles begin to develop. Each oocyte experiences division forming a secondary oocyte which can be released during ovulation. It will only complete the meiosis cycle if fertilized by a sperm.

- **SPERMATOGENESIS** is the process by which spermatocytes are derived from spermatogonia cells. Each primary spermatocyte divides into two secondary spermatocytes. Subsequently each spermatocyte divides into two spermatozoa. As these mature they develop into sperm cells.

Biochemistry

- Males - Hormonal control of testicular function: At the onset of puberty, the hypothalamus releases gonadotropin releasing hormone (GnRH) which stimulates the anterior pituitary to secrete follicle stimulating hormone (FSH) and luteinizing hormone (LH). FSH aids spermatogenesis by stimulating the Sertoli cells. LH stimulates the release of testosterone by the cells of Leydig. Testosterone functions in development of sexual characteristics and functions and, as an anabolic hormone, stimulates protein synthesis.

- Females - Hormonal control of oogenesis: GnRH from the hypothalamus stimulates the anterior pituitary to release FSH and LH. FSH stimulates growth of the follicle while LH stimulates growth of the corpus luteum. androgens are formed and converted to estrogen, which acts on the anterior pituitary to increase FSH and LH and supports growth of endometrium. The follicle begins to secrete inulin which negatively feeds back to the anterior pituitary to stop producing FSH. After ovulation, if fertilization occurs, the corpus luteum secretes progesterone to support growth of the endometrium. If fertilization does not occur, hormone levels decrease, the corpus luteum is destroyed and the endometrium is discharged during menstruation.

TOPIC C – EDUCATION & COMMUNICATION

1. Components of the educational plan

a. Targeted setting/clientele

(1) Cultural competencies and diversity

- **CULTURAL COMPETENCY** is an act of awareness and acknowledgement that value systems vary across cultural strata and how cultural groups make decisions. It is necessary in dietetic practice to be aware of cultural competence, appreciate its importance, but also to practice it. There are a number of models available to incorporate the tenets of cultural compentency. Irrespective of the model selected, core elements such as awareness, acknowledgement, skill development and inductive reasoning should be utilized in the process.

- Cultural competency is associated with diversity and diverse cultures. **DIVERSITY** is the process of including the opinions and perspectives of underrepresented minority groups. Diversity includes valuing and respecting differences regarding age, gender, sexual orientation, ethnicity, race, religion, lifestyles, personal values, etc. Diversity must be prevalent and valued before cultural competency is achieved.

(2) In-service education (students, health and rehabilitative service providers)

- **IN-SERVICE EDUCATION** is a continuous process to upgrade and reinforce desired behaviors in employees who work in a facilityor business or those who represent it as health and service providers. It may be conducted by persons within the institution or by outside experts. Topics, attendance and programs should be documented as part of the department's continuing quality assurance efforts.

- All new employees should be offered a well-planned **ORIENTATION PROGRAM.** This familiarizes and acquaints a new employee to the organization, the department and job responsibilities. A good orientation program will increase productivity because the employee will be able to carry out the responsibilities of the job in a timely fashion, and learn proper ways to carry out the requirements of the position.

(3) Patient/client counseling

- The goal of the client interview is to collect valid data (eating and lifestyle patterns, medical status, activities) while maintaining a positive and open environment conducive to disclosure of lifestyle information, as well as feelings and emotions (self-esteem, self-confidence, anxiety, anger, confusion, uncertainty). In an interview, the nutrition therapist's goal is to build rapport with the client and develop a trusting relationship. In this way the therapist can effectively coach the client in the process of self-management.

- The environment is an important aspect of the process. Comfort, privacy and confidentiality should be assured, and interruptions from other people and the telephone calls or computer messages should be avoided. Usually, client and counselor sit on chairs to talk as a desk may be perceived as a barrier. The counselor should record notes soon after each session.

(4) Other (e.g., on-the-job training, telemedicine/telehealth, e-learning)

- **ON-THE-JOB TRAINING** usually takes place in the setting in which the job will be performed. It often is done through simulation or demonstration, with the trainee replicating the process. Sometimes, computer assisted instruction or audiovisual aids are used as the first part of the instruction.

- **TELEMEDICINE** is an application of clinical medicine where information is consultatively communicated through interactive audiovisual media. Telemedicine can be simple as in discussion over the telephone or complex as videoconferencing to conduct real-time consultations. Telemedicine is the use of telecommunication and information technology to deliver clinical care.

- While telemedicine refers to delivery of clinical services, **TELEHEALTH** refers to both clinical and non-clinical services including research, education and administrative.

- **E-LEARNING** consists of all forms of electronic learning and instruction. It pertains to out-of-classroom and in-classroom education through technology. The e-learning process includes webinars, computer-based learning and virtual education.

b. Goals and objectives

- **GOAL SETTING** is a process of identifying changes in behavior that are mutually agreeable to client and counselor. The goals should be clear, measurable and attainable behaviors toward which the client works. **LONG-TERM GOALS** should be significant and relevant enough to be motivational. They are best accomplished through a series of short-term goals. **SHORT-TERM GOALS** are the steps in the behavioral process necessary to attain the desired outcome.

- Each person is unique and each personal goal should reflect this uniqueness. A counselor or teacher can facilitate goal setting but cannot determine its content.

- Guidelines for goal setting include the following:

  ➢ Be positive. For example, a goal for the client might be to eat one more fruit each day, as opposed to saying, "Don't eat fried foods."
  ➢ Be sure the goal is within the client's control.
  ➢ Include the client in the goal-setting process. Ask, for example, "How much time can you spend walking every day?"
  ➢ Be specific. For example, "Weigh portions of meat and eat no more than 6 ounces of meat a day" is a better goal than "Eat less meat."

- During the first visit, the dietitian's assessment should identify the client's stage of change phase, in order to help set goals and facilitate change.

- To provide better advice, service or care, the dietitian communicates to the client what he or she hopes to accomplish with the interview. The professional can alleviate fear and uneasiness by informing the client of what to expect during the initial interview and during successive sessions. The client should be an active participant and be encouraged to ask questions or restate objectives to ensure that he or she understands what is going to happen. Successful goal setting depends on agreement about the problem. If the process of self-management is to be effective, the client must be allowed to set the outcome goals, with the guidance of the counselor.

- Client self-sufficiency or self-management is the long-term goal of most nutrition counseling. **SELF-EFFICACY** is when a client believes in his/her ability to make and sustain changes. The degree of independence developed will depend on the severity of the client's condition, the client's willingness to make changes, the barriers to changes and the counselor's skill in encouraging the client to take responsibility for independent living skills.

- Goals should be selected on the basis of identified problems that will promote positive behavioral change. Clients should be asked what kind of changes they would like to make and why they believe the changes are important. Goals should be set according to highest priority and as one is achieved, the client should move to the next.

- Both short and long term goals should be set. They should help to promote success by being realistic and achievable. The counselor should help the client to set one or two goals and to develop action plans to achieve them. Too many goals or goals that are too ambitious or global are not attainable and create feelings of failure rather than of success.

Behavioral objectives

- **BEHAVIORAL OBJECTIVES** identify specific, realistic outcomes that a person/organization wants to attain. Objectives may be written in the cognitive, affective and psychomotor domains. These objectives must be determined before educational methods and techniques are selected. Objectives should be measurable and confirmed by behavior. A well-stated objective identifies performance, condition and criterion elements.

- **PERFORMANCE ELEMENTS** state what the learner will be able to do (e.g., able to identify all forms of simple sugar) upon completion of the learning activity.

- **CONDITION ELEMENTS** describe setting, cues and equipment associated with the behavior and determine which resources will be provided or withheld (e.g., able to plan an appropriate dinner menu without looking at diet instructions).

- **CRITERION ELEMENTS** set the level of achievement, the standard by which performance is measured (e.g., able to correctly reassemble a vegetable shredder in five minutes or less).

- Behavioral objectives are written with verbs that allow assessment of action. These verbs may also follow a learning theory-based classification in Bloom's classic *Taxonomy of Educational Objectives.*

VERBS COMMONLY USED IN BEHAVIORAL OBJECTIVES

Health AND Safety Behaviors

Clean	Cover	Eliminate	Go	Taste	Wear
Clear	Drink	Empty	Sanitize	Uncover	
Close	Eat	Fill	Stop	Wash	

Creative Behaviors

Alter	Design	Organize	Rearrange	Restate	Simplify
Ask	Explain	Paraphrase	Regroup	Restructure	Synthesize
Change	Generalize	Predict	Reorder	Revise Rewrite	Vary
Combine	Modify	Question	Rephrase		

Logical AND Judgmental Behaviors

Analyze	Compare	Decide	Evaluate	Generate	Plan
Appraise	Conclude	Deduce	Explain	Induce	Structure
Combine	Contrast	Defend	Formulate	Infer	Substitute

Discriminative Behaviors

Choose	Describe	Distinguish	Isolate	Omit	Point
Collect	Detect	Identify	List	Order	Select
Define	Differentiate	Indicate	Match	Pick	Separate

Social Behaviors

Accept	Answer	Contribute	Forgive	Participate	Talk
Agree	Argue	Cooperate	Group	Permit	Thank
Aid	Assist	Disagree	Help	Praise	Volunteer
Allow	Communicate	Discuss	Name	React	

Language Behaviors

Abbreviate	Call	Pronounce	Sign	Summarize	Write
Accent	Edit	Read	Speak	Tell	
Alphabetize	Outline	Recite	Spell	Translate	
Articulate	Print	Say	State	Verbalize	

Study Behaviors

Arrange	Classify	Follow	Map	Quote
Categorize	Compile	Gather	Mark	Record
Chart	Copy	Label	Name	Search
Cite	Diagram	Locate	Note	Sort
Circle	Find	Look	Organize	Underline

Mathematical Behaviors

Add	Count	Extrapolate	Integrate	Record	Tally
Calculate	Derive	Extract	Multiply	Solve	Verify
Check	Divide	Graph	Number	Subtract	
Compute	Estimate	Group	Plot	Tabulate	

Laboratory Science Behaviors

Alpha	Convert	Grow	Limit	Replace	Transfer
Apply	Decrease	Increase	Operate	Report	Weigh
Calibrate	Demonstrate	Insert	Plant	Set	
Conduct	Dissect	Keep	Prepare	Specify	
Connect	Feed	Lengthen	Remove	Time	

c. Needs assessment (external constraints, competing programs, illness)

(1) Individual

- **NEEDS ASSESSMENT** helps to establish a starting point for any type of educational program. This assessment helps the instructor or counselor understand the level of understanding and prior knowledge of the employee or client, so there is no time wasted.

- Preparation of an educational intervention should be guided by the findings from an assessment of learner needs. Various assessment methods are available. Selection is dependent on instructional resources (time, funding, expertise), program objectives and student characteristics. Needs assessment activities are project-driven and may range from a lengthy, intensive process to a very focused, brief survey.

- A **PRE-ASSESSMENT (PRE-TEST)** is a diagnostic evaluation performed prior to instruction for the purpose of placement and classification of individuals according to their personal characteristics, current knowledge, skills, abilities, aptitudes, interests, personality, educational background and psychological readiness to learn.

- **ASSESSMENT** should determine any constraints to learning, such as the learner's physical and psychological readiness, communication barriers such as reading level or language, financial status, and possible problems resulting from illness and dietary changes.

- Written or computerized **TESTS** can be used to determine current knowledge of an individual. These may take the form of achievement tests, performance tests, checklists, inventories or objective or essay tests. Questions may be true/false, multiple choice, fill-ins, matching, short answer or essay. Examples include food intake surveys, planning meals for a patient with diabetes and selecting low-sodium choices from a list.

- **DIRECT OBSERVATION** of specific activities may be used to determine skill level in operating a piece of equipment, ability to take anthropometric measurements or evaluation of meal choices by a patient. Observers may be present or hidden from the activity in progress, depending on the anonymity desired. Examples include evaluating eating habits by viewing food in the refrigerator and on shelves in the home or evaluating how a person operates a commercial dish machine.

- Clients and/or employees can be presented with real-life situations and asked to work through the scenario. This **ROLE-PLAYING** or **SIMULATION** technique may be used to create a situation to test an individual's decision-making ability in handling day-to-day problems. Emergencies or unusual incidents can be simulated using a computer or video, and the learner can practice responding to a specific situation. Computerized simulations can also be used as a testing technique. Examples include practice handling customer complaints or teaching women to breastfeed.

- **DEMONSTRATION** is a technique in which behaviors (skill level, habits) are exhibited and/or assessed. The client or employee may perform tasks in the presence of an evaluator. Actions that need to be corrected provide the basis for a teaching plan.

I. PRINCIPLES OF DIETETICS (12%)

(2) Group

- When involved in group counseling situations (e.g., orientation, in-service training and professional development), the instructor should do a needs assessment to determine what knowledge the employees already have, what knowledge deficits exist, who can best address these issues and what the best delivery format will be. This information should be ascertained prior to presenting the information. Training and development activities promote quality services and productivity. They also enhance morale and job satisfaction.

- Many techniques of assessment of individuals can be used in a group setting. In a group setting, however, use of pre-assessment questionnaires or pre-tests may be helpful.

- If there is a possibility to form several groups, pre-assessing knowledge/attitude in advance may be helpful. Group dynamics can play a role in group learning and can be a divisive factor to a successful outcome. Individuals also learn from others in the group.

d. Content: community resources, learning activities/methodology, references and handouts, audiovisual specifications

- The content of programs are determined by the following:
  - ➢ Available facilities dictate teaching methods, materials and visuals used and number of learners.
  - ➢ Language of instruction, location, availability of transportation, times programs and services are offered, and accessibility for those with disabilities influence ability to participate and must be considered when planning programs.
  - ➢ Available resources impact program planning. Resources may include personnel and their skills, financial support, audiovisuals and educational materials, technology, federal, state, and local programs and voluntary health agencies. Agencies such as the American Heart Association and the American Cancer Society provide community-based programs, as do local colleges and universities, religious institutions, healthcare institutions and support groups. The educator should help the client or employee identify internal and external resources and should match clients with available community programs.

- Individuals who are experts, or who have personal experience related to the program subject, may be asked to speak to a class or group. Hearing about a subject from different people increases student interest and demonstrates that there are a variety of resource people available from which one can learn. A good resource person has information and ability beyond the expertise of the group leader and can serve as a role model for students.

Learning activities/methodology

- Learner needs, resource availability and instructor skill should influence the choice or blend of strategies.

- Instructional activities may consist of one, more than one, or a composite of the following strategies:
  - ➢ In **LECTURES,** the presenter does most of the talking to students. Techniques may

include visuals and questions. The lecture method is an efficient way to deliver information and is useful if the educational goal is to acquire knowledge.

➤ **LABORATORY/EXPERIENTIAL** strategies emphasize direct experience with materials pertinent to the area of study (e.g., food models to learn portion control). Techniques may include field trips (e.g., to the supermarket). This method is useful if the educational goal is to develop skills or compare products.

➤ A **DISCUSSION SEMINAR** provides opportunities for interaction between the instructor and students. It is useful when learners have emotional or intellectual resistance to the information being presented because it brings their resistance to light. Discussion encourages application, problem solving, immediate feedback and exploration of varied perspectives. Discussions may also be a useful strategy to evaluate the ability to think and/or communicate ideas.

➤ **QUESTIONS AND ANSWERS** permit an exchange between learner and teacher. By asking questions, learners can have concerns addressed directly. Questions from teachers should explore student ideas rather than elicit "right" answers. Question and answer sessions increase the effectiveness of lecture techniques.

➤ **SUPPORT GROUPS** teach one another by sharing experiences and modeling appropriate behavior. This method encourages discussion and problem solving. It is difficult to communicate a great deal of information in support groups, but they are useful in creating a positive and supportive environment in which to learn and try new behavior.

➤ **ROLE-PLAYING/SIMULATION** may be based on enactment of real-life situations without risk if the learner's actions are inappropriate. The learner is asked to respond, demonstrating his or her ability to handle a situation. The objectives are to make a connection between theory and practice, to engage in critical thinking and to develop problem solving and coping skills. Video simulations bring the situation to the learner and provide additional opportunities to stop the video and discuss specific actions or reactions.

➤ **DEMONSTRATION** involves acting out or showing a learner an intellectual skill, attitude or motor skill. This method is most effective if the learner is given an opportunity to repeat the demonstration. At that time, errors can be corrected and the learner can develop confidence in the skill.

➤ **SELF-PACED** learning rate rests with the student who works at his or her own pace, convenience and ability. This method offers individualized experience with less failure and is an excellent technique for teaching adults and those with special needs. However, individual work may need careful monitoring to ensure that students don't go "off-task" or continue with a number of significant errors.

➤ **COMPUTER-ASSISTED** learning is self-paced and non-threatening unless the user has a fear of computers. Computers provide immediate feedback to the learner, which improves motivation. The cost of equipment and the availability of software may be limiting factors.

- **PROBLEM-BASED LEARNING (PBL)** is a case-driven, learner-centered, small group approach that has been shown to foster critical thinking, problem solving, self-directed learning skills and to enhance knowledge acquisition and retention. The PBL process proceeds from the concrete to the abstract with a problem vignette as the initiating action. Learners draw from their existing knowledge base to form hypotheses and offer ideas about the presenting situation. Problem-solving and reasoning activities occur until additional information is needed. This information, depending upon its type, may be obtained in two ways.

➢ Factual knowledge that would normally be obtained from a chart, interview or examination is available from the small group facilitator, who holds a "data sheet" about the problem.

➢ Gaps in the knowledge base, termed **LEARNING ISSUES**, are studied independently in self-directed learning sessions. Information obtained from the facilitator and from independent study is applied to the problem to continue the problem solving cycle. **PROBLEM CLOSURE** includes a comparison of the student derived management plan with the optimal problem outcome and an assessment of self-performance and group dynamics.

- **DISTANCE EDUCATION** is based on communication technologies that have allowed instruction to extend beyond the traditional classroom. Advantages of distance education are that students can work at their own pace, considering their work and personal schedules and avoid limitations placed by geographic distances, transportation problems, resource availability or physical disabilities.

➢ Both synchronous and asynchronous modes of delivery are effective in distance education. Simultaneous communication between educators and learners is **SYNCHRONOUS INSTRUCTION**, while delayed delivery communication is **ASYNCHRONOUS.** Compressed video systems, two-way audio and video networks and computer software that support virtual classrooms have been successfully used to deliver instruction ranging from single classes to entire degree programs. Educators using distance-learning technologies must master the nuances associated with delivering courses via distance education, in addition to expert application of teaching techniques. For example, distance education training programs should address special methods to personalize the class, overcome the absence of nonverbal communication, promote class interaction, administer assessment activities and prepare adequate audiovisual and study guide materials. The personalization is often accomplished in a "chat room" wherein students and teachers can have meaningful on-line discussions.

- **CONTINUING EDUCATION** is a process of self-directed learning, generally beyond the work site, to remain technically competent and meet emerging education needs. It is necessary to maintain registration as a dietitian or diet technician. Continuing education of all health team members helps maintain the quality of care by keeping practitioners up-to-date on current technology and research. Education can also promote recognition of dietitians as experts by other health team members. Continuing education supports the dietitian's commitment to lifelong learning.

References and handouts

- All instructional aids should enhance the learning experience and be appropriate to the audience, the topic and the budget. Learning styles vary and many individuals learn better when provided with auditory support, visual images or practice situations. Computer-generated slide presentations are popular instructional aids.

- Printed materials such as textbooks, training manuals and handbooks can be both reference sources of information and sequenced mediums of instruction. They are best used in conjunction with workbooks, self-study forms and other materials, that allow the learner to demonstrate his or her understanding of the information. Printed handouts written especially for a target population (e.g., pregnant teens) using familiar language, drawings and examples are very useful. Today's educators stress the importance of printed materials that help learners, of all ages, explore and discover their own ideas and ways to solve problems instead of materials that stress giving the "right" answers on tests.

- If material created and published by others is reproduced in whole or in part in a program, the developer should first get permission to use it (describing the intended use to the creator) and credit should be given to the source. Often **PERMISSION FEES** to reproduce copyright materials are charged. For example, reproducing the *Exchange Lists for Meal Planning* requires a permission fee payable to The Academy of Nutrition and Dietetics or The American Diabetes Association. Many publishers waive permission fees or charge nominal fees for material used for educational purposes. The © symbol means material is copyrighted and cannot be copied or reproduced in any way without permission of the copyright holder.

- Information published by the government or governmental agencies is developed at taxpayer expense. It is in the "public domain" and may be reproduced without permission or fees. Examples include MyPlate and *Dietary Guidelines for Americans*. There is, however, a fee charged to reproduce the *Recommended Dietary Allowances/DRI.*

Audiovisual specifications

- Audiovisual materials support information presented in written or oral form. Audiovisual resources include slides, films, videos, overheads, computer (*Power Point* presentations), flip charts, photographs, posters and food models. Materials should be previewed to assure appropriateness and to exclude sexual, racial, ethnic and age biases.

- After viewing, discuss the information in the audiovisual to be sure it has meaning for the group and that it contributes to their learning.

- Well made audiovisuals provide consistent, high quality images that can be repeated in a variety of settings as adjuncts to teaching activities or as independent devices of instruction (for large and small groups, training programs, orientation, individual and group counseling, etc.)

- Self produced video or slide presentations are effective because learners enjoy seeing familiar settings and people and can relate to the situation.

- Through audiovisuals, a teacher can present information dramatically (e.g., microscopic shot of contaminated cutting board, graph showing fatalities from various causes), impressing students and improving retention.

- Videos are especially useful because the popularity of television and videos in the home has made didactic instruction boring to individuals used to seeing colorful, action-packed presentations supported by sound and music.

- **AUDIOVISUAL INSTRUCTION** (audiotapes, videotapes, CDs, DVDs) also extends the availability of informative and entertaining experts and personalities.

- CD's or referrals to websites often accompany print material for classroom or self-study use.

- When developing visuals, use the following tips:
  - ➢ Make sure materials are readable or visible to everyone in the audience.
  - ➢ Present numbers in graphs when possible, to show comparisons.
  - ➢ Limit copy on slides to keywords. Present only one message per visual.
  - ➢ Use black, dark blue or dark green for words on flip charts. Red is hard to read and should be used for emphasis only. Alternating colors increases readability.
  - ➢ Print in large letters and use upper and lower case to increase readability.
  - ➢ Use clear graphic images that support messages. Materials should be appropriate for the given situation.

- Literally, millions of nutrition information documents are available from Internet resources. Government agencies place nutrition resources on web sites for easy access. Electronic discussion groups and web sites devoted solely to food and nutrition interests provide information as well as access to experts. Legal issues such as copyright ownership, licensure to "practice" online, as well as rights and fees for intellectual property have been developed, although there are areas where legal usage are not yet clearly defined.

e. Evaluation criteria

- Before setting criteria, the three "w" questions should be answered.
  - ➢ The purpose—why?
  - ➢ The timing—when?
  - ➢ The specific outcomes—what?

- Evaluation strategies may consist of an assessment of participant reactions to programs, measures of change in an organization, measures of behavioral change and learning in the cognitive, affective and psychomotor domains. Evaluation may be norm or criterion referenced. **NORM REFERENCING** compares students with the norm of a group. **CRITERION REFERENCING** measures performance toward a defined objective or standard.

- Test items and methods should reflect the objectives of the educational program.
  - ➢ In a classroom, the instructor should evaluate the learning that has taken place at various intervals in the term. This is often accomplished by establishing an objective standard of what the person is expected to know at the completion of parts and/or all of the instruction. (Criterion Referenced)
  - ➢ It can also be accomplished by comparing an individual student's performance to the average performance of the group. (Norm Referenced)

f. Budget development

- For each program to be developed, adequate financial resources must be assured.

  - ➢ The person responsible for the program should look for all possible sources of revenue.
  - ➢ Based on the revenue projection, a budget can be outlined. All cost centers need to be considered including materials, personnel, room rental, food service, promotion, etc.

> The program has to be justified.
> If an individual or group is going to support the program, the instructor should be able to show that it is cost-effective and that it may eventually generate income and/or a cost or mission-related benefit.

g. Program promotion

- A successful educational program should attract as many eligible clients/students as possible. To do this, the program has to be known by the target audience.

- The type(s) of promotion you use will depend on the educational service being offered.

- If an in-service is being offered, the promotion can take the form of personal contact or e-mail with the people you specifically want to be present.

- It can also consist of flyers sent to individual members or posting the information in strategically located areas of the workplace.

- If a program is being offered to people in the local community, flyers can be posted on local bulletin boards, or car windshields, distributed in supermarkets and outpatient clinics. If there are sufficient funds, radio and television promotions spread the message.

- Reaching the number of people you want to expose to your message and the number of times the message is seen is very important. It often takes multiple reminders before people sign up for programs.

- The message has to contain the program goals, must be relevant to the target audience and it must be clear and consistent.

- Websites, social networks and personal contacts are also excellent promotional tools.

2. Theories of educational readiness

- There are many theories in the field of educational readiness, motivational behavioral change and the orientation to learning. Readiness, in the learning process, includes the works of major theorists/behavioralists including Maslow, McClelland, Herzberg Bruner, Piaget, Montessori, Rogers and Skinner. (See Domain III A, c 4 for motivational learning theories, etc.)

- Piaget and Bruner theorized that readiness in learning requires internal mental functions that include insight, memory perception and processing of information. Maslow and Rogers theorized that certain cognitive and affective needs have to be met before learning could occur. Skinner demonstrated that stimuli, in the external environment, could produce behavioral changes toward a desired goal.

- Learning is a process whereby the individual: 1) acquires information for a particular purpose or end product (task or goal); 2) to change behavior or behavioral patterns; 3) desires knowledge or information for its own sake, or; 4) creatively uses information. Any one or combination of these processes constitutes learning.

- Learners need to be at the maturation, environmental, affective and/or cognitive level, according to some theorists, to benefit from the learning process. If any of these are not present, or impaired, learning readiness is minimized. For example, if the learner is under extreme stress due to health issues, the environment is not conducive to good learning.

- In dietary counseling, there are often factors that affect learning; i.e., stress due to illness, noise or other distractions, language barriers, etc. Often teaching is best in stages, including written, and/or audio-visual materials, to reinforce learning with opportunities to ask questions or express concerns at the next learning session.

- Adults are generally task or problem-centered learners. They want to see how the information can be applied to solving life and work issues. Their readiness and need to learn can be motivated by personal life experiences, health concerns or desire to improve work performance.

3. Implementation

a. Communication

(1) Interpersonal

- Creating an environment for learning facilitates education. For group or individual counseling, the environment should provide a private setting without interruption, comfortable seating that allows for appropriate distance between individuals, proper lighting, comfortable temperature and good ventilation. For groups, make sure the speaker and all members can easily be seen and heard.

- Even more important than establishing this physical environment is the attention given to a psychological environment. A psychological environment conducive to learning is characterized by a climate of mutual respect, collaboration, mutual trust, supportiveness, openness and authenticity, pleasure and humaneness.

- **COMMUNICATION** refers to all methods that convey feeling or thought between persons. Effective communication requires clear presentation, concise wording, accurate messages, descriptive words and visuals, clearly presented tables and figures, reasonable units of presentation (not too much or too little), relevant and current information, formats appropriate for the presentation (oral/written), and presentation and examples appropriate for the audience and purpose.

- Formal means of communication within organizations include regular staff meetings, reports and newsletters, in-service education, videos, magazines, memorandum or e-mail communication and sales meetings. Informal means of communication include networking, bulletin boards, memos and voice mail.

- **WRITTEN COMMUNICATIONS** by letter, fax message, e-mail, memo or minutes of meetings can be used to document conversations, meeting procedures and outcomes; set forth proposals; document agreements; suggest actions to be taken; present points of view; communicate grievances; give commendations and recommendations; and clarify meaning. Written communications can be public or confidential. Be careful what is put in writing or sent as an electronic commmunication as it may become a legal document. Never send a memo written while angry or with real or implied threats.

- To keep communication channels open between the learner(s) and the dietitian, the dietitian should create a supportive environment using both verbal and nonverbal communication techniques. The dietitian should be sensitive to cultural aspects of interpersonal relations. For example, different cultures have different ways to respect authority or modesty. Eye contact, in some cultures is not acceptable; while in others it is expected and appreciated. A handshake or any touching is not acceptable in others.

(2) Group process

- **GROUP DYNAMICS** is the interpersonal forces that affect group behaviors. Forces such as status, trust and competition can improve or interfere with the communications process.

- There are four developmental phases of group dynamics. They are not necessarily sequential; groups move back and forth.

  ➤ In the **INDIVIDUAL-CENTERED, COMPETITIVE PHASE**, each individual establishes him or herself in the leadership hierarchy and finds a role in the group.
  ➤ In the **FRUSTRATION AND CONFLICT PHASE**, hostility and blame focus on the leader and others when frustration is not relieved. The individual feels no personal responsibility for attaining group goals.
  ➤ In the **GROUP HARMONY PHASE** cohesiveness develops. Members are generally supportive but tend to avoid conflict and negative reactions. There is more concern with group needs than with individual needs, which may be repressed.
  ➤ In the **GROUP-CENTERED PRODUCTIVE PHASE** members are concerned for others but do not avoid conflict. Members accept responsibility for personal behavior and become more tolerant of others' values and behavior.

Group process

- Meaningful involvement and participation improve productivity and accomplishment of personal and group goals. When a person feels discounted or lacks influence, he or she may attack, complain, look for a scapegoat or try to monopolize the group to get increased attention. If members of a group disagree on an action, there is likely to be poor support for implementing the action. When group members do not feel safe, they often withhold information, thus distancing themselves from the group.

- **CONGRUENCE** is the accurate match between words and behavior. When someone shouts that he or she is not angry, there is a lack of congruence. To maintain communication, both sender and listeners must maintain congruence. Informal groups tend to form when individuals who do not agree with an action get together separately to discuss it and plan strategy. When informal subgroups form, the unity of an entire group may be threatened as the need for self-actualization supersedes group goals.

CHARACTERISTICS OF EFFECTIVE GROUPS

➢ The reason for the group is clear to all.
➢ A competent leader keeps discussion focused and facilitates participation.
➢ The atmosphere promotes work being done.
➢ There are guidelines for making decisions (vote, majority, quorum, etc.) Every member feels free to contribute.
➢ Members have learned to cope with conflict.
➢ There are established standards of behavior including how freely emotion will be expressed.
➢ Members realize that their needs will be met and there is an obligation to share time to meet the needs of others.
➢ Members respect confidentiality, encouraging an atmosphere of trust.

Group roles

- **TASK-ORIENTED ROLES** include an initiator, contributor, information-seeker, information-giver, coordinator, energizer, orienter, historian and/or policy-tracker.

- **MAINTENANCE ROLES** include that of harmonizer, standard-setter, observer and/or follower.

- **INDIVIDUAL ROLES** include that of aggressor, blocker, recognition seeker, dominator, help seeker and/or special interest advocate.

Group size

- As group size increases, members have less direct involvement and participation. In large groups, individuals tend to direct communications to an individual of high rank, often the leader or speaker, rather than interacting with each other.

- Large groups tend to break into subgroups, forming factions and allegiances. Groups of 8 to 30 function more like a class than an interactive group. Dividing large groups into smaller task-oriented or discussion groups that report back to the full group encourages more participation.

- In groups of 3, 2 members tend to pair up and the other may feel attacked or neglected. A group of 4 to 8 is ideal for group counseling and therapy.

Group leadership

- The group leader is responsible for responding to the needs of the group and defining the initial purpose of the group. The leader facilitates participation of each individual.

- Some research shows that autocratic leadership sometimes produces greater quantitative results whereas democratic leadership produces better morale and qualitative results. Autocratic leaders are sometimes called **DIRECTIVE LEADERS**. Autocratic leaders tend to make independent decisions and try to manipulate others to agree or to approve ideas and/or actions.

- Group leaders need to assess their own control needs and facilitation skills. Group leading is a skill that can be developed but there are considerable variations in style and skill.

- An effective group leader needs to do the following:

  - Help individuals recognize and cope with someone who tries to monopolize group time.
  - Involve quiet or non-participating members.
  - Recognize and interpret body language.
  - Recognize that some learn without being very verbal.
  - Select appropriate groups.
  - Encourage feelings of safety and belonging.

Types of group leadership

- **KURT LEWIN** (1944) supported the concept of **DEMOCRATIC LEADERSHIP**. Lewin's key concepts were as follows:

  - Democratic behavior cannot be taught by autocratic methods.
  - Democratic leadership improves group efficiency.
  - Group discussion clarifies issues better than do lectures.
  - Member participation is more likely to result in behavior change.

- **DREIKURS** (1959) promoted using a family council to solve family problems--an application of group process. Democratic leadership is also called **NONDIRECTIVE LEADERSHIP** by Dreikurs. Effective democratic leaders:

  - Respect and trust group members.
  - Exhibit confidence that the group will meet its goals.
  - Encourage each member's problem-solving skills.
  - Accept each member's contribution and make it relevant.
  - Listen empathetically.
  - Test understanding and recap what is said.
  - Link contributions of different members.
  - Are able to accept criticism.
  - Make group members feel safe.
  - Can use influence to arouse emotion or quiet unrest.

Avoiding groupthink

- **GROUPTHINK** occurs when members of a group agree on an issue to avoid conflict or judgment of colleagues. Groupthink stifles creativity and preserves the status quo. To avoid groupthink:

  - The facilitator should encourage critical evaluation and accept criticism of him or herself.
  - The facilitator should assume an impartial stance instead of stating preferences and expectations.
  - The organization should set up several groups to evaluate policies and procedures and then compare findings.

➤ Before reaching a final consensus, group members should discuss the issues with qualified associates who are not part of the decision-making process.

➤ Experts should be brought in to challenge the group.

➤ At least one member of the group should be assigned to play the role of "devil's advocate" at each meeting.

➤ Feasibility and effectiveness should be considered in subgroups and then differences negotiated.

➤ There should be a "second chance" meeting to allow members to express doubts or reservations before a final decision is made.

b. Interviewing

(1) Techniques of questioning: open-ended, closed, leading

- **OPEN-ENDED QUESTIONS** are broad questions that allow freedom of response. They allow the client to explore an issue instead of offering a simple "yes" or "no" response. Open questions can start with "What," "How," or statements such as "Tell me more" and "Please, be more specific." Examples include: "What obstacles will you face when you try to implement these new behaviors?" "Tell me more about your concerns related to exercise."

- **CLOSED-ENDED QUESTIONS** are more restrictive and are usually answered with a "yes," "no" a short response. These questions do not encourage exploration and can lead to a dead-end in the counseling process. However, closed questions can be appropriate when obtaining specific data or focusing a client's response. Examples include: "Were you able to follow your food plan when traveling last week? Who purchases and prepares food at home? What foods do you usually eat between meals?"

- **LEADING QUESTIONS** can be used when the nutrition therapist understands the nature of the problem, has specific suggestions and feels comfortable assuming responsibility for helping the client work with a problem. Leading questions or comments are sometimes counter-productive in counseling. They may reveal the therapist's bias or assumptions, which may then lead to a distorted answer by the client. For example, asking what a client eats for breakfast may be considered a leading question because it assumes the client eats breakfast and may make the client alter his/her answer.

- **AFFIRMING** is when a counselor tells a client that what he or she is doing normal and understandable given the circumstances thus supporting the client's efforts to change behavior.

- **ALIGNMENT** is a supportive statement telling a client that the counselor understands and is with him or her in difficult times.

- **CONFRONTING** is a technique that challenges a client's statement with the intention of identifying inconsistencies between words and behaviors or actions and beliefs. It is a descriptive statement of a client's mixed messages or an identification of something that has been distorted by the client. Failure to confront, when appropriate, limits the effectiveness of the counseling process. However, confrontation that leads to an argument or makes a client defensive is not productive, so this technique should be used with caution.

- **DISCREPANCY** is when a change results in both positive and negative consequences. This strategy identifies conflicting feelings and provides an opportunity to evaluate a situation from multiple perspectives.

- **DOUBLE-SIDED REFLECTION** is a statement from the counselor describing a discrepancy between the client's current and previous words that provides an opening to examine behavior.

- **EMPATHY** is a technique by which the counselor accepts a client's feelings of turmoil about making changes or concern for a client's pain or difficulty.

- **MOTIVATIONAL INTERVIEWING** is a counseling style designed to achieve the willingness to change within a client/patient.

- **NEGOTIATION** is a strategy where client and counselor interaction allows for a compromise designed to achieve a specific goal.

- **NORMALIZATION** is a statement indicating that the client's behavior is perfectly within reason and normal, which validates the client's reaction to a specific situation.

- **REFLECTIVE LISTENING** is identifying what the client is feeling and stating that feeling.

- **REFRAMING** is a strategy in which the counselor changes the client's interpretation of the same basic data that he or she has given and offers a new viewpoint.

c. Counseling

(1) Techniques: motivational, behavioral, other

<u>Motivational techniques</u>

- When working with individuals struggling with behavior change, it is important to express empathy by reflective listening and understanding that the client's expressing ambivalence and reasons that block change is normal.

- Develop discrepancy and recognition that modifying any behavior has multiple consequences, both advantages and disadvantages.

- Avoid defensiveness or arguments by reducing confrontation and changing strategies if a client becomes defensive.

- Invite new perspectives to deal with resistance.

- Support self-efficacy and affirm client's ability to carry out change. Compliment freely about successes.

- Motivating techniques are intended to help the learner succeed in changing behavior. Threats are generally not motivating (e.g., "lose weight or you will have a stroke") and may provoke fear and stress rather than positive behavior changes. Effective motivating techniques support values and outcomes that truly matter to the client. Motivations are both internal and personal, and it is a therapist's job to help the client identify the appropriate motivating forces.

- **REWARDS** are positive consequences of behavior and may be used to reinforce positive eating behaviors. Rewards may be praise, improved appearance, better lab values, reduced pain or any positive consequence.

- **CONTRACTS** are written understandings between the counselor and the client that identify target behaviors. The contract specifies the role of both the counselor and the client in reaching mutually agreed upon goals, the reinforcement to be used, the frequency of reinforcement and who will provide the reinforcement.

- **FEEDBACK** is responding to the client's behaviors. Assume the client is making the best possible choice he or she can at the moment. Positive feedback can be reinforcement for desired behavior. For example, the client expresses disappointment in the food record she submits to the therapist. You might note that on four out of the seven days that she met her goal for fruits and vegetables. Behavioral changes will be maintained only if the learner sees positive results and satisfying outcomes.

Counselor motivation

- Healthcare workers' personal needs may affect the way they help others in what they say and do. It is important for a future RD or DTR to understand his or her reasons for entering the field. Some common personal needs are to help others, to have contact with people, to fulfill a personal commitment and to earn a living.

- Motives and needs that can negatively influence a helping situation include the following:
  - ➢ **NEED FOR CONTROL** or **NEED TO BE NEEDED:** Feeling needed or depended upon may cause the helper to extend a relationship beyond what is appropriate.
  - ➢ **NEED FOR POWER:** Feeling powerful can result in giving too much advice, taking too much control, or making threats for noncompliance.
  - ➢ **NEED TO BE LIKED:** Excessive need to be liked may cripple a counselor's ability to be honest with a client.
  - ➢ **NEED FOR PRESTIGE:** The need for prestige may color a counselor's ability to contend with failure and to report findings objectively.

Behavioral techniques

- The **INNOVATION-DECISION PROCESS** (Rogers-Shoemaker Change Process) is a sequence of events:
  - ➢ **Knowledge:** The individual is exposed to the innovation's existence and learns about it.
  - ➢ **Persuasion:** The individual forms a favorable or unfavorable attitude toward the innovation.
  - ➢ **Decision:** The individual engages in activities that lead to a choice to accept or reject the innovation.
  - ➢ **Confirmation:** The individual continues with the innovation or may reverse the previous decision if exposed to conflicting messages.

- The **HEALTH BELIEF MODEL** suggests that people are likely to follow health recommendations if they are motivated and if they believe that they are susceptible to illness; that the occurrence of the condition will have a serious impact on their lives; that following a particular set of health recommendations will be beneficial; and/or that the health recommendations will provide psychological benefits.

- In this model, prior beliefs and attitudes influence interpretations, effective learning is incremental, reinforcement is valuable, behavior is habitual and learning includes both knowledge and skills. By identifying a person's status on each variable in the health belief model, an educational diagnosis is made. This leads to formation of an educational plan directed toward modifying beliefs.

- The health belief model assumes the following:

  ➢ Clients bring their own set of beliefs, attitudes, motives, experiences, knowledge and expectations to the situation.
  ➢ Learning proceeds best when it is incremental.
  ➢ Behaviors that are reinforced or rewarded tend to be learned and repeated.
  ➢ Behavior patterns that affect health are learned early in life and are difficult to change.
  ➢ Learning has both a cognitive and a skill component.

- **STEWART'S BEHAVIORAL CHANGE PLAN** has three sequential steps:

  1. Divide nutrition information into a sequence of small manageable steps.
  2. Involve the client in planning the nutrition behavior change.
  3. State each change within a total nutrition instruction plan.

- Adults usually use one of three approaches to healthcare:

  ➢ **TRADITIONAL APPROACH**: This approach leads to change only if there is a symptom of illness or a disease exists. The individual seeks a physician to diagnose and cure the condition. This is the pattern for many acute conditions that develop suddenly and can be cured by specific medication.
  ➢ **PREVENTIVE APPROACH:** The focus is upon identifying risk factors and making behavior changes to prevent or minimize risk.
  ➢ **WELLNESS APPROACH:** The focus is making positive lifestyle choices to enhance physical and mental well-being. This approach can retard onset of chronic disease.

Individual counseling

- Understanding personal needs and motivations clarifies interpersonal relationships, including those in counseling and supervision. Needs should not be evaluated as good or bad, but by how they influence helping relationships. Helpers should establish systems for reevaluating their needs throughout their professionals careers.

- Individuals must be assured of confidentiality in group or individual counseling. The counselor must assure privacy and keep client records secure. Disclosure of names, conditions or other information shared by the counselor without the client's permission is a breach of professional ethics. Written records should be kept of each session. Counseling and all other interventions should be documented as to date and actions taken and shared with other members of the healthcare team as appropriate.

- The consultative process begins when a person seeks help in solving a problem, answering a question, making a decision or changing behavior. Steps of the consultative process are as follows:
  1. Develop rapport using appropriate interviewing techniques.

2. Gather information about the present situation during the interview and observation.

3. Set realistic short-term and long-term goals agreed to by the client and the counselor.

4. Introduce an intervention that will move the patient toward the desired goal (e.g., teach skills, control the stimulus, give positive reinforcement, model).

5. Provide follow up (reinforce successes; modify whatever is unsuccessful).

- If the counselor sees that the helping situation has become negative and is not reparable or that the client's priority needs cannot be met by the counselor's skills, the client should be referred to another counselor (dietitian, psychologist, physician, licensed clinical social worker, medical social worker, etc.)

- The counselor/teacher should determine what information the client needs to know to accomplish his/her objectives. For example, the counselor might determine if the client is eating appropriate portion sizes by asking specific questions related to measuring.

- Specific skills to be developed may require demonstration by a person with that skill and practice by the learner. For example, how does one give an insulin injection, measure blood sugar levels, breast-feed or operate a piece of food service equipment? Observation of the skill demonstrated by the learner confirms attainment of the basic skill. Further practice increases proficiency.

d. Methods of communication

Appropriateness of communication

- Use language materials appropriate for the client's educational level. Avoid professional jargon. Assess what the client knows before beginning counseling.

- Patients under extreme physical or mental stress (as when hospitalized for an illness) may not be receptive to counseling at that time. Express concern and arrange for counseling at a later date when nutrition intervention has a higher priority. Often a physician telling a patient that a dietary change is essential will increase receptivity.

- Sensitivity to the client's religious beliefs and cultural habits is essential for successful counseling. Financial resources and availability of kitchen facilities may influence the types of foods emphasized during counseling.

- Timing is essential to counseling. A client must be physically, psychologically and emotionally ready for counseling, otherwise the counseling will not be successful. Often timing of counseling is influenced by participation of family, caregivers or others who cook for or feed the patient. A shared undertaking of priorities for nutrition care promotes support of goals and compliance with the plan.

(1) Verbal/non-verbal

- **VERBAL COMMUNICATION** uses spoken words that are heard by one or more people. Techniques for good verbal communication include the following:

  ➢ Discuss problems descriptively rather than judgmentally.

➢ Describe situations as problems to be solved rather than as errors.
➢ Offer alternatives as suggestions rather than dictates.
➢ Treat clients as equals and treat everybody with respect.
➢ Be empathetic.
➢ Be aware of cultural and individual sensitivities (e.g., calling a person by his or her first name and making assumptions about sexuality or lifestyle.)

- **NONVERBAL COMMUNICATION** reflects feelings through facial expression, tone of voice, posture, eye contact, gestures and touch. The professional should maintain control of nonverbal communication to create a supportive environment and communicate interest, respect and concern. Non-verbal responses support effective communication. Techniques of non-verbal communication include the following:

  ➢ **Eye contact**: Look directly at the individual in a relaxed but serious way when listening or talking.
  ➢ **Body posture**: Posture should be relaxed, leaning forward slightly, facing the learner with hands in lap. Use occasional hand or arm movements to emphasize points.
  ➢ **Gestures**: Use occasional affirmative head nods, smiles and responsive expressions. Avoid sweeping gestures, which suggest power and may be threatening.
  ➢ **Vocal quality**: The voice should be pleasant, interested, conversational yet precise, and free of excessive slang, jargon or technical language.
  ➢ **Personal habits**: Avoid distracting habits like playing with hair or objects or tapping fingers.

- Non-verbal cues for Americans include:
  ➢ Shaking the head "no" while making an affirmative statement diminishes the meaning of the spoken words
  ➢ Tugging at one's collar exhibits discomfort or feelings of being trapped.
  ➢ Evading eye contact indicates uneasiness at being direct.
  ➢ Hands placed on hips demonstrate anger or feelings of dominance.
  ➢ Locked or crossed arms are defensive mechanisms or closed posture.
  ➢ Pointing or wagging of the index finger indicates a judgmental demeanor.
  ➢ Wide eyes with raised eyebrows may signify guilt or shock.
  ➢ Covering the mouth with the hand reveals a feeling of regret for something said or restraint about saying something.
  ➢ Clenched fists indicate indignation or conflict.
  ➢ Clenched jaw suggests outrage or defiance.
  ➢ Bouncing, swinging or crossed legs show excitement or anger.

- **FEEDBACK** is a listener's response after interpreting another's message. Listening is an active skill that assists in gathering data conveyed by sound (words, music, etc.) Effective listening builds trust and reduces misunderstanding.

- **To listen effectively:**
  ➢ Give your complete attention.
  ➢ Stop talking.
  ➢ Put the talker at ease.
  ➢ Show the speaker you want to listen.
  ➢ Remove distractions.

➢ Show empathy – listen to understand, not to reply.
➢ Do not interrupt.
➢ Be patient.
➢ Hold your temper.
➢ Restrict argument and criticism.
➢ Ask questions. Be nonjudgmental.
➢ Analyze content of main ideas.

Effective communication skills and techniques

- **RAPPORT** is a getting acquainted process designed to develop an empathetic and friendly working relationship. Rapport is established through **PACING**, the process of accepting a person as he or she is. Pacing is accomplished through open-ended questions, attentive silence, positive/open non-verbal behaviors, rephrasing and paraphrasing and encouragement to talk. The interviewee should be put at ease and relieved of anxiety. Keeping a client waiting for a long time increases anxiety and reduces rapport. Calling a client or employee by his or her preferred name, appropriate to the situation, increases rapport. For example, a teenager may be "Jane," a 78 year-old woman "Mrs. Smith."

- **MIRRORING** is a method of nonverbal pacing that imitates a person's movements. Mirroring must be unobtrusive. It can be very effective in situations where rapport is difficult.

- **EMPATHY** is the ability to accept another's feelings of turmoil and communicating a desire to understand what clients or employees are feeling. Empathic remarks do not have to agree with the other person but should demonstrate the desire to understand. Empathic listening, sometimes without words, communicates that you want to understand. People appreciate empathy but resent attempts to be manipulated by insincere responses.

- **JUDGMENT** and **BIAS** are opinions, conscious or unconscious, personal or professional, that may affect the way an individual sends and receives messages in a communication situation.

(2) Written

- **WRITTEN COMMUNICATION** is part of every nutrition professional's daily routine. It requires careful choice of word and format. It can be handwritten such as a letter, a memo, a note in an employee's record, documentation in a patient's chart or through various forms of technology such as word processing, e-mail, etc.

- **CHARTING** is an established format of communication that is available to all members of a healthcare team, written in language or code that is clearly understood by all. Notations on a patient's chart are used as a legal documentation of care.

- **E-MAIL (ELECTRONIC MAIL)** is a quick, accessible and fast way to communicate. It is a form of written communication, and as such, it can easily be archived. Archived materials are often used to back up arguments in a dispute. It may also not be the most efficient forum for discussion. There are other digital venues that may be more appropriate (e.g., chat rooms, blogs.) Some dietitians use e-mail to counsel clients, especially those who live in remote areas and cannot get to see the dietitian in person. E-mail allows 24-hour communication. When used for professional purposes, e-mails should be written as one would write a letter and e-mail communications and addresses should be professional with proper spelling and presentation. Those who do use e-mail for this purpose must be aware of legal, ethical and professional issues related to Internet communications. Emails provide a record of communication that can become legal documents. Email does not convey emotion as one can hear on the telephone, and one cannot see other non-verbal communication.

- **FACSIMILE (FAX)** is a method of transmitting reproductions of messages, photographs, charts, graphs and other hard copy media over telephone lines. It requires special equipment at the transmitting and receiving points. Some computer software permits faxes to be sent and received via modems. Ethically, no one should read a fax communication addressed to another person. As many people use shared fax machines, confidentiality cannot be assured.

(3) Media (e.g., print, electronic, social media)

- **OVERHEAD PROJECTORS** and **LCD PROJECTORS** are very effective teaching tools. However, the user must pay attention to the suggestions made in the section on instructional media because technology is not effective if it is not properly used or if it does not work.

- Use **INSTRUCTIONAL MEDIA** effectively when teaching classes, conducting individual counseling, making a presentation or training a group of employees.

  ➢ The material should be able to be seen by everyone in the room; it should be simple, conveying one idea at a time.
  ➢ Use few words and standardized lettering.
  ➢ Have a backup plan in the event you cannot use the media you planned.

- **VOICE MAIL** is a system to leave telephone messages and communicate with individuals and/or groups through assigned voice mailboxes. Voice mail allows 24-hour communication, but receiving the message is dependent upon regularly checking the voice mailbox. Messages should be clear and the caller's name and return telephone numbers said slowly and clearly.

- **TEXTING** is a way of communicating short written messages to users of smart phones. Text messages can be useful for confirming or changing appointments or sharing information or photos via phone.

- **MASS MEDIA** include television, radio, newspaper and magazines. Most people get nutrition information from mass media sources. By supplying the media with credible information, RDs boost the quality of reporting and the accuracy of the public's information about nutrition. To make the most of mass media as a means of communication, the professional should:

  ➢ Monitor the popular press, radio and television, especially those programs and publications that are popular among your clients or target audiences.
  ➢ Communicate with the media in meaningful terms (e.g., talk about food not nutrients; give examples from local hospitals or healthcare programs).
  ➢ Respond quickly when asked for information. If you do not know answers to questions, call someone who does or give the reporter a referral.
  ➢ As a speaker, send a quick, clear message; prepare carefully, dress appropriately.
  ➢ Write letters or make calls to compliment reporters and to clarify mistakes.
  ➢ Respect deadlines.

- **PRINT MEDIA** includes newspapers, magazines and other forms of communication that are traditionally on paper.

- **ELECTRONIC MEDIA** includes websites, mobile applications (apps), e-books, e-magazines and other methods of distributing content via computers and mobile devices such as smart phones and tablet PCs (e.g., iPad).

- **SOCIAL MEDIA** includes electronic communications, such as Facebook, Twitter, Google+ and other social media sites. See Domain 3 for information on social networking in the section on media relations.

(4) Technology (e.g., informatics)

- **INFORMATICS** is the acquisition, processing, storage and dissemination of information by a microelectronics-based combination of computing and telecommunications.

  ➢ Other methods of technologic communication include: cell phones, closed-circuit television, satellite communications, remote learning and/or conferencing, such as video conferencing or classes, on-line courses using *Blackboard* or other programs that do not necessarily use video, social networking, chat rooms, blogging and others. When using any of these devices for professional purposes, ethics and professionalism should be employed.

- **HEALTH INFORMATICS** is comprised of information science, computer science and healthcare. It deals with the resources, devices, and methods required to optimize the acquisition, storage, retrieval, and use of information in health and biomedicine. Health informatics tools include computers, clinical guidelines, formal medical terminologies, and information and communication systems. User controlled health informatics may include such things as Apps such as MyFitnessPal, devices like FitBit, and other similar tools and applications to monitor and mange one's own health.

4. Evaluation of educational outcomes

a. Measurement of learning

(1) Formative

- **FORMATIVE EVALUATION** is a diagnostic tool and takes place during development, planning and/or instructional phases of the educational program. Formative tests help determine weaknesses in the instructional plan so that improvements can be made.

(2) Summative

- **SUMMATIVE EVALUATION** analyzes the results of an educational program after it is fully operational. Summative tests evaluate the degree of achievement of program objectives.

- **PRODUCT EVALUATION** concentrates on specific products such as test scores, work samples and self-reported measures. The internal workings of a situation and how effects are achieved are reviewed in a **PROCESS EVALUATION**.

- **QUALITATIVE EVALUATIONS** are descriptive and concerned with capturing depth and experience detail. **QUANTITATIVE EVALUATIONS** are based on results from tests, questionnaires and surveys that yield numeric results.

- **OUTCOME-ORIENTED EVALUATION** is when the evaluation directly measures each major objective. For example, if the objective states that the learner will be able to safely and correctly operate a piece of equipment, pen and paper evaluation would not be appropriate. Observing the learner operating the equipment is the appropriate evaluation strategy.

- **COMPETENCY-BASED EVALUATION** is a demonstration that a person has achieved a specified level of knowledge, skill, behavior or attitude. Merely completing a specific course or treatment program does not demonstrate a person's competency. For example, the situation-based questions on the RD exam are designed to test competency and ability to apply what has been learned in the classroom and educational programs.

- **PROCESS-ORIENTED EVALUATION** evaluates the learning situation or teaching program but does not indicate learning is actually occurring. It is useful to evaluate or compare teaching methods, for example, comparing videotaped diet instructions to instructions given personally by dietetics staff.

- **VARIATIONS/COMBINED EVALUATION** are other evaluations that combine elements of process and outcome evaluation. The educator can measure participant behavior changes and responses to various teaching methods.

- Direct and indirect measures can be used to assess effectiveness. Ongoing evaluation helps the instructor determine progress toward learning objectives and adjust instruction according to learner needs.

- **PRE-TESTS** determine knowledge, attitude and/or behavior before instruction takes place.

- **POST-TESTS** evaluate the effectiveness of instruction by measuring the change of knowledge, skill behavior or attitude from the pretest level.

- Low rates of dropouts and good attendance indicate successful programs. High dropout rates may indicate a need for screening clients for readiness or reevaluation of instructional strategies used. Follow-up assessment at three months, six months or one year post-instruction provides valuable information about educational effectiveness.

- The timing of an assessment should be appropriate to objectives. Are desired behavioral changes short or long-term goals? Evaluations must be conducted at appropriate times for results and actions to be measured and valid.

- Evaluation techniques should be appropriate for the stated objectives and the learner's educational, physical and social characteristics. For example, evaluating a dietetics student's interview of a client is an inappropriate evaluation if the current objective is for the student to list the steps and outline the material for a patient interview.

- Problems in evaluation often result from improperly written objectives. If performance is not stated in measurable terms, conditions are omitted or criteria are missing, it is difficult to create a test situation that measures effectiveness or accuracy.

- Actual costs should be evaluated against the projected budget. Cost areas to be evaluated include developmental and instructional time, materials and supplies, equipment, testing devices and personnel. Costs such as publicity, phones, travel, rent and insurance should also be considered. Developmental and instructional costs divided by the number of clients served by the program provide an INSTRUCTIONAL COST INDEX for the program.

$$\textbf{Instructional Cost Index} = \frac{\textbf{Total Development + Instructional Cost}}{\textbf{Number of Clients}}$$

- Evaluation should be based on the institutional objectives for offering the program. For example: Was institutional visibility improved? Are more community members using the institution? Is patient length of stay appropriate?

- Evaluations of presentations usually include comments from the participants. Was the instructor prepared? Was the program well organized and sequenced? Were the educational strategies appropriate for the audience? Were educational materials of good quality and relevant to the population? Was the facility comfortable?

- The evaluation process includes documentation of process and outlines including recording results in both the clients' records and the department's records as a quality assurance measure. Are scores on rating of services cards improving? Is plate waste more or less after menu changes?

Evaluation of group behavior

- Having observers present may alter the behavior of group participants.

- Evaluating group behavior requires trained observers who can identify key roles of group members. It is best to work from videos of group sessions since there is opportunity to slow actions, especially when multiple things are happening in a group process.

- Recording forms keep a running account of disagreements, agreements, decisions, topics, unresolved issues and so forth. Observers note how group members deal with issues. Task oriented groups can use reaction sheets at the end of a meeting to assess the success of a meeting and how members feel personally about the group.

- Whether it is a formal or informal work group, each group displays unique patterns of interaction as members get to know and trust each other, becoming more comfortable. Group participants and facilitators should develop the following skills: functioning as initiators, information and opinion seekers, clarifiers, coordinators, orienters, supporters, harmonizers, tension-relievers and gatekeepers. A group may be convened for many reasons and each dictates a different format. A meeting may be called for exchange of information, brainstorming, problem solving, instruction, education, training, sharing of experiences or ideas, decision-making, planning, evaluation or recreation.

Evaluation tools

- Several evaluation tools are available to the educator. The educational experience should be carefully reviewed to ensure selection of the most appropriate tool since each has unique characteristics, uses, advantages, limitations and rules for construction.

- **OBJECTIVE TESTS** include multiple-choice, recall, matching and true-false tests. Multiple-choice tests include items with one right answer, a best answer, association types, analogy types and reverse (or the most incorrect) responses. Recall tests may be simple recall, identification, recall to a problem or situation and listing or enumeration. Matching tests may require item identification, term and definition pairing or combining problems and solutions. True-false test construction may require evaluation of a single statement or cluster of phrases. Modified true-false tests may require justification or alteration of items marked false.

- Essays and other subjective tests assess higher mental processes than objective tests. Essay test items elicit restricted and unrestricted responses. Unrestricted responses reveal depth and scope of knowledge, originality and critical thinking. The restricted response is related to more specific areas and stresses organizational skill.

- Evaluation of advanced information or assessment of depth of knowledge may be accomplished by oral examinations. These exams are subjective and vary with the situation. A specialized type of oral examination, the **TRIPLE JUMP EXAMINATION** has been used to evaluate problem-based learning formats because it incorporates the hypothesis-generating, problem-solving and independent study components that comprise a problem-based format.

- **PRACTICAL EXAMINATIONS** are useful for evaluating learning that has been hands-on or experiential because actual performance is assessed. When tasks are organized into discrete units for the purpose of assessing specific objectives or abilities, the format is also called an **OBJECTIVE STRUCTURED CLINICAL EXAM (OSCE)**. Practical examinations require careful construction to be an accurate reflection of the learning situation and need highly standardized materials for use or observation by the students. The practical examination is not limited to its original use in evaluating laboratory knowledge. It is also appropriate when assessing any performance based activity that can be broken into stages, e.g., nutrition assessment, nutrition counseling, food service operation activities and one that employs complex tools such as computer images, laboratory and x-ray reports, spread sheets and food service equipment.

- **DISCUSSIONS** can evaluate thinking and depth of knowledge. A discussion develops thinking skills when participants challenge one another for reasons and examples and present counter arguments. These skills are also revealed when participants discuss worthwhile materials, present relationships between the subject under discussion and other relevant experiences and general principles and ask relevant questions.

- **CONCEPT MAPS** are drawings that show the mental connections made among concepts. Learners may compare their maps with peers and the instructor to develop meta-cognitive skills. Educational programs that require conceptual learning with high theoretical content can benefit from concept map evaluation.

- A **PORTFOLIO** is a collection of evidence that demonstrates the acquisition of skills, knowledge, attitudes, understanding and achievement. Portfolios are useful for both formative and summative evaluations; they could be labeled a "learning resume." Portfolios are not intended to be a stand-alone evaluation tool, but to complement additional evaluation techniques. Portfolios may vary in scope, organizational strategy and appearance, but to document proficiency in knowledge and skills four types of documentation have been identified. These include:

- ➤ **ARTIFACTS** are actual samples of student work.
- ➤ **REPRODUCTIONS** are examples that lend a permanent nature to typically transient events, e.g., photographs.
- ➤ **ATTESTATIONS** are documents about the learner's performance that are written by someone other than the learner.
- ➤ **PRODUCTIONS** are statements prepared for the portfolio that identify knowledge and skills gained as displayed in the portfolio, e.g., captions on pictures or an essay about the value of a specific experience that is shown in the portfolio.

- **UNOBTRUSIVE MEASURES** may be useful in evaluating the effects of educational programs. Examples include the rate at which mats wear out near exhibits, checkout frequencies of specific library resources and repurchase of specific products (e.g., disposable cups).

- **SELF-EVALUATION** may consist of journals and records, checklists, self-reported attitudinal scales and self-critiques of role-play or simulation activities. Self-evaluation can also assess personal continuing education needs.

5. Client information

a. Records

- **RECORDS** are a systematic documentation of a patient'/client's individual healthcare history. The medical record is comprised of both the physical chart and the totality of the information for each patient's/client's health history. Due to the nature of the personal data contained in a medical record, there are many ethical and legal issues surrounding confidentiality relative to third party access, appropriate storage and disposal.

b. Confidentiality

- **CONFIDENTIALITY** is the assurance that private personal information will not be revealed to anyone who is not directly been authorized to receive that information. All medical and financial information is confidential.

- Confidentiality and privacy of health information is set by The federal Health Insurance Portability and Accountability Act (HIPAA), implemented in 2003. These standards only apply to health records maintained by healthcare providers, health plans and health clearinghouses and only if the facility transmits records in electronic form.

- Forms may be signed to permit the sharing of medical or other information to specific individuals, family members, insurers or agencies.

- The Code of Ethics of the AND requires that members maintain the confidentiality of information about clients, patients, etc.

- Business contracts often require that the person receiving information about business practices, procedures, plans, finances or other information maintain confidentiality and not disclose that information to other parties. Failure to maintain confidentiality can have severe legal consequences and financial penalties.

6. Documentation

- The Joint Commission on Accreditation of Healthcare Organizations (JCAHO) requires documentation of dietetics services. The information is necessary for evaluation of medical nutrition therapy and any legal issues that may arise.

- Documentation is a method of communicating with other health professionals as to patient tolerance of food, counseling and other education provided. Records can be used for research, to confirm referrals, or to obtain reimbursement for services.

- Insurance companies require documentation of nutrition services given on an outpatient basis to assess whether or not dietetics services were effective.

- Documentation of employee training and education is necessary for safety issues, keeping the staff informed of current policies and procedures and the correct use of all equipment.

7. Orientation and training

- All new employees should be offered a well-planned **ORIENTATION PROGRAM.** This familiarizes and acquaints a new employee to the organization, the department, and the job responsibilities. A good orientation program will save productive time because the employee will be able to carry out the responsibilities of the job in a timely fashion and learn proper ways to carry out the requirements of the position.

- **TRAINING PROGRAMS** differ from orientation programs in that training programs should teach or improve skills and concepts. A primary objective of training is to keep skills at a good level or to improve performance to acceptable levels. Training programs should also be established for employees you think may have the potential to be promoted. Retraining may be necessary for current employees who are not performing at a high enough level or if the job or equipment has changed since initial employment.

TOPIC D – RESEARCH

RESEARCH is learning about unobserved phenomena by studying and interpolating relevant data on observed phenomena.

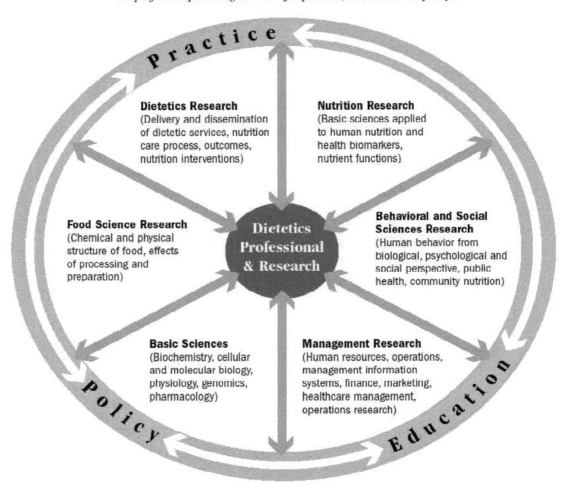

Research: Foundation of the Dietetics Profession

The American Dietetic Association believes that research is the foundation of the profession providing the basis for practice, education and policy.

Practice

Dietetics Research
(Delivery and dissemination of dietetic services, nutrition care process, outcomes, nutrition interventions)

Nutrition Research
(Basic sciences applied to human nutrition and health biomarkers, nutrient functions)

Food Science Research
(Chemical and physical structure of food, effects of processing and preparation)

Dietetics Professional & Research

Behavioral and Social Sciences Research
(Human behavior from biological, psychological and social perspective, public health, community nutrition)

Basic Sciences
(Biochemistry, cellular and molecular biology, physiology, genomics, pharmacology)

Management Research
(Human resources, operations, management information systems, finance, marketing, healthcare management, operations research)

Policy

Education

Dietetics is the integration and application of principles derived from the science of nutrition, biochemistry, physiology, food management and behavioral and social sciences to achieve and maintain people's health.

Scientists from many disciplines contribute to the categories of research used by the dietetics professional. Descriptors of each category of research found in the wedges are for illustrative purposes and not intended to be limiting, as there are other emerging areas of research.

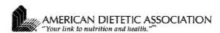

AMERICAN DIETETIC ASSOCIATION
"Your link to nutrition and health."

Reprinted with permission of The Academy of Nutrition and Dietetics.

1. **Types of research and research design**

- The purpose of research is to gain and/or verify information. The researcher must be able to use scientific methodology to explore and formulate concepts, design studies, collect and evaluate data and write clear and concise conclusions based on the results of the research.

- For a comprehensive review of research in dietetics practice, refer to Elaine R. Monsen and Linda Van Horn (ed.), *Research: Successful Approaches* 3rd edition, Academy of Nutrition and Dietetics, Chicago, IL, 2008.

Types of research

- **BASIC RESEARCH** is also called "pure" or "fundamental" research. This type of research is done not with a specific goal, but to increase a body of knowledge and explore the unknown; for example, examining the structure of vitamin antioxidants. In basic research, all variables are subject to rigorous controls as in laboratory studies. In applied research involving human subjects, there are more independent variables, making control harder to achieve.

- **APPLIED RESEARCH** takes known information, goods and/or services and attempts to substantiate, solve problems or rework existing concepts, information and products. Applied research is used to support operational decision making. General steps to conduct applied research are:
  1. Identify problem and assess need. Research may evolve from problems encountered in practice; from desires to increase effectiveness, test concepts published in the literature or from interest in applying techniques from other disciplines to the practice of dietetics. The focus should be on one component that is feasible to study in the setting. The research should start with a simple question.
  2. Search the literature. Review both current scientific literature and classic articles. A critical review of previous studies can be the basis of solid research. Contact people interested in and/or experienced in the research area.
  3. Develop a hypothesis. A **HYPOTHESIS** is a supposition, arrived at by inductive reasoning, which declares a probable outcome of a study and acts as a guide to the kind of data to be collected and the methods of analysis. The object of research is to test the hypothesis. Many studies use a null hypothesis. A **NULL HYPOTHESIS** is a statement that there is no relationship between the variables (as one changes the other stays the same) or that there is no difference between groups (e.g., between those who did receive services and those that did not).
  4. Design the study to test the hypothesis. An experimental study design must describe sample selection, assignment to treatment groups, interventions, equipment or measurement instruments to be used, where and how data will be gathered, plans for data analysis and a schedule of activities. A proposal may be submitted to solicit funds to conduct the research or to obtain approval of the instructional review board.
  5. Conduct a pilot study to refine the study design and examine preliminary data.
  6. Begin the study.
  7. Gather the data.
  8. Analyze and evaluate data using appropriate statistical methods.
  9. State conclusions, applications and areas needing additional study.
  10. Disseminate (publish) the research study.

- Both basic and applied research are necessary in the development of information and knowledge in the field. For example, the structure of a vitamin (identified in basic research) was used to develop synthetic vitamins. Applied research is used to analyze and clarify associations between risk factors and disease.

- In conducting research, there are 6 general steps to integrate scientific principles:
  1. Define the problem.
  2. Determine the probable causes.
  3. Determine alternative solutions.
  4. Select the best solution.
  5. Test the solution.
  6. Evaluate.

Types of research design

- The research design is based on the question(s) to be studied. Time, space, number of subjects, ethical considerations and available resources determine research design.

Quantitative research

- **QUANTITATIVE STUDIES** collect numerical data or statistics.

- In **EXPERIMENTAL RESEARCH** design, all factors are held constant except those manipulated by the experimenter to determine cause and effect on the experimental group and to compare those results to the control group. Essential components of experimental research include:

  ➢ Randomized selection of subjects from a fairly homogenous population (population refers to the entire group from which subjects can be selected.) **RANDOM** means that everyone in that particular population has an equal chance of being chosen (e.g., random selection of all 9th graders in the city of Portland, Oregon). The subjects selected are the sample.

  ➢ Randomized assignment of subjects to a treatment (experimental) group or control (comparison) group.

  ➢ The **CONTROL GROUP** may be given routine, traditional care and/or medication. An untreated group is used as control only if there is no recognized treatment. The control group may be given placebos to keep subjects and sometimes researchers, unaware of the group to which they were assigned. See "blind" and "double blind" studies.

  ➢ The **DENOMINATOR** for a performance measure, is the sample of cases that will be observed to determine conformance to medical review criteria. Number of patients (universe or sample) who have a specific condition or procedure.

  ➢ The **NUMERATOR** for a performance measure, is the cases in the denominator group that experience events specified in the medical review criterion as evidence of guideline conformance.

  ➢ Careful observation and factual recording of outcomes following or are concurrent with intervention or treatment of both groups is required.

  ➢ **TREATMENT** is the independent variable or cause of the outcome. Treatment may be experimental intervention or control treatment.

  ➢ **REPEATED-MEASURE DESIGNS,** also called **WITHIN-SUBJECT DESIGNS,** expose the same persons to multiple treatments rather than assigning different treatments to different groups. The variations in response to different treatments are measured. The time between treatments is planned to eliminate delayed response to earlier treatments. For example, the researcher gives the patient the same medication but in different dosages, and blood pressure is measured as a response to the dosage variable.

> **CASE MIX** is the distribution of a group of patients into categories reflecting differences in patients' diagnoses/conditions.

> For a **CASE REPORT,** data gathered on one subject forms a design. **CASE SERIES** deals with more than one subject. The researcher classifies subjects by similar diagnoses and determines which variables are significant in the care and treatment of future subjects with the same diagnoses.

- **CROSS-SECTIONAL STUDIES** are based on data collected on a group of subjects at a single time (e.g., testing all 14-year-old males in a particular school system to determine average body weight of that group.)

- **TIME-SERIES DESIGNS** consist of observations over time of a single group (such as an annual survey) or across groups at a single time. This design is useful in identifying and tracking trends.

- **RANDOMIZED CLINICAL TRIAL** is a clinical trial in which treatments are randomly assigned to the subjects. The random allocation eliminates bias in the assignment of treatments to patients and establishes the bases for statistical analysis.

- **LONGITUDINAL STUDIES** follow the same sample group over a prolonged period. Baseline measurements made at the beginning of the study are compared with measures taken at a later date or at various intervals (e.g., testing heights of the same 100 boys each year from birth through age 18).

- **PROSPECTIVE STUDIES** begin with the belief that a particular behavior or variable will create a particular outcome; that is, if a certain dietary action will later cause a particular outcome or disease. An example is the Framingham study of dietary change to reduce incidence of heart disease.

- **RETROSPECTIVE STUDIES** look at manifestations of an outcome and then attempt to uncover causes or relationships by going back in time; such as, a view of past dietary practices of individuals who have developed kidney stones.

- **QUASI-EXPERIMENTAL RESEARCH,** also called **OBSERVATIONAL RESEARCH,** resembles experimental research but does not have a control group. Each subject serves as his/her own control. It may be used when all independent variables cannot be easily manipulated. It is characterized by partial control such as the inability to truly randomize treatment assignments.

- **COHORT (FOLLOW-UP) STUDY** follows the experimental group over a period of time to observe and record the experiences of its members. The investigator is the only person who records and reports. Cohort studies test a hypothesis but do not involve investigator in manipulation of variables. A **COHORT** is a group of persons with a similar characteristic or factor of interest that is followed over an extended period of time. Cohort studies are used to study diseases and the impact of lifestyle characteristics. Many subjects are needed to compare incidences between groups with different exposures. Some cohort studies involve hundreds of thousands of individuals.

- **CASE CONTROL STUDIES** are used to explore individual histories by comparing prevalence of exposure to factors of interest in individuals who have a disease with others without a disease. These studies are less expensive than cohort studies and are particularly useful in studying the etiology of rare diseases. Problems with case control studies include determining whether a factor was the cause or result of the disease, difficulty or bias in recalling information and the comparability of cases and controls.

- **NON-EXPERIMENTAL RESEARCH DESIGNS** may include historical, descriptive, case control and correlation studies. These types of research observe or document present and past information. No direct manipulation of cause and effect is possible, although outcomes may be inferred. An example would be a study of food intake patterns of Colonial Americans found in journals, diaries and letters, with inference to nutritional deficiencies suffered by that population.

Qualitative research

- **QUALITATIVE RESEARCH** can be characterized as a systematic approach using methods of inquiry that capture the subjective experience and its meaning for the individual using the subject's own language and narrative summaries. Generally this type of research is used to investigate human behavior.

- **GROUNDED THEORY RESEARCH** collects observations from real-life situations in order to develop theoretical propositions.

- **ETHNOGRAPHIC STUDIES** deal with identifying cultural behavior for a particular societal group from the perspective of individuals of that group. Participant observation and interviewing is the cornerstone of ethnography.

- **FOCUS GROUPS** are informal groups of about 5 to 12 people who are asked to share their concerns, experiences, belief, opinions or problems. Focus group interviews provide qualitative information that help managers develop a plan of action. They are less expensive to conduct than individual interviews and can result in information of a sensitive nature that might otherwise be difficult or costly to obtain.

- **PHENOMENOLOGICAL RESEARCH** explores the meaning of events and interactions to ordinary people in particular situations. Those who do this research deal with varied cognitive, subjective perceptions of reality and do not assume they know what things mean to the people they are studying.

Other research

- **EPIDEMIOLOGICAL RESEARCH** is used to develop focuses on the priorities for healthcare planning by studying disease patterns, frequency of disease (incidence and prevalence) and potential etiological and risk factors. This method of research may use vital statistics, records, screening tests and surveys to qualify the extent and identification of diet and nutrition-related problems within a population and suggest associations among factors.

- **CLINICAL TRIALS** are studies that are interventions to evaluate treatments and their effectiveness. In clinical trials there is an entire reference population, which can be divided into an eligible group and an ineligible group. Among those eligible and willing to participate, the group is divided into participants and non-participants in the trial. Among the participants, there is further segmentation into the treatment group and the control group with random selection between groups. In clinical trials the study is stopped if an intervention, procedure, food or medication puts and individual or group at health risk.

- **MEDICAL NUTRITION THERAPY PROTOCOL** is a plan or set of steps, developed through a consultative process by experts and practitioners. This plan incorporates current professional knowledge and available research, and clearly defines the level, content and frequency of nutrition care that is appropriate for a disease or condition to be followed in a study. This type of research establishes the evidence for or against continuation of certain practices.

Principles of research

- **CONTROL OF VARIANCE** is important. Variance items to consider include variables, the measurements collected in research and the characteristics of persons that vary within the study population.

- **DEPENDENT VARIABLES** are the outcome variables of interest (e.g., serum cholesterol).

- **INDEPENDENT VARIABLES** are those variables that are thought to influence the dependent variable and that are manipulated by the study design (e.g., fiber intake).

- The **SAMPLE SIZE** is the number of subjects. The sample size must be large enough to provide adequate data for statistical correlation. When the group is small, the findings cannot be extrapolated to larger populations.

Types of samples

- **RANDOM SAMPLE** is drawn from the entire target population. All members of the target population have an equal probability of being included in the sample. Random sample studies are likely to represent the target population and can be used to make generalizations if the sample is large enough.

- **STRATIFIED RANDOM SAMPLES** are taken when a larger group is divided into subcategories, or strata, according to one or more characteristics. Subjects are selected randomly from within the stratum being examined (e.g., females within specified ZIP codes with median incomes of X dollars).

- **SYSTEMATIC SAMPLING** is a procedure for selecting a probability sample when lists of the population are readily available (e.g., every eighth member on a mailing list is selected for a sample).

- **CLUSTER SAMPLE** is a procedure that first samples a larger group and then specific subgroups or units (e.g., triglyceride values of RNs in Illinois; triglyceride values of RNs in urban hospitals in Illinois).

- **ACCIDENTAL SAMPLES** occur when subjects are readily available but not screened for characteristics. This is a non-probability, non-random sampling method (e.g., first hundred individuals willing to sample a food in a grocery store taste test).

- In a **CORRELATED SAMPLE** homogeneous pairs (siblings, twins, individuals matched by diagnosis, etc.) are identified and assigned to separate test groups.

- In **INDEPENDENT SAMPLES,** no relationship exists between individuals in two or more groups.

Control of bias

- **BIAS** is a distortion of results caused by some factor other than those under study. Bias can mask the true relationship between the factors and the outcome.

- Possible psychological effects of testing on researchers and/or subjects can be alleviated by a **BLIND STUDY** in which subjects do not know if they are in the treatment or control group. In a **DOUBLE BLIND STUDY,** neither subjects nor research staff know if subjects are in the treatment or control group. A double blind study design is harder to administer but eliminates bias as a variable. It is more difficult to do feeding or food studies that are blind or double blind than pharmaceutical studies, which are typically blind studies.

- Subjects who volunteer for research studies are typically highly motivated and anxious to comply and respond correctly. This anxiety and need for approval is called **EVALUATION APPREHENSION.** The integrity of the study is compromised if the subjects know whether they are in the treatment or control group.

- Sometimes results are tainted because subjects respond to what they believe are expectations or simply because they are participants (even if assigned to the control group). This is called the **PLACEBO EFFECT.** For example, an inert sugar pill (placebo) that looks like the medication is taken by a control group, while an experimental group takes a similar looking active drug. The subject taking the placebo often reports positive effects even though he or she has taken a inert medication.

Control and nonequivalent control groups

- Selection of an appropriate control group depends on the hypothesis. Controls should be representative of the population under study. Nonequivalent control groups include:
  - ➢ **MATCHED GROUPS** occur when experimental and control groups are similar in size and number and may constitute naturally occurring assemblies, but the subjects have not been randomly assigned from a population to either the experimental or the control group.
  - ➢ **SELF-SELECTION** occurs when subjects choose to be in an experimental (treatment) group. Results of treatment effects are blurred because subjects may be particularly motivated to seek treatment.

Accuracy and precision of method

- **COMPLIANCE** means strict adherence to the study design. A research study needs a high level of compliance because deviations from the standard research protocol affect the results. Common types of noncompliance include dropout or attrition rate, failure to comply with protocol and change in motivation, lifestyle, etc. Noncompliance rates are increased in long and demanding studies.

- **ACCURACY** is a quantitative measure of the validity of an instrument. For example, one cup of flour has a specific standard weight in grams but measured cups of flour may differ (slightly) from that number of grams. Accuracy requires specific techniques, measures and calibrations.

- **PRECISION** is a quantitative measure of the reliability of an instrument, described by the amount of variation that occurs randomly. (Measurement and reporting are discussed in later sections.

Ethical considerations

- Ethics are important in the choice of topics, study populations, methodologies, interventions, data collection procedures and research summaries, including reports of data sampling errors.

- Any present or potential conflicts of interest must be stated (stock in company, consultant to company, etc.) by the researcher.

- Sources of funding for research must be reported. A lot of research is supported by industry that provides funding to provide a research base on which to position products, etc. The researcher has an ethical obligation to state the funding source and publish all findings, both positive and negative findings. Funders may resist publication of failed efforts or products.

- Procedures to ensure confidentiality and prevent identification of study participants must be established for record keeping, data storage, data retrieval, follow-up, computing and reporting. For example, code numbers or initials should be used instead of names to identify subjects; faces in photos should be blocked.

- Care must be taken to report all research data, both positive results and negative results. It is unethical to skew the selection of study participants, to report only part of the findings, or fail to report the response rate.

- **HUMAN SUBJECTS REVIEWS** should evaluate ethical conduct and the potential risks and benefits of a study. Ethical guidelines protect the rights, privacy and well-being of study subjects. For example, medications or nutrients known to cause birth defects would not be given to pregnant women. Institutions generally require all subjects to sign an **INFORMED CONSENT** document that describes the nature of the study, expectations and all potential risks before participation in a study. Participants receiving placebos must sign an informed consent, since they do not know whether they will be in a control or an experimental group.

- A **SUBJECT AT RISK** is an individual who might be exposed to the possibility of physical, psychological or other harm as a consequence of participating in research that goes beyond accepted methods to meet needs. Risk is a matter of professional ethics and judgment. Risks (real or potential) must be clearly identified and made known to every subject.

- An oversight or advisory committee must be available to review procedures related to subject privacy, confidentiality and well-being. A review board should review protocol to ensure ethical conduct and to evaluate potential risks and benefits. If potentially dangerous side effects or results begin to appear in a study, either the researcher or the review board may intervene to stop the study and avoid possible damage to subjects.

FORMAT OF A RESEARCH PUBLICATION

- **Title:** A clear, descriptive title will facilitate referencing after publication.
- **Abstract:** An **ABSTRACT** is a short description of the research study that includes objectives of study, a brief description of methodology, results, and principle conclusions. Abstracts are usually limited to 250 words.
- **Introduction:** The introduction presents the problem and provides background information, including purpose of study, hypothesis, and review of literature.
- **Methods:** This section describes research design, instrumentation, and method of data collection. Selection and description of subjects and methods of data analysis are included.
- **Results:** This section includes statistical results, response rates of subjects, reasons for incomplete data and dropout rates, description of study population, and examination of variables.
- **Discussion:** This section includes the researcher's interpretation of results, which can be compared or contrasted with similar studies or previous data, and generalizations (inferences) that can be made. Limitations of the study should be stated.
- **Future research:** The researcher may have encountered problems that warrant future study. This section is not usually required but is suggested in some research formats.
- **Key references:** Books, articles, interviews, etc. are listed in correct scientific citation form.
- **Appendices:** Appendices include samples of tests, questionnaires, or other information used in the research

---

RESEARCH EVALUATION CHECKLIST

REQUIREMENTS:
- The researcher has clearly stated what the problem was and the specific area being observed.
- The researcher has indicated exactly how the problem was observed.
- The researcher has precisely described the subject group.
- Data are accurately reported using appropriate statistical methods.

OTHER CONSIDERATIONS:
- Prior research was reviewed.
- Appropriate length of time of observation.
- Appropriate number of subjects.
- Data presented showing the relationship between the subjects and the research done on them.
- Identification of other outside variables, either direct or indirect, that may have interfered with the results of the study.
- Extent that data are significant in demonstrating a relationship between cause and effect of the research. Results lend themselves to being extrapolated to a larger population.
- Results of the study show that the numerical data and analysis lead to a proper conclusion.
- References appropriate, current and in correct format.
- Researcher offers other possibilities for future research on this topic (optional)

2. Statistical evaluation, interpretation and application

Evaluation of research literature

- Most major journals are published by professional organizations. Other sources are Internet research sites such as The National Library of Medicine; indices, such as *Applied Science and Technology Index*; abstracts and annual reviews, such as *Biological Abstracts*; and unpublished dissertations and theses. Research presented in professional publications usually has been peer reviewed for proper research methodology prior to publication.

- **PEER REVIEW** is the primary method that the science community uses to monitors itself. Experts in the field who have first-hand knowledge of the research topic conduct peer reviews. They critically review the research for scientific accuracy, cohesiveness, clarity and contribution to the knowledge in the field.

- **NON-PEER REVIEW** is conducted by individuals who do not necessarily have professional expertise in the area, but are connected to the review process by other factors. For example, students may serve on an editorial board for alumni publications that print accepted articles but do not send them out for peer review.

- Summaries of research articles or selected parts of research are often printed or shared via the Internet or in product publicity. This is largely unmonitored and may reflect the bias of the reviewer or a commercial interest rather than the facts confirmed by journal peer review.

- **REVIEW OF RESEARCH** is a summary of seminal and significant research on specific topics. The reviewer is not in a position to determine if the data are accurate. Reputations can be destroyed and/or grant moneys confiscated when falsified data are discovered. The scientific community demands and expects correct data. If the study is replicated using the same information and the results differ, the initial researchers must justify their conclusions.

- **META-ANALYSIS** of research literature is an approach which summarizes the statistical results of controlled empirical studies and clinical trials, particularly when the individual research sample size is too small to be statistically significant or when investigators disagree over the findings. By combining the results from multiple studies, researchers may estimate the strength of the relationship between two variables of interest or test the overall significance level by combining probability levels from studies with similar hypotheses.

- Controversial studies are usually replicated numerous times before the scientific community will take a position, especially if the results are to be given as advice to the public. Studies that are in conflict with each other may be presented with the understanding that the issue is being studied by a number of researchers and that no conclusions can be made at the time. For example, if studies on caffeine used adult male subjects, can we say the results would be the same if the subjects were female? No, testing would be required to determine the effects of caffeine on adult females.

- **STATISTICAL METHODS** are used to describe data (e.g., mean, variance) and to infer results to a larger population (significance tests).

  - ➤ The **CHI-SQUARE TEST** is used to show the relationship between two categorical variables (e.g., treatment A and treatment B).
  - ➤ **MCNEMAR'S TEST** compares two correlated samples (e.g., patients matched by diagnosis and receiving the same treatment).
  - ➤ The **T-TEST** is used to determine how significant the differences are between the mean scores of two groups or samples.
  - ➤ The **PAIRED T-TEST** is usually used in an investigation in which a continuous response measure is observed before and after the subject receives a treatment, or in which observations of two groups are linked by pairing.
  - ➤ **ANALYSIS OF CO-VARIANCE** is generally a more efficient statistical significance test than the T-Test when the response measure is related to the initial measure, as are the data. In analysis of covariance, the slope of linear regression of initial data is compared to the slope of linear regression of resulting data.
  - ➤ The **PEARSON PRODUCT MOMENT CORRELATION CO-EFFICIENT** is the most common effect size indicator of correlational studies. Cohen applied general descriptive terms to small ($r=0.10$), medium ($r=0.30$) and large ($r=0.50$) effect sizes. Effect sizes relate the sample group to the overall population and support the validity of the research.
  - ➤ **Z-SCORES** convert scores from two or more different tests into standard units. The Z-score tells how many standard deviations a value lies above or below the mean of the data set to which it belongs.
  - ➤ The difference between **ONE-SIDED SIGNIFICANCE TESTS** and **TWO-SIDED SIGNIFICANCE TESTS** rests with the hypothesis. If the hypothesis specifies in advance that the treatment group is different (either positively or negatively) from the control group, the test is one sided; if no direction is given, it is two sided. Usually a two-sided test should be used.

Validity and reliability

- **VALIDITY** means the ability of a test or an instrument to measure what it intends to measure. For example, exam questions on standardized tests must be evaluated for validity before they count in scored tests.

- **EXTERNAL VALIDITY** is the extent to which one can generalize the study conclusions to populations and settings.

- **RELIABILITY** is the extent to which the measurement can be replicated. It means consistency of results by a measuring instrument when applied to the same specimen repeatedly by the same or different persons. For example, recipes specifying 400 grams of flour.

- **REPLICATION** is the attempt to reproduce the method and results of earlier research to determine validity of the original study. Successful replication confirms the original results and demonstrates reliability.

Interpreting results

- To interpret results, the researcher must first analyze or summarize data and draw conclusions. Then the researcher must make decisions based on those conclusions. Researchers should state limitations of the research; such as, the sample is not representative of a larger population of cases, or generalizations may need to be confirmed by further studies.

Descriptive statistics

- **FREQUENCY DISTRIBUTIONS** are arrangements of numbers on a graph showing the number of times that a given score or group of scores occurs. Distribution organizes data systematically to give researchers an indication of the nature of the data.

- **MEASURES OF CENTRAL TENDENCY** indicate the location of a distribution on the measurement scale. Measures of central tendency are averages that tend to be centrally located in the distribution. The most commonly used indices of central tendency are as follows:

  - **MODE** is the most frequently occurring score.
  - **MEDIAN** is the middle value in the set of data. If there are an even number of scores, (e.g., 20) extrapolate a middle figure by averaging the middle two scores.
  - **MEAN** is the arithmetic average of the total combined scores or values. A single extremely high or low score will have more direct effect on the mean than on the median. The formula for computing the mean (μ) is to divide the sum (Σ) of the samples (x_i) by the number of samples (N):

$$\mu = \frac{\sum X_i}{n}$$

Where: μ = mean
x_i = i value of the X variable (i.e., score)
n = number of scores or subjects
$\sum x_i$ = sum of X values ($X_1 + X_2 + \ldots + X_n$)

| SAMPLE FREQUENCY DISTRIBUTION TEST ||
Score	Frequency
10	1
9	1
8	4
7	4
6	5
5	0
4	3
3	1
2	1
1	0
0	0
Total = 126	**N = 20**

Mode = 6 (most frequently occurring score) Median = 6.5 (the score that half the examinees score at or below. If there is an even number of scores, (e.g., 20) extrapolate a middle figure by averaging the middle two scores. Since half of the test-takers scored 7 or above and half scored 6 and below, the median score is 6.5. Mean = 6.3 N = total number of scores or subjects

- **VARIABILITY** is the degree to which scores vary.

- **RANGE** is the difference between the highest and lowest scores.

- **STANDARD DEVIATION (SD)** is a measure of variability in relation to the mean. It is usually used with a normal bell-shaped distribution. The arithmetic mean is drawn, and the SD on either side (+ or -) of the mean shows the distances between individual scores and the mean. In the normal distribution, 95% of scores will fall within ±2 SD.

THE NORMAL FREQUENCY DISTRIBUTION (3 SD)

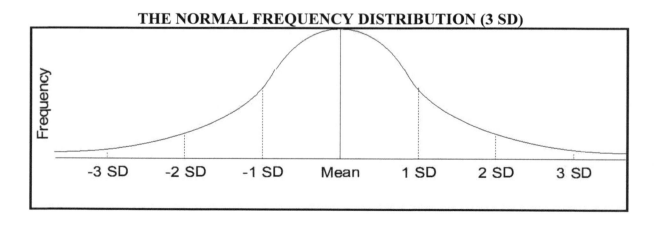

- If the distribution is bell-shaped (i.e., has normal or **GAUSSIAN DISTRIBUTION**) the SD is a good descriptor. A median score that is less than a mean score suggests that the distribution has a positive skew. A positive skew has a "tail" on the right. A "tail" to the left (**SKEWED DISTRIBUTION**) indicates the median score is greater than the mean and is negatively skewed. A few values that are very large or very small can distort the skew. If so, the median is a better measure of central tendency than the mean.

- **STANDARD ERROR (SE)** measures the confidence level relative to the population (sample) size and describes the variation relative to that population (sample) size. It is calculated by dividing the sample SD by the square root of the sample size.

- **CONFIDENCE LEVEL** is the level at which there is confidence that the sample estimate is within one, two or three standard error(s) of the parameter. It is calculated using the estimated value and its standard error. For example, one is 68% confident that the sample is within one standard error, 95% that the sample is within two standard errors or 99% that the sample is within three errors of the parameter.

- The range of percentage of confidence is called **CONFIDENCE INTERVAL.** At the 68% confidence level, the confidence interval would be 45-55%.

- **SIGNIFICANCE LEVEL** is the probability level below which the null hypothesis is rejected. If a difference is "not statistically significant," the mean difference may be zero.

Variable/dispersion measurements and scales

- **VARIABLES** are the measurement points collected in research.

- **MEASURES OF DISPERSION** are intervals or distances on the score scale that indicate how the scores are spread or dispersed.

- **NOMINAL SCALES** are variables that group different categories with names, not numbers; no answer is ranked higher or lower than any other (e.g., male/female, yes/no responses).

- **ORDINAL SCALES** are categorical variables that are ranked in a continuum (e.g., performance evaluation ratings, test scores).

- **RATIO SCALES** are variables in which the categories have equal value between scores (e.g., degrees on a thermometer, grams on a scale).

- **LIKERT SCALES** are a set of items to which the subject expresses an opinion or attitude and agrees or disagrees to a particular extent (e.g., strongly agree, agree, neither agree or disagree (neutral), disagree, strongly disagree). Likert scales can be used in assessing attitudes and opinions (e.g., quality of hospital food).

- **CONTINUOUS SCORES** take on any value of the measurement scale under consideration (e.g., energy intake, height, weight, temperature).

- **DICHOTOMOUS SCORES** fall into mutually exclusive groups (e.g., race, gender, presence or absence of disease, stage of cancer).

Inferential statistics

- **CORRELATION** is the relationship between two variables. The **CORRELATION CO-EFFICIENT** describes the strength in the relationship between the two variables. A high correlation between variables does not necessarily imply a cause and effect relationship.

- **REGRESSION** is used to determine the association between two or more variables and to make predictions based on their linear relationship.

Interpretation of current research/data

- When drawing conclusions from research data, one needs to recognize the limitations of the study design and execution (violations of research protocol, sources of bias, subject violation, sample size, response rate, compliance, subjects lost to follow-up, missing values).

- The outcome of research is a determination of whether the original hypothesis is supported by analysis of the data.

  The **NULL HYPOTHESIS (H_0)** is a statement that no relationship (e.g., difference or effect) exists between the variables and that any difference observed is a result of a sampling error. The most frequently used levels of significance are at the .05 and .01 levels. If the null hypothesis (H0) is true and accepted, or false and rejected, the decision in either case is correct. If it is true and rejected (a false positive) it is a **TYPE I ERROR**. If it is false and accepted (a false negative), it is a **TYPE II ERROR.**

TESTS OF HYPOTHESES

	Accept H0	**Reject H0**
H0 is true	Correct decision	Type I error
H0 is false	Type II error	Correct decision

- The **P VALUE** is the probability of rejecting the null hypothesis when it is true. The criterion for "Deemed Unlikely" is the probability that such a difference could occur by chance when there is really no true difference.

- **TABLES** are a systematic method for presenting numerical results. Tables often group data into intervals for presentation (e.g., children aged 1-5, 6-10 and 11-15).

- **FIGURES** are all illustrations except tables and graphs. Figures are not used to express precise numerical data.

- **GRAPHS** (scatterplots, histograms, bar charts, pie charts, etc.) are visual representations used for showing trends and relationships. Graphs are easily understood by the general public are frequently used in newspapers and magazines when numbers need graphic or visual support. Many computer programs can generate graphs from data tables.

- A **HISTOGRAM** places values along the horizontal axis and frequency along the vertical axis and draws vertical bars for each value or group of values. The result is a vertical or horizontal bar chart (e.g., amount of iron in beef, chicken and fish).A **PIE CHART** is a circle divided to show how 100% of a unit is allocated among various areas (e.g., distribution of all of calories consumed, or sources of all of agency's income).

- A **LINE GRAPH** shows a general trend of one or more items over time, charted by connecting points (e.g., growth chart).

- A **STATISTICAL MAP** compares geographical regions on the basis of one or more factors, (e.g., frequency of particular diseases among states).

- A **PICTOGRAPH** uses drawings to compare or present data (e.g., silhouette of man showing relative amounts of lean tissue, fat, water, etc).

- A **SCATTERPLOT** places one variable on the vertical axis and another variable on the horizontal axis. Then each case is put in a cell (usually marked with a dot) according to the two variables on the graph (e.g., age at onset of pregnancy and weight of infant born, which might confirm that teenagers tend to have more low-birth-weight babies).

Application of research to dietetic practice

- Data can have practical use when applied to study specific populations or used to document a researcher's practice. If a study were carried out with relatively few violations or omissions, the results may be applicable to the larger population.

- Meaningful recommendations can only be made if the study shows that changes will make a significant difference.

- Research results should be reported to the profession through publications that have juried or peer reviewers. If selected for publication, research can be duplicated and validated by professional peers. Until research is peer reviewed, published, and independently replicated, judgments should be withheld. The popular press often asks dietitians to comment on new research findings and reporters may encourage extrapolation of limited research findings to the whole population.

- Significant research may change or modify concepts, attitudes, procedures, or educational approaches in the field of dietetics. All properly done scientific research adds to the body of knowledge and information.

- The AND conducts research on a routine basis. For example, the member database and studies that collect cost-benefit information on nutrition services provide opportunities for all and members to participate in Academy-based research.

- Dietitians are being encouraged to conduct **OUTCOMES RESEARCH** with which positive results with patients/clients and cost savings of Medical Nutrition Therapy can be documented. This is especially important for reimbursement purposes.

3. Evidence-based research

- **EVIDENCE-BASED RESEARCH** is research that has been judged by experts to have merit and to adhere to specific criteria. Research articles included in the AND Evidence Analysis Library meet the following criteria: English language publication; human subject research; peer-reviewed publication; meet specific inclusion criteria (within range of years of publication, ages of subjects, size of sample, etc.) established for the specific question to be addressed.

- **EVIDENCE-BASED DIETETICS PRACTICE** is the use of systematically reviewed scientific evidence in making food and nutrition practice decisions by integrating the best available evidence-based research with professional expertise and client values to improve outcomes.

- Peer reviewed literature based on research that was correctly gathered and results interpreted correctly are examples of evidence-based research. Much medical research is in peer reviewed journals but it is difficult to find evidenced- based research on many management, communications or culinary topics.

- In using evidence-based research one must go back to the original source as it is often misinterpreted when reported in other publications or on the internet.

TOPIC E - MANAGEMENT CONCEPTS

Because Management is the focus of Domain III, all management content is consolidated in that Domain to avoid repetition.

Domain II - Nutrition Care For Individuals and Groups

Domain II = 50% of the test.

TOPIC A –SCREENING and ASSESSMENT

1. **Nutrition screening**
   a. Purpose
   b. Selection and use of risk factors and evidence-based tools
   c. Parameters and limitations
   d. Methodology
   e. Participation in interdisciplinary nutrition screening teams
   f. Cultural competence

2. **Nutrition assessment of individuals**
   a. Dietary intake assessment, analysis and documentation
   b. Medical and family history
   c. Physical findings
      (1) Anthropometric data
      (2) Nutrition focused physical exam
   d. Medication management
      (1) Prescription and over-the-counter medications
      (2) Medication/food interactions
   e. Diagnostic tests, procedures, evaluations
      (1) Assessment of energy requirements
      (2) Biochemical analyses
   f. Physical activity habits and restrictions
   g. Economic/social
      (1) Psychosocial and behavioral factors
      (2) Socioeconomic factors
      (3) Functional factors
   h. Educational readiness assessment
      (1) Motivational level and readiness to change
      (2) Educational level
      (3) Situational: environmental, economical, cultural

3. **Nutritional assessment of populations and community needs assessment**
   a. Community and group nutritional status indicators
      (1) Demographic data
      (2) Incidence and prevalence of nutrition-related status indicators
      (3) Prevalence of food insecurity
   b. Development and maintenance of nutrition screening and surveillance systems
      (1) National, state, and local reference data (e.g., NHANES, BRFSS, YRBSS)
   c. Availability of community resources
      (1) Food and nutrition assistance programs
      (2) Consumer education resources
      (3) Health services

(4) Studies on food systems, local marketplace, food economics
(5) Public health programs

TOPIC B – DIAGNOSIS

1. Relationship between nutrition diagnoses and medical diagnoses
   a. Pathophysiology
   b. Identifying medical diagnoses affecting nutrition care
   c. Determining nutrition risk factors for current medical diagnoses
   d. Determining nutrition factors for groups

2. Data sources and tools for nutrition diagnosis
   a. Organizing assessment data
   b. Using standardized language

3. Diagnosing nutrition problems for individuals and groups
   a. Making inferences
   b. Prioritizing
   c. Differential diagnosing

4. Etiologies (cause/contributing risk factors)
   a. Identifying underlying causes and contributing risk factors of nutrition diagnoses
   b. Making cause and effect linkages

5. Signs and symptoms (defining characteristics)
   a. Linking signs and symptoms to etiologies
   b. Using subjective (symptoms) and/or objective (signs) data

6. Documentation

TOPIC C – PLANNING and INTERVENTION

1. Nutrition care for health promotion and disease prevention
   a. Identification of desired outcomes/actions
      (1) Evidence-based practice for nutrition intervention
      (2) Evaluation of nutrition information
      (3) Food fad
      (4) Health fraud
   b. Determination of energy/nutrient needs specific to life span stage
   c. Implementing care plans
      (1) Nutrition recommendations to promote wellness
      (2) Communication and documentation

2. Medical nutrition therapy
   a. Identify desired outcomes and actions
   b. Relationship of pathophysiology to treatment of nutrition-related disorders
      (1) Critical care and hypermetabolic states
      (2) Eating disorders

II. NUTRITION CARE FOR INDIVIDUALS AND GROUPS (50%)

   (3) **Food allergies and intolerance**
   (4) **Immune system disorders, infections and fevers**
   (5) **Malnutrition: protein, calorie, vitamin, mineral**
   (6) **Metabolic, endocrine, and inborn errors of metabolism**
   (7) **Oncologic and hematologic conditions**
   (8) **Organ system dysfunction**
   (9) **Orthopedic/wounds**
  c. **Determine energy/nutrient needs specific to condition**
  d. **Determine specific feeding needs**
   (1) **Oral**
    (a) **Composition/texture of foods**
    (b) **Diet patterns/schedules; diagnostic test meals**
    (c) **Modified diet products and food supplements**
    (d) **ADAptive equipment**
   (2) **Enteral and parenteral nutrition**
    (a) **Formulas and calculations**
    (b) **Routes, techniques, equipment**
    (c) **Complications**
   (3) **Complementary care, herbal therapy**
  e. **Implementing care plans**
   (1) **Nutrition therapy for specific nutrition-related conditions**
   (2) **Basis for quality practice [evidence-based guidelines, standardized process (NCP), regulatory and patient safety issues]**
   (3) **Counseling**
   (4) **Communication and documentation**
   (5) **Discharge planning and disease management**

3. **Implementation and promotion of national dietary guidance (e.g., MyPlate, *Dietary Guidelines for Americans*)**
  a. **Legislation and policy development**
  b. **State and community resources and nutrition related programs**
   (1) **Block grants to states**
   (2) **Federal and state funded food and nutrition programs**
   (3) **Community interventions**

4. **Development of programs and services**
  a. **Identification and attainment of funding**
  b. **Resource allocation and budget development**
  c. **Provision of food and nutrition services to groups**

TOPIC D - MONITORING and EVALUATION

1. **Monitoring progress and updating previous care**
  a. **Monitoring responses to nutrition care**
  b. **Comparing outcomes to nutrition interventions**

2. **Measuring outcome indicators using evidence-based guides for practice**
  a. **Explaining variance**

II. NUTRITION CARE FOR INDIVIDUALS AND GROUPS (50%)

      b. Using reference standards
      c. Selecting indicators

3. Evaluating outcomes
      a. Direct nutrition outcomes
      b. Clinical and health status outcomes
      c. Patient-centered outcomes
      d. Healthcare utilization outcomes

4. Relationship with outcomes measurement systems and quality improvement

5. Determining continuation of care
      a. Continuing and updating care
      b. Discontinuing care

6. Documentation

II. NUTRITION CARE FOR INDIVIDUALS AND GROUPS (50%)

TOPIC A – SCREENING and ASSESSMENT

1. Nutrition screening

- **NUTRITION SCREENING** is the process of discovering characteristics known to be associated with dietary or nutritional problems.

a. Purpose

- The purpose of screening is to systematically identify clients who may be at nutritional risk and who require additional assessment. If done correctly, it will help to determine the specific care needs of the patient/client or population.

  - In many hospitals, today, the initial screen is performed on one form by nursing for all health disciplines (patient-centered care.) In this model, the screening form has had the input of all departments.

  - The nutrition part of the screen should determine baseline data and outlier information, which can have an impact on nutrition risk.

b. Selection and use of risk factors and evidence-based tools

- Screening factors should be based on the population served and may be specific to a facility. Methods of screening are determined by availability of previous medical records, immediate medical condition, potential forongoing care or client's ability or willingness to cooperate. Transient populations (i.e., homeless) must be screened and offered treatment during a single appointment.

- Common screening factors include information found in the medical record. Medical, social and diet history (from client or other persons when appropriate), pertinent biochemical data, anthropometric measurements and clinical observation will provide sufficient data to identify those clients requiring additional assessment.

- Initial screening should cover the following areas: physical ability to obtain and consume foods, food tolerance/intolerance, diet history, current height and weight and weight history, alcohol use/abuse, current diagnosis, polypharmacy and potential food/nutrient interactions.

- The Academy of Nutrtion and Dietetics defines Evidence-Based Dietetics Practice as "the use of systematically reviewed scientific evidence in making food and nutrition practice decisions by integrating best available evidence with professional expertise and client values to improve outcomes. Evidence-based guidelines are systematically developed statements based on current scientific evidence to assist the practitioner and patient decisions about appropriate healthcare for specific clinical conditions." and members may access this information from the AND website.

c. Parameters and limitations

- Screening identifies clients at nutritional risk so nutrition intervention can be implemented early or before more serious problems develop. Screening may decrease length of a hospital stay, reduce complications and lower medical costs. Although useful, basic screening techniques may miss subtle indicators of problems and/or may not be repeated often enough to catch changing problems or altered values. If in-depth assessment and nutrition intervention are not required initially, serial screenings often help to identify changes in lab values, problems and nutritional status (e.g., postsurgical

II. NUTRITION CARE FOR INDIVIDUALS AND GROUPS (50%)

trauma). Screening should help to identify priorities in the care of the client or population group. Based on available resources, implementation of nutrition care should follow.

d. Methodology

- Risk factor data may be obtained by several methods based on the needs of each specific client or facility. Interviews with clients or significant others may be conducted by a dietitian, dietetic technician registered, healthcare worker or other trained interviewer. This interview can be considered a structured intervie w because most of the interview questions are generated in reference to a nutrition screening form. Completion of a self-report form, usually in a checklist format, is another method to obtain nutrition screening data. An evaluation protocol, such as a weighted scoring system, may be developed to interpret the client generated responses so that appropriate and cost sensitive follow-up care is planned.

- Since nutritional screens are intended to be an efficient method to assess the amount of nutrition intervention required, many screening protocols rely on obtaining information found only in the hospital chart or medical record. The efficiency of this method depends on being able to easily locate the pertinent information in the medical record. Direct client input increases the time spent, but may be necessary if the chart does not provide adequate information. All aspects of the screening process should be periodically evaluated. All patients and/or populations should be monitored for continuity of care, reassessment of needs and future planning.

- Nutrition screening may be conducted by completing a nutrition screening equation that provides a mathematical formula based on a few key screening factors to predict nutritional risk.

- A **SUBJECTIVE GLOBAL ASSESSMENT** is a nutrition screening method that combines the efficient medical record review with direct client involvement. Assessment is based on client history and physical examination. The patient's perception of his or her ability to accomplish self care is identified. Items related to weight change, dietary intake, gastrointestinal symptoms and functional capacity are located in the medical record and the client is observed for the presence of muscle wasting, loss of subcutaneous fat and edema. Clients are subjectively rated as well nourished, moderately malnourished or severely malnourished. Appropriate nutrition assessment and intervention activities are based on this rating.

- Screening methods may be specific to age group. For example, the **NUTRITION SCREENING INITIATIVE** is specifically developed for the elderly. To promote the effective use of resources, the **PEACH SURVEY** (the Parent Eating and Nutrition Assessment for Children with Special Health Needs Survey) was developed to screen young children (birth to five years) with or at risk for developmental problems. Parents completing a survey, provide data. This survey with form is available in the *Journal of the Academy of Nutrition and Dietetics*, Vol. 94 #10, October 1994: 1156-1158.

e. Participation in interdisciplinary nutrition screening teams

- In the current patient focused environment, a trained member of the healthcare team, usually a member of the nursing department, conducts the initial screening. It is vital for the nutrition staff to have input on the specific questions to be asked and to train the interviewers.

- Dietitians should be active members of the patient's/client's healthcare team to work together to provide the best care possible.

f. Cultural competence

- With current changes in demography in many areas, the dietitian should become aware of possible use of traditional therapies, cultural taboos and language difficulties. In order to be most effective, practitioners should familiarize themselves with local culture and develop an awareness of culturally appropriate, respectful and relevant interactions.

- Information on food patterns of various world religious groups is in Domain IV.

2. Nutrition assessment of individuals

- The AND has developed a standardized **NUTRITION CARE PROCESS** for dietetics professionals, which is a "consistent structure and framework used to provide nutrition care…" The process is meant to support and promote individualized care, can be used for patients/residents in healthcare facilities and for clients in many community settings. The process manages activities, uses problem solving and critical thinking skills, and is a quality improvement tool. Use of the standardized process helps the profession generate data to help validate nutrition care. The traditional SOAP or other methods of charting can be used in this process, but a new template called, **ASSESSMENT, DIAGNOSIS, INTERVENTION, MONITORING AND EVALUATION (ADIME)** can be used.

- Steps in the nutrition care process include:
  - Nutrition assessment
  - Nutrition diagnosis
  - Nutrition intervention
  - Nutrition monitoring and evaluation

The Nutrition Care Process and Model

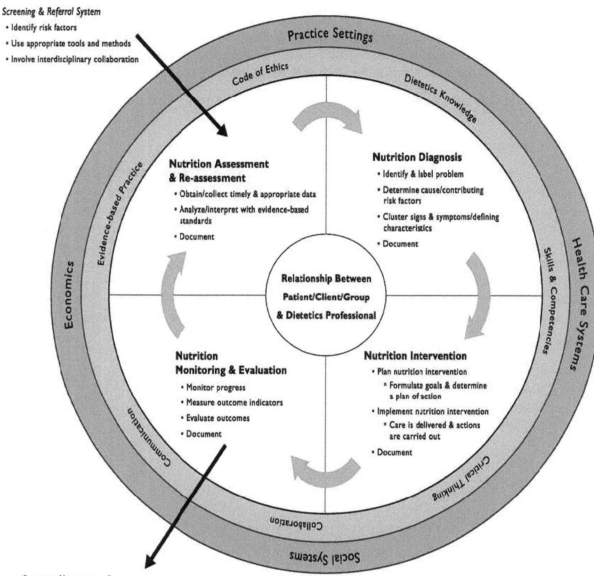

Screening & Referral System
- Identify risk factors
- Use appropriate tools and methods
- Involve interdisciplinary collaboration

Practice Settings

Code of Ethics

Dietetics Knowledge

Evidence-based Practice

Economics

Nutrition Assessment & Re-assessment
- Obtain/collect timely & appropriate data
- Analyze/interpret with evidence-based standards
- Document

Nutrition Diagnosis
- Identify & label problem
- Determine cause/contributing risk factors
- Cluster signs & symptoms/defining characteristics
- Document

Relationship Between Patient/Client/Group & Dietetics Professional

Nutrition Monitoring & Evaluation
- Monitor progress
- Measure outcome indicators
- Evaluate outcomes
- Document

Nutrition Intervention
- Plan nutrition intervention
  - Formulate goals & determine a plan of action
- Implement nutrition intervention
  - Care is delivered & actions are carried out
- Document

Communication

Collaboration

Social Systems

Critical Thinking

Skills & Competencies

Health Care Systems

Outcomes Management System
- Monitor the success of the Nutrition Care Process implementation
- Evaluate the impact with aggregate data
- Identify and analyze causes of less than optimal performance and outcomes
- Refine the use of the Nutrition Care Process

Reprinted with permission.

II. NUTRITION CARE FOR INDIVIDUALS AND GROUPS (50%)

- **NUTRITION ASSESSMENT** includes collection of nutritional adequacy information, (diet history, detailed nutrient intake), health status (anthropometric, biochemical, physical and clinical conditions and physiological and disease status.) In addition, functional and behavioral status (social, cognitive, psychological, emotional factors, quality-of-life measures and change readiness.) Once collected, the components have to be evaluated and reviewed in order to identify problem areas to make a nutritional diagnosis. Data must be compared to established standards appropriate for the population. Dietary data may be compared to the DRI/RDA. Laboratory data are compared to the normal ranges of values accepted by the institution. Computers offer mechanisms to process and assess data; for example, computerized medical records can monitor medications and flag changes in laboratory values that have been affected by medications. The interpretation of data is limited by the potential for error. Non-nutritional factors, improper techniques or poorly calibrated equipment may cause false positives. False negatives may result from underlying nutritional problems masked by a disease state, medications, improper technique or poorly calibrated equipment. Once a patient/client has been identified at moderate or high risk, additional information must be collected to possibly support a diagnosis of malnutrition.

a. Dietary intake assessment, analysis and documentation

Dietary intake assessment

- **DIETARY INTAKE** is usually compared to standards like the Dietary Reference Intakes/Recommended Dietary Allowances or a food group system. For metabolic and research studies, food intake must be carefully measured, weighed and calculated. Nutrient deficiency is determined using standardized procedures (growth measurements, triceps skin fold, bone mineralization, etc.) and evaluating symptoms.

24-hour recall (pattern)

- The foods eaten in the last 24 hours (or on a usual day if the previous day was not typical) are listed and the amount consumed is estimated. Recalls are not useful if patient has had limited choices or prescribed meals were provided. The list may be written or oral, with answers recorded. Recalls provide general intake patterns, but people tend to misestimate portions and underreport consumption of alcohol, fats and sweets.

Food frequency questionnaire (profile)

- The client is furnished with a list of foods or food groups and is asked how often he or she eats those foods. A **FOOD FREQUENCY QUESTIONNAIRE** is used to provide a general profile of usual intake. Food lists may encompass a wide variety of foods or be limited to a specific food type depending on the nutrient or food intake information required. Some food frequency questionnaires also ask for estimates of portion size.

- Some crosschecks may be incorporated such as asking how much milk is drunk daily and how many quarts or other containers are purchased each week.

Diet history (3-7 day History)

- A **DIET HISTORY** is a record of shopping, cooking, eating patterns, and food intake and identifies intolerance or allergies, use of supplements, problems chewing or swallowing, economic or social factors influencing intake, changes in appetite and so forth.

- A common diet history method includes the **FOOD RECORD**. The client keeps a record of the food consumed (time and amount) over a period of time, usually three to seven days. The task of keeping a food record promotes awareness and often improves food choices. Both client and counselor use food records for evaluation of choices. Food records are generally used for outpatients and counseling clients.

- Dietary intake data should include:

  - Appetite and intake including appetite or taste changes; factors affecting chewing or swallowing problems (dentition status, dysphagia); feeding independence (paralysis, amputation); ability to shop for food, vitamin, mineral, herbal or other nutrition supplementation.
  - Eating patterns or typical patterns (daily and weekend including ethnic and favorite foods), dietary restrictions (understanding of and compliance with these restrictions), frequency of eating away from home, use of fad diets.

Interviews/verification

- **DIRECT OBSERVATION** is usually done on an inpatient basis. The clinician observes what the patient actually eats. This is most useful for calorie counts or when a record of protein intake is needed. Care must be taken to subtract uneaten food from the amount served. Observing that nobody else ate any food on the tray (i.e., visitors or another person in room) is important for accuracy.

- Direct observations can also be done if there are home visits, when contents of the refrigerator, pantry or food store register receipts can be assessed.

Data interpretations and limitations

- Dietitians should be aware that both food intake data and energy expenditure, as reported by individuals, might be underreported or overreported. Few individuals can accurately remember all foods consumed and even fewer can correctly estimate portions consumed. A "large" portion of pasta to one person may be ½ cup, but to another the "large" portion may be 2 cups.

- Food data tables are based on standard serving sizes that are very modest. Typical portions served have become larger in recent years. Most restaurants serve portions 2–4 times that of a standard portion, yet the individual believes this serving to be one portion. Also, there is a known tendency to underreport consumption of alcohol, sweets and snacks, etc.

- Records of food sold for human consumption in the United States far exceed estimates of foods consumed by the total population.

b. Medical and family history

- A **MEDICAL HISTORY** includes the chief medical complaint, diagnosis, review of systems, presence of chronic illness, risk of complications, allergies, pertinent medications, alcohol and drug use, bowel habits, present or past illness, surgical history and family medical history. In addition it includes the chief nutrition complaint, cognitive abilities and mental and emotional health.

- Medical histories help the dietitian understand patient/client nutrition related problems, such as recent significant weight loss, changes in taste, dehydration and so forth.

c. Physical findings

measure sub Q fat Stories

(1) Anthropometric data

- **ANTHROPOMETRICS** are physical measures of body size, contour and indicators of body composition. Height and weight are the most important and accessible anthropometrics for all population groups. For children less than 3 years of age, skinfold thickness and head circumference are useful measurements. The 50th percentile is considered standard for these measures. Measurements between the 15th and 85th percentiles are considered average whereas measurement between the 5th and 15th suggest moderate depletion; below the 5th percentile indicates severe depletion. In children, heights and weights should be recorded on a standard growth grid, which will provide a record of a child's gain in height and/or weight as the child grows. This grid can also compare the child's measurements to those of other children at the same age. Since these measures are indicators of growth and development in infants and children, investigation is needed if there is a drop off or acceleration of growth rate. Measurements below the fifth percentile or above the 95th percentile for infants and children are clearly outside the norm and require further investigation, interpretation and followup.

Height

- An individual's height in inches can be measured directly by using a stationary measuring rod or stadiometer if a person is able to stand. Height can also be measured (length by tape measure) in a recumbent position or by body segment lengths when traditional measurements are not feasible. Recumbent length measurements are appropriate for infants and children younger than 2 or 3 years of age. Sitting heights may be used for children disabled people who cannot stand.

- **ARM SPAN MEASUREMENT** may be taken to determine the approximate height of adults who are bedridden or unable to stand. Arm span is primarily long bones and correlates well with height at maturity. Aging or osteoporosis minimally affects arm span measurement. The measure from the patient's sternal notch to the longest finger on the dominant hand is doubled, estimating height. This procedure may be difficult and unreliable for persons with contracture or spinal deformity.

- **KNEE HEIGHT** can also be measured to estimate stature in adults, who are unable to stand or stand straight, using formulas. The formula uses a knee height measurement in related to years of age. (Note: Exam candidates should know that these techniques are used, but probably would not be expected to memorize specific height formulas.)

- **Directions for taking this measure:** The left leg should be used wherever possible for this measurement. The patient should be placed in a supine position with the left knee and ankle positioned at a 90° angle. Apply the caliper with the fixed part under the heel and the sliding blade over the anterior surface of the thigh, proximal to the patella and with the caliper shaft parallel to the tibia shaft to measure knee height.

Weight

- **ACTUAL BODY WEIGHT (ABW)** reflects a weight measurement, usually in pounds, at the time of the examination. This measurement may be influenced by a person's fluid status.

- **USUAL BODY WEIGHT (UBW)** is a report of a recent, typical weight. The report is dependent on the client's memory. But usual body weight is important to know when a person is ill in order to determine if there has been a recent weight loss or gain.

- In cases of unintentional weight change, a result of 85% to 95% usual body weight (UBW) indicates mild depletion; 75% to 84% UBW indicates moderate depletion; and less than 75% UBW indicates severe depletion. To determine percentage of weight change:

  [handwritten: Wt loss: 85-95% = mild; 75-84% = moderate; <75% = severe]

$$\% \text{ UBW change} = \frac{(\text{UBW} - \text{ABW}) \times 100}{\text{UBW}}$$

- Weight may be obtained using chair scales, bed scales, standing scales or baby scales for infants. To obtain accurate weights, use scales that are properly calibrated. Valid assessment of weight status requires obtaining reliable weight measures. Heavy clothes and shoes, soiled diapers, casts and braces may invalidate weight measures. Failure to consider time of day, amount of clothing and timing of meals during routine weighing protocols yields unreliable results, compromising weight status assessment.

- Body weight may also be estimated from equations that include knee height and mid-arm circumference measurements (MAC). Formulas have been developed from ages 6-18, 19-59 and 60-80 years with accuracy ranging from 7.5 to 14.5kg. Weights for 60-80 year-olds may be calculated with the formulas shown below.

  Black Female 60 - 80 years (1.50 KH) + (2.58 MAC) - 84.22

  White Female 60 - 80 years (1.09 KH) + (2.68 MAC) - 65.51 k

  Black Male   60 - 80 years (0.44 KH) + (2.86 MAC) - 39.21

  White Male   60 - 80 years (1.10 KH) + (3.07 MAC) - 75.81

Body frame

- Frame size may be estimated by either a wrist circumference or elbow breadth measurement. The designation of body frame size allows the determination of optimal weight for height to be modified for a more accurate estimation.

- **WRIST CIRCUMFERENCE** is found by measuring the smallest part of the wrist distal to the styloid process of the ulna and radius. The r-value can then be established by calculation. The r-value is then used to classify the body frame size as small, medium or large for males and females.

$$r = \text{ratio of height to wrist circumference}$$

$$r = \frac{\textbf{Height in centimeters}}{\textbf{Wrist circumference in centimeters}}$$

Frame Size Estimates
Based on wrist measurements in inches

	r Value	
Frame Size	**Women**	**Men**
Small	>10.9	>10.4
Medium	10.9 -9.9	9.6 -10.4
Large	<9.9	<9.6

- An additonal method to determine the body frame size is to measure the wrist with a tape measure and use the following chart to determine whether the person is small, medium or large boned.

Women:
  Height under 5'2"
  - Small = wrist size less than 5.5"
  - Medium = wrist size 5.5" to 5.75"
  - Large = wrist size over 5.75"
  Height 5'2" to 5' 5"
  - Small = wrist size less than 6"
  - Medium = wrist size 6" to 6.25"
  - Large = wrist size over 6.25"
  Height over 5' 5"
  - Small = wrist size less than 6.25"
  - Medium = wrist size 6.25" to 6.5"
  - Large = wrist size over 6.5"

Men:
  Height over 5' 5"
  - Small = wrist size 5.5" to 6.5"
  - Medium = wrist size 6.5" to 7.5"
  - Large = wrist size over 7.5"

- Since **ELBOW BREADTH** is less affected by adiposity and is highly correlated with muscle size and lean body mass, it provides a more accurate estimation of skeletal size than wrist circumference. Measure the distance between the two prominent bones on either side of the elbow. A tape measure or ruler may be used, but for the most accurate results, use of calipers or a Frameter is recommended. The Metropolitan Life Insurance Company developed charts to estimate frame size from these measures.

Skinfold measurements

[handwritten: not accurate w/ extreme high body weight]

- **SKINFOLD THICKNESSES** are measurements estimating subcutaneous fat stores, which can be used to estimate body fat. The validity of this measurement relies on the accuracy of the measurement and repetition of the measurements over time. As obesity increases, the accuracy of this measurement decreases. This measurement can be a good indicator of calorie reserves; however, fat stores can remain normal in moderately malnourished individuals. In addition to using skinfold measurements in conjunction with other anthropometric indices, skinfold data should be compared with percentile standards from multiple body sites or collected as serial measurements over time to provide the most thorough and accurate assessment of nutritional status. The amount and rate of change in body fat can help establish the presence and severity of protein-energy malnutrition (PEM). Triceps, biceps, subscapular and suprailiac skinfold measurements, using calipers, are most commonly used.

[handwritten left margin: +NPTE Review uses calipers]

- **CALIPERS** are instruments used to measure skinfold thickness at selected sites (e.g., mid-upper arm triceps) to estimate body fat. Circumferences of outer arm and skinfold measurements are used to estimate skeletal muscle mass. The measurement is evaluated at different body points against reference standards for age and sex. Excess fat in the abdomen ("apple shape" or **ANDROID**) is a greater health risk (particularly for heart disease) than fat in the hips and thighs (a "pear shape" or **GYNOID**) body.

Other circumference measurements

- Circumference measurements are performed because fat distribution is recognized as an indication of disease risk. If excess body fat around the abdomen is out of proportion to total body fat, it is considered to be a risk for illnesses associated with obesity and the metabolic syndrome.

- **WAIST CIRCUMFERENCE** is a commonly used circumference measure to assess abdominal fat content. The Centers for Disease Control (CDC) have determined that the measurements may not be useful if a person is less than 5 feet tall or has a BMI of > 35. The CDC has also determined that measurements in men of > 40 inches or in women of > 35 inches are independent risk factors for disease when the waist measurement is out of proportion to total body fat. It has been shown to be another simple, but accurate, indicator of risk by the World Health Organization International Task Force on Obesity and was first published in *NIH Guidelines on the Treatment of Obesity in Adults*, 1998. Waist circumference should be measured on the standing patient, midway in the mid-axillary line between the lowest rim of the rib cage and the iliac crest - not at the maximum point or at the umbilicus. Current research indicates waist circumference is a better marker of abdominal fat than waist-to-hip ratio.

*[handwritten left margin: CDC:
- Not accurate
If: <5ft or
BMI >35
- Risk:
men >40"
Women >35"]*

- **WAIST-TO-HIP CIRCUMFERENCE RATIO** (**WHR**) is an older method than waist circumference and is not frequently used. It is now used to measure excess fat deposition patients with HIV.

- Body circumference measurements taken at various body sites are used to estimate skeletal muscle mass (somatic protein stores) and body fat stores. Data is less reliable in individuals with poor upper body development.

- **MIDARM** or **UPPER ARM CIRCUMFERENCE (MAC)** estimates skeletal mass and fat stores. It estimates skeletal mass and fat stores. It is measured in centimeters on the upper arm at the midpoint between the tip of the acromial process of the scapula and the olecranon process of the ulna. It is not a sensitive indicator when used alone but is commonly used to calculate arm muscle circumference.

- **MIDARM MUSCLE** or **ARM MUSCLE CIRCUMFERENCE (MAMC),** *[muscle]* determined from midarm muscle circumference and **TRICEPS SKINFOLD (TSI)** measurements, provides an index of skeletal muscle mass but does not account for bone mass differences in percentage of fat based on sex, or for age variation based on sex. The measurement is insensitive to small changes in muscle mass; however, it does provide a quick approximation of muscle mass and is minimally affected by edema. MAMC may be determined by an arm anthropometry nomogram using TSF and MAC or by using the following (multiply result by 10 for MAMC in millimeters.

$$\text{MAMC (cm)} = \text{MAC (cm)} - [3.14 \times \text{TSF (cm)}]$$

- **TOTAL UPPER ARM AREA (TUAA)** *[Area]* is a value used to determine upper arm fat area. Total upper arm area can be derived from this formula:

$$\text{TUAA (mm}^2) = \frac{\text{MAC}^2 \text{ (mm)}}{4 \times 3.14 \text{ (or 12.57)}}$$

- **UPPER ARM MUSCLE AREA (UAMA)** is good indication of lean body mass, skeletal protein reserves and protein energy malnutrition (PEM). UAMA indicates more marked changes than does MAMC, may be a more physiologically related indicator and is used in calculating upper arm fat. For bone-free arm muscle area, subtract 10 (for males) and 6.5 (for females) from the results of the UAMA formula.

$$\text{UAMA (mm}^2) = \frac{[\text{MAC (mm)} - (\text{TSF (mm)} \times 3.14)]^2}{4 \times 3.14 \text{ (or 12.57)}}$$

[accounts for bone mass/sex]

- **UPPER ARM FAT AREA (UAFA)** *[Fat]* can be calculated using the following formula. It is uncorrected for bone-free value. This calculation may better indicate changes in fat stores than TSF. The UAFA formula is:

$$\text{UAFA (mm}^2) = \text{TUAA (mm}^2) - (\text{UAMA (mm}^2)$$

- **HEAD CIRCUMFERENCE** measurements are used for children under three years of age to mainly to assess non-nutritional abnormalities. Malnutrition has to be very severe to affect this measurement.

Growth charts

- Growth charts are used in clinical and research settings to assess the nutritional status and general health and well-being of infants, children and adolescents. The charts can be used to measure growth of these population groups from birth through age 20, by plotting height and weight each time the individual has a physical examination. It is usually recommended that once infants reach their growth channel (depending on genetics and birth weight from 3 months to 1 year) it is healthiest for them to continue their growth within the same channel.

- Using improved statistical procedures and national survey data from NHANES II and III growth charts were published in June 2000 with BMI for age charts for both boys and girls. To access the growth charts see: **www.cdc.gov/growthcharts**. There are also growth charts for children who are WIC clients and for children of several ethnicities.

Body composition measurements

- **UNDERWATER WEIGHING** is the classic measure (also called **HYDRODENSITOMETRY** and water displacement). Another method is **BIOELECTRIC IMPEDANCE,** which measures body fat, using low intensity electrical current. It is considered a reliable measurement of body composition in comparison to both BMI and height/weight measurement. It is a non-invasive and portable method considered to be safe. **DUAL ENERGY X-RAY ABSORPTIOMETRY (DEXA)** provides a measurement of total fat distribution and bone mineral density in most people, except the extremely obese or those whose hydration status is not normal. Deposition of intraabdominal and subcutaneous fat is also assessed by **COMPUTED TOMOGRAPHY** (**CT SCAN**) and **MAGNETIC RESONANCE IMAGING (MRI),** which can also be used to measure skeletal and visceral organ size. Each test has limitations and all results are estimates.

- Body composition components include the following:
  - ➢ **LEAN BODY MASS (LBM)** is the active fat-free body cell mass that largely determines basal metabolic rate, energy and nutritional needs. Exercise helps maintain and develop LBM.
  - ➢ **BODY FAT** reflects the number and size of **ADIPOCYTES** (fat cells) making up the adipose tissue. In adult men, body fat should be 14-28% of total body weight; in women, 15-29%, varying with age, climate, exercise and fitness. About half of body fat is subcutaneous (insulating) fat, which can be measured by fat folds using calipers. Body fat acts as an insulator, prevents excessive heat loss and protects visceral organs from shock.
  - ➢ **BODY WATER** varies with relative leanness/fatness and with age, hydration and health status. It is generally about 60% of body weight. LBM contains more water than any other body tissue except blood.

- **BONE MINERAL MASS** is primarily skeletal structure, accounting for about 6% of total body weight. Calcium in bones makes up about 2% of total body weight.

(2) Nutrition-focused physical exam

- The purpose of this exam is to assess for signs and symptoms of malnutrition and/or specific nutritional deficiencies.

- Dietitians have been performing nutrition-focused physical examinations for many years, but many dietitians believed that they should not touch a patient. Currently, dietitians are performing many more examinations for the nutrition-focused physical exam.

- Steps include inspection, a visual assessment of the body to see if there are any changes from normal.

Not currently practiced

take vital signs. Some perform indirect calorimetry and
...s to help them assess energy requirements and evaluate

...pate) the body. Percussion can be used to assess the
...ving feeding routes or to detect fluids in the lungs. A
...ntify bowel sounds.

...luate range of motion and assess the patient's/client'

...ained to do dysphagia screening and also do head, neck

- For many years, dietitians have made clinical observations as seen in the following chart:

CLINICAL OBSERVATIONS IN NUTRITIONAL ASSESSMENT

Subject	Observations	Potential Nutrient Involved
Hair	Dull, thin, color and texture change, pluckable, dry	Zinc, protein, protein calorie malnutrition (PCM), copper
Face	Pale, swollen, dermatitis around lips and nostrils, cheilosis (cracks @ mouth corner)	Riboflavin (B2), protein, niacin, other B vitamins (B3)
Eyes	Pale conjunctiva, fissures at corners, gray spots (Bitot spots), keratomalacia*	Vitamin A, B vitamins, ascorbic acid, iron
Tongue	Swollen, edematous, magenta tongue	Riboflavin, niacin, other B vitamins (B2)
Gums	Soft, bleeding, spongy	Ascorbic acid
Nails	Pale, brittle, ridged, spoon-shaped	Iron
Legs	Muscle pain (especially calves), edema	Protein, thiamin (B1)
GlANDs	Enlarged thyroid or parotid	Protein, iodine, selenium, Zn
Musculoskeletal	Bowed legs, knock knees, enlarged joints, hemorrhages, wasted muscles, loss of fat	PCM, vitamin D, ascorbic acid, calcium
Neurological	Confusion, psychomotor changes, irritability, weakness, sensory loss	Thiamin (B1), B12, riboflavin (B2)
Skin	Dermatitis, pale, dry, scaly, delayed wound healing, petechial hemorrhages	Niacin, vitamins A and K, ascorbic acid, essential fatty acids

d. Medication management   keratomalacia – a softening & ulceration of the cornea of the eye (Vit A deficiency)

(1) Prescription and over-the-counter medications

- Part of a good nutrition assessment is to identify all prescription and over-the-counter medications and any complementary/alternative therapies the client uses or has used. Many people think over-the counter medications are harmless, but all have the potential to interact with prescription medications, food and alternative therapies.

- ＊ Dietitians should monitor intake of vitamins, herbs, and supplements in addition to medications, to assure awareness of potential interactions.

(2) Medication/food interactions

- Drug/medication/nutrient interactions can be caused or complicated by a variety of issues. A person's nutritional status, body composition, illness, intake of alcohol, illegal

II. NUTRITION CARE FOR INDIVIDUALS AND GROUPS (50%)

substances, herbs, supplements, and allergies are some causes of these interactions. In addition, some people do not take medications according to prescribed instructions, for example, with meals or a certain number of hours before or after meals. Some people are overmedicated because they have prescription medications from several physicians without anyone having checked other medications. This is called **POLYPHARMACY.** Some people, especially the elderly, may forget to take medication, or that they have taken the medication, and take it again.

- Medications can alter food intake by depressing or stimulating appetite, for example, by altering taste or causing nausea. Drugs can alter digestive processes by changing acidity of the digestive tract; raising or lowering secretion of digestive juices; or changing gastrointestinal motility (transit time). Foods can interfere with intended drug actions by slowing absorption time or by contributing pharmacologically active substances. Foods can alter metabolism and/or excretion of drugs, for example, by changing urine acidity or reabsorption mechanisms in the kidney. Many drugs can be excreted in breast milk so lactating women should avoid use of both non-prescription and prescription drugs unless specifically advised by a physician.

- There is an increased amount of certain drugs in the bloodstream (e.g., cyclosporine, statins) when taken with grapefruit juice, which contains **NARINGENIN,** a flavonoid that inhibits metabolic enzymes. (@ site of the liver)

- Milk and milk products inhibit absorption of tetracycline.

- Vegetables rich in vitamin K can inhibit oral anticoagulants. Patients require instruction to avoid these foods when taking prescribed medications. The information should also be included on the medication label. monitor

- Taste alterations occur as unpleasant aftertaste, decreased or heightened sensation. Common examples of medications that cause taste alterations are Colace, Lopid, Cisplatin, Flagyl and Dilantin.

- Appetite changes can cause unplanned weight loss or gain along with nutritional imbalances and sometimes growth retardation in children. Examples of drugs that cause appetite loss include Plaquenil, Proleukin, Apresoline, and Ritalin. Antidepressants, antipsychotics and anticonvulsants can increase appetite. Eat before taking?

- Some drugs cause gastrointestinal irritation and ulceration, gastritis, and may lead to serious gastric bleeding with long-term use. These include such drugs as non-steroidal drugs (NSAID) such as aspirin and ibuprofen. Constipation or diarrhea may be caused by codeine and morphine. Some antibiotics can cause diarrhea because of destruction of intestinal bacteria.

- Other medications may cause depressed tissue levels of vitamins and minerals; for example, Phenobarbital and Dilantin can cause depressed levels of ascorbic acid, biotin (B7) folate, or vitamin D and may depress absorption of vitamin B12, folate, vitamin B6 and vitamin K. cobalamin B9 Pyridoxine

- Monoamine oxidase inhibitors, such as dopamine, tyramine, phenylethylamine and (MAOI) histamine may, in some people, cause a hypertensive crisis. Aged cheeses, smoked meats, soy sauce, tenderized and marinated meats, fava or broad bean pods and snow pea pods, sauerkraut and other pickled vegetables, such as kim chee, meat and yeast extract,

severe increase in BP that can lead to a stroke or damage to (180+ / 120+) blood vessels mm/Hg concentrated yeast extracts, miso, soy sauce, tap beer and Korean beer and overripe and spoiled fruits may cause the crisis. Use other alcoholic beverages and cola in very small amounts and with extreme caution.

- Aspirin, anti-malarial drugs (e.g. quinine sulfate) and sulfonamides (e.g. sulfasalazine) should not be taken by people who are prone to vitamin K deficiency, or by people who have the genetic deficiency of G6PD (glucose-6-phosphate dehydrogenase.)

e. Diagnostic tests, procedures, evaluations

(1) Assessment of energy requirements

- Energy is needed to support basal metabolism, physical activity and digestion of food.

Factors affecting energy needs

- **BASAL METABOLIC RATE (BMR)** is a measure of the energy needed to support the body at rest in a post-absorptive state, a **THERMONEUTRAL STATE** (comfortable room temperature) in a supine (lying down) position. It is performed upon awakening, before any physical activity, 12 hours after eating (including tea, coffee, nicotine.) This is approximately 60-70% of total energy used by the body. The amount of energy used for basal metabolism depends mainly on lean body mass and is higher in individuals with more lean body mass. The **BASAL ENERGY EXPENDITURE (BEE)** is the measurement of the basal metabolic rate. It is usually expressed as kcal/kg body weight/hour or kcal/24 hours.

  - Age growth influence metabolic requirements. Infants have the highest BMR, based on energy per pound of body weight. Basal energy needs decrease during childhood and increase again during adolescence, but never to the level of infancy. Adults generally need 30 – 40 calories per kg of body weight. During adulthood, energy needs decrease about 2-3% per decade after age 30.
  - Sex variations in energy needs stem from differences in lean body mass. Females need 5-10% fewer calories than males because females have a higher amount of fat tissue, which is less metabolically active.
  - Height influences basal energy needs. Tall, thin people have a higher BMR because of a larger body surface area.
  - Environment influences BMR. Exposure to cold increases heat production, producing a condition known as **NONSHIVERING THERMOGENESIS.**
  - Persons who are **FEBRILE** (with elevated temperature) or experiencing an infectious state will have a higher BMR. For each degree Fahrenheit above normal body temperature, there is a 7% increase in energy needs. For each degree Celsius, there is an increase of 13%.
  - Pregnancy (during second and third trimesters) requires an increase of calories over a woman's non-pregnant needs, as does lactation.
  - Athletes have increased energy needs depending on the intensity and duration of their sport. In general, they also have proportionately more muscle mass, which is more metabolically active.
- **THYROID FUNCTION TESTS** are indirect measures of BMR. **PROTEIN-BOUND IODINE (PBI)** is the form in which thyroid hormone, bound to plasma protein, is transported in

the blood. PBI provides a good index of thyroid function. A normal concentration of 5-mcg/100 ml of plasma increases to 8-mcg/100 ml of plasma in hyperthyroidism.

- Because obtaining a truly basal metabolic measurement is impractical in most settings, the **RESTING METABOLIC RATE (RMR),** is a more appropriate term for metabolic rate or energy expenditure in the awake, resting, post-absorptive state. Criteria are not as controlled regarding food intake and physical activity, so the RMR is somewhat higher than the BMR. The **RESTING ENERGY EXPENDITURE (REE)** measures the RMR and is usually expressed as kcal/kg body weight/hour or kcal/24 hours.

- There are almost 200 published guidelines for estimating the resting energy expenditure such as the non-protein energy requirements of hospitalized patients. There is controversy as to which is best because some overestimate and some underestimate actual caloric needs. One of the most common methods is the **HARRIS-BENEDICT EQUATION** This formula, used since 1919) is specific for sex, height, weight and age but is not recommended for obese people because it has shown higher error when compared with others in use.

    REE kcal (men) = 66.5 + (13.75 x wt. in kg) + (5.0 x ht. in cm) -(6.78 x age in years)
    REE kcal (women) = 655 + (9.56 x wt. in kg) + (1.85 x ht. in cm) – (4.68 x age in years)

- The **MIFFLIN-ST. JEOR EQUATION,** is another equation (published in 1990) for estimating energy needs for adults 19-78 years of age. This is recommended for general use and has shown less error than the Harris-Benedict equation when used for obese individuals.

    REE kcal (men) = (10 x weight in kg.) + (6.25 x ht. in cm) – (5 x age in years)+5
    REE (women) = (10 x weight in kg.) + (6.25 x ht.in cm) – (5 x age in years) – 161

- An abbreviated version for persons of normal height and weight is:
    REE (women) = weight in kg x 0.95kcal/kg x 24 hours
    REE (men) = weight in kg x 1 kcal/kg x 24 hours

- The **IRETON-JONES EQUATION** is recommended for hospitalized patients with a variety of clinical conditions because it has been validated and found to be especially useful for obese patients and critically ill or injured patients. This equation uses more specific information than the other two.

    For spontaneously breathing patients:

    $$EEE = 629 – (11 \times age) + (25 \times wt\ in\ kg) – (609 \times obesity^2)$$

    For ventilator dependent patients:

    $$EEE = 1784 – (11 \times age) + (5 \times wt\ in kg) + (244 \times sex^3) + (239 \times T^4) + (80 \times B^5)$$

    [1] EEE = estimated energy expenditure (kcal/day)

    [2] Obesity = >30% above IBW or BMI > 27 (present= 1, absent = 0)

    [3] (male = 1, female = 0);

    [4] T = dx of trauma:(present = 1, absent = 0)

    [5] Burn dx (present = 1, absent = 0)

- For essentially healthy people, use an activity percentage factor plus additional calories for anabolism if there is weight loss. If an individual has fever or stress, use the fever or stress percentages instead of the activity factor.

- Additional calories for activities are based on a percentage of the REE. Energy expended during physical activity is voluntary. Exercise is the main variable in caloric requirements of individuals. The energy cost of a physical activity can be expressed as a percentage of the REE.

- The REE may overestimate basal energy needs, especially for persons with lower basal energy needs. The 2002 National Academy of Sciences report on Dietary Reference Intakes (DRI) for Macronutrients includes formulas for the Estimated Energy Requirements (EER) for each age group.

FACTORS INCREASING REE	Percent to Add
Activity	
Sedentary (rest, personal care, sitting, walking slowly)	20%
Light (housework, light gardening, childcare, painting)	30%
Moderate (walking briskly, yard work, doubles tennis)	40%
Heavy (shoveling snow, jogging, singles tennis)	50%
Anabolism	
Moderate weight loss	5%
Severe weight loss (<75% UBW)	10-15%
Stress	
Minor surgery (tonsillectomy, dental, etc.)	10-15%
Major surgery (abdominal, orthopedic, etc.)	20-40%
Major burns	50-100%
Fever	
Per degree above normal Celsius	13%
Per degree above normal Fahrenheit	7%

- To estimate energy needs, use the person's weight and degree of physical activities as the total energy needs:

Sedentary	25-30kcal/kg
Moderate activity (e.g. routine walking)	35kcal/kg
Heavy activity (e.g. some sports)	40kcal/kg

These values should be adjusted for age: decrease total by 100kcal for every 10 years of age over age 30.

- **THERMIC EFFECT OF FOOD (TEF)** is the energy required for food processing (digestion, absorption, transport and storage of the nutrients.) This food intake effect is

II. NUTRITION CARE FOR INDIVIDUALS AND GROUPS (50%)

sometimes referred to as the SPECIFIC DYNAMIC ACTION (SDA) of food. The TEF can be estimated as 10% of the calories needed for basal and activity needs. Although the thermic factors of protein and fat and some spices are higher, mixed diets are estimated at the 10% level.

- To calculate total energy needs, add the calories required for activity and special needs (e.g., pregnancy, illness or growth) to the calories that are required for the TEF and the calories that are required for maintaining resting energy expenditure (REE). When dealing with food calories, which are really kilocalories (kcal), the more familiar term "calorie" is usually used.

Calculation methods

Standard weight

- Evaluation of a patient's weight and weight changes may be one of the single most important tools in determining nutritional status. Whenever possible, actual current measurements should be used.

- Several methods can be used to determine weight for height and compared with reference or standard values.

  ➢ IDEAL WEIGHT FOR HEIGHT is <u>not used</u> as a reference standard anymore. Tables such as the Metropolitan Life Insurance Tables or the NHANES I and II percentiles are not considered to be as accurate a predictor of risk for chronic disease and malnutrition as the BMI.

  ➢ One can estimate DESIRABLE BODY WEIGHT (DBW), using the HAMWI METHOD.

Hamwi (rule of thumb) Method

Males = 106 lb. for 5 ft., plus 6 lb. per inch over 5 ft.
or 106 lb. minus 6 lb. per inch under 5 ft.

Females = 100 lb. For 5 ft., plus 5 lb. per inch over 5 ft.
or 100 lb. minus 5 lb. per inch under 5 ft.

✱ Add 10% for large-framed subjects.   *frame size by wrist circumference*
Subtract 10% for small-framed subjects.   *of elbow breadth (p.192-193)*

Subtracting 10% for the lower end and adding 10% for the higher end determines the desirable weight range.

- The comparison of desirable weight, usual weight and actual weight (ABW), and weight change are additional indicators of nutritional risk. The following equation determines percentage of DESIRABLE BODY WEIGHT (DBW):

$$\% \text{ DBW} = \frac{\text{ABW X 100}}{\text{DBW}}$$

Weight/height ratio, body mass index (BMI)

BODY MASS INDEX (BMI or QUETELET INDEX) defines the level of adiposity based on the relationship of weight to height. It does not take frame size into account, has the least correlation with body height and the greatest correlation with independent measures of body fatness for all adults. BMI can be calculated using the formulas, or the dietitian may use a nomogram based upon height and weight. The following chart translates BMI into relative health risk. Body mass index tables are available at: **www.cdc.gov/healthyweight/assessing/bmi/index.html**

BODY MASS INDEX (BMI).

$$BMI = \frac{\text{Weight in kg}}{(\text{height in meters})^2}$$

Classification	BMI	Health Risk
Underweight	< 18.5	Moderate
Normal Weight	18.5 – 24.9	Normal
Overweight	25.0 – 29.9	Increased
Obese Class I	30.0 – 34.9	High
Obese Class II	35.0 -39.9	Very High
Extreme Obesity	40.0 +	Extremely High

BMI	19	20	21	22	23	24	25	26	27	28	29	30	31	32	33	34	35	36	37	38	39	40	41	42
	NORMAL						OVERWEIGHT					OBESE										EXTREME OBESITY		
Height (Feet-Inches)	Weight (Pounds)																							
4'10"	91	96	100	105	110	115	119	124	129	134	138	143	148	153	158	162	167	172	177	181	186	191	196	201
4'11"	94	99	104	109	114	119	124	128	133	138	143	148	153	158	163	168	173	178	183	188	193	198	203	208
5'00"	97	102	107	112	118	123	128	133	138	143	148	153	158	163	168	174	179	184	189	194	199	204	209	215
5'01"	100	106	111	116	122	127	132	137	143	148	153	158	164	169	174	180	185	190	195	201	206	211	217	222
5'02"	104	109	115	120	126	131	136	142	147	153	158	164	169	175	180	186	191	196	202	207	213	218	224	229
5'03"	107	112	118	124	130	135	141	146	152	158	163	169	174	180	186	191	197	203	208	214	220	225	231	237
5'04"	110	116	122	128	134	140	145	151	157	163	169	175	180	186	191	197	204	209	215	221	227	232	238	244
5'05"	114	120	126	132	138	144	150	156	162	168	174	180	186	192	198	204	210	216	222	228	234	240	246	252
5'06"	118	124	130	136	142	148	155	161	167	173	179	186	192	198	204	210	216	223	229	235	241	247	253	260
5'07"	121	127	134	140	146	153	159	166	172	178	185	191	198	204	211	217	223	230	236	242	249	255	261	268
5'08"	125	131	138	144	151	158	164	171	177	184	190	197	204	210	216	223	230	236	243	249	256	262	269	276
5'09"	128	135	142	149	155	162	169	176	182	189	196	203	210	216	223	230	236	243	250	257	263	270	277	284
5'10"	132	139	146	153	160	167	174	181	188	195	202	209	216	222	229	236	243	250	257	264	271	278	285	292
5'11"	136	143	150	157	165	172	179	186	193	200	208	215	222	229	236	243	250	257	265	272	279	286	293	301
6'00"	140	147	154	162	169	177	184	191	199	206	213	221	228	235	242	250	258	265	272	279	287	294	302	309
6'01"	144	151	159	166	174	182	189	197	204	212	219	227	235	242	250	257	265	275	280	288	295	302	310	318
6'02"	148	155	163	171	179	186	194	202	210	218	225	233	241	249	256	264	272	280	287	295	303	311	319	326
6'03"	152	160	168	176	184	192	200	208	216	224	232	240	248	256	264	272	279	287	295	303	311	319	327	335
6'04"	156	164	172	180	189	197	205	213	221	230	238	246	254	263	271	279	287	295	304	312	320	328	336	344

Adapted from: George Bray, Pennington Biomedical Research Center, *Clinical Guidelines on the Identification, Evaluation, and Treatment of Overweight and Obesity in Adults: The Evidence Report*, National Institutes of Health, National Heart, Lung, and Blood Institute, September 1998.

- When weight loss is desired, setting a weight loss goal of 1 or 2 BMI units is appropriate and can result in reduced health risks.

- **SIGNIFICANT WEIGHT LOSS** is defined as ≥ 1% to 2% in 1 week, ≥ 5% in 1 month, ≥ 7.5% in 3 months, and ≥ 10% in 6 months. An unplanned or recent weight loss of 10% or more is a risk factor for malnutrition, while weight loss exceeding 20% is a high risk factor for surgical patients.

- If body parts have been amputated, other methods (e.g. knee-height formula) of estimating healthy body weight must be used.

- Calculating total energy needs requires knowledge of client weight, activity level, sex and possibly height. Manual calculations or short-cut nomograms that have been devised to replace mathematical calculations by locating and connecting information on a chart, may complete the calculation. There are a large number of computer programs that allow energy needs to be determined after the pertinent client data is entered. These computerized options range from hand-held computerized calculators, to personal

II. NUTRITION CARE FOR INDIVIDUALS AND GROUPS (50%)

computer programs, to components of larger, system-wide packages (e.g. a program that measures Respiratory Quotient and identifies substrate utilization). All methods are based on the concept that total energy needs are the sum of basal, thermic effect of food and activity energy components. If data is entered accurately and all other parameters are equal, computerized methods are more accurate and less time consuming.

- Important operating features of computerized diet analysis systems include computer hardware requirements, cost of the software package, user's manual and help screen availability. Instructions should also include methods used to search for and enter foods to be analyzed, viewable information during data entry, ease of editing the food list and the dietary standards with which analyses are compared. Database manipulation availability and data entry features should be assessed prior to purchase.

- The United States Department of Agriculture (USDA) maintains computerized nutrition databases that can be accessed on the Internet. Standard USDA nutrient databases and those used for government surveys, such as the National Food and Nutrition Survey, (NFNS) and per capita, per day data on nutritional content of the United States food supply are other sources of nutrient information.

(2) Biochemical analyses

Lab values related to nutritional status

- Biochemical tests of nutritional status are minimally influenced by other factors such as exercise, infection, stress or trauma. Age, sex, heredity, menstrual cycle, hydration or disease should be considered, and ranges of normal values used for interpretation. Some biochemical tests reflect immediate nutrient intake; others reflect long-term intake.

- Laboratory data are obtained from an examination of blood, urine, tissue, feces, bone or fluid losses from the body. Test results are compared on the written report to standardized or normal values used by the testing laboratory. Dietitians are expected to know some key normal values, but reports of laboratory analysis always indicate the values that are not within normal limits.

- Laboratory tests are often ordered in groups, called panels. The Centers for Medicare and Medicaid (CMS) use the term, **BASIC METABOLIC PANEL (BMP)** (mini panel) to define the components of each test for reimbursement purposes. The BMP usually includes: glucose, serum sodium and potassium, carbon dioxide or bicarbonate, serum chloride, blood urea nitrogen, (BUN) calcium and creatinine. This is similar to the CHEM 7 panel, which does not include calcium. The **COMPREHENSIVE METABOLIC PANEL (CMP)** includes the components of the BMP plus albumin, total protein, alkaline phosphate (ALP), alanine transaminase (ALT), aspartate aminotransferase (AST),calcium serum, direct bilirubin, Gamma-GT (gamma-glutamyl transpeptidase), LDH (lactic dehydrogenase), serum phosphorous, total bilirubin, total cholesterol, total protein, uric acid. This is similar to the CHEM 20 panel. Common serum chemistry panels that include electrolytes, phosphorous, total cholesterol and triglycerides and in addition to many tests in the basic and comprehensive metabolic panels, urinalysis and **COMPLETE BLOOD COUNT (CBC)** are necessary for dietitians in making a nutritional diagnosis and formulating a plan for implementation of care.

- **NITROGEN BALANCE** measures the net changes in the body's total protein mass. The body protein mass is constantly being catabolized and renewed. Nitrogen balance is the difference between nitrogen intake and output. During catabolism, the difference is negative; during anabolism, the difference is positive; when in balance, the difference is zero. An estimate of nitrogen balance can be made by measuring urine urea nitrogen, comparing it to nitrogen intake for the same period and adding a factor of 4 for non-urea nitrogen loss (losses in feces, skin and respiration).

  NITROGEN INTAKE = $\dfrac{\text{protein in g consumed by patient in 24 hr}}{\text{6.25g protein}}$

  N BALANCE = N intake (g/24 h) – N output (g urinary urea [g/24h] + 4.0 g)

  If nitrogen output is expressed in terms of urinary nitrogen, the 4.0 correction factor is changed to 2.0.

- When nitrogen intake is greater than nitrogen output, there is a **POSITIVE NITROGEN BALANCE.** The patient is in a state of **ANABOLISM,** with synthesis of body tissue protein exceeding breakdown of tissue protein. Positive nitrogen balance is common during growth, weight gain and pregnancy. When nitrogen intake equals nitrogen output, there is **NITROGEN BALANCE.** The buildup of tissue protein is equal to the breakdown of tissue protein, and so dietary protein intake meets needs. When nitrogen intake is less than nitrogen output, there is a **NEGATIVE NITROGEN BALANCE.** The patient is in a state of **CATABOLISM,** with breakdown of tissue exceeding synthesis of tissue protein. Negative nitrogen balance is common when there is weight loss, severe trauma or burns. When catabolic, dietary protein should be increased to replace losses and promote anabolism.

TESTS FOR VISCERAL PROTEIN

Test	Half-Life	Indication	Influences	Normal Values
Serum albumin (albumin accounts for over 50% of total serum proteins and changes slowly)	16-21 days	Prolonged protein deficiency	Elevated in dehydration or in patients receiving transfusions; depressed values in patients with liver disease and fluid overload, protein-losing enteropathy, burns, cancer, tuberculosis, nephrotic syndrome, pregnancy; levels affected by chemotherapy, steroids, and malabsorption. Not a good indicator of PEM because of its long half-life and because plasma albumin is replenished by extravascular albumin, which is higher than plasma albumin, when plasma albumin is low.	Normal = 3.5 -5.0g/dL Mild depletion = 2.8 - 3.4g/dLModerate = 2.1 - 2.7g/dL Severe = < 2.1 g/dL
Serum transferrin	8-10 days	Predictor of visceral protein status and iron depletion	Elevated in iron deficiency; decreased with protein-energy deficiency, chronic disease and liver dysfunction, fluid overload, pregnancy and vitamin A deficiency.	200-400mg/dL
Transthyretin (TTHY) also called prealbumin or thyroxine-binding prealbumin (TBPA)	2 days	Sensitive indicator for short-term protein therapy--responds to repletion in 2-3 days	Iron status, trauma, infection, recent dietary protein intake. Decreased in liver disease, protein-losing enteropathy, nephrotic syndrome and hemodilution.	19-43 mg/dL(lower values indicate deficit of protein or energy)
Retinol-binding protein (RBP)	10-12 hours	Quick response to repletion	Decreased in stress, vitamin A and zinc deficiencies, hyperthyroidism, nephrotic syndrome, liver disease, protein losing enteropathy, hemodilution. Elevated in chronic renal disease.	2.1-6.4 mg/dL
C Reactive Protein (CRP)	Increases within 4-6 hours of trauma	Monitors progress of stress reactions	When CRP begins to recede, anabolic period has begun and more intensive nutrition support can begin. TTHY levels increase as CRP levels decline.	Normal value is 0. In inflammation it increases dramatically.
Insulin-like growth factor1 (IGF-1)	About 4 hours	Rapidly responds to changes in protein-status, independent of inflammatory process efficacy of nutrition support	Concentration is affected by hepatic, renal, and some autoimmune diseases and estrogen use. Not currently in wide use in clinical settings. levels may be affected in burns and thrombosis.	95-395 mcg/L
Fibronecten (FN)	About 15 hours	Current research indicates possible use as an indicator of nutritional status and a possible of the efficacy of nutrition support	Not as affective by acute stress as other markers, but may be important for assessment of patients under acute stress because it has a short half-life. Has a role in wound healing so serum levels may be affected in burns and thrombosis.	220-400mg/dL

Tests of red blood cells/iron status

- **HEMATOCRIT (HCT)** is the volume of red blood cells in the ~~~le~~ blood. Elevated levels may indicate dehydration or polyc~~~~~ate generalized anemia, over-hydration or hemorrhage. Normal values are 39-49% for men and 33-43% for women. Normal hematocrit levels are lower during pregnancy and higher in newborns.

- **HEMOGLOBIN (HGB)** is an iron-containing molecule that carried oxygen in red blood cells. The amount of hemoglobin in blood is determined by the concentration of red blood cells. Low levels can indicate generalized anemia, protein-calorie malnutrition or hemorrhage. Normal values are 14-17g/dL for men and 12-15g/dL for women. Black men and women tend to have lower hemoglobin levels than white men and women. Normal hemoglobin levels are lower during pregnancy because plasma volume increases causing hemodilution. Normal levels are higher in newborns.

- **MEAN CELL VOLUME (MCV)** describes red blood cells in terms of individual red cell size. MCV is the volume of the average red blood cell. Elevated levels may indicate macrocytosis from folate or B_{12} deficiency. Low levels indicate microcytosis from iron deficiency, high iron need, malabsorption or blood loss. Normal values are 80-94 cu/microns.

$$MCV = \frac{\text{Hematocrit value (HCT)}}{\text{Red Blood Cell Count (RBC)}}$$

- **TOTAL IRON-BINDING CAPACITY (TIBC)** is the total amount of iron that can be carried in the plasma by transferrin. Transferrin is normally 20-40% saturated, so serum iron levels are about one-third the level of total iron-binding capacity. Less than 16% saturation is consistent with iron deficiency. Normal values are 240-450 mcg/dL. Levels above 450mcg/dL indicate iron deficiency. In 30% -40% of persons with iron deficiency anemia, TIBC is not elevated.

- **RED CELL DISTRIBUTION WIDTH (RDW)** refers to the variation in red blood cell size distribution. A wide variation in size, ranging from very small to large, has been shown to be an early indicator of a nutritionally induced anemia. In the presence of other normal red cell indices, an increased RDW can be an early sign of iron deficiency. Normal values are usually considered to be < 16%. RDW is also useful for detecting mixed nutritional deficiencies (e.g. with iron and folic acid) that may present a normal MCV. However, the complete clinical situation should be considered because a high RDW may be related to non-nutritional causes such as a recent transfusion or significant increase in reticulocytes.

Test of lean body mass

- **CREATININE HEIGHT INDEX (CHI)** is a biochemical test to estimate body muscle mass. Provided that renal function is normal, there is no rapid muscle catabolism (such as in trauma or surgery) and fluid intake is adequate. A client's urinary excretion rate is compared to the expected excretion rate for an individual of similar height and sex.

$$\% \text{ CHI} = \frac{\underline{\text{Actual milligrams of urinary creatinine for 24 hours x100}}}{\text{Standard milligrams of 24-hour urinary creatinine}}$$

Normal range	90% to 100%
Moderate deficit	<80%
Severe deficit	<60%

Refer to tables for standard and reference values for men and women of different age groups.

Collection and interpretation

- Caution should be exercised in using one specific laboratory value to make a nutritional diagnosis.

- Variations in laboratory results may be biological or analytical in origin. Biological variation refers to intra-and inter-individual variation in age, sex, weight, reproductive status, alcohol and tobacco use, exercise, genetic factors, posture and altitude. For example, collection after exercise will decrease iron and lipid levels compared to collection after rest. Time of day may influence laboratory results such as the specific gravity of urine.

- Analytical errors may be pre-or post-collection. Pre-collection analytical errors include equipment breakage, inadequate sample volume, using the wrong patient, poor sample transport conditions and contamination. Post-collection analytical errors include equipment failure and comparison against the wrong reference population.

- Interpretation of laboratory data in the elderly may be difficult. Reference ranges for lab testing in the elderly are lacking and variations within the elderly population limits reference values. Interpretation may be complicated by the presence of multiple chronic diseases and medications. Laboratory values that do not change with age include hepatic function tests (AST, ALT, GGTP, serum bilirubin), coagulation tests, serum electrolytes, total protein, calcium, phosphorus, serum folate, blood pH, $PaCO_2$, serum creatinine, thyroxine, hematocrit, hemoglobin, RBC indices and platelet count. Examples of laboratory values that do change with age include a slight decline in serum albumin, increased uric acid, decreased creatinine clearance, slight increase of TSH and T_3, decreased white blood count and a minimal increase in blood glucose.

f. Physical activity, habits and restrictions

- Intensity and duration of activity patterns can provide information related to body composition and metabolism. Less intense activities use less energy per unit of time due to involvement of fewer muscle cells. The greater the duration of an activity the greater the energy utilization.

- Active lifestyles are consistent with good health. The current thinking is that everyone should do 60 minutes or more of moderate activity each day to promote health, optimal weight and fitness.

II. NUTRITION CARE FOR INDIVIDUALS AND GROUPS (50%)

- High exercise intensity relies more heavily on glucose as a fuel; glycolysis is accelerated and glycogen from muscles is used. Low exercise intensity, with adequate oxygen and oxidative enzymes, relies on a mixture of fat and carbohydrate as fuel. As exercise intensity decreases and duration increases, fat is a more important source of fuel. Trained endurance athletes utilize fat because lipoprotein lipase activity is higher in trained muscle and intramuscular triglycerides can be more utilized more efficiently.

g. Economic/social

- Assessment must be set within the context of ethnic background, family size and income, living and cooking arrangements, occupation, mode of travel, educational level, value systems, age, etc. Actions recommended must be attainable, within the client's economic means, and appropriate to cultural values and level of education and must, first and foremost, be acceptable to the client.

(1) Psychosocial and behavioral factors

- Psychological status has a profound impact on food intake by affecting eating behavior and the emotional environment. Treatment of behavioral disorders may influence nutrient needs due to side effects of medications and abnormal activity patterns (ranging from lethargic to frenetic behavior). Measures of psychological assessment have been shown to be useful to determine nutrition intervention.

- The **MINI-MENTAL STATE EXAMINATION** assesses attention, memory, and language. Depression may be gauged by the **BECK DEPRESSION INVENTORY** and special surveys to assess depression in the elderly are useful.

(2) Socioeconomic factors

- Nutrient intake is affected by socioeconomic factors. An inadequate income, lack of knowledge and skills in food preparation, inability to purchase food, living alone, cooking for one and factors related to low income such as inadequate cooking facilities are socioeconomic variables that may adversely affect nutritional status.

- In addition to affecting observable, tangible results, socioeconomic factors may influence the validity of nutritional assessment data provided by patients. For example, caregivers may not accurately report their children's intake if embarrassment or fear prohibit their revealing an inadequate diet. Limited ability to read or write, often not disclosed, reduces reporting. Nutrient intake problems span the entire socioeconomic spectrum; therefore, the dietitian should not assume dietary adequacy for affluent clients.

- Cultural and religious food patterns are an important part of many people's daily diets. The dietitian should be culturally/ethnically aware of the major role these patterns have in daily meals. (See Food Patterns of Selected Cultural Groups in Domain IV.)

Lifestyles

- The dietitian should, whenever possible, support clients who have adopted non-traditional lifestyle practices based on strong beliefs, unless those practices are harmful to health.

(3) Functional factors

- The assessment of **FUNCTIONAL FACTORS** is performed to ascertain the ability of people to carry out tasks necessary to adequately care for themselves. This includes assessments of adequate strength, activities of daily living (ADL) and the environment in which the person lives.

- The assessment can be performed by standard assessment tools, such as the Subjective Global Assessment, strength testing, and/or direct observation of the patient's ability to perform certain tasks, such as shopping, climbing stairs and cooking.

h. Educational readiness assessment

(1) Motivational level and readiness to change

- **MOTIVATION** is an indicator of an individual's readiness to learn. It is what causes a person to take action. Motivation arouses and instigates behavior, gives direction and purpose to behavior, supports positive behaviors and/or leads to choosing or preferring a particular behavior. It is concerned with what an individual will do rather than with what he or she can do.

- **BEHAVIOR MODIFICATION** is the alteration or extinction of previously learned behavior (thinking, feeling or doing) to encourage the development of new, positive behavior. For example, improving an overweight person's self-esteem by developing his or her musical talent may be a primary educational objective.

- Principles of behavior modification are as follows:

  - ➤ The principle of **CLASSICAL CONDITIONING** is based on laboratory experiments. The best-known experiment involved Pavlov's dogs. The dogs salivated when events occurred (a bell ringing) that had regularly and repeatedly come before the *Riley* presentation of food. **IVAN PAVLOV** theorized that consistent repetition of stimuli (the bell) could elicit a particular and conditioned response (salivating). *Dwight/Jim*
  - ➤ The principle of **OPERANT CONDITIONING** maintains that behaviors that are followed by satisfying consequences or removal of negative stimuli are more likely to occur in the future than are those with less satisfying consequences.
  - ➤ **EDWARD THORNDIKE** tested this theory and formulated the Law of Effect describing response-consequence conditioning of rewards, reinforcement and punishment.
  - ➤ **B.F. SKINNER** continued in Thorndike's tradition, explaining behavior on the basis of principles of operant or instrumental conditioning. Skinner developed a way to observe behavior in discrete units that could be recorded and evaluated as action-response-reinforcement. Toilet training of children with rewards of treats or praise for using the toilet is a common example. Skinner's behavioristic approach has been widely used in classrooms, mental hospitals, prisons, clinics and the workplace. In some situations, it may be unduly manipulative.

- The principle of **COGNITION** is that an individual's perceptions of external events, rather than the events themselves, influence behavior. Beliefs, attitudes, opinions and self-image can influence the change process. Cognitive restructuring may be needed to modify negative, self-defeating or pessimistic thoughts about themselves or their ability to adopt a potential treatment or program. Examples of negative cognition are: "I can't lose weight," or "It doesn't matter whether I'm fat because no one likes me anyway."

- **STAGES OF CHANGE MODELING** describe the processes of health behavior change. Prochaska and others have studied groups of people trying to change high-risk lifestyle behaviors, such as smoking, and increasing exercise or losing weight. The researchers have found that participants are more successful in changing behaviors over the long term when strategies are more closely matched to their stage of change. Thus the nutrition therapist can identify the client's stage for change and use strategies that are appropriate for that stage. The majority of people with dietary problems are within the first three stages of change. The traditional approach assumes readiness to change and may be one of the reasons many intervention programs fail. Prochaska, J.O., et al, work is described in "In Search of How People Change", *American Psychology, 1992: Vol 47(9), 1102-1114*. The six stages Prochaska identifies are:

  1. In the **PRE-CONTEMPLATIVE STAGE** clients have not accepted or personalized the health risks involved and do not recognize the need for change.

  2. Clients in the **CONTEMPLATIVE STAGE** believe they have a problem but are not sure where to start. They intend to start but are not committed to a specific date or action.

  3. The **PREPARATION STAGE** is where clients are ready to make changes but have not taken action yet. Clients need to find a goal or a strategy he/she finds acceptable and achievable.

  4. In the **ACTION STAGE** clients have taken steps to change and are modifying behavior.

  5. The **MAINTENANCE STAGE** requires increased coping skills and support for continual change.

  6. In the **RELAPSE STAGE** clients need renewed commitment and motivation because they have lost interest or become discouraged. The goal is to renew efforts. (If there is no relapse, behavioral change is successful; if there is relapse, there is often a return to the pre-contemplative stage.)

- **SANDOVAL**, et.al. has modified the stages to apply to nutrition counseling.

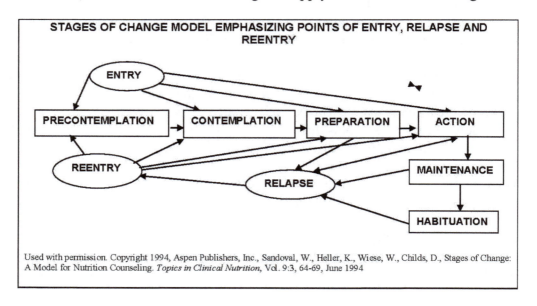

STAGES OF CHANGE MODEL EMPHASIZING POINTS OF ENTRY, RELAPSE AND REENTRY

Used with permission. Copyright 1994, Aspen Publishers, Inc., Sandoval, W., Heller, K., Wiese, W., Childs, D., Stages of Change: A Model for Nutrition Counseling. *Topics in Clinical Nutrition*, Vol. 9:3, 64-69, June 1994

(2) Educational level

- **LITERACY** is an individual's ability to read, write and speak English, to compute and solve problems at levels of proficiency necessary to function on the job and in society, to achieve one's goals and to develop one's knowledge and potential.

- **FUNCTIONAL LITERACY** is relative, depending upon the society. Generally, functional literacy refers to the ability to read and write at a level sufficient to participate actively and independently in activities within a society. In some countries, this may mean the ability to read and write one's name. Vocabulary, knowledge and comprehension are usually used to determine functional literacy.

- Grade reading level of materials can be tested through readability tests. Low-level reading materials for adults are usually written at a sixth-grade level. Computer programs that determine the reading level of texts are available.

- Defining literacy for persons whose first language is not English is challenging. Some will be highly literate in one language but not in another. Also, low literacy does not necessarily imply low intelligence. Some people with low literacy hold jobs and function well and competently. Many who cannot read English do not acknowledge that and develop compensatory behaviors, so that low literacy is not evident. A typical behavior is to bring written information home and have another person read or explain it or assist in completing a task or filling out a form.

- The average level of educational attainment in the United States is grade 12.7. Materials such as newspapers, forms that people need to fill out, street signs and public notices have a readability level between 8th and 12th grade. Large type, plenty of white space, and pictures or illustrations facilitate clients' learning, especially for those with low reading levels.

- Because some individuals may have low literacy, signs warning of dangers should be universal symbols of warning and/or be colors/shapes that are recognizable as dangers. Safety procedures should be practiced, not only provided in written form.

- Assessing a client's ability to read and comprehend printed material will guide the selection of teaching aids and materials provided. Rudolph Tuesch used grade levels to identify the degree of complexity of written materials through use of a readability formula. The **TUESCH FORMULA** and its subsequent versions establish the reading level that is required to read certain materials. The formula focuses on word length, word frequency and sentence length. The theory behind Tuesch's formula is that the more complicated the text (more syllables, more long words and longer sentences), the higher the level of literacy required.

THE SMOG READABILITY FORMULA

How to Test for Readability

To calculate the SMOG reading grade level, begin with the entire written work that is being assessed and follow these steps:

1.   Count off 10 consecutive sentences near the beginning, in the middle, and near the end of the text.
2.   From this sample of 30 sentences, circle all of the words containing three or more syllables (polysyllabic), including repetitions of the same word, and then total the number of words circled.
3.   Count the number of polysyllabic words in the 30 sentences and look up the approximate grade level on the chart.

SMOG CONVERSION TABLE*

Total Polysyllabic Word Counts	Approximate Grade Level (+/-1.5 Grades)
0-2	4
3-6	5
7-12	6
13-20	7
21-30	8
31-42	9
43-56	10
57-72	11
73-90	12
91-110	13
111-132	14
133-156	15
157-182	16
183-210	17
211-240	18+

* Developed by Harold C. McGraw, Office of Educational Research, Baltimore County Schools, Towson, Maryland. Source: Making Health Connections Work, NIH Publication Number 89-1493, USDHHS, NIH, National Cancer Institute, 1989.

- It is best for translations to other languages to be done by individuals who are familiar with the language (and dialect, where possible), culture and subject matter and who are able incorporate appropriate cultural terms and images.

(3) Situational, environmental, economic, social, cultural

- Cultural, socioeconomic, language and physical needs must be taken into account when setting goals.

- Nutrition therapists often deal with individuals who have multiple medical and therapeutic needs. The most critical needs for management and control of an existing condition should be determined. For example, information about low-fat foods is valuable for almost all clients, but when faced with uncontrolled diabetes mellitus, a client needs dietary information geared specifically to management of this particular condition. It is important for the therapist to help the client focus on the most crucial needs first.

- Environmental, societal, occupational and behavioral factors affect health. Younger adults may be most interested in health promotion activities designed to improve appearance, weight and increase energy and stamina. Older individuals are generally more interested in disease prevention than are individuals under age 30. Clients are more interested in preventing problems that they perceive are personal risks to them because of family history, lab tests or known risk factors. Pregnant women, for example, are at a "teachable moment" for health promotion.

- Clients' needs must be evaluated within the context of their families. Counselors ought to consider the following questions: To what degree is special meal preparation feasible? Who is responsible for that preparation? What financial resources are available? Will treatment deprive other family members of important items or activities? Will other family members be supportive of treatment (e.g., weight loss diet)? Is the client's condition influenced by the family situation (e.g., anorexia nervosa, obesity and alcoholism)? Are there family habits that influence the client's needs (e.g., working mother, cultural or religious beliefs about health or food)?

- Some clients need nutritional assistance to facilitate rehabilitation. In assessing a client's rehabilitative needs, the nutrition therapist might ask the following questions: "How will nutrition affect the success of the rehabilitative process? What are the priorities for rehabilitation? Is diet a part of the immediate needs? For example, a high-protein, high-vitamin diet will promote healing after surgery.

- Nutrient needs during the life cycle vary. Knowing the average or approximate age of an audience helps the nutrition therapist prepare information specific to his/her clients' needs. For example, when asked to speak to a group of women, one will want to know if the audience is young mothers, single working women, students or older women as different groups have differing interests and concerns.

- The population being addressed should determine the presentation format, instruments, examples, and so forth, as well as the topics used for educational programs

- **BARRIERS** block understanding. Only after individuals are aware of the beliefs that influence how they perceive others can they alter communication to safeguard against these factors becoming barriers to understanding.

- Common **ATTITUDINAL BARRIERS** include negative perceptions of intelligence, experience, culture, language, age and status. Ways to compensate for barriers are to paraphrase or restate what a person has said, de-emphasize status distinctions, use clear language and concrete examples and make empathic responses. Sometimes it is useful to develop peer counseling situations or use translators if there is great "distance" between teachers and learners. For example, often individuals who have lost weight are very successful leading weight control groups; community nutrition programs may prefer hiring professionals of the same ethnic background as the clients. Fewer barriers and easier rapport are generally found among individuals of the same culture or with a shared problem or interest.

- Instructional adaptations are necessary for learners with disabilities. Learners who have visual, auditory, emotional and social impairments and physical, speech and learning disabilities may require very specific adjustments in instruction and evaluation activities.

- All learners with disabilities should be encouraged to become actively involved in the learning process. Learners with visual impairments benefit from: clear verbal instructions and material, especially audio cassettes that can be replayed; key words in outline form in large print 18-point font sizes or larger; short, concise instructions; involvement of other senses such as touch or smell; and repetition to reinforce key points.

- Learners with auditory impairments benefit from: instructions in American Sign Language; speaking slowly in natural and articulated tones; reduction of distracting or interfering sounds; printed material, preferably provided in advance; involvement of other senses such as sight, touch or smell.

- Learners with speech or language disorders benefit from: extra time for verbal expression and comprehension; evaluation with games, puzzles, food models and other methods that do not require verbal response; speakers using normal voice tone and short sentences; choices to indicate response rather than questions requiring open-ended responses.

- Learners with physical disabilities benefit from: evaluation and reduction of barriers and obstacles, especially for those with impaired mobility; communication with physical, occupational or rehabilitation therapists to identify needs; handouts and tapes to reinforce instruction; consideration of physical limitations on an individual basis.

- Learners with social and emotional impairments benefit from: close cooperation with appropriate members of the healthcare team; discussion of inappropriate behaviors in a non-threatening manner; positive reinforcement of appropriate behaviors; familiar persons in the room that provide comfort and support; well documented observations.

- Adults with learning disabilities benefit from: appropriate strategies to improve visual or auditory perceptions; clear, concise, ordered instruction; repetition; show and tell methods that involve several senses; elimination of distractions; plenty of time for instruction and evaluation.

3. Nutritional assessment of populations and community needs assessment

- A COMMUNITY is a group of individuals that can be defined by location, function, shared interest or social cohesion.

- The traditional community agency role was a "waiting mode" in which professionals waited for clients; now more are in a "seeking mode" in which professionals extend services to previously untreated, high-risk persons. A community agency with a nutrition component focuses clinical concern on a population rather than on individuals. It considers interactions of people and their environment, including biologic and social phenomena; identifies alternatives by locating and developing existing resources and strengths in the community; directs its efforts toward prevention and health promotion; teaches self-care but still provides nutritional supervision and management.

- Assessment is a necessary prerequisite step that identifies problems and prioritizes programs and services.

a. Community and group nutritional status indicators

- The local public health department often has statistical information that may be helpful to a community nutrition program in assessing the needs of the local population.

- Nutrition risk status includes maternal and infant mortality rates, or the number of low birth weight infants born locally; the prevalence of obesity, the number of new immigrants, unique health-related practices, age of the population, socioeconomic data, illness identified with poor nutritional status.

(1) Demographic data

- **DEMOGRAPHICS** deal with age, race, sex, living arrangements, population density, birth rate and death information, compiled from numbers, counts, etc., by categories.

- Changes in this data may be important signals to the public health community that there is new need for services.

(2) Incidence and prevalence of nutrition-related status indicators

- Individuals with known risk factors, chronic diseases or lab values that predict future risks should be evaluated for potential drug/nutrient interactions, malnutrition or other consequences related to the specific risk factor.

- Specific ethnic and cultural groups may have increased or decreased incidence of particular diseases as a result of heredity or habits. Demand for services for young children and the elderly depends on numbers within specific age groups.

(3) Prevalence of food insecurity

- **FOOD INSECURITY** occurs when individuals or households have difficulty providing enough food for each person due to lack of resources. Food insecurity includes the inability to purchase enough food to avoid hunger or enough healthful food.

- The term **FOOD DESERT** refers to areas where there is a limited supply of fresh, affordable, wholesome food. Some low income urban areas have few grocery stores and limited transportation so residents rely on venues that primarily sell snacks, packaged goods and fast food and offer limited healthful options.

- Specific needs populations (e.g., homeless, low-income, AIDS patients, transient populations), are more likely to have high medical and nutrient risks but are difficult to reach. Numbers and needs can be assessed through the use of existing support services (shelters, clinics, food banks) or schools (free lunch program) or SNAP program. Collaboration with social service agencies and religious institutions extends availability of nutrition services. Needs may fluctuate seasonally.

Special needs populations

- The team approach is recommended for assessment of populations with special needs. The team may include physicians, geneticists, biochemists, dietitians, psychologists, nurses, speech and occupational therapists, social workers and others. Nutritional assessment of persons with developmental disabilities includes the same components as for the general population. However, behavioral, communication, cognitive, dental, motor and feeding skill assessments are also integral components in the assessment, planning and evaluation process. Feeding observations are useful when oral-motor or feeding delays are present. Dietary assessment tools specifically targeted to the disabled have been developed.

- The **EDUCATION OF ALL HANDICAPPED CHILDREN ACT** mandates education for all children aged 6 to 21 years in the least restrictive environment. As a result, special provisions for serving children with special needs are mandated according to the National School Lunch Program, School Breakfast Program, Civil Rights and Rehabilitation Act of 1973. Child nutrition programs also must follow the regulations in the Americans with Disabilities Act of 1990. The most frequent requirements for the school food service program to serve the special needs child include menu modification related to texture, calories and nutrients; environmental considerations, and working with special education teachers and parents. The law also requires provision of comprehensive nutrition services to special needs children aged 3-5 and recognizes nutritionists as the qualified health professionals to provide this care. This law is now known as **INDIVIDUALS WITH DISABILITIES EDUCATION ACT (IDEA).**

NUTRITION-RELATED HEALTH RISKS AND PROBLEMS AT VARIOUS STAGES OF LIFE

Group Risks and Problems

Group	Risks and Problems
Pregnant women	Pre-pregnancy underweight or overweight; inadequate or excessive weight gain; anemia; gestational diabetes, pre-eclampsia; frequent pregnancies; under age 18; low nutrient intake; excess nutrients from supplements; consumption of alcohol or drugs causing fetal alcohol syndrome or birth defects; smoking; **PICA** which is eating non-food items such as plaster, paper, clay or laundry starch.
Infants/children	Failure to thrive; overfeeding; obesity, underfeeding; premature introduction of regular food or cow's milk; lack of fluoride; inadequate iron; inadequate exercise leading to obesity; infant diarrhea, constipation; **NURSING BOTTLE SYNDROME;** the sucking on bottles with milk or juice at bedtime erodes baby teeth and causes malformations of developing teeth because the liquid forms an encouraging medium for growth of decay-causing bacteria.
Adolescents	Excess or inadequate calories, sodium, fat; iron-deficiency anemia; malnutrition; fad diets; eating disorders; inappropriate dieting or sports nutrition practices; substance abuse; teen pregnancy; inadequate calcium intake, especially by girls; obesity; supplements among boys.
Adults and Elderly	Hypertension, hyperlipidemia, elevated blood cholesterol; diabetes mellitus; excess or inadequate calories; excess alcohol or drugs; inactivity; malnutrition; low iron, calcium, potassium, vitamin D, fiber; osteoporosis; constipation; dental problems; drug-nutrient interactions; excess supplementation; poor eating habits; inability to secure or prepare food due to lack of transportation, mobility, funds or social isolation; the elderly take more prescribed medications that are likely to cause gastrointestinal upsets or changes in flavor; diminished senses of taste and smell in the elderly often decrease appetite and the enjoyment of food; changes in motor skills may decrease ability to cook and eat; digestion is less efficient and small frequent meals are desirable.

NUTRITIONAL FACTORS INVOLVED IN COMMON HEALTH PROBLEMS

Health Problem	Probable Nutrition Cause or Result
Anemia	Inadequate iron and/or folate intake; malnutrition in children
Cancer (experimental AND epidemiologic data for some forms)	Excessive fat intake; low fiber intake: obesity; vitamin and mineral deficiencies or excesses; alcohol
Cirrhosis	Malnutrition; excessive alcohol intake
Constipation	Inadequate fiber or fluid intake; high fat intake; reaction to medications
Dental caries	Excessive, frequent consumption of concentrated sweets; lack of fluoride; poor hygiene
Diabetes (type 2)	Obesity; excessive carbohydrate/caloric Intake; sedentary lifestyle
Diverticulosis	Inadequate fiber intake
Hypercholesterolemia	Obesity; excessive intake of total fat, saturated fat and cholesterol
Hypertension	Obesity; excessive caloric intake; excessive sodium intake (in sodium sensitive individuals)
Infection	Malnutrition; poor hygiene
Obesity	Excessive caloric intake; excessive fat intake; sedentary lifestyle
Osteoporosis	Inadequate calcium or vitamin D intake
Underweight, growth failure	Malnutrition, inadequate calories; malabsorption; poor feeding practices

b. Development and maintenance of nutrition screening and surveillance systems

- **NUTRITIONAL MONITORING** measures changes in the populations' nutritional status over time.

- A **SURVEY** is a collection of data that provides the analysis of some aspect of an area or a group.

- **SURVEILLANCE** is an approach to collecting data on a populations' health and nutritional status in which data collection occurs on a regular and repeated basis.

(1) National, state, and local reference data (e.g., NHANES, BRFSS, YRBSS)

National surveys and national surveillance systems

- **NUTRITIONAL SURVEILLANCE** involves frequent, continuous examination and reporting of nutrition-related parameters. The **NATIONAL NUTRITION MONITORING AND RELATED RESEARCH PROGRAM (NNMRP)** was passed in 1990. The comprehensive plan was developed and approved to unify the planning and coordination of data collection and analysis coordination for the large number of federal agencies that monitor nutrition related information of the United States population. In addition, it is meant to identify health related problems and trends and to develop program strategies to address the public health concerns that may be diet related. Public policy and nutrition research priorities are often based on these data. The United States Department of Agriculture (USDA) and The Department of Health and Human Services (DHHS) work jointly to coordinate and implement activities. Among concerns mentioned in several of the reports issued, are the percentage of overweight children and adults in the population, the continued intake of total fat and saturated fat above recommended levels, anemia in selected segments of the population and food insecurity.

National surveys

- **TEN-STATE NUTRITION SURVEY (1968-1970)** was the first survey to evaluate the nutritional status of a large segment of the population (about 24,000 families). The survey was conducted by the Department of Health, Education, and Welfare (DHEW), now the Department of Health and Human Services (DHHS.) In each of the ten states from geographically diverse regions, families with incomes below the poverty level in 1960 were selected for participation, on a random basis. The objectives of the survey were to find the location and prevalence of serious hunger, malnutrition and other health problems in the population being studied. The survey examined nutritional status on the basis of dietary intake, anthropometric, clinical, biochemical and dental assessment. Demographic information on all family members was also obtained. Results of the Ten-State Nutrition Survey were as follows:
  - ➤ Malnutrition or increased risk of malnutrition existed in a large proportion of the population, especially among low-income persons. It was more common in African Americans and Hispanics than whites.
  - ➤ Social, cultural and geographic differences affected nutritional status.
  - ➤ There was more evidence of unsatisfactory nutritional status among adolescents 10-16 years old than in other age groups.
  - ➤ Obesity was prevalent among adult females, especially African American women, and among children and adolescents. In some age groups, 50% of women were obese.
  - ➤ Low hemoglobin levels indicated widespread iron deficiency.
  - ➤ Protein intake was generally adequate.
  - ➤ Young people in all groups had a high incidence of low vitamin A levels, with the greatest number among Hispanics living in Texas.
  - ➤ There was some evidence of ascorbic acid deficiency, mostly among males and the elderly.
  - ➤ There was evidence of poor riboflavin status among African Americans and young people of all ethnic groups.
  - ➤ Poor dental health and low levels of dental care were common.

Food consumption surveys

- **UNITED STATES DEPARTMENT OF AGRICULTURE (USDA) HOUSEHOLD FOOD CONSUMPTION SURVEYS,** also called **NATIONWIDE FOOD CONSUMPTION SURVEYS** were conducted at approximately 10-year intervals since 1936 to find out the kinds and amounts of foods people eat. The major objective of these individual intake studies is to describe food consumption behavior and determine adequacy of food and nutrient intakes. The data are used to develop national nutrition policies related to food production, food safety, food assistance, marketing and nutrition education. Family food plans and other publications of the USDA are based on these surveys.

- The **CONTINUING SURVEY OF FOOD INTAKES BY INDIVIDUALS (CSFH)** has been conducted on a yearly basis beginning in 1985. Results of these surveys showed vast changes in food availability and in eating behaviors during ten-year periods. In 2000, the USDA and DHHS merged the CSFII with NHANES and it is now called the **NATIONAL FOOD AND NUTRITION SURVEY (NFNS)**. The **DIET AND HEALTH KNOWLEDGE SURVEY (DHKS)**, began in 1989 was a telephone survey that followed up the CSFII. **"WHAT WE EAT IN AMERICA"**, is the dietary portion of the new survey, since 2002. Results are often published in the popular press.

  Annual surveys

- **HEALTHY EATING INDEX (HEI)** is a summary measure of overall diet quality; compared to the *Dietary Guidelines for Americans*, designed to access and monitor the dietary status of Americans. It is a program that was developed in 1995 by the **CENTER FOR NUTRITION POLICY AND PROMOTION (CNPP)**, a division of the USDA.

National surveillance systems

- The national surveillance systems are coordinated by The **CENTERS FOR DISEASE CONTROL AND PREVENTION (CDC.)** They are statistical service programs that provide data to state and local health agencies concerning low-income populations of children and pregnant women who are enrolled in publicly funded nutrition related programs. States that receive this information use it for program planning. The populations used for these studies are self-selected because they participate in these programs, so they may represent the nutritional status of all individuals in the community.

  - The **PEDIATRIC NUTRITION SURVEILLANCE SYSTEM** (PEDNSS) started in 1974. This system monitors indications of nutrition status such as short stature, under or overweight, anemia, low birth weight, and methods of feeding infants. The data is compared with information from a reference population to estimate prevalence.
  - The **PREGNANCY NUTRITION SURVEILLANCE SYSTEM** (PNSS) started in 1979. This system monitors pre-gravid underweight and overweight, prenatal weight gain and anemia. Since 1987, self-reported data on smoking and alcohol consumption are used to examine the dose effect of these on infant birth weight. It also monitors method of feeding infants.
  - The **BEHAVIORAL RISK FACTOR SURVEILLANCE SYSTEM** (BRFSS) monitors personal risk behaviors in each of the 50 states. Data collected relates to health status, access to healthcare, tobacco and alcohol use, injury control (use of seat belts), use of prevention services (immunization and mammography), HIV/AIDS, dieting practices, frequency of intake of dietary fat, fruits and vegetables, treatment for high blood cholesterol. The survey is conducted on adults aged 18 or older by telephone.. States use the information to plan public health programs on nutrition and health.
  - The **YOUTH RISK BEHAVIOR SURVEILLANCE SYSTEM** (YRBSS) started in 1990, is sponsored by National Center for Chronic Disease Prevention and Health Promotion (NCCDPHP)of the Centers for Disease Control (CDC). It is an annual survey of high school age students in all states and the District of Columbia, the US Virgin Islands

and Puerto Rico. The survey collects demographic information; smoking and alcohol use; weight control practices, exercise and eating practices information.

Reference data (e.g., National Health and Nutrition Exam Survey)

- Data provide a research base and a basis for community assessment, prioritizing resource allocation, program planning, legislation and evaluation of change.

- The usefulness of collected data is limited to the population studied. Extrapolating to other populations may not be appropriate. Data are based on a large sample, but they can be used as an indicator of potential problems and trends for a select community.

- Dietary adequacy cannot be related to a fixed cut-off point, such as percentage of DRI/RDA. No single point accurately separates the well nourished from the undernourished. DRI/RDAs are often set for the "average" person and are therefore, in excess of the needs of many individuals. They are set high to allow for individual variations. The guidelines accompanying the DRI/RDAs states that "the RDAs should not be used to assess the adequacy of individual diets," although this is commonly done.

- It is difficult to directly associate nutrient intake with development of chronic disease.

- Data are limited by lack of information about the nutrient composition of foods, by lack of accurate assessment techniques for many nutrients and by poor estimates and reports of amounts of foods actually consumed.

- **TREND ANALYSIS** is the tracking of trends with information gathered at more than one time. Trend analysis can examine how programs or events affect eating behaviors or nutritional status, or it may track trends by reuse of questionnaires to monitor responses or concerns at different times. Business and industry also monitor trends in consumer interests, nutrition concerns, sales of food items and so forth. For example, the Food Marketing Institute publishes an annual survey of consumer shopping habits, attitudes and other trends.

- Vital and health statistics include the following:

  - ➤ **MORBIDITY** is the number of individuals with a disease in a given area.
  - ➤ **MORBIDITY RATIO** is the ratio of sick to well in a given area, expressed in terms of the population, usually per 100,000.
  - ➤ **MORTALITY** is the death rate. It measures frequency of death for a specific time period (often 1 year) in relation to the total population. Examples of morbidity and mortality statistics are neonatal and infant mortality rates and the incidence of morbidity or mortality due to coronary heart disease, diabetes, hypertension or alcoholism.
  - ➤ **EARLY PERIODIC SCREENING, DIAGNOSIS AND TREATMENT** (EPSDT) is a program that will reimburse for nutrition screening, assessment and counseling of low-income children up to age 21 through Medicaid. WIC records and local health departments are sources of these data.

- **NATIONAL HEALTH AND NUTRITION EXAMINATION SURVEY I (NHANES I)** (1971--1975) was conducted by the Department of Health Education and Welfare (DHEW), now known as the Department of Health and Human Services (DHHS), as part of a continuing program to obtain information on the health of Americans. NHANES I provided a surveillance system that measured nutritional status and enabled changes to be monitored. It was the first nationwide health survey to include nutrition in the United States. It consisted of a true sample of the population, so findings could be applied to the entire U.S. population. The survey was designed to determine the nutritional status of a sample of the population between 1 and 74 years of age. The evaluation of nutritional status was based on clinical examinations, biochemical tests, anthropometric measurements, dietary intake data based on a 24-hour recall and food frequency questionnaires. Nutrient intakes were compared with the RDA, reported as a percentage of the standard. Data groups were divided into "below poverty level" and "above poverty level."

from 1975

- Key results of NHANES I were:

  - ➤ There was more evidence of low iron intake than of other nutrients, especially among children age 1-3, adolescents age 12-17, women age 18-44, low-income white females age 65 and over and African American females in both income groups.
  - ➤ Most groups met recommended levels for calorie intake. Fat represented 37% of calories.
  - ➤ Most people had adequate intakes of protein, but men age 55-65+ in the low-income group and all men over age 65 had lower levels, as did females age 15-17 and over age 55. Women age 35-44 and over age 55 also had lower intakes.
  - ➤ Generally, the intake of other key nutrients was adequate, but some groups had low intakes of calcium, vitamin A and ascorbic acid.
  - ➤ It was estimated that 28% of adult females and 19% of adult males were obese.

- **NATIONAL HEALTH AND NUTRITION EXAMINATION SURVEY II (NHANES II)** (1976–1980) had a target population of individuals 6 months to 74 years old. Larger proportions of young children (6 months to 5 years old) and the elderly (69 to 74 years old) were studied. Evaluation of nutritional status was based on the same assessment tools as in NHANES I.

- Differences from NHANES I were:

  - ➤ Anemia was investigated in detail because of the results of NHANES I.
  - ➤ Special studies of plasma zinc and copper were included.
  - ➤ More information about intake of vitamin and mineral supplements was gathered.
  - ➤ Data about participation in government food programs were collected.
  - ➤ Data for vitamin A were taken only for the 3-11-year-old age group, because vitamin A did not seem to be a problem for older age groups in NHANES I.
  - ➤ Analyses of thiamin and riboflavin were omitted because of problems in determining urinary values.

- Key results of NHANES II were as follows:

  - ➤ Serum iron levels were higher for males than for females and higher for white females than for African American females. The highest prevalence of iron deficiency was in children ages 1-2, girls and women during childbearing years and adolescent boys.
  - ➤ On any given day, 66% of women ages 18-30 consumed less than the recommended amount of calcium.

II. NUTRITION CARE FOR INDIVIDUALS AND GROUPS (50%)

- Serum zinc was higher in males age 15 and over than in females. Whites age 3-74 had higher levels than African Americans. Non-poverty males had higher values than poverty males, but no differences were seen in females. Data on serum zinc levels were inadequate for assessing zinc status, but were useful in identification of groups at risk.
- Men reduced energy intake from 2,700kcal at age 23-24 to 1,800kcal at age 65-74. Women reduced energy consumption from 1,600kcal to 1,300kcal over the same period.

- The **HISPANIC HEALTH AND NUTRITION EXAMINATION SURVEY (HHANES)** (1982-1984) collected health and nutritional data on the three largest subgroups of Hispanics including Mexican-Americans residing in the Southwestern states of Arizona, California, New Mexico, Colorado and Texas; Cuban-Americans from Dade County, Florida; and Puerto Rican residents of the New York City metropolitan area. Data collection methods included physical examinations and interviews, diagnostic testing, anthropometric measurements and laboratory tests. The purpose of the HHANES was to obtain basic data on specific chronic conditions in addition to basic health and nutritional information. The only finding that differed from the general population was that children aged 2 to 5 years showed a greater prevalence of low height for age.

- **NATIONAL HEALTH AND NUTRITION EXAMINATION SURVEY III (NHANES III) (1988-1994)** targeted four population groups: children aged 2 months to five years; persons aged 60 years and older; black Americans; and Mexican-Americans. The five main goals of NHANES III were:

  - to estimate the national prevalence of selected diseases and risk factors;
  - to estimate national population reference distributions of selected health parameters;
  - to document and investigate reasons for secular trends in selected diseases and risk factors;
  - to contribute to an understanding of disease etiology; and
  - to investigate the natural history of selected diseases.

  Issues emphasized were child health, health of older Americans, occupational health and environmental health, including exposure to pesticides and amount of carbon monoxide in the blood.

  - Information gathered from NHANES III was used by the Food and Drug Administration to change food fortification regulations. It also was used by the National Cholesterol Education Program to evaluate public education activities, by the Healthy People programs to evaluate 33 of the health objectives and by the National Center for Health Statistics to revise child growth charts. Specific interview questions allowed the study of food security issues.
  - Diagnostic procedures unique to the third NHANES included bioelectric impedance, and bone density measurements using dual-energy x-ray absorptiometry. There was no upper age limit in this study, which was helpful in studying age related nutritional issues.

- NHANES surveys have been conducted on a continuous basis at approximately 5-year intervals. In addition to the valuable nutrition intake data, they also provide a health profile of the nation's population. The **NHANES** that began in 1999, became a continuous survey, and has a goal of studying 5000 people each year. It is linked to related government population surveys such as The **NATIONAL HEALTH INTERVIEW SURVEY (NHIS)** and the CSFII. Data from this study, known as the **NATIONAL FOOD AND NUTRITION SURVEY (NFNS)** will be available more quickly but will not be comparable to previous NHANES studies.

Guidelines for interpretation

- Consider the subjects studied (humans, animals, cultured cells, bacteria, etc.) and the methodology.

  - ➤ Causal relationships cannot be determined by typical nutritional surveys, but must have longitudinal data.
  - ➤ Consider limitations inherent in the study design or dietary survey method. For example, studies of a few individuals cannot be applied to all people; studies on adult males cannot be applied to females or children. Surveillance systems provide continuous monitoring of nutritional status of individual groups, especially high-risk groups. Major components are nutritional assessment, measuring changes over time and presenting data to policy makers in a timely fashion.
  - ➤ Keep in mind that there is a tendency to underreport food/nutrient intake because foods reported as consumed are calculated as standard amounts and many people consume much larger portions. Few surveys require actually weighing/measuring food.

Other

- The **NUTRITION SCREENING INITIATIVE** is an effort supported by about 30 organizations including and that provides screening procedures and screening checklists for the elderly. The process begins with a self-administered screening tool or checklist. The first screen, Level 1, can be administered by a community member, social worker or healthcare professional, to individuals with identified early warning signs. The Level 2 screen is a history obtained by a physician, nurse or dietetics professional. It includes medical diagnosis, chronic illnesses, medication, dentition, bowel habits, alcohol/drug abuse, eating disorders, emotional or psychological conditions and height and weight. Advice may be given to encourage self-help to improve diet or lifestyle. Referrals to social service and healthcare professionals are provided when need is indicated.

c. Availability of community resources

- Community agencies provide varied services based on eligibility for services, geographic location, cost of services and referral mechanisms.

- There are many organizations that provide help to community agencies. The services range from data collection, help in planning programs, help in identifying the community needs to location of financial resources.

- Local and federal public health departments offer help with demographic information and location of local organizations.

- These organizations range from local WIC programs, schools, hospitals, to services for the homeless, services for the chronically ill, disabled people and the elderly.

II. NUTRITION CARE FOR INDIVIDUALS AND GROUPS (50%)

Community service agencies

- Community service agencies can work with patients or clients to help them get special services including meals, help with shopping, appliances, etc. This can aid in better patient outcomes.

COMMUNITY SERVICES

Problem Category	Agencies that Provide Services
Educational	Child day-care facilities School systems Vocational training programs Department of Mental Retardation Veterans Administration Bureau of Indian Affairs Migrant opportunity programs Community action programs
Economic	Employment services Vocational training programs Rehabilitation programs Welfare, including food assistance programs Religious and other voluntary organizations Bureau of Indian Affairs Social Security
Medical	Hospitals Health departments: state, county, city School nurses Local physicians Veterans Administration Hospital Indian Health Service Other local health services
Social	Child Care facilities School systems Legal Aid Local Service and religious organizations Mental health services Migrant opportunity programs Welfare
Transportation	Local service and religious organizations Migrant opportunity programs
Environment	State and county health departments Public service and utility companies Local government officials Agricultural extension programs
Food	County and city welfare departments, including food assistance programs Local volunteer and religious organizations School lunch Food banks, pantries

(1) Food and nutrition assistance programs

Food stamp program

- The **Supplemental Nutrition Assistance Program (SNAP)**, formerly the Food Stamp Program, is a federal entitlement program established in 1964 to provide more food buying power to low income individuals or families through monthly allotments of stamps that can be used to obtain food. USDA administers the program. An **Entitlement Program** is a government-funded program that allows anyone who meets eligibility standards to receive benefits.

- Recipients of **SNAP** use an Electronic Benefit Transfer (EBT) card similar to a credit card, to purchase food and food products for human consumption from businesses that are approved to accept the cards. This includes the purchase of hot foods to carry out (e.g., cooked chicken) purchased from approved vendors. Seeds and plants for home gardens may also be purchased. A household may not use the SNAP card to purchase alcohol, tobacco, vitamins, medicine, pet food and non-food items, such as soap or paper goods. To qualify for the program, households must meet eligibility criteria and provide proof of their statements about household financial circumstances.

- Eligibility and allotments are based on income, household size, assets, housing costs, work requirements and other factors. Most households must have gross monthly incomes below 130 percent of the poverty line and net monthly incomes at or below 100 percent of the poverty guidelines for their household size. Households with elderly or persons with disabilities are subject only to the net income test. **Net Income** is the income of the entire household that counts in figuring SNAP minus the deductions for which the household is eligible. Most households may have up to $2000 in countable resources (cash, bank accounts, car, stocks/bonds and so forth). Households may have $3000 if at least one person is age 60 years or older.

- Single, able-bodied adults with no dependents must be employed at least 20 hours per week to be eligible for SNAP. Unemployed people cannot receive SNAP benefits for longer than 3 months. Undocumented aliens are not eligible for SNAP.

Title III Nutrition Services

- **Title III Elderly Nutrition Program Of The Older Americans Act** includes Congregate Meals and Home Delivered Programs. The nutrition program established a national feeding program for the elderly known as the **Congregate Meals Program**, which is administered by the **Department Of Health and Human Services (DHHS)**, the **Administration On Aging (AOA)** and state and local agencies on aging.

- Title III programs are intended to keep seniors living independently in their communities rather than in extended care settings at government expense. The congregate meals program provides free or low-cost meals to the elderly or handicapped, who cannot afford to eat adequately, lack preparation skills, or are alone. A meal must meet at least one-third of DRI/RDAs. The program must serve at least one hot meal at least five days a week, and also must provide social interaction and referrals to social and rehabilitation services. Congregate programs are housed at senior centers, religious facilities, housing projects, schools or restaurants. Some programs offer transportation services.

- Another component of Title III is **Home Delivered Meals** for elderly or handicapped individuals who are too ill or otherwise unable to get to congregate meal sites. This service may be requested after hospital discharge. Most home delivered programs deliver two meals per day—one hot and one cold. Each meal must provide one-third of the DRI/RDAs.

- The **SENIOR FARMERS' MARKET PROGRAM (SFMP)** provides low income seniors with coupons that can be used to buy fresh, locally grown vegetables and fruit at farmers' markets, community supported agriculture programs (CSA) and roadside stands.

CHILD NUTRITION PROGRAMS

- Child nutrition programs include school breakfast and lunch programs and special milk programs. Child nutrition programs are administered by the USDA Food Nutrition Services (FNS) and include the following:

School Breakfast and Lunch Program

- **TEAM NUTRITION** is a nationwide program that is an initiative of the USDA Food and Nutrition Service to support the Child Nutrition Programs through training and technical assistance for food service, nutrition education for children and their caregivers, and school and community support for healthy eating and physical activity.(**www.fns.usda.gov/TN**)

- **SCHOOL BREAKFAST PROGRAM** provides a nutritious breakfast to children. The eligibility criteria for providing free or reduced-price meals are the same as for school lunch. Not all schools that offer school lunches have breakfast programs. Breakfasts must provide one-fourth to one-third of RDAs. A breakfast should include milk, fruit, bread or cereal and, when possible, a serving of protein rich food (e.g., cheese, egg, peanut butter). Studies show that children who participate in this program have higher achievement test scores than eligible non-participants.

- **THE AFTER SCHOOL SNACK PROGRAM** provides snacks to children who are enrolled in after school educational and enrichment programs through age 18. Income eligibility is met on the same basis as school lunch and breakfast programs.

- **CHILD CARE FOOD PROGRAM** provides nutritious meals to children enrolled in child-care centers or daycare homes. It sets standards for types and amounts of foods served.

- **SUMMER FOOD SERVICE PROGRAM** provides free nutritious meals for low-income children during school vacation at day camps where at least 50% of the children are from households below 185% of the poverty level.

- This USDA milk program helps schools, child care centers, homes and summer camps (not participating in other federally supported child nutrition programs) by reimbursing for milk served to children.

Special Supplemental Nutrition Program for Women, Infants and Children (WIC)

- The **SPECIAL SUPPLEMENTAL FOOD PROGRAM FOR WOMEN, INFANTS AND CHILDREN (WIC),** provides supplemental foods and nutrition education to pregnant, postpartum and breast-feeding women and to children, up to age 5, who are considered to be at nutritional risk. This program is administered by USDA and gives cash grants to agencies that offer services. Nutritional risk can be medically based, such as anemia, underweight, obesity, maternal age, HIV infection or a history of high-risk pregnancy. Diet based risks include GI disorders, renal, cardio-respiratory disorders, poor dietary patterns, or conditions that put the applicant at risk for medical or nutritional problems, such as alcohol and substance abuse.

- Benefits are provided to participants through local health agencies and clinics, which must also provide participants with appropriate ongoing healthcare services and nutrition education. Nutritional risk is determined by a local health professional who evaluates risk using federal guidelines. Each state may work within the federal guidelines to establish its own nutritional risk criteria based on state nutrition and health policies. Records of height, weight and blood tests for iron deficiency are maintained for each participant.

- WIC foods are designed to supplement the diets of participants. Foods provided are high in protein, calcium, iron, ascorbic acid and vitamin A. Iron-fortified formula is provided for infants. WIC funding is limited and some programs must set priorities for service to those most in need because funds do not permit serving the entire eligible population. Many WIC programs offer breastfeeding classes to their prenatal population.

All components identified from NHANES data.

- The WIC Program has lowered medical costs, increased gestation periods, produced higher birth weights and lowered infant mortality.

Child and Adult Care Food Program

- The **CHILD AND ADULT CARE FOOD PROGRAM (CACFP)** was established to assure nutritious meals for children up to age 12, the elderly, and certain handicapped people who take part in non-profit, licensed or approved day care programs. Centers receive funding from the federal government for two meals and one snack per participant, and one additional meal or snack, if the individual is in attendance for eight hours or more.

Commodity Distribution Program

- **COMMODITY SUPPLEMENTAL FOOD PROGRAM (CSFP)** provides commodity supplemental foods to low-income, children ages 5-6 and women who are 6-12 months postpartum, non breastfeeding and seniors over age 60. At times, butter, cheese and other commodities are distributed through senior centers and food banks. Some states have income guidelines and identification as nutritionally at risk to meet eligibility requirements for the program. Individuals may not participate in both CSFP and WIC programs.

Expanded Food and Nutrition Education Program

- The **EXPANDED FOOD AND NUTRITION EDUCATION PROGRAM (EFNEP)** provides nutrition aides and paraprofessionals from the community to work in low income areas to teach food and nutrition to peers. EFNEP is a program provided by USDA's Cooperative Extension Service.

Area Agency on Aging

- The **AREA AGENCY ON AGING (AAA)** is part of a network across the United States that is committed to meet the nutritional needs of the elderly. The program was established through the Older American's Act and is administered by the United States Administration on Aging (AOA). Regional Agencies on Aging oversee the State Agencies on Aging (SAA) and the Elderly Nutrition Program (ENP.) The nutrition program is the basis of the Older American's Act, which included four purposes of the program. Many elderly persons do not eat because:

  ➤ They can't afford to buy food or enough food.
  ➤ They lack the skills to choose foods and prepare nourishing and well-balanced meals.
  ➤ They have limited mobility, which may impair their capacity to shop and cook for themselves.
  ➤ They have feelings of rejection and loneliness, which reduce the incentive necessary to prepare and eat a meal alone.

- Seniors, especially those with low incomes, are provided with nutritionally sound meals that meet the *Dietary Guidelines for Americans*, served at specific centers or in their homes. The programs include the Title III program and the Meals on Wheels Programs.

- Program nutritionists use the Nutrition Screening Initiative as a screening tool and perform risk profile assessments. They also offer nutrition education.

Community resources as source of nutrition information assistance

- The **AGRICULTURAL RESEARCH SERVICE OF USDA CONSUMER AND FOOD ECONOMICS RESEARCH DIVISION** compiles food consumption data and conducts food consumption surveys, such as NHANES.

- The **HUMAN NUTRITION INFORMATION SERVICE (HNIS)** performs research on the nutritive value of food and human nutrition to improve professional and public understanding of the nutritional adequacy of diets and the national food supply. It collects and disseminates technical, educational and non-print material on food use, food management and human nutrition problems. It supports **NATIONWIDE FOOD CONSUMPTION SURVEY** and maintains the on-line database of nutrient values in food.

- The **COOPERATIVE EXTENSION SERVICE (CES)** is the educational agency of the Department of Agriculture, funded by the USDA, state governments (through their land grant colleges) and county governments. CES agents provide advice and information to the public.

U.S. Department of Health and Human Services (DHHS) Public Health Service

- The **NATIONAL INSTITUTES OF HEALTH (NIH)** supports nutrition research as it relates to health maintenance, human development through the life cycle, disease prevention and disease treatment. An example is the Diabetes Control and Complications Trial DCCT, 1995.

- The **NATIONAL CANCER INSTITUTE (NCI)** is the lead federal agency for cancer prevention and control.

- The **NATIONAL HEART, LUNG AND BLOOD INSTITUTE (NHLBI)** studies the role of nutrition in heart and lung disease. It conducts community-based, media intensive, education field trials for cardiovascular health. It also conducts the **NATIONAL CHOLESTEROL EDUCATION PROGRAM (NCEP)**

- **FOOD AND DRUG ADMINISTRATION (**FDA) ensures the safety, quality and accuracy of labeling of most foods and food additives. It conducts research into the quality of food, factors affecting bioavailability, sufficiency of the food supply, toxic products resulting from food processing, methodologies for the analysis of nutrients, metabolites in foods and acute and chronic toxicity of essential nutrients. It monitors and provides surveillance activities that provide information about the nutrient composition of foods; food labeling; and public knowledge, attitudes and preferences concerning foods. Nutrition information and education are part of the responsibility of the FDA. Labeling on food products is the largest source of nutrition information available to the public. The FDA regulates and monitors information on most nutrition labels. The exception is products containing meat and poultry, which are regulated by the USDA.

  - The FDA produces publications (*FDA Consumer* and *The FDA Model Food Code*), slide shows, tabletop exhibits and movies on nutrition for the public, health professionals and educators. District FDA offices have nutrition personnel to answer questions from professionals and consumers.

  ### (2) Consumer education resources

- Voluntary health agencies, such as the American Cancer Society, the American Diabetes Association, the American Heart Association and the March of Dimes are sources of educational materials, speakers and current information for health professionals and consumer information. They may offer limited funding for programs or conduct or sponsor research. Many dietitians volunteer to serve on committees to support the work of voluntary health agencies. Churches, alcohol and drug abuse programs and disease related organizations all provide information and may provide referral systems, support groups and/or programs.

- Professional organizations such as The Academy of Nutrition and Dietetics, the American Public Health Association and the American Association of Family and Consumer Sciences certify and maintain professional standards, provide consumer and professional information and educational materials and support research.

- Foundations such as the Robert Wood Johnson Foundation and the Kaiser Foundation fund health and nutrition-based research and projects.

- Business and industry, including trade associations, food vendors and retail market chains, are potential funding sources for communities grant programs. They may offer facilities, materials and/or speakers to programs at low cost. Examples include the National Dairy Council, the Food Marketing Institute, Abbott Laboratories, Mead-Johnson and the National Cattlemen's Beef Association.

- Information from business and industry typically reflects the specific concerns of the business or industry producing the materials. Before use, the dietitian should evaluate materials for balance (e.g., all nutrient data are included even when potentially negative) and accuracy of the message. The current trend is to form coalitions and partnerships between business and industry and professional organizations to extend and fund nutrition messages. The AND and the Society for Nutrition Education have industry partners that provide funding for the design, production and distribution of messages developed by both professional organizations.

- Training facilities, community colleges, universities, healthcare facilities, community nutrition programs involved with local nutrition initiatives, and nutrition-related activities including feeding programs, vending machine policies, school nutrition curriculum and school health programs are also consumer education resources.

Resource allocation and budget development

- **Financial:** Money may be available for community services from federal, state or local government, private granting foundations or organizations. Fundraising activities by institutions, community groups or churches often support community nutrition programs.

- **Personnel:** Plans should consider personnel availability, skill levels and costs.

- **Facilities:** Plans should consider size, equipment, arrangement, location, accessibility and availability. Some businesses will donate the use of facilities as a community service.

(3) Health services

- Health services resources include numbers of beds and occupancy rates of hospitals and extended care facilities; numbers served by community agencies; and numbers and geographic distribution of doctors, dietitians, public health nutritionists and nurses, school nurses, social service workers and health educators.

- Community services include public health clinics, hospital outpatient clinics, public transportation, food assistance programs, public health programs, community-based programming (YMCAs, boys and girls clubs, community and senior centers, day care) and all things available to members of the specific community. To evaluate community services, examine availability and types of services, eligibility/enrollment requirements, geographic location, cost of services, referral mechanisms and accessibility to the handicapped.

(4) Studies on food systems, local marketplace, food economics

- "A **FOOD SYSTEM** is a set of interrelated functions that includes food production, processing and distribution; food access and utilization by individuals, communities and populations; and food recycling, composting and disposal." (Boyle and Holben, *Community Nutrition in Action,* Thomson Wadsworth, p.359, 2010.)

II. NUTRITION CARE FOR INDIVIDUALS AND GROUPS (50%)

- The availability of food, type of markets (supermarkets, small grocery stores, convenience stores, farmers markets, food cooperatives, health/organic food stores), food costs and food standards (compliance with local/state food standards) all can be studied to assess the local food supply.

- According to several recent studies, there are many people in the United States who are food insecure, some with hunger and some without hunger. Many of these people have to use food pantries and emergency kitchens to have access to food. Those who are eligible for SNAP or other food assistance programs, are somewhat less insecure. People who are food insecure usually have more health problems because of lack of proper nutrition. The people who are food insecure, but not hungry, may not be able to afford foods with adequate nutrients, and this may lead to chronic disease later in the lifespan.

- People with limited incomes that are above the poverty line may have to make choices between paying the rent and buying food or paying for medication. These people may not be eligible for assistance and may be too proud to ask for help.

- Food security is an area that has been of concern because of the number of people who have no access to cooking facilities or refrigeration. Food safety education has been added to the programs of many community agencies that provide health and nutrition education, as well as programs that provide food services.

- The federal government has recently taken action by passing legislation **TITLE III OF THE PUBLIC HEALTH SECURITY AND BIOTERRORISM PREPAREDNESS AND RESPONSE ACT OF 2002**, to increase the security by expanding regulations, revising guidelines for food producers and importers and increasing funding for the agencies that oversee food systems. Issues addressed include microorganisms and bioterrorism.

- Federal agencies with oversight responsibilities for food systems include **DEPARTMENT OF HOMELAND SECURITY (DHS)** through **The FEDERAL EMERGENCY MANAGEMENT ADMINISTRATION (FEMA)** ; **UNITED STATES DEPARTMENT OF AGRICULTURE (USDA)** and its agency, the **FOOD SAFETY INSPECTION SERVICE (FSIS)** ; **DEPARTMENT OF HEALTH AND HUMAN SERVICES (HHS)** and its agencies, **CENTERS FOR DISEASE CONTROL AND PREVENTION (CDC)** and The **FOOD AND DRUG ADMINISTRATION (FDA)** through The **CENTER FOR SAFETY AND APPLIED NUTRITION (CFSAN)**; and industry through the **FOOD MARKETING INSTITUTE (FMI)** and the **GROCERY MANUFACTURERS OF AMERICA (GMA).**

(5) Public health programs

Public health programs and practices

- The planning process puts problems and resources into a framework that provides for the best use of resources. Public health programs provide services based on health problems within the community. When problems are identified, goals, objectives, priorities and interventions are determined.

- The **PROBLEM STATEMENT** must clearly describe the scope, nature and population affected with the nutrition problem. For example, "iron-deficiency has been found in 20% of the preschool children in the five lowest income neighborhoods of the city" is a problem statement. Needs or problems may be determined by a population's expressed desire for programming; by failure to achieve a predetermined health standard; by results of surveys, surveillance and so forth.

- **GOALS** are broad statements of what an organization hopes to accomplish over a specific period of time. Goal planning involves:

  - ➢ Identifying and clarifying organizational mandates, missions and values.
  - ➢ Assessing the external environment, including strengths, barriers, threats and opportunities.
  - ➢ Identifying strategic issues facing the organization.
  - ➢ Formulating plans to manage the issues in terms that are realistic, measurable and attainable.

- **OBJECTIVES** are specific statements detailing how the general goal will be obtained or what the expected outcome will be. Objectives are always concrete, measurable and attainable, and they may include measures of quality, quantity, cost and time. Types of objectives include long-term, short-term, departmental, administrative, instructional, production, clinical, educational, personal or professional. Objectives should be specific enough to show the degree to which an objective has been attained. An instructional objective is to provide one-half hour of individual or group counseling to 25% of those who attend the diabetes clinic during the months of July through September.

- **PRIORITIES** must be set to maximize use of resources. Because resources are likely to be limited, human, financial and material resources should be allocated based on careful study and analysis. Objective criteria should be determined to rank priorities. Personal interests and political or peer pressure should be avoided when setting priorities. Examples of factors that can be used in establishing priorities include:

  - ➢ Availability of funds. (Can we afford it?)
  - ➢ Availability of suitable personnel. (Does the staff have the skills to do it or can they be trained to do it?)
  - ➢ Number of people affected by the action or inaction. (Benefit for 1% of group versus 50%.)
  - ➢ Seriousness, propriety and legality of situation. (Extent of risks.)
  - ➢ Need for immediate action. (Can this wait?)
  - ➢ Anticipated success of action. (Revenue source, publicity for organization, etc.)
  - ➢ Existence of scientific knowledge and techniques. (Is information or technology available to succeed?)

- Develop a list of alternative solutions to the problem (e.g., limiting factors, resources required, possible outcomes, benefits). Begin the program when staff has been trained, space and equipment secured, materials prepared, program advertised and so forth. Establish a plan to measure outcome/results against goals. This will indicate not only successes but also opportunities for improvement.

- Public health programs require continuing evaluation during the implementation phase to evaluate all elements of nutrition care delivery.

- Media can be used to publicize programs or for health promotion messages. Television and radio (public service announcements, talk shows, personal interviews) or newspapers are some examples. Community-based programs are generally publicized in local media seen or heard by target audiences. Use the local library or call the media to get names of

II. NUTRITION CARE FOR INDIVIDUALS AND GROUPS (50%)

editors or producers to contact, deadlines, photo or slide requirements, etc. Posters, flyers or announcements in supermarkets, community centers, laundromats or anywhere people from the target audience gather are inexpensive ways to publicize programs. Referral services should be used to provide cost effective services.

- Intervention should result in changes in knowledge, skills or attitude. Interventions can be accomplished via group or peer counselors to reduce the time and cost of professional services. All types of intervention need monitoring and evaluation.

  - ➢ **Knowledge**: The client needs an education program. Assess the extent and limits of current knowledge. For example, the client has the required skills, resources and motivation but needs special knowledge about an identified problem.
  - ➢ **Skills:** The client needs practice. For example, the client has the required knowledge but needs practice in food purchasing, handling, storage or menu planning. Practice should be observed and evaluated.
  - ➢ **Attitudes**: The client needs to modify his or her behavior. Assist the client to develop desirable changes in attitude and modify behavior to achieve a health outcome.

- Program services should meet the assessed needs of target populations. Criteria for selecting a target population include the following:

  - ➢ The group is at high risk for nutrition or diet-related problems (e.g., low-income, homebound elderly).
  - ➢ There is a high incidence of problems in the group (e.g., pregnant women with low birth weight infants in previous pregnancies).
  - ➢ There is evidence that nutrition intervention will help solve particular problems (e.g., elite athlete workshops).
  - ➢ Experts and authorities agree that nutrition management of the problem will be an effective intervention (e.g., teenagers with hyperlipidemia).
  - ➢ A group or an organization will validate the nutrition message (e.g., pregnant women in Lamaze class).

Public health studies

- Public health services focus on the health and well being of population groups. Knowledge is drawn from nutritional, biological, behavioral, social and managerial sciences to treat physical, mental, social and economic conditions detrimental to health. Community nutrition services are provided to improve the nutritional status of the population served. Nutrition is included in preventive, diagnostic, curative and restorative services and should be integrated with medical and social services.

- **EPIDEMIOLOGICAL STUDIES** define and explain the interrelationships of factors that determine disease frequency and distribution in a community. Many such studies are conducted by the National Center for Health Statistics. Other important epidemiologic studies are the Framingham Heart Study and the Nurses Health Study.

- **INCIDENCE** refers to the number of new cases of a disease during a specific period of time. **PREVALENCE** refers to the number of existing cases of a disease at a particular time. Prevalence is used to plan, monitor and evaluate healthcare programs.

Programs

- Community health organizations' service limits are based on other social and medical services available for client referrals.

- Clinical care may be offered for acute health problems, may offer a range of services (such as blood tests, electrocardiograms, prescriptions) and have physicians and other members of a healthcare team at one location. Often clinics are set up on specific days for special purposes (diabetes clinic, well-baby clinic, etc.) to provide cost-effective coverage for medical needs with specialists available on particular days.

- Group education is useful when resources (time, money, staff and facilities) are limited. Clients may benefit from support of other group members.

- Referral resources typically include prenatal care, well-child services, special medicine clinics, family planning clinics, substance abuse treatment programs, exercise programs and food assistance programs.

- Consultation and technical assistance may be provided by other public health professionals (nurses, physicians, dentists, social workers, psychiatrists, educators, family and consumer science specialists, etc.) working with dietitians to plan, implement and evaluate community health programs.

- Training programs may be geared for target lay audiences, volunteers, paraprofessionals or professionals, for example, child-care programs for teen mothers, education for hospice workers.

Monitoring

- **NUTRITIONAL SURVEILLANCE** involves planning and implementing continuous data collection to evaluate key indicators of nutritional status. An example is the NHANES survey.

- A **REFERRAL SYSTEM** extends the network of services available to solve clients' problems and generates new clients for the dietitian through referral by others in the healthcare network.

- A **NUTRITION REFERRAL DOCUMENT** should include:
  - ➤ Client identification, age, sex, address and telephone number.
  - ➤ Name, address, telephone number and agency of person making referral.
  - ➤ Reason for referral and the type of service needed.
  - ➤ Diagnosis and diet prescription (if applicable).
  - ➤ Place where referral report is to be sent.

- The role of each team member should be known to all in order to maximize communication and quality of care. Community health dietitians should know availability and cost of other professional services in order to refer appropriately.

TOPIC B – DIAGNOSIS

- A nutrition diagnosis helps the dietitian set realistic and measurable expected outcomes, select appropriate interventions, and track the patient's/resident's/client's progress. It is not a medical diagnosis and describes changes in nutritional status and the cause of these changes. The nutrition diagnosis uses words like ineffective, increased/decreased, altered, impaired, acute/chronic, risk. It should be linked to the problem diagnosis by words such as "related to", or "as evidenced by". The relationships may be pathophysiological, cultural, environmental, situational, psychosocial, and so forth. It should also include an evidence statement to show the method of determination of the diagnosis. The AND has developed standard nutrition diagnostic terminology. Dietetics professionals are asked to chart diagnoses in the form of a Problem (diagnostic label), Etiology (cause/contributing risk factors), and Signs and Symptoms (defining characteristics), known as a **PES STATEMENT**.

1. Relationship between nutrition diagnoses and medical diagnoses

- A **MEDICAL DIAGNOSIS** is "The determination of the nature of a disease" *(Stedman's Concise Dictionary for the Health Professions, 3rd Ed. 1997, Williams & Wilkins.)*

- A **NUTRITION DIAGNOSIS** is an identified nutrition problem that dietitians are responsible for treating and where the primary intervention is nutrition related. It is based on the assessment; which helps to identify the possible diagnoses. Data should be grouped and studied to help identify the nutrition diagnostic code, and the nutrition diagnosis. Critical thinking and clinical judgment are required in order to arrive at the proper diagnosis. Diagnoses can be the nutrition problem that is current, or it can be calling attention to the risk of one developing. (*see International Dietetics & Nutrition Terminology (IDNT) Reference Manual: Standardized Language for the Nutrition Care Process, Second Edition, The Academy of Nutrition and Dietetics, 2009* for terminology and nutrition diagnosis codes.)

a. Pathophysiology

- **PATHOPHYSIOLOGY** is the disruption of normal body functions that is seen in disease.

b. Identifying medical diagnoses affecting nutrition care

- Dietitians must understand the pathophysiology in order to make a proper nutrition diagnosis, because many diseases have a major impact on a person's nutritional status and this must be taken into account when assessment is performed.

c. Determining nutrition risk factors for current medical diagnoses

- Sometimes behavioral issues regarding food cause the symptoms of the disease, and while the disease most likely will not be cured, symptoms will be diminished if nutrition issues are addressed. Treating nutrition problems identified in a patient/client that are the direct result of the disease process may help to bring about a positive outcome.
- Care must be taken to differentiate the nutrition diagnosis from the medical diagnosis because the nutrition diagnosis is static. It can change over time as the patient's /client's medical condition changes. In addition, a nutrition diagnosis is contingent upon nutrition being the primary treatment - the dietitian is the primary caregiver.

d. Determining nutrition factors for groups

- A community needs assessment is used to evaluate what the health and nutritional needs of the community are. It can help to identify health risks that the people in the community face.
- Completion of this assessment can diagnose the nutritional needs of the community and help the community nutritionist develop programs designed to alleviate some of the prevalent health and nutritional risks.

2. Data sources and tools for nutrition diagnosis

a. Organizing assessment data

- Nutrition assessment is the first step in the nutrition care process.
- When analyzing information from assessment data, biochemical and medical test results, medical procedures, anthropometric measurements, physical examination findings, food and nutrition histories and client histories are used.
- By thorough analysis of this data, the dietitian can see if a significant nutrition problem exits.
- Data can be obtained from many sources such as the referring healthcare provider or agency, the interview with the patient/client and/or family, the medical record and so forth.
- The data from the nutrition assessment is of great importance to help identify the nutrition diagnosis from a list of possible diagnoses prepared as data are studied. The dietetics professional must bear in mind that the nutrition diagnosis identifies a nutritional problem that the dietitian is generally responsible for treating independently.
- Data are collected by category on a worksheet and tentative nutrition diagnostic codes are placed near each abnormal finding. In that manner, the organized data will allow the dietitian to find the nutrition diagnosis best suited to the patient/client.

b. Using standardized language

- Using standardized language and process does not mean giving standardized care. The standardized language can be the basis for collecting evidence that nutrition care improves outcomes.
- Standardized language is an excellent communication tool and helps to measure outcomes in a reliable manner.

3. Diagnosing nutrition problems for individuals and groups

a. Making inferences

- **CRITICAL THINKING** identifies and evaluates evidence to guide decision-making and/or come to a conclusion by inference. It is a process with many steps and requires a person to use in-depth analysis of evidence to make these decisions. The process involves making judgments as to the merit of certain information. Experience enhances the critical thinking process.

b. Prioritizing

- After looking at all the evidence and setting forth several possible nutrition diagnoses, the dietitian should look at all the evidence to evaluate the most important issues.

c. Differential diagnosing

- **DIFFERENTIAL DIAGNOSING** is the determination of which of many problems with similar symptoms is the correct diagnosis for this patient/client. Making a differential diagnosis requires comparisons and contrasts of all findings.

4. Etiologies (cause/contributing risk factors)

a. Identifying underlying causes and contributing risk factors of nutrition diagnoses

Using an organized structure that focuses on nutritional problems, factors relating to the existence of a pathophysiological, psychosocial, situational, developmental, cultural and/or environmental problems should be considered. Underlying causes such as over or underweight, specific data from an intake assessment, and nutrition knowledge and beliefs will aid the dietitian in making a correct nutritional diagnosis.

b. Making cause and effect linkages

- In order to make a nutrition diagnosis, one must have information that shows how the specific diagnosis was chosen. The diagnostic label identifies the problem; the underlying cause is the etiology. Once the etiology is identified, a nutrition intervention that should resolve the problem can be identified. The statements are linked by the PES terminology, relating the problem to the etiology that is based on the signs and symptoms (evidence.)

5. Signs and symptoms (defining characteristics)

a. Linking signs and symptoms to etiologies

- The evidence for the diagnosis is the signs and symptoms (S/S). The S/S are linked to the nutrition diagnosis and etiology in a **PES STATEMENT**: The diagnosis is the Problem (P); "related to" the Etiology (E) "as evidenced by" the S/S.

b. Using subjective (symptoms) and/or objective (signs) data

- The symptoms and signs data are used to show why the nutrition diagnosis was chosen correctly.

6. Documentation

- Documentation should be completed in a timely fashion. Documentation for followup assessments should address the status of the nutritional therapy goal or desired outcomes, a review of the nutrient intake analysis, a revision of the nutrition plan and statements supporting any changes in nutritional therapy and/or nutritional diagnosis.

- Documentation activities occupy a significant amount of dietitians' time. Studies have shown better healthcare team response when the documentation style is a brief, focused, clinical communication.

- Implementation of the electronic medical record is associated with increased use of automated clinical documentation methods. As lengths of inpatient stay decrease and outpatient services increase, automated methods assist office staff to document required information in a limited time.

- Many healthcare facilities document via computerized patient records. This keeps the record clear and available at all times, and avoids poor handwriting for orders and other important patient information. Fewer documentation errors are found using this method and it is easier to track outcomes and collect data.

- Regardless of the charting method used, all written documentation should follow these guidelines:

  - Be legible.
  - Write in black ink without any "white out"; errors should be crossed out with a single line, dated and initialed and noted as an error.
  - All entries should be dated and signed, with name and credentials.
  - Record only pertinent facts, no criticisms or personal opinions.
  - Record information chronologically and succinctly.

- The AND Standardized Language Committee developed some questions to ascertain the validity of the PES Statements.

  - Can the dietetics professional resolve or improve the nutrition diagnosis?
  - Is there any nutrition intervention that would deal with the etiology and resolve or improve the problem? Or, can the intervention reduce or eliminate the signs and symptoms?
  - Does the nutrition assessment data support the proposed PES Statement?
  - Is the etiology listed "root cause" an issue that can be addressed by the dietetics professional?
  - Will measuring the signs and symptoms tell the dietetics practitioner if the problem is cleared or improvement is shown?
  - Are the signs and symptoms mentioned precise enough to be measured and evaluated for change?
  - If there is a choice between two nutrition diagnoses from different domains, choose the intake nutrition diagnosis.

TOPIC C – PLANNING and INTERVENTION

- **NUTRITION INTERVENTION** is the third step in the Nutrition Care Process (NCP). This step has two parts: the planning process and the implementation process.

Planning process

- The planning process should address each identified problem, giving highest priority to those of greatest importance. It includes patient/client family, and other staff involvement, review of practice guides and policies, setting goals and definition of the specific nutrition intervention strategy.

Implementation process

- This is the action phase of the plan. Assessment data is used to implement the activities and interventions that will help the patient/client meet established goals and objectives. This process may help to identify the parts of the plan that need to be changed.

Nutrition intervention terminology

- The **STANDARDIZED NUTRITION INTERVENTION TERMINOLOGY** is organized into four classifications: food and/or nutrient delivery; nutrition education; nutrition counseling; and coordination of nutrition care. Each classification contains a list of subclasses and is meant to be used by all dietetics professionals in areas of practice where nutrition intervention occurs.

- Nutrition interventions should be individualized and followed-up to determine if the intervention is occurring. In this phase, strategies may have to be adjusted, if the goals of treatment are not being met.

- Nutrition education, and nutrition counseling are separated intentionally because they are separate strategies. Nutrition education is instructive, while counseling seeks to change behaviors.

1. Nutrition care for health promotion and disease prevention

a. Identification of desired outcomes/actions

(1) Evidence-based practice for nutrition intervention

- The AND defines **EVIDENCE BASED PRACTICE (EBP)** as "an approach to healthcare wherein health professionals use the best evidence possible, i.e. the most appropriate information available to make decisions for individual patients. EBP values, enhances and builds on clinical expertise, knowledge of disease mechanisms and pathophysiology. It involves complex and conscientious decision-making based not only on the available evidence but also on client characteristics, situations and preferences. It recognizes that healthcare is individualized and ever changing and involves uncertainties and probabilities."It defines **EVIDENCE-BASED DIETETICS PRACTICE (EBP)** as "…use of systematically reviewed scientific evidence in making food and nutrition decisions by integrating best available evidence with professional expertise and client values to improve outcomes." (*Scope of Dietetics Practice Framework, Section 4B, Definition of Terms, 2005.* **www.eatright.org**)

- EBP requires a critical thinking process. The dietitian must ask many questions and know current information regarding the best available evidence for each case. The AND has an evidence library on its website, which is free for members. New information is added frequently.

(2) Evaluation of nutrition information

- An evidence base should be used to back the information.

  - ➤ Is there a reference list from scientifically acceptable research journals?
  - ➤ Has the research been duplicated in studies conducted on reasonably sized groups?
  - ➤ Is the only support of claims from satisfied users?

II. NUTRITION CARE FOR INDIVIDUALS AND GROUPS (50%)

- The author's credentials should be valid for this type of research.

  - ➢ Is there a credentialed author, or a credible group funding the research?
  - ➢ Is the information peer-reviewed?
  - ➢ Is the author biased by financial gain from the results?
  - ➢ Are there full disclosures of funding and/or conflict of interest?

- Information should be correct, complete and current.

  - ➢ Are proper statistics used?
  - ➢ Is the sample size adequate?
  - ➢ Is the sample properly selected?
  - ➢ Are references current?

(3) Food fad

- American consumers are offered an ongoing supply of food fads and approaches to weight reduction. Many programs promise fast results with minimal effort. These promises create unrealistic expectations. Some diets are potentially harmful, but most people do not sustain such diets long enough for harm except financial waste. Some current fad diets restrict carbohydrates, promote high protein and fat intakes, or make claims for expensive or unique products that are useless or have no valid scientific evidence to substantiate claims.

- Faddists often sell products or books and may not tell or know the truth and science of nutrition. Dietitians should speak up and present sound advice when faddist information is presented to the public in presentations, print, books, internet, television or social media.

- General criteria for evaluating popular diets:

  - ➢ They should provide adequate amounts of all nutrients. Weight reduction diets may be deficient in calories and essential nutrients. Low calorie diets should include supplements if necessary.
  - ➢ They must contain foods that are readily available, reasonably priced and adaptable to family meals or restaurant eating.
  - ➢ They should provide adequate fiber and sufficient fat for satiety.
  - ➢ They should not eliminate any group of foods.
  - ➢ They must be maintainable for prolonged time.
  - ➢ They should not attribute "magical" curative powers to any particular foods, food groups or supplements.
  - ➢ They should help develop long-term, healthful eating habits.

(4) Health fraud

- Many consumers are concerned about their health and try to eat well. There is an abundance of research in professional and lay literature about the constituents of a healthy diet. Some of the information is confusing and misleading; this leaves the road open to health fraud.

- Promoters of health fraud do it deliberately, for financial gain. Some offer health remedies that don't work and some offer programs that have not had enough research to prove their worth. Products offered range from health remedies, to items that improve appearance and/or well being.

- Print and electronic media often disseminate popular diets and research updates before preliminary findings can be confirmed. The dietitian should be aware of the popular press so those client questions can be answered. Maintaining contact with the local press positions dietitians as preferred sources of information.

- The Internet is a popular site for research. While much of the information found on the Internet is scientifically sound, there are many sites that have misleading and fraudulent information. Consumers have to be taught how to determine what appropriate health information is.

  ➢ When buying products promoted for good health, *caveat emptor* applies. Federal requirements for supporting some of the science for the array of health products on the market may not exist, so some claims can be very misleading.
  ➢ If it sounds too good to be true, it probably is not true. Claims of miracle cures or easy weight loss are often fraudulent. Questionable claims include curing insomnia, hair loss, stress, improving memory or eyesight or slowing aging.
  ➢ Dietary supplements encompass vitamins and minerals as well as herbals and botanicals. Supplements are concentrates and extracts that can provide amounts in great excess of normal diets.
  ➢ Excessive dosages of some herbal supplements can cause miscarriages and high dosages of many botanicals are untested.
  ➢ Multivitamins may help some people. Pregnant women, elderly, and those on inadequate diets benefit from multivitamins or fortified cereals, but dosages higher than DRIs may be harmful.
  ➢ Less is known about herbals and botanicals than vitamins and minerals. There are no standards for herbals or botanicals that set safe or effective doses. They can be marketed for medical effects but are largely unregulated. Some regulations are in development. The United States Office of Dietary Supplements is currently running research on many of the popular herbals and botanicals.
  ➢ High doses of some dietary supplements may be harmful and can interfere with some prescribed drugs. Excesses of vitamins A, D, niacin, B_6, iron and folic acid cause harm, as do ma huang, guar gum, willow bark, comfrey, chaparral, arnica, belladonna and pennyroyal.
  ➢ "Natural" is not synonymous with "safe." Natural can be toxic. Few herbal remedies bear warning labels.

- For good health, eat a variety of foods. Foods contain protective compounds and are the best source of nutrients for health. The National Council against Health Fraud (**www.ncahf.org**) and Quackwatch (**www.quackwatch.com**) are two websites that have information on a variety of health frauds. Also check current position papers of the Academy of Nutrition and Dietetics.

b. Determination of energy/nutrient needs specific to life span stage

- Information regarding energy is presented earlier in Domain II and in Domain I.

c. Implementing care plans

(1) Nutrition recommendations to promote wellness

<u>**Nutritional adequacy**</u>

- Menu planning should be done to assure provision of adequate calories and nutrients to individuals served. MyPlate or other food plans usually form the basic meal plan. Individuals have medical conditions, risk factors, or food intolerances that should be considered as meals are planned. Nutritional values of menus can be calculated using food composition tables or computerized nutrient databases.

<u>**Client acceptance, diet patterns, schedules**</u>

- Serving nutritionally adequate food is not enough. Menus should be planned with client preferences mind. Food habits must be respected and foods provided at mealtimes must be reasonable and acceptable to clients.

- The nutrition care plan is adapted for specific nutrition related problems and consists of a nutrition assessment, the identification of nutrition problems, the setting of objectives of nutrition care, nutrition intervention activities (including education) and evaluation of the nutrition care. The objectives and interventions should be patient-centered and individualized. An important aspect of this process is to help the individual understand that he or she will have to be an active participant in the nutrition care.

- Generally, advice for maintaining a healthful diet is based on three meals and one or more snacks. Lifestyles and work schedule may require meals at irregular or atypical times.

<u>**Sociocultural, ethnic, and religious factors**</u>

- Cultural patterns of food behavior are based on food availability, education, economics, geography, agricultural and marketing practices, beliefs about health and safety, history, tradition and symbolic meanings (religious, political, social) attached to foods. Preferences of ethnic groups served should be incorporated into menus to promote acceptance. Menu planning should include foods suitable for those whose religious beliefs require particular foods and should omit foods and food combinations that are to be avoided for cultural or religious reasons.

(2) Communication and documentation

<u>**Communications**</u>

- A client on a new diet (even if a general one to promote wellness) needs basic information or needs to review his or her long term diet and make appropriate changes to promote health and wellness.

- *Dietary Guidelines for Americans* provides general guidance for selecting a diet that promotes health. They are not adjusted for patients with special dietary needs such as illness or food intolerance. Individual needs should be addressed through assessment and counseling.

- Accessibility to the nutritional care plan allows the entire health team to understand the rationale for nutritional care and the means by which it will be provided. One of the most effective methods for planning care is the **INTERDISCIPLINARY TEAM CONFERENCE**. The interdisciplinary team conference allows each discipline to share its assessments and to gain greater understanding of the total needs. Communicating nutritional care plans allows the entire health team to participate in the nutritional care and to reinforce the patient's education whenever there is an opportunity. Dietitians should be confident of their abilities in patient/healthcare personnel interaction. In addition to their scientific and technical competence, dietitians are expected to be skilled communicators.

Documentation

- Documentation is necessary for determining the effectiveness of program or treatment and for cost-benefit or cost-effectiveness analysis. Documentation includes:
  - ➢ Recording the process and outcome of intervention in the medical record or the client file.
- Documenting progress toward achievement of program or treatment objectives by changes in biochemical parameters, anthropometric measures and food patterns.
  - ➢ Recording the process and outcome of training or counseling.
  - ➢ Documenting changes in behaviors by frequency of clinic visits, observation of food choices, frequency of referrals to other healthcare professionals and referrals from other healthcare professionals to dietitians.

- Regardless of the setting for client/patient care, appropriate documentation techniques should be followed. These include all relevant information including all benchmark information, tests results, plans for care and follow-up, and evaluation mechanisms.

- Care plans must be reassessed to monitor a physical condition and rescreening should be done periodically. The client should keep a record of behavior (e.g., record food eaten) in order for the dietitian to monitor intake. Weight, growth charts and biochemical tests should be repeated at predetermined intervals to monitor the condition being assessed, to assure positive outcomes.

2. Medical Nutrition Therapy

- **MEDICAL NUTRITION THERAPY (MNT)** is an essential to comprehensive healthcare. Individuals with a variety of conditions can improve their health and quality of life by receiving medical nutrition therapy. During an MNT intervention, RDs counsel client behavioral and lifestyle changes required to impact long term eating habits and health.

- Medical nutrition therapy includes:
  1. Performing a comprehensive nutrition assessment determining the nutrition diagnosis;
  2. Planning and implementing a nutrition intervention using evidence-based nutrition practice guidelines;
  3. Monitoring and evaluating an individual's progress over subsequent visits with the RD.

- RDs provide MNT and other nutrition services for a variety of diseases and conditions including:
  - Cardiovascular diseases: hypertension, dyslipidemia, congestive heart failure
  - Diabetes: Type 1, Type 2, gestational
  - Disease prevention: general wellness
  - GI disorders: celiac disease, cirrhosis, Crohn's disease
  - Immunocompromise: food allergy, HIV/AIDS
  - Nutritional support: oral, enteral, parenteral
  - Oncology
  - Pediatrics: infant/child feeding, failure-to-thrive, inborn errors of metabolism
  - Pulmonary disease: COPD
  - Renal disease: insufficiency, chronic failure, transplantation
  - Weight management: overweight/obesity, bariatric surgery, eating disorders
  - Women's health: pregnancy, osteoporosis, anemia

- MNT is not the same as the nutrition care process. MNT is one specific type of nutrition care. The NCP format can and should be used for all types of nutrition care, including MNT, because it is a standardized format.

a. Identify desired outcomes and actions

- Desired outcomes are identified through outcomes research. In contrast to previous thinking, current theory holds that the most effective intervention may be identified through study of clinical, economic, social and ethical studies. **OUTCOMES RESEARCH** measures the impact of an intervention on health and resource use. Interventions with positive results are expanded to other areas by translating the outcome findings into practice guidelines. Insurance companies look for outcomes research to determine the value of reimbursing for nutrition services. It is very important for dietitians to do this type of research, not only for reimbursement, but to assure quality care.

- **PROCEDURES** are prescribed methods to accomplish actions, including specific tasks, materials, equipment and other resources. Procedures (and criteria used) to document productivity and promote quality assurance are included in various and publications.

- **POLICIES** are written guidelines establishing standards and rules. For example, a policy may outline where and when documentation is required.

- **RISK MANAGEMENT** is a program established through policies and procedures to minimize risk and liability. Risk management includes protection against malpractice and personal liability. A particular concern is maintaining confidentiality of medical records. An example of risk management is a policy on when to feed and not to feed by tube in terminal illness.

- A company or healthcare facility may have a manager of risk management who determines needs for liability insurance. For example, a nutrition services department may be asked to document potential side effects of very low-calorie diets to determine if specific insurance may be necessary to cover potential complications.

- **TREATMENT EVALUATION RISK MANAGEMENT** is the weighing of risks and benefits of a specific treatment before an action is taken. For example, determining if the need for weight loss justifies delay of surgery.

II. NUTRITION CARE FOR INDIVIDUALS AND GROUPS (50%)

b. Relationship of pathophysiology to treatment of primary nutrition-related disorders

(1) Critical care and hypermetabolic states

Trauma

- **TRAUMA** is a critical injury, such as extensive burns or bone fractures, that creates extreme physiologic and psychological stress. Generally, physical trauma increases needs for calories, protein, vitamin C and zinc. Individual nutrition support plans should include replenishing catabolic losses, meeting anabolic needs for healing and providing emotional support.

Surgery

- The objectives of dietary management for surgery are to improve the preoperative nutritional state of the patient in preparation for the stress of surgery, to hasten recovery and to maintain good nutrition and rapid healing in the postoperative period.

- If there is time because the surgery is elective, a high-protein, high-kcal **PREOPERATIVE DIET** is given to optimize patient nutritional status. Calories may not have to be increased for obese patients.

- The night before surgery, all food is usually withheld so that the patient goes to surgery with an empty stomach. Food aspiration is a potential problem with anesthesia.

- **POSTOPERATIVE DIET** regimes depend on the type and extent of surgery. After major or gastrointestinal surgery, patients usually have nothing by mouth (NPO) for 24-48 hours. The diet typically progresses from clear liquids, to soft or light diet and then to a general diet when gastrointestinal motility has resumed, and the patient is able to eat. High-protein, vitamin and mineral rich diets promote healing. If surgery involves the GI tract, further modifications may be necessary.

Burns

- The goals of treatment of burns are to promote wound healing, to prevent infection and weight loss and to restore fluid and electrolyte balance to prevent shock. Provide a high-kcal, high-protein, high-fluid diet that is liberal in vitamins, especially vitamin C and zinc. Tube feeding or TPN may be necessary if the patient is unable to take sufficient quantities of fluid and food by mouth.

- The first 24-48 hours should concentrate on fluid and electrolyte replacement. The greatest intravascular loss occurs during the first 8 hours. Therefore, where possible, about half of the total amount of volume needed for the first 24 hours should be administered during the first 8 hours. Serum sodium, body weight and osmolar

  concentrations are used to monitor fluid status. Feeding should begin as soon as fluid is stabilized. The preferred method of nutritional support is enteral feeding, but parenteral support may be necessary for some patients. Very early enteral feeding has been used successfully to minimize the catabolic response.

- Protein intake of burn patients should be 20%-25% of total calories when burns cover 10% or more of total body surface area; 15% of total calories with burns of 1-10% of total body surface area. Recommended non-protein calories to nitrogen ratios are 100:1 and 150:1 respectively. Monitor BUN, serum creatinine and hydration status for patients on high protein diets. The burn patient may suffer protein loss from protein catabolism, increased urinary nitrogen excretion, and loss of protein through wound exudates. In addition, people with thermal injuries are prone to infections.

- Fat intake should be 25 to 30% of calories for enteral feedings. Parenterally fed burn patients should receive no more than 2.5g of fat/kilogram body weight per day. Fat is a less effective source of energy than glucose for burn patients because fat can be immunosuppressive. Decreased carnitine levels associated with burns decrease the transport of long-chain fatty acids and can lead to hyperlipidemia. The type of the lipid is important; diets within the aforementioned parameters should contain omega-3 fatty acids, which may improve the immune response and the tube feeding response.

- Carbohydrate intake should be approximately 60% of total calories. To ensure glucose oxidation, glucose should be provided at a rate less than or equal to 5-7mg/kg/minute in parenteral feeding. The maximum calorie load given should be no more than approximately 100% above the REE.

- Caloric needs may increase as much as 100% above the REE, which is the maximum load the body can handle. Weight maintenance is the goal until after the acute phase has passed.

- Formulas have been developed to determine energy and protein needs, and protein losses of burn patients. In addition, indirect calorimetry methods are used to assess energy expenditure and substrate utilization.

(2) Eating disorders

- Treatment for disordered eating requires nutritional intervention in conjunction with psychological and medical treatment. The first treatment priority is to stabilize the patient and correct fluid and electrolyte imbalance. The second priority is caloric adjustment to move weight toward the normal range. Food plans tailored to the individual include calories to meet requirements based on height, weight, sex and age; vitamin and mineral supplementation; structured eating situations to help the client experience "normal" eating; and avoidance of trigger foods that may lead to bingeing or purging.

- In **ANOREXIA NERVOSA**, clients have an intense fear of gaining weight or becoming fat, and a preoccupation with food. Restrained eating is often coupled with extreme exercise patterns that lead to weight maintenance below 15% of expected weight, a distorted body image and "feeling fat" even when emaciation is evident. There is moderate to severe weight loss, muscle weakness and fatigue, with glycogen depletion leading to muscle tissue breakdown. Physiological changes include **AMENORRHEA** (absence of at least 3 menstrual cycles), **ORTHOSTATIC HYPOTENSION** (drop in blood pressure when standing, causing dizziness and sometimes fainting), **BRADYCARDIA** (abnormally low heart action), lowered core temperature, **LANUGO** (growth of fine, neonatal type hair on skin), decreased thyroid function, **HYPOTHERMIA** (lowered body temperature) and delayed gastric emptying. The immune function is compromised, with nutrient deficiencies, electrolyte imbalances and protein-calorie malnutrition (PCM). Victims are at a high risk for osteoporosis due to the amenorrhea, low calcium intake, low weight and decreased estrogen levels. Death can result from self-imposed starvation. Anorexia nervosa is more common in females than males, especially among teenagers and young adults. Some young athletes (particularly gymnasts and ballet dancers) are encouraged by their coaches to be very thin and light. This practice can lead to anorexia nervosa.

- Anorexia nervosa is an emotional and psychological disorder with nutritional results and requires therapy by professionals. Hospitalization including IVs or tube feeding may be necessary for anorexia nervosa. However outpatient therapy is the preferred treatment modality because of the increased cost associated with hospitalization. Only patients with outpatient treatment failure or severe medical and nutritional problems are hospitalized.

- With **BULIMIA NERVOSA** clients have episodes of binge eating, followed by **PURGING** (vomiting, use of laxatives or diuretics), fasting or excessive exercise to control weight. Presence of hydrochloric acid in the esophagus and mouth can cause parotid gland enlargement, heartburn and dental erosion. Bleeding or torn esophagus, bloodshot eyes, dehydration, bloating, flatulence and constipation also may occur. If serious electrolyte imbalance occurs, low potassium levels can cause cardiac arrhythmia. Dentists identify many bulimics because frequent vomiting causes dental erosion.

- **EATING DISORDERS NOT OTHERWISE SPECIFIED (EDNOS)** - People diagnosed with EDNOS make up about 50% of those diagnosed with eating disorders. They exhibit some symptoms of either anorexia nervosa or bulimia nervosa. They may indulge in binge eating behaviors (without the purging), similar to bulimia, they may meet all guidelines for a diagnosis of anorexia, except the amenorrhea, or they may be people of normal weight who do not binge, but who do purge after a normal sized meal. Those who have EDNOS may develop anorexia or bulimia nervosa if left untreated.

- **BINGE EATING DISORDER** is defined as eating an amount of food larger than most people would eat in a discrete period of time. The individual usually has a feeling of lack of control over the experience. It occurs about twice a week for six months or longer and does not involve regular purging or fasting or excessive exercise. Weight cycling does occur.

- Indirect calorimetry has shown the resting energy expenditure of anorexia nervosa patients increases more during refeeding than anticipated from calculations with standard formulas. Therefore, refeeding regimens greater than three to four thousand kilocalories may eventually be required. The initial diet prescription is usually in the range of 1200-1400kcal/day, with daily increases of 100-200kcal every few days.

(3) Food allergies and intolerance

- Food sensitivities and adverse reactions may cause systemic, gastrointestinal, respiratory or dermatological symptoms that may be mild or severe in intensity. To manage dietary allergies and sensitivities, exclude the offending food from the diet. Forms of food preparation in which the allergen may be used should be controlled. When the offending food allergen is not known, elimination test diets for allergy may be used. A food diary is maintained to determine which foods cause adverse reactions. Food labels should be examined carefully to prevent ingestion of offending foods. Foods most likely to cause IgE-mediated allergic reactions include cow milk, eggs, fish and shellfish, nuts (especially peanuts), soy, wheat and cinnamon.

POTENTIAL SYMPTOMS OF FOOD SENSITIVITY

Type	Symptoms
Dermatologic	Redness, itching, rashes, hives
Gastrointestinal	Nausea; vomiting; swelling of lips, neck or throat; abdominal cramps and pain; bloating; gas; fecal blood loss; malabsorption
Respiratory	Sneezing, itching, nasal congestion and inflammation of tissues of respiratory system, irregular breathing
Systemic	Anaphylaxis, pallor, irritability, headaches, low blood pressure, cardiac arrhythmias

---

- An **EGG-FREE DIET** is a general diet that eliminates eggs in all forms (cookies, soups, custards, French toast, ice cream, mayonnaise, breaded meats, muffins, egg noodles and All-natural Simplesse®). On labels, watch for albumin, dried egg solids, globulin, ovoglobulin, livetin and vitellin.

- An **EGG, WHEAT AND MILK-FREE DIET** is a general diet with omission of all eggs and egg products, wheat and wheat products and milk and dairy products. Soymilk supplements may be given. Ry-Krisp™, cornmeal, oatmeal, rice and barley cereals, rice flour and tapioca are the permitted grain products.

- A **CORN-FREE DIET** eliminates corn, cornmeal, corn cereals, corn-based products such as corn solids, corn starch, corn syrup, vegetable starch, dextrose, corn oil, corn alcohol, corn sugar and modified food starch.

- A **MILK-FREE DIET** is a general diet with the omission of milk and milk-based products. It is similar to a lactose-free diet. Soy milk substitutes, soy-based cheese and lactose-free supplements may be given. On ingredient lists, watch for casein, a milk protein that may be added to lunch meats and other products in food processing, and the words DMS (dried milk solids), lactalbumin, whey and whey solids. Emphasize non-milk calcium sources. Milk allergy is not analogous to lactose intolerance. A person allergic to milk is usually allergic to the protein and may not be lactose intolerant.

- A **WHEAT-FREE DIET** is a general diet omitting all forms of wheat, including flour, wheat germ, wheat bran, modified food starch, graham flour, semolina, farina and couscous. Food labels should be examined carefully because wheat is used as a binder in many prepared foods. Grains allowed include Ry-Krisp, cornmeal, oats, rice, barley and tapioca.

TERMINOLOGY RELATED TO ALLERGIES

ADVERSE REACTION	A clinically abnormal response believed due to an ingested food or food additive
ALLERGY	An adverse reaction following exposure to an inhaled, ingested or injected substance that results in a response from the immune system
ANAPHYLACTIC REACTION	Anaphylaxis-like food reaction as a result of non-immune release of chemical mediators; can mimic the signs and symptoms of food hypersensitivity
ANAPHYLAXIS	Specific, often severe, sensitivity to a substance acquired on a prior exposure
ANTIBODIES	Molecules of proteins formed by the human body in response to antigens
ANTIGEN-ANTIBODY COMPLEX	Combination of an antibody and a food protein that has been absorbed in the body; also called Immune Complex
ANTIGENS	Molecules that stimulate the immune system to produce a response
ASYMPTOMATIC SENSITIVITY	A response with antibody formation but no symptoms
COLIC	Irritability and discomfort of infants due to allergic response to milk; characterized by crying, poor sleeping and abdominal pain
ECZEMA	Scaly skin rash with red and/or white bumps that itch; scratching to relieve itching can cause bleeding and infections; eczema is also called **ATOPIC DERMATITIS**
FOOD ALLERGY	A severe immune response to a food protein with release of histamine that can be mild, severe, or even fatal
FOOD HYPERSENSITIVITY	An immunological hypersensitivity or truly allergic reaction resulting from the ingestion of a food or food additive
FOOD IDIOSYNCRASY	A quantitatively abnormal response to a food or food additive; such response differs from its physiological or pharmacological effect and resembles a hypersensitivity reaction, but there is no immune mechanism

FOOD INTOLERANCE	A physiologic response to an ingested food or food additive that is not proved to be immunological in nature; this category includes idiosyncratic, pharmacological, metabolic or toxic food reactions
FOOD POISONING	An adverse reaction after food ingestion as a result of a natural toxic constituent of the food or contamination of the food by microorganisms and/or their toxins
FOOD SENSITIVITY	A general term for an adverse reaction to an ingested food or food additive
FOOD TOXICITY	A general term suggesting an adverse reaction after the ingestion of a food or food additive as a result of a direct non-immune action
IMMUNE SYSTEM	All organs, cells and molecules that respond (both positively and negatively) to environmental substances
IMMUNOGLOBIN E (IGE)	The specific antibody that attaches to cells and causes rapid-onset reactions
MAST CELLS	Cells containing mediators that are receptive to IgE and attach to it
MEDIATORS	Chemicals in various cells that are receptive to reactions, thus bringing on symptoms
METABOLIC FOOD REACTION	A metabolic response to ingested good or good additives in the host recipient
MUCOSA	Inner layer or cells of the gastrointestinal tract that are closes to the lumen
PHARMACOLOGICAL FOOD REACTION	A reaction to chemicals, including food additives, in ingested food
PLACEBO	Substance without known physiological effect that is used to mimic a real substance being tested, such as inert substances in pill form or food without a common ingredient (e.g., custard made with egg and milk substitutes that looks like regular custard)
SYMPTOMATIC SENSITIVITY	Detectable antibodies to an allergen (food or an inhaled or ingested substance) that cause symptoms upon exposure
URTICARIA (HIVES)	Raised lumps or welts that are very itchy

- Gluten sensitivity (intolerance) is not a food allergy. Gluten sensitivity is related to celiac disease and involves more than wheat restriction. (See Celiac Disease, Gluten-sensitive Enteropathy.) Gluten intolerance results in destruction of villi of the intestines, interfering with absorption of nutrients and causing severe GI and other symptoms.

- Adverse food reactions may be confused with food allergy. Some individuals are sensitive to sulfites, nitrates, artificial color (FD&C Yellow #5—Tartrazine) and may have severe reactions. For those with such reactions, label reading is essential and care must be taken to avoid potential sources of these substances. For example, textured vegetable protein, hydrolyzed proteins and meat extracts contain forms of glutamate. Labeling law requires that all foods containing MSG, tartrazine, sulfites or nitrites must declare this on the ingredient list.

- Pharmacological substances that occur naturally in food may also cause adverse reactions. Some individuals are sensitive to:

  - Caffeine: Coffee, tea, cola beverages and other sodas, over-the-counter medications. Histamine: Beer, fish, wine, chocolate, sauerkraut.
  - Tyramine: Cheese, pickled herring, avocado, oranges, bananas, tomatoes.
  - Serotonin: Bananas, tomatoes, plums, avocado, pineapple.

DIAGNOSIS OF FOOD SENSITIVITY

Reliable Tests	**Procedures**
Oral Challenge	The patient is on a hypoallergenic diet and given a test dose of suspected food in capsule form. Patient response is measured The test may be open, blind or double-blind. The elimination diet followed by an oral challenge test is a reliable form of diagnosis.
Skin testing	Dilute extract of food is placed on scratched or punctured site of patient's skin. This test is more accurate for non-food allergies (e.g. pollen) and needs to be followed by an oral challenge test, as there are many false positives for allergies.
Radioallergosorbent Extract Test (RAST)	A patient's blood sample is mixed with food on a paper disk to measure the formation of antibodies. This test is expensive and less accurate than other tests, but is useful if the patient is very sensitive and a true reaction needs to be avoided.
Enzyme-linked	ELISA test procedures are similar to RAST testing procedures, but do not use radioactive substances to measure the formation of antibodies. ELISA
Immunosorbent Assay (ELISA)	Tests are generally less expensive than RAST tests.
Unreliable Tests	
Cytotoxic testing (Leukocyte antigen testing, Brian's Test)	White blood cells are mixed with plasma and examined under a microscope upon exposure to a food sample.
Neutralization testing (Provocative testing)	Food extract is injected under the patient's skin. As symptoms develop, additional injections are made to neutralize symptoms.
Sublingual testing	Drops of food or allergen are placed under the tongue and symptoms observed and recorded.

(4) Immune system disorders, infections and fevers

- Diets for those with infections should be high in kcal, protein, carbohydrate, sodium chloride and fluid. In acute fever, it may be necessary to give a clear liquid diet and maintain hydration. With recovery, the patient is gradually advanced from soft foods to those of regular consistency. Small, frequent feedings are better tolerated than large meals.

- Increase kcal intake 7% per degree Fahrenheit of fever.

- Individuals who are infected with **HUMAN IMMUNODEFICIENCY VIRUS (HIV)** may be in different stages of the disease. As medical science gains a better understanding of the disease, people are being diagnosed and treated earlier. There may be few or no noticeable symptoms, but some unnoticed and subclinical changes such as loss of lean body mass with no change in total body weight, increased susceptibility to food and waterborne bacterial diseases and vitamin B_{12} deficiency may occur.

- **ACQUIRED IMMUNE DEFICIENCY SYNDROME (AIDS)** Individuals are considered to have AIDS when they are diagnosed with a minimum of one well defined, life threatening clinical problem that is clearly related to HIV immunosuppression. Opportunistic infections caused by bacteria, fungi, viruses or protozoa are often present. Symptoms include diarrhea, weight loss, fever and malabsorption. These infections are often related to decreased CD4 levels of about 200. CD4 is a part of the T-helper lymphocyte cells of the immune system. They protect against infection, are sensitive to nutritional factors and are a marker for the progression of AIDS. **CACHEXIA** (muscle wasting) results from decreased food intake and increased needs due to fever, sepsis and malabsorption. Weight maintenance and proper nutrient intake should be encouraged to improve quality of life and to optimize resistance.

- In AIDS there is often fat and lactose intolerance. Diarrhea and **ORAL THRUSH** (sores in the mouth) can impair food ingestion, digestion and absorption. Nutrition plans should promote optimal nutrition, particularly additional calories and protein, to increase resistance to infection. High intakes of B vitamins, thiamin, niacin and B_{12}, and antioxidants A, C, E, selenium and beta-carotene may help strengthen immune function and slow the progression of the disease.

- The diet should be modified for consistency and nutrient content according to symptoms. Usually small, frequent, high calorie/high protein meals are tolerated. Vitamin and mineral supplements and/or supplemental beverages are given. Scheduling of drug infusions after meals can increase food intake. As the disease progresses, soft or pureed foods may be necessary.

- Enteral feeding often leads to intractable diarrhea. A diagnostic determination of the cause of diarrhea and malabsorption is necessary. Antibiotics and antidiarrheal medications, low fat, low lactose, low fiber diet modifications and increased fluid consumption can also minimize diarrhea. Relatively low dose enteral feeding should be continued only if it does not produce diarrhea. Total parenteral nutrition (TPN) is then the only therapeutic nutrition treatment and, if instituted, must be continued until death.

- People with AIDS often turn to complementary or alternative therapies. Many are unproven for AIDS and may affect care they are receiving. Some therapies interfere with drugs and cause drug resistance and complicate other medical therapies.

- Rigorous hand washing and safe food handling techniques are important to minimize or prevent opportunistic infections. Individuals with AIDS should never consume potentially hazardous foods such as raw oysters, sushi, undercooked meat or raw eggs.

(5) Malnutrition: protein, calorie, vitamin, mineral

Protein and energy

- **PROTEIN CALORIE MALNUTRITION (PCM)** also called **PROTEIN ENERGY MALNUTRITION (PEM)** is a state of impaired nutritional status caused by a deficiency of protein, calories or both.

- **KWASHIORKOR** is prolonged protein insufficiency in the presence of adequate calories results in loss of visceral protein and decreased cellular immunity. Characteristics include distended abdomen, fatty liver, puffy hands and feet, skin sores and failure to resist infection.

- **MARASMUS** is prolonged lack of calories and prolonged protein insufficiency results in loss of muscle and fat stores. Depression of both somatic and visceral protein can occur. Characteristics include low weight, wasted muscles, reduced hormones and low body temperature.

- **FAILURE TO THRIVE** is growth retardation due to inadequate ingestion or use of food/nutrients by infants, children and the aged. Both organic and non-organic failure to thrive is seen. Organic failure to thrive is sometimes the result of severe central nervous system damage, a birth anomaly or disease. Lack of nurturing and touch are most likely to cause in non-organic failure to thrive, but the condition may be reversed with physical care and feeding.

- Treatment of protein-calorie malnutrition is a **HIGH PROTEIN, HIGH KILOCALORIE DIET**, which provides for the nutritional rehabilitation of the protein-calorie malnourished patient, alleviates weight loss or tissue wasting in conditions where normal levels of protein and calories will be insufficient (such as in infectious hepatitis) and promotes healing. This diet is used for catabolic states and will promote liver regeneration and replenish glycogen stores. Poor growth is inherent in certain syndromes, such as in patients with severe central nervous system damage.

- For severely malnourished patients, judicious feeding, slowly progressing to a high-protein, high calorie diet must be followed to build tolerance for increased digestive and metabolic processes. Otherwise, refeeding syndrome can develop.

- A typical high protein, high-calorie diet for an adult may include 1,000 or more calories per day as calorie-dense supplements in addition to full meals and snacks as tolerated. The diet should provide a minimum of 1.5g of protein per kg body weight for adults. Infants and children may need up to 4g per kg of body weight per day.

- The diet is essentially a regular one supplemented with high protein foods. Additional servings of milk, meat and eggs may be used with special high protein, high calorie liquid supplements. When calories must be increased to extremely high levels, the diet will be high in fat, when possible, because fat provides greater calorie density and a lower volume of food can be consumed.

- The relationship between non-protein calories and protein/nitrogen needs careful consideration. A high protein diet without enough calories from non-protein sources will cause much of the nitrogen to be wasted. The optimal kilocalorie to nitrogen ratio is 100-200kcal per gram of nitrogen intake.

Other vitamin and mineral deficiencies

- **OSTEOPOROSIS** is a bone disorder characterized initially by abnormal porosity as a result of decrease in the bone mass. The primary defect is degeneration of the cellular matrix that holds the bone structure. Osteoporosis is a disorder resulting from an imbalance between bone resorption and bone synthesis. Studies have shown that it is caused by a disturbance of calcium metabolism in association with inadequate calcium intake, hyperadrenocorticalism, hyperthyroidism, hyperparathyroidism, scurvy, various malignancies, immobilization or rheumatoid arthritis. Persons drinking fluoridated water have a lower incidence of osteoporosis because fluorine improves calcium balance by delaying the excretion of calcium. Weight bearing exercise, such as walking, is important to improve muscle tone and stimulate the bone surface to bind calcium.

- Osteoporosis is especially common in older women with prolonged poor calcium intakes. It causes hunched back and weak bones that fracture easily. It is best prevented by adequate calcium intake and physical activity. Estrogen and calcium supplementation may be prescribed after menopause to reduce release of calcium from bones. There is current concern about the increasing prevalence of osteoporosis and research on ways to avoid it. Dietary modifications (food and supplements), hormonal replacement and medications (Evista®, Fosamax®, Actonel®) to preserve bone are being widely used. Women are advised to be tested for bone density prior to menopause to determine osteoporosis risk and begin treatment if necessary.

- **OSTEOMALACIA** is the adult form of rickets. It is characterized by demineralization of bone or bone softening that is associated with insufficient vitamin D and mineral availability.

- **RICKETS** is caused by a disturbance in calcium-phosphorus metabolism and/or lack of vitamin D. It is essentially a disease of defective bone formation, manifesting itself in many ways, such as delayed closure of the fontanelles, (softening of the skull and bulging of the forehead) and poor muscle tone, which results in a potbelly appearance of the abdomen. Soft, fragile bones, leading to bowing of the legs; enlargement of the wrists, knees and ankle joints; and bending at the junction of the rib joints, forming the "rachitic rosary" and projecting the sternum, giving the appearance of a "pigeon breast" are other symptoms.

  - ➢ **VITAMIN D RESISTANT RICKETS** is probably hereditary and requires supplementation.
  - ➢ **CONDITIONED RICKETS** is the result of other diseases.
  - ➢ **LATE RICKETS** (late in childhood) is associated with malabsorption syndrome or renal acidosis.
  - ➢ **RENAL RICKETS** is caused by kidney failure.

DEFICIENCY/TOXICITY OF VITAMINS

FAT-SOLUBLE VITAMINS

Vitamin	Symptoms of Deficiency	Symptoms of Toxicity
Vitamin A retinal, retinol acid, provitamin A,(carotenoids) such as carotene	**XEROPHTHALMIA**: Night blindness, epithelial cells become dry and keratinized, conjunctiva and cornea become dry and blindness may result; **HYPOVITAMINOSIS A**: cessation of bone growth, tooth or bone deformities; anemia, keratin in follicles	**HYPERVITAMINOSIS A**: Decreased clotting time; fatigue; hair loss; jaundice; muscle soreness, rashes, itching, peeling skin; bone and joint pain; liver and spleen enlargement; nausea, weakness; severe headache; cessation of menstruation; brittle nails
Vitamin D calciferol, cholecalciferol, dihydroxy-vitamin D 1, 25 dihydroxycholecalciferol	**RICKETS** in children, **OSTEOMALACIA** in adults; bowed legs, misshapen bones, enlarged wrists and knees, potbelly in children, deformed bones in adults: poor tooth formation; high secretions of parathyroid hormone; muscle spasms	Withdrawal of calcium from bones; kidney stones; calcification of kidneys, soft tissue and blood vessels; excessive thirst and urination
Vitamin E alpha-tocopherol, betatocopherol, gamma tocopherol, alpha tocotrienol	Red cell breakage, anemia; unlikely except in children with cystic fibrosis or neuromuscular abnormalities; some reports of fibrocystic breast disease; fibrosis; neuromuscular abnormalities; alpha-tocopherol is the most active form, other forms are calculated in alpha-tocopherol units	Interference with anticlotting medication; headache; a few cases of fatigue, skin rash and abdominal discomfort reported when over 600mg/day consumed
Vitamin K phylloquinone, naphthoquinone, menadione is synthetic form	Hemorrhaging, prolonged blood clotting time	Megadoses interfere with anticoagulant drugs; RBC hemolysis; jaundice

DEFICIENCY/TOXICITY OF VITAMINS and MINERALS

WATER-SOLUBLE VITAMINS

Vitamin	Symptoms of Deficiency	Symptoms of Toxicity
Vitamin C (ascorbic acid) supplements may obscure some laboratory tests, including glucose testing	**SCURVY**: Hemorrhages of gums, under skin, into joints; anemia; slow wound healing; psychological depression; joint pain; atherosclerotic plaque	Nausea, headaches, rashes, hemolytic anemia, aggravation of gout, diarrhea; risk of kidney stones; body can become dependent on high vitamin C levels resulting in **REBOUND SCURVY** if supplementation is stopped abruptly
Thiamin (B$_1$)	**BERIBERI**: Loss of appetite; nausea; vomiting; constipation; loss of knee and ankle reflexes; depression; confusion; feeling of persecution; enlarged head; edema in "wet" beriberi; muscle wasting in "dry" beriberi; heart failure; more common in alcoholics	Rapid pulse, weakness, headache, insomnia
Riboflavin (B$_2$)	**ARIBOFLAVINOSIS:** **CHEILOSIS** (fissures at corners of mouth); sore, magenta-red tongue; photophobia; eye lesions, skinrash	Not seen
Niacin (nicotinic acid, nicotinamide or niacinamide)	**PELLAGRA**: severe diarrhea; painfully sore mouth and GI tract; dark, peeling dermatitis; mental derangement, delirium; more common on very low-protein diets; pellagra sometimes called disease of the 4 D's--diarrhea, dermatitis, dementia, death	Diarrhea, nausea, vomiting, inflamed tongue, fainting, dizziness, low blood pressure. Nicotinic acid causes itching, burning and flushing, abnormal heartbeat, gastrointestinal distress; other forms of niacin may not cause flushing
Vitamin B$_6$ (pyridoxal, pyridoxamine or pyridoxine)	Sideroblastic anemia, weakness, lack of coordination; convulsions in infants; greasy dermatitis; inflamed mouth with ulcers and rash on face in adults; abnormal electro-encephalogram; kidney stones most common as result of medications (e.g., drugs for tuberculosis, oral contraceptives)	Depression, fatigue, headaches; pyridoxine can induce neurological disorders, ataxia and severe sensory neuropathy
Pantothenic acid	Vomiting, GI distress, insomnia, fatigue, burning feet syndrome	Occasional diarrhea, water retention
Folate	Macrocytic anemia; red, sore tongue; diarrhea; weight loss; weakness; depression; irritability; paranoia; birth defects higher in pregnant women ingesting low folate levels	Diarrhea, insomnia, irritability; can obscure symptoms of pernicious anemia (vitamin B$_{12}$ deficiency)

DEFICIENCY/TOXICITY OF VITAMINS and MINERALS

**WATER-SOLUBLE VITAMINS,
cont.**

Vitamin	Symptoms of Deficiency	Symptoms of Toxicity
Vitamin B$_{12}$	**PERNICIOUS ANEMIA** (same macrocytic anemia as folate deficiency: numbness of hands and feet, poor coordination, severe mental disorders); usually from lack of intrinsic factor; most common in strict vegetarians	Decreased renal function; kidney stones in susceptible persons
Biotin	Pallor, drowsiness, muscle pain, nausea, loss of appetite, scaly dermatitis, motor weakness; has been reported in total parenteral nutrition (TPN); usually seen with excessive consumption of raw eggs, since raw eggs have a biotin blocker called AVIDIN	Not seen

DEFICIENCY/TOXICITY OF MINERALS

MAJOR MINERALS

Mineral	Symptoms of Deficiency	Symptoms of Toxicity
Calcium	May contribute to rickets, osteomalacia, and osteoporosis (stunted growth, bone loss); TETANY low blood calcium, increased excitability of nerves, uncontrolled contracting of muscles	Decreased renal function; kidney stones in susceptible persons
Chloride	Growth failure, poor appetite, more alkaline blood, behavioral and learning problems, muscle cramps	Vomiting
Magnesium	Poor appetite, nausea, muscle tremors, poor coordination, weakness, confusion, convulsions, hypocalcemia, hypokalemia, depressed pancreatic hormone secretion, difficulty in swallowing	Not seen
Phosphorus	Muscle weakness	Large intake may lower calcium absorption, but wide range of ratios causes no adverse effects in children and adults; HYPERPHOSPHATEMIA associated with calcification of soft tissues
Potassium	Can be fatal; weakness, lethargy, change in heart rhythm, muscle paralysis; can result from diuretic therapy	Occurs from supplements, renal failure; muscle weakness, cardiac arrhythmia
Sodium	Rare; excessive sweat losses cause nausea, giddiness, muscle cramps, fatigue, appetite loss	Hypertension in susceptible persons

II. NUTRITION CARE FOR INDIVIDUALS AND GROUPS (50%)

DEFICIENCY/TOXICITY OF VITAMINS and MINERALS

TRACE MINERALS

Mineral	Symptoms of Deficiency	Symptoms of Toxicity
Chromium	Abnormal glucose tolerance, associated with coronary artery disease	Rare; occupational exposures damage skin and kidneys
Copper	Rare, including anemia, skeletal changes	Amounts over 10mg/day can be toxic; vomiting, diarrhea; **WILSON'S DISEASE** with excess copper deposition
Fluoride	Tooth decay	**FLUOROSIS** (discolored teeth), nausea, itching, vomiting
Iron	**ANEMIA**: hypochromic, microcytic; fatigue, paleness, shortness of breath on exertion; lowered immunity, impaired cognitive and learning ability in children, itching, reduced ability to regenerate body temperature; **PICA**: eating clay or other non-food substances and ice	Infections; individuals genetic defect develop **HEMOCHROMATOSIS**, with **HEMOSIDEROSIS**; both are caused by excessive iron storage and lack of excretion; overdose can be fatal
Selenium	No symptoms in humans except low blood levels (anemia)	Digestive system problems; loss of hair and nails; amounts greater than 200mcg may produce chronic toxicity; fatigue, odor of garlic on breath, tooth damage
Zinc	Growth retardation, anorexia, loss of taste acuity, delayed sexual maturation, scaly skin and dermatitis, mental depression, deficiencies in immune response, hair loss, chronic diarrhea, photophobia, altered hormonal functions; atherosclerosis, impaired cell division	Supplements can result in toxicity, i.e., anemia, heart muscle degeneration, diarrhea, elevated white blood cell count, renal failure, reproductive failure, muscle pain, drowsiness, raised LDL, lowered HDL, reduced sense of smell and taste, impaired folate absorption

- **(6) Metabolic, endocrine, and inborn errors of metabolism**

DIABETES MELLITUS

- **HYPERGLYCEMIA** is elevated plasma glucose, and is present in all but the mildest cases of diabetes. Symptoms of hyperglycemia include increased urination, thirst, fatigue and weight loss. Untreated hyperglycemia can lead to diabetic ketoacidosis. The normal plasma glucose level is 70-100mg/dL.

- **HYPOGLYCEMIA** results from a sudden decline in the blood glucose level and requires immediate treatment. In hypoglycemia, plasma glucose levels are below 70mg/dL. It is caused by poor blood sugar regulation. While common in those with diabetes, hypoglycemia is sometimes seen in people without diabetes. When insulin is given, hypoglycemia may occur if food intake is inadequate at the time of peak insulin activity or if increased exercise causes insulin increase. Regulate amount and type of insulin and food intake.

- Hypoglycemia is sometimes called insulin reaction.

  - **Causes:** Unusual exercise, insufficient consumption of food, excessive insulin due to decreased need or inaccurate insulin administration.
  - **Symptoms:** Sweating, impatience, double vision, hunger, pallor, palpitation, headache, light-headedness, confusion, tiredness, dizziness, emotional instability, unconsciousness, seizures.
  - **Treatment:** Immediate consumption of a carbohydrate source, such as fruit juice, hard candy, sugar, sweetened carbonated beverage. In more severe cases, seek emergency aid, administer intravenous glucose or glucagon immediately, and then give oral glucose after the patient responds to intravenous treatment. The "15/15 rule" is to give 15g carbohydrate, wait 15 minutes and test blood glucose again. There is a danger of over treating if testing is done before the glucose can be absorbed. If mild, the patient should eat or drink carbohydrate-containing food. If more advanced, the patient needs 10-20g of rapidly absorbable sugar followed by a second dose 15 minutes later. Those with diabetes should carry glucose tablets, which are quickly absorbed and metabolized.
  - Hypoglycemia sometimes occurs with sulfonylureas such as Glyburide (Micronase® DiaBeta®) Tolbutamide (Orinase®) and glipizide (Glucotrol®).The normal hormonal response to hypoglycemia is release of the counter-regulatory hormones: glucagon, epinephrine, cortisol and growth hormone.

Diagnostic tests and monitoring

- The **DIABETES CONTROL AND COMPLICATIONS TRIAL (DCCT)** found a strong link between glycemic control and developing fewer complications of diabetes. Management, therefore, requires teamwork among all healthcare providers. Careful coordination of medical nutrition therapy (MNT), medications, exercise, blood glucose monitoring and self-management education is vital in order to achieve goals, and lifestyle changes that lead to the following outcomes:
  - Maintaining normal or as near normal blood glucose levels as possible.
  - Providing the optimal nutrition for the individual, including adequate calories for the specific life cycle stage or other illness.
  - Achieving optimal lipid levels.
  - Preventing and/or treating the acute complications of insulin treatment.
  - Preventing and/or treating the chronic complications of diabetes.

- **SELF-MONITORING OF BLOOD GLUCOSE (SMBG)** is encouraged for persons with diabetes to improve self-management skills. Blood sugar levels are frequently checked and recorded, usually 4 or more and up to 8 times each day. Testing is done with reagent strips (Dextrostix®, Chemstrip®) using finger-prick blood samples read by a glucometer. Results may indicate a need to adjust the disease management program (insulin and/or diet). Some patients have **INSULIN PUMPS** that allow insulin to be released into the bloodstream (based on monitored blood sugar values) in either basal or bolus amounts without injections.

- **FASTING PLASMA GLUCOSE (FPG)** is the preferred test for diagnosis because of its ease of administration, convenience, acceptability to patients and lower cost. It is done after not eating for at least 10 hours. Diagnosis for type 1 and type 2 diabetes is based on two fasting blood glucose tests of greater than 126mg/dL (7.0 mmol/L). Impaired fasting homeostasis is indicated if the fasting glucose is greater than 110mg/dL and less than 126mg/dL. Normal fasting glucose is less than 110mg/dL.

- **ORAL GLUCOSE TOLERANCE TEST (OGTT)** is another method used for diagnosing diabetes. The patient should not be ill or taking medication or vitamin supplements that may affect the test. For the test, a standard glucose drink (Glucola®) containing 75g of carbohydrate is given. If the patient weighs less than 50kg, then 50g is given; if the patient weighs 50-100kg, then 75g is given; if the patient weighs more than 100kg, then 100g is given. Blood glucose is tested at the beginning, at ½, 1, 1½ and 2 hours after the carbohydrate load. Normal pre-prandial fasting glucose levels are less than 110mg/dL.

- **RANDOM BLOOD GLUCOSE TEST** can be taken at any time of the day. A diagnosis for type 1 and type 2 diabetes is a level of greater than 200mg/dL plus symptoms such as excess urination, thirst or unexplained weight loss.

- **GLYCATED HEMOGLOBIN (GHB)** tests reflect the exposure of hemoglobin and other proteins to circulating glucose. Because glucose attaches to protein in a slow, concentration-dependent and irreversible manner, glycated hemoglobin tests reflect average plasma glucose concentrations over time. Glycated hemoglobin can be measured by different methods that look at different components of the product. Hemoglobin A1C (HbA1c) is one measure of glycated hemoglobin. It is an integrated measure of long-term (2-3 months) glycemia. For non-diabetics, the normal range is 4-6%, the goal for diabetics is <7%. If blood glucose is high, the level will be high. This level is not used to adjust daily insulin doses nor should it be used for diagnosis.

- **GLYCATED SERUM PROTEIN (GSP)** measures mostly glycated albumin that has a faster half-life than hemoglobin. It is used in situations where A1C tests cannot be measured or may not be useful, such as in hemolytic anemias. The GSP may be valuable in assessment of a treatment regimen because it provides an index of glycemic status over the preceding 1-2 week period. It is not considered equivalent to the A1C test.

- **GLUCOSURIA** is when glucose spills into urine because the sugar concentration exceeds the renal threshold (160-180mg/100 ml). The presence of glucose is shown by use of indicator paper (Tes-Tape®), paper stick (Clinistix®) or tablet in urine (Clinitest®).

- **KETONURIA** is a condition characterized by ketone bodies in urine (acetoacetic acid, betahydroxybuteric acid and acetone) that indicates incomplete oxidation of fatty acids. Diabetics should test for ketones in urine on a regular basis during illness and when glycemic levels are steadily above 240mg/dL (13.3 mmol/L). Ketonuria can also be present when body fat is being used for fuel in the absence of dietary carbohydrates.

- For the individual who is on a plan that involves **CONVENTIONAL INSULIN THERAPY,** (a specific number of insulin injections per day), consistency in the timing and amount of food eaten is essential.

- For the individual whose plan involves **INTENSIVE DIABETES MANAGEMENT** (three or more insulin injections per day or use of an insulin pump), meal plans are more flexible in both timing and consistency. Individuals are taught to adjust insulin dosages to actual food intake or timing of the meal, although consistency in timing and amount of food eaten helps to improve glycemic control.

Criteria for diabetes testing in asymptomatic, undiagnosed individuals

- **type 1 Diabetes:** Testing presumably healthy individuals for the presence of any immune markers, outside of a clinical trial setting, is not recommended at this time.

- **type 2 Diabetes:** In asymptomatic, undiagnosed individuals, screening for diabetes should be considered in all individuals at age 45 years and above and, if normal, it should be repeated at three-year intervals.

- Testing should be considered at a younger age or be carried out more frequently in individuals who:

  - Are overweight [BMI) $\geq$25kg/m[1]].
  - Have a first-degree relative with diabetes (e.g. children, parents, grandparents.)
  - Are members of a high-risk ethnic population (African American, Hispanic, Native American, Asian.)
  - Delivered a baby weighing > 9 lb. or were diagnosed with gestational diabetes mellitus.
  - Are hypertensive ($\geq$140/90).
  - Have an HDL cholesterol level $\leq$35mg/dL and/or a triglyceride level $\geq$250mg/dL.
  - On previous testing, had glucose levels above normal limits.
  - Have other clinical conditions associated with insulin resistance (e.g. PCOS).

DIAGNOSTIC BLOOD GLUCOSE LEVELS	
	Plasma Glucose mg/dL
Normal fasting	PG < 110
2 hour	PG < 140
Diabetes fasting	PG $\geq$126
2 hour	PG $\geq$200
Casual plasma glucose (CPG)	PG $\geq$200
Impaired fasting glucose	PG 100 - 125
Impaired glucose tolerance, at 2 hours	PG 140 -199

CLASSIFICATION OF DIABETES

type 1

(formerly called Insulin Dependent Diabetes Mellitus (IDDM), juvenile onset diabetes, ketosis-prone diabetes, brittle diabetes, adult onset diabetes, maturity diabetes, ketosis-resistant or stable diabetes)

Abrupt onset, at any age, mostly diagnosed before age 30; low or absent endogenous insulin; dependent on exogenous insulin for life; ketosis prone; often underweight at onset; possibly due to virus (i.e. mumps); genetic tie in some, environmental; classic "P" symptoms of hyperglycemia—polydipsia, polyuria, polyphagia. 5%-10% of all diagnosed cases of diabetes.

type 2

(formerly called Non-Insulin-Dependent Diabetes Mellitus (NIDDM) or, in younger adults and children, Mature Onset Diabetes in the Young (MODY)

Gradual onset; most older than 30 at diagnosis, but currently occurring more often in younger adults and children (MODY), serum insulin levels elevated, depressed or normal; not prone to ketosis; may require insulin or oral hypoglycemic agent; many can be controlled by diet alone; most often overweight or obese (especially intraabdominal) at onset (about 80%); largest percent have genetic ties; most prevalent form of diabetes (about 90-95% of cases).

Secondary Diabetes

(diabetes occurs as a result of other disorders or pancreatic disease, hormonal, drug or chemical-treatments)

Associated with certain conditions or syndromes: induced, insulin receptor abnormalities, certain genetic syndromes, other causes unknown; level of hyperglycemia consistent with diagnosis of diabetes.

Gestational Diabetes Mellitus (GDM)

Diabetes brought on by the extra hormonal and growth demands of pregnancy. It can predict later diabetes, but usually ceases for the mother after the infant is born. Glucose intolerance that has onset or recognition during pregnancy; is associated with increased perinatal risk, including congenital complications and development of diabetes later in life, affects about 4% of pregnant women.

Impaired Glucose Homeostasis

Not a clinical entity, but is a risk factor for DM and CVD.

Meal plans

- A careful assessment of current nutritional practices is an important first step in determining the individualized diet plan and lifestyle changes that should to be recommended. In order to cause minimum disruption to a person's life, it is important to determine the daily routine and schedule, including usual waking time, usual meal and snack time, school, or work schedule, exercise practices, and bedtime.

- Calorie determination is made based on what the person is currently eating, insulin management or medication plans, reasonable weight goals and desired outcome goals.

- Often weight loss is desirable. As little as a 5-10 pound weight loss in type-2 diabetics may produce positive clinical outcomes.

- Depending on the individual's lifestyle, motivation and educational background, diets may be planned using simple guidelines such as MyPlate or more complex plans using the *Exchange Lists for Meal Planning*, counting approaches such as carbohydrate counting, total available glucose (TAG) or the calorie point system. All food plans should help the client select appropriate foods specific to his/her needs, including caloric levels, where necessary.

- Glycemic controls for adults who have diabetes include an A1 C of <7.0%; preprandial capillary plasma glucose of 90-130mg/dL, peak postprandial capillary glucose <180mg/dL.

Glycemic index

- The **GLYCEMIC INDEX** measures how a carbohydrate containing food raises the blood glucose. Foods are ranked related to how they compare to a reference food: glucose or white bread. A food with a high index raises blood glucose more than a food with a medium or low index. Meal planning with this program requires choosing foods with a low or medium index or if a food with a high index is chosen combining it with a low index food. The Glycemic index of a food is lower when it is eaten as part of a meal than when eaten alone. There are some very nutritious foods that have a higher index than some foods with a lower index. The nutritious higher index foods should not be omitted from the diet. Rather, they should be combined in a meal with lower index foods.

Planning guidelines for diabetic food plans

- The diabetic food plan should provide:
  - ➤ Sufficient calories to achieve and maintain reasonable weight.
  - ➤ Carbohydrate intake based on individual goals (usually about 45-55%). In an individual with well controlled diabetes, sucrose restriction is not justifiable on the basis of glycemic effect, but some nutritive sweeteners may adversely affect LDL cholesterol levels.
  - ➤ Protein at 12-20% total calories, (the same as for a non-diabetic, about 0.8g/kg/day). Dietitians are using the high protein diet in the treatment of some clients with type 2 diabetes mellitus with good results. The calorie distribution is 40% carbohydrate, 30% protein and 30% fat. However, some research has shown that in patients whose diets contained more than 20% protein over a period of time had a higher incidence of albuminuria.
- Fat: Type 1 diabetics at a healthy weight and with normal lipid profile should follow the recommendations for the NCEP Total Life Style Change Diet. For type 2 patients, the percentage of fat calories should be linked to desired outcomes reduced total dietary fat if weight loss is necessary. If LDL reduction is the target, a NCEP Step II Diet is suggested. If there is insulin resistance or other problems that may be the result of a high carbohydrate diet, consideration should be given to a diet containing about 40% of calories from carbohydrate, about 40% of calories from fat, with less than 10% from saturated and the increase from monounsaturated fat.
  - ➤ Fiber: 20-35g of dietary fiber per day, same as for general population.

- Sodium same as for general population.
- Sugar substitutes such as aspartame (Equal®), acesulfame K (Sunette®), sucralose (Splenda®), and saccharin are safe to consume by all people with diabetes. During pregnancy, because saccharin can cross the placenta, the other sugar substitutes are better choices.
- Alcohol for occasional, moderate use with physician's permission, blood glucose will not be affected by moderate alcohol use if diabetes is well-controlled.
- Vitamin and mineral supplements are not needed by the majority of people with diabetes unless medications or lab values indicate need for specific nutrients.

- In diabetes mellitus, risk for coronary heart disease is two to four times greater in both men and women, regardless of age, and a heart healthy diet is advised. More restrictions are necessary if hypertension is present.

Calculating a diabetic diet

- A meal pattern should be developed based on the patient's normal eating habits, unless they need improvement. Positive habits and preferences should be preserved as much as possible. The diet order or prescription usually provides the total daily calories. It may indicate the percentage of carbohydrate distribution among meals and snacks, based on the type of insulin to be given. To develop a realistic meal plan that fits the patient's lifestyle, include the patient in the planning process. To calculate a diet using the exchange system, follow these steps:

  - Using recommended number of calories, determine grams of CHO, PRO and fat.

    Total calories x percent carbohydrate = CHO calories ÷4 = grams CHO
    Total calories x percent protein = PRO calories ÷ 4 = grams PRO
    Total calories x percent fat = fat calories ÷ 9 = grams fat

    Example:
    1,500 calories with 55% CHO, 20% PRO, 25% fat
    CHO grams = 1500 calories X 55% of diet at 4 calories/g = 206g CHO
    PRO grams = 1500 calories X 20% of diet at 4 calories/g = 75g
    PRO Fat grams = 1500 calories X 25% of diet at 9 calories/g = 42g fat

  - Determine the nutritional needs for milk per day and whether the patient will drink milk. Generally plan 2 cups for adults and 3 to 4 cups for pregnant and lactating women or children. Calculate with the appropriate type of milk (skim, 2%, etc.)
  - Estimate the number of servings from the vegetable and fruit groups; include a minimum of five total servings from these two groups, preferably more.
  - Add the grams of carbohydrate, protein and fat from the three groups: milk, vegetable and fruit.
  - Divide the remaining grams of carbohydrate by 15 to determine the remaining number of starch/bread exchanges.
  - Assign the number of meat exchanges by subtracting the total protein already provided from the milk, vegetable and starch allowances and dividing the remaining grams by 7. Counselors calculate using lean (3g fat per exchange) or medium-fat meats (5g fat), based on patient's habits.

- ➤ Assign the number of fat exchanges based on the amount of calories and fat left; most individuals should have a minimum of three fat exchanges per day.
- ➤ After determining the exchanges, formulate a sample meal plan. Use foods preferred by the patient to illustrate how the plan is to be used. The patient should demonstrate understanding by selecting a diet using the plan.

- **CARBOHYDRATE COUNTING** is a meal planning method that can add variety to food choices and flexibility to the meal plan. Carbohydrate is the main nutrient in food that affects blood glucose (sugar) levels. In MyPlate, foods in the starch, fruit and milk groups and "empty calorie" contain carbohydrates. In the Exchange Lists, foods from the starch, fruit, milk and vegetable exchanges are the carbohydrate foods.

  - ➤ One carbohydrate choice = 15g of carbohydrate = 1 starch, fruit, starchy vegetable, or milk. Some carbohydrate foods count as 2-4 carbohydrate choices.

  - ➤ Carbohydrate counting is becoming more popular with people who have diabetes because it is, for some, easier to manage and foods that do not contain carbohydrate do not have to be counted. Depending on how diabetes is managed, the starting point is about 45-60 grams of CHO at a meal. The dietitian should help clients work this type of diet within their insulin management program. Protein and fat should be included in each meal to balance the meal. Review carbohydrate counting in *Count Your Carbs: Getting Started*, available from and or the American Diabetes Association.

- **CALORIE POINT SYSTEM** is a simplified method to compute the intake of calories on a daily basis. Each calorie point is equal to 75 calories and each portion size has a set number of calories.

- Eating a specific amount of carbohydrate at each meal and at snacks can help control blood glucose levels. The number of carbohydrate choices per meal is adjusted by calorie needs and the amount of carbohydrate the body can use without raising blood glucose above target ranges. For those on insulin, doses can be adjusted to match the carbohydrate eaten. Although counting carbohydrate is the first priority, advice should be given about control of fat and types of fat because individuals with diabetes have a higher risk of cardiovascular disease.

- **FOOD EXCHANGES**, developed by the American Diabetes Association and The Academy of Nutrition and Dietetics (now AND), simplify the selection of a balanced diet. Foods with similar carbohydrate, protein and fat content are grouped into exchange lists. There are exchange lists for breads and starches, meats and meat substitutes, milk, fruits, vegetables and fats. Many people with diabetes mellitus are expected to know exchanges (assuming appropriate literacy and learning ability) and be able to plan and calculate diets based on exchanges. Some weight control programs, such as Weight Watchers, also use food exchanges for planning.

- Dietitians should know exchanges and be able to calculate diets based upon them. See *Choose Your Foods: Exchange Lists for Diabetes*, available from the American Diabetes Association or AND.

Medications

- **INSULIN** is a protein extracted from animal (pig or cow) pancreas or bioengineered from bacteria or fungal cells and biosynthetic human insulin analog. Insulin must be administered by injections because as a protein it is denatured by hydrochloric acid in the stomach and digested, leaving it unavailable for use in the body. Type, dosage and frequency are highly individualized. The standard potency is U-100 (100 units/ml). Insulin must be kept refrigerated.

- **HUMAN INSULIN (HUMULIN)** is the insulin of choice. Human insulin has been made synthetically 1984, and most newly diagnosed patients begin on this type of insulin. It can be replicated by DNA technology. It is available as short, intermediate or long acting. It is usually absorbed more quickly than animal insulin, peaks earlier, has a shorter duration time and has lower potential for antibody formation.

INSULIN ACTION

(Time of onset, peak AND duration may vary from individual to individual.)

Insulin Type	Appearance	Onset (min)	Peak (min)	Duration (hr)
Rapid Acting				
Lispro (Humalog)	Clear	5-15	30-90	3-5
Aspart (NovoLog)	Clear	<5-15	30-90	3-5
Glulisine (Apidra)	Clear	5-15	30-90	3-5
Short Acting				
Regular	Clear	30-60	2-4	5-8
Intermediate acting				
NPH	Cloudy	120-240	4-10	10-16
Long acting				
Determir (Levemir)	Cloudy	120-240	No peak	20-24
Glargine (Lantus)	Cloudy	120-240	No peak	18-24
Combinations				
70/30 (70% NPH, 30% regular)		30-60	Dual	10-16
75/25 (75% neutral protamine lispro, 25% lispro)		30-60	Dual	10-16
70/30 (70% neutral protamine aspart, 30% aspart)		30-60	Dual	10-16

- **ORAL HYPOGLYCEMIC AGENTS (OHA)** lower elevated blood glucose and are used for treatment of type 2 diabetes. **SULFONYLUREAS** are classified as first generation and second generation. They lower the blood sugar level and reduce glycosuria by stimulating the pancreatic beta cells to secrete endogenous insulin. Over a long time, they can cause the beta cells to be unable to produce any insulin and they may cause weight gain and hypoglycemia. First generation include Tolbutamide (Orinase®), Tolazamide (Tolinase®) and Chlorpropamide (Diabinese®). Second generation include Glyburide (Glynase Prestabs®) and Glipizide (Glucotrol®), extended release Glipizide (Glucotrol XL®) and Glimepiride (Amaryl®). The newer ones are more potent, require smaller dosages and are metabolized in the liver to inactive metabolites. Onset and duration vary considerably.

- **MEGLITINIDE** responds to glucose levels by improving insulin secretion. It binds to a different site than the sulfonylureas. It has a very fast onset, is short acting, and can be taken immediately before meals. It decreases the risk of hypoglycemia between meals and during the night. It is on the market as Repaglinide (Prandin®) and Nateglinide (Starlix®). The effect of Nateglinide is dependent on the presence of glucose.

- **BIGUANIDES** lower blood glucose by decreasing the release of glucose in the liver, making cells more sensitive to insulin and lowering insulin resistance. They do not stimulate insulin secretion. They require the presence of insulin, exogenous or endogenous, to be effective. Metformin (Glucophage®) is a biguanide drug taken 1-3 times daily and can be taken alone or combined with other diabetes drugs. It does not cause hypoglycemia and, at the beginning of therapy, may cause a small amount of weight loss. It improves lipid levels but should not be used for patients with renal or active liver disease. Other biguanides include metformin extended release (Glucophage XR®), a liquid metformin (Riomet®.) Metformin is also available in combination with several sulfonylureas such as glipizide (Metaglip®.) Side effects include gastrointestinal distress in about 50% of patients. It should be taken with meals to minimize distress.

- **ALPHA GLUCOSIDASE INHIBITORS** slow or inhibit the body's absorption of carbohydrates. Acarbose (Precose®) and Miglitol (Glycet®) are alpha glucosidase inhibitor drugs. They do not cause hypoglycemia or weight gain, but can cause transient GI disturbances, so therapy should be very low dose to start.

- **THIAZOLIDINEDIONES (TZDs)** act by decreasing insulin resistance in the muscle and adipose tissue, which helps the muscles and adipose tissue to take up glucose. They tend to increase HDL cholesterol and often help to decrease triglycerides. Side effects include weight gain and edema, which are more prevalent in patients who take this drug with insulin. People who have advanced forms of congestive heart disease or hepatic impairment should not use TZDs. Two newer forms of TZDs, Roseglitazine (Avandia®), and Pioglitazone (Actos®), are less likely to cause liver toxicity than Rezulin (troglitazone), which was recalled in March 2000.

- Combination therapy with insulin and hypoglycemic agents may be used if glucose is poorly controlled with either oral agents or insulin alone.

- **HYPOGLYCEMIA** (low blood sugar) is the most common side effect of sulfonylureas. Gastrointestinal problems, primarily nausea or diarrhea, are most commonly reported with Glucophage® and Precose®. Side effects are dose-related.

Youth

- Children and adolescents with diabetes mellitus require careful evaluation and counseling in order to deal with multiple physical, social and emotional needs. Calories are based on the nutrition assessment.

- The child and parent/caregiver requires education as to the meal plan, exercise guidelines, hypoglycemia and hyperglycemia treatment, modifications for short-term illness, blood glucose monitoring and plans for continuing care.

- The dietitian's role is usually assessment, education counseling and followup, typically every 3-6 months. Education may include topics of label reading, bag lunches, holidays, birthday parties, sports, snacks, adjusting mealtimes, fast food choices, healthy snacks, etc. Children and adolescents with diabetes should be encouraged to take as much personal responsibility for their food choices and care as their developmental stage allows.

Pregnancy

- **GESTATIONAL DIABETES MELLITUS (GDM)** is a form of diabetes that occurs only during pregnancy due to the increased metabolic demands of mother and fetus. Diagnosis is usually made by screening all pregnant women between the 24th and 28th week of pregnancy.

  - In the pregnant woman with diabetes, the diet should provide enough calories and nutrient requirements for pregnancy.
  - Weight gain should be on a similar curve as the non-diabetic pregnancy.
  - The diet should be carefully designed and controlled to avoid hyperglycemia and ketone formation in the blood, which is associated with an increased risk of fetal complications.
  - The patient should monitor and record blood glucose data, so the dietitian can help her plan her meals wisely.
  - The percentage of macronutrients should be calculated on a case-by-case basis and evaluated frequently based on the careful monitoring of blood glucose, ketonuria and weight gain.
  - Generally, foods high in total carbohydrate are limited (about 40-45% of total calories), with frequent small feedings during the day, to keep blood glucose controlled and possibly avoid the need for insulin injections, but this may not be good for all women with GDM. The breakfast meal should contain the least amount of CHO (about 30g) at breakfast.
  - If exogeneous insulin is necessary, it should be human insulin. Appropriate exercise is also helpful in control of GDM.

- Pregnant women with diabetes typically give birth to larger babies. This can complicate delivery so labor may be induced before term.

- Women with type 1 or type 2 diabetes, who become pregnant, remain classified as type 1 or type 2, but their diabetes does not subside after pregnancy. These women require stricter control than GDM.

- Women with diabetes may breastfeed. Careful monitoring and support is necessary because breastfeeding may make blood glucose control more difficult. Many women with gestational diabetes return to non-diabetic state after delivery.

Exercise

- Individuals with diabetes should discuss their exercise program with a physician or diabetes counselor. Education is usually required regarding the potential of hypoglycemia and insulin in people with type 1 diabetes, and the need for extra carbohydrate or fluid adjustments. Blood glucose monitoring is indicated to maintain appropriate control. Proper footwear is important for those with diabetes because of increased potential for infection.

- For everyone, exercise results in improved fitness, flexibility, endurance, muscle strength, and usually helps those with diabetes improve insulin sensitivity. It also promotes psychological wellbeing.

- Physical training can increase insulin sensitivity of muscle tissue in type 2 and improves lipoprotein values. For those with diabetes, exercise can improve cardiovascular fitness, minimize cardiovascular complications of diabetes and reduce hypertension. Exercise can assist in weight control and management. Extra calories and carbohydrate are not added for type 2 patients.

- Hypoglycemia can be a problem for both type 1 and type 2 patients who take insulin or oral hypoglycemic medication. Because repletion of liver and muscle glycogen can take from 24 to 30 hours, hypoglycemia can occur any time after exercises are completed.

  ➤ Hypoglycemia can occur after high-intensity exercise as a result of the counter regulatory hormones.
  ➤ Hyperglycemia can also result from exercise, especially when people exercise at a higher level of intensity than is normal for them. This is due to a marked increase in counter-regulatory hormones and utilization of glucose may not be equal to the released hepatic glucose.

- Exercise should not be started if blood glucose levels are higher than 250-300mg/dL.

  ➤ Generally, carbohydrate should be adjusted for exercise, based on glucose levels, at the onset of the exercise regimen. In type 1, 15g of dietary carbohydrate is added for every 1-1½ hours of vigorous exercise.

- Strenuous exercise is contraindicated for people with very poor metabolic control, especially if ketosis is present. Exercisers with diabetes should increase their fluid intake. When exercising, all individuals with diabetes should carry identification (name and diabetic condition) and a source of readily available carbohydrate to avoid emergencies and to direct medical attention for proper treatment.

Blood glucose monitoring

- Blood glucose control is the most important factor in preventing or delaying complications of diabetes. Factors that cause blood glucose to rise include insufficient insulin, inadequate oral medication, excessive carbohydrate intake, the presence of other hormones (e.g., glucagon), stress, illness or infection. Blood glucose levels drop because of too much insulin or oral hypoglycemic agent, not enough food, an unusually high amount of exercise, delayed or skipped meals and from some medications.

- Patients should regularly check blood glucose with the frequency and type of monitoring determined in consultation with the counselor. The blood glucose records are used to coordinate the diabetes management plan, meet nutrition therapy goals, evaluate and modify the meal plan as necessary.

Emergencies

- The RD plays a key role in "sick day management" of the person with diabetes. When individuals with diabetes are ill, they should continue taking insulin or OHA, test blood glucose frequently, test urine for glucose and ketones, increase fluid intake and try to eat normal amounts of carbohydrate unless their blood sugar is over 250mg/dL. If blood sugar is high, less carbohydrate may be eaten. Often it is necessary to eat smaller, more frequent meals and eat softer foods. Insulin needs increase with fever. If regular foods cannot be eaten, carbohydrate calories can be obtained from liquid sources. Generally 1½ cups of fluid per hour and 15g carbohydrate every half hour should be consumed.

- **KETOACIDOSIS** results from insufficient insulin through deliberate or unavoidable omission of prescribed insulin or a greatly increased need.

- Patients are usually thirsty, polyuric, weak and short of breath. They have typical gasping for breath ("air hunger") called **KUSSMAUL'S BREATHING**, and sometimes nausea and altered consciousness.

- Both hyperosmolar coma and lactic acidosis are variants of ketoacidosis from the point of view of therapy and pathophysiology. Lab findings in ketoacidosis include: increased glucose, acetoacetate, amylase and creatinine; decreased pH, bicarbonate, pCO_2 and sodium.

- Uncontrolled diabetes with severely elevated blood glucose levels may lead to ketosis, ketoacidosis and **DIABETIC COMA**. Symptoms include: thirst, dry mouth, flushed face, progressive drowsiness, nausea, vomiting, abdominal pain, cold and dry skin, characteristic "fruity" breath (ketoacidosis), difficulty breathing, headache, dizziness, extreme weakness, glucosuria and ketonuria.

- Diabetic ketoacidosis (DKA), is more likely to occur in persons with type 1 diabetes and can be fatal if untreated.

- **HYPEROSMOLAR HYPERGLYCEMIC NONKETONIC SYNDROME (HHNK)** is seen in those with undiagnosed or mild diabetes, usually in the elderly, who experience a precipitating stress such as acute pancreatitis or myocardial infarction. It is also a potential complication of enteral feedings or total parenteral feeding. The resulting hyperglycemia, 600-3,000mg/dL, leads to hyperosmolarity and osmotic diuresis. The consequence is dehydration and hypovolemia, leading to compromised blood flow and thrombotic complications. The disorder is distinguished from diabetic coma by the absence of ketoacidosis. Treatment is by adequate fluid intake and blood glucose control.

- **LACTIC ACIDOSIS** is characterized by more severe acidosis and compensatory deep breathing compared with ketoacidosis. It is caused by insufficient oxygen to the tissues, inducing a switch from aerobic to anaerobic metabolism. It can also be a side effect of medication.

- Ketoacidosis, hyperglycemic hyperosmolarity and lactic acidosis must be treated quickly, as these conditions may be fatal if untreated.

  - Inject insulin immediately. Regular insulin is then given intravenously at least every six hours or by continuous infusion.
  - Replace fluid electrolyte intravenously, including normal saline, potassium and sometimes bicarbonate. As hyperglycemia and glucosuria diminish, 5% glucose is added.
  - As the condition improves, give oral replacements such as salted broth, juice and water to replenish fluid, sodium, potassium and other electrolytes.

- The **SOMOGYI EFFECT** is hypoglycemia followed by rebound hyperglycemia caused by the release of counter-regulatory hormones, especially as insulin activity declines.

- The **DAWN PHENOMENON** is early morning hyperglycemia (usually between 4 a.m. and 9 a.m.). People who experience this phenomenon should eat more food at bedtime or consideration should be given to changing the type of insulin taken at bedtime.

Complications of diabetes

- Chronic complications include retinopathy, peripheral and autonomic neuropathy, vascular diseases, gastropathy, nephropathy and increased risk of infection. The ten-year Diabetes Control and Complications Trial (DCCT) found that intensive management and improved blood glucose control in type 1 patients, reduced retinopathy by 76%, neuropathy by 60% and reduced albuminuria.

- Complications can often be postponed or minimized by good control of blood sugar. Kumamoto and UKPDS Studies in type 2 patients demonstrated that intensive management and improved blood glucose control in diabetes patients reduced complications.

INBORN ERRORS OF METABOLISM

- **INBORN ERRORS OF METABOLISM** are metabolic disorders that are recessive genetic traits. They are caused by the absence or limited activity of a specific enzyme or cofactor. Many diseases of this type have been identified and are treated mainly with medications and medical nutrition therapy that is specific to the disorder. Most infants are tested for these diseases at birth because quick diagnosis can improve outcomes in most of these children.

- **GALACTOSEMIA** is an inborn error of metabolism characterized by an inability to convert galactose to glucose due to a lack of enzymes: Galactokinase 1phosphate uridyl transferase or Uridine diphosphate galactose 4-epimerase. Untreated galactosemia results in mental retardation, cataracts, liver failure and death.

  - **Treatment:** Eliminate galactose from the diet. Eliminate milk and all dairy products and dates, papaya, bell peppers, persimmons, tomato and watermelon which contain galactose. Use galactose-free formula (ProSobee®, Isomil®, Neomullsoy®, Soyalac®, or fortified soymilk to replace milk during the first year. Label reading is of utmost importance and the restriction is lifelong.

- **GLYCOGEN STORAGE DISEASE** is an inborn error of metabolism resulting in deposition of either too much or too little glycogen in tissues. There are several types of this disease (Type I-IV) and treatment depends on the specific problem, which may be due to a deficiency of one or more of the following enzymes—glycogen synthetase, glucose-6-phosphate, branching enzyme, debranching enzyme, myophosphorylase and/or hepatophosphorylase.

  ➤ **Treatment:** Eliminate fructose, sucrose, lactose and galactose. Starches are not restricted unless they contain contraindicated sugars. Children need glucose or corn starch/polycose nocturnal infusions to maintain normal blood sugar levels. Limit saturated fatty acids and cholesterol because patients are at risk for hyperlipidemia.

- **LACTOSE INTOLERANCE** is caused by an inability to tolerate foods containing lactose due to lactase deficiency. Lactase deficiency is more common in Blacks and Asians than in Caucasians. Lactase deficiency can be induced by omission of milk and dairy foods in the diet over time. The body begins to produce less lactase, thus causing lactose intolerance.

  ➤ **Treatment:** A **LACTOSE-FREE DIET** eliminates milk and all foods containing lactose. If not chosen carefully, this diet may be deficient in calcium, vitamin D and riboflavin since milk products are eliminated. A severe congenital form of lactase deficiency results in persistent diarrhea and failure to thrive. Symptoms often seen secondary to this disease include regional enteritis, ulcerative colitis and gluten-induced enteropathy that may subside as the medical pathology improves.

  ➤ Some persons may tolerate a small amount of lactose or are able to consume lactose-containing foods if consumed in the form of specially designed milk (Lact-Aid milk ™), if the lactase enzyme has been taken in pill form or lactase drops have been added to milk.

  ➤ Some persons who have this disease may be able to tolerate hard cheese or small amounts of lactose containing foods eaten during the day. For example, while a person may not be able to tolerate an 8-ounce glass of milk, he/she may be able to tolerate 2 ounces over cereal or in coffee. The diet protocols must be individualized.

- **PHENYLKETONURIA (PKU)** is an inborn error of metabolism in which the amino acid phenylalanine cannot be metabolized to tyrosine. The largest majority of those affected have a deficiency of phenlalanine hydroxylase. The others have a deficiency of dihydropteridine reductase or do not make the biopterin synthetase group of enzymes.

  ➤ **Treatment:** Infants are tested in the hospital (by blood test) to determine if they can metabolize phenylalanine. If PKU is present, a special formula is given to avoid toxic effects of high blood phenylalanine levels. There are many formulas available for PKU, such as Phenex-1 and 2, Phenyl-Free 2. Foods that are high in phenylalanine, which is an essential amino acid, are supplemented on an individualized basis and closely monitored, in order to give a sufficient amount of phenylalanine to meet growth needs of infants and toddlers.

  ➤ Food products containing aspartame (including NutraSweet®, which contains phenylalanine) are eliminated. There is no reason for sugar substitutes since there is a high need for carbohydrates as calories.

  ➤ Pregnant women with PKU must carefully follow their diet to avoid birth defects. They should be on diets low in phenylalanine.

OTHER METABOLIC AND ENDOCRINE DISORDERS

- **ADRENOCORTICAL INSUFFICIENCY (ADDISON'S DISEASE)** is an atrophy of the adrenal cortex with loss of hormone production. It is treated with hormones and a high protein, moderate carbohydrahigh salt diet. Sodium excretion is high and dietary potassium may be restricted. To avoid hypoglycemia, frequent meals, with between-meal feedings are served. About one-third of patients also have diabetes.

- **HYPERTHYROIDISM** is an endocrine disorder caused by excessive secretion of the thyroid hormone or as a result of overmedication with potent thyroid drugs, hyperactivity of thyroid or a tumor. Symptoms are goiter with thyroid enlargement, nervousness and loss of weight. The treatments are surgical and pharmacological rather than nutritional.

- **NON-DIABETIC HYPOGLYCEMIA** is not a disease but a symptom of improper carbohydrate metabolism. It may occur in the diabetic patient (from not eating or from too much insulin) but may also be caused by other disorders or conditions (e.g., recent abdominal surgery, medications, alcohol that blocks glucose production by the liver, salicylate in aspirin, tumors of the pancreas or adrenal insufficiency). It is usually defined as blood glucose below 70mg/dL and is documented by a five-hour glucose tolerance test. In people without diabetes, the oral glucose tolerance test (OGTT) may induce abnormal responses. Physicians may test blood levels when symptoms occur.

- There are many misdiagnoses of hypoglycemia based on symptoms of stress or anxiety. **REACTIVE HYPOGLYCEMIA** or **FUNCTIONAL HYPOGLYCEMIA** occurs after a meal, due to imbalance of food and insulin. Insulin remains present after food is gone. **FASTING HYPOGLYCEMIA** can result from periods without food or from alcohol or medication.

  - **Symptoms:** Sweating, weakness, hunger, rapid heartbeat, shakiness and confusion are produced by a compensatory increase in epinephrine secretion as the body attempts to increase hepatic glycogenolysis to offset falling blood glucose levels.
  - **Treatment:** The diet should provide adequate calories while controlling the carbohydrate and protein intake. Carbohydrate counting or the exchange lists can be used. The meal plan is divided into five or six meals, with some protein and fiber at each meal and reduced simple sugars. Often caffeine and stimulants are eliminated from the diet. Liquids high in sugar should be avoided because they are absorbed rapidly and cause rapid swings in blood sugar levels.

- **METABOLIC SYNDROME** (formerly called **SYNDROME X**) is a cluster of metabolic disorders that include obesity, glucose intolerance, hypertension, dyslipedemia and insulin resistance. It is characterized by abdominal obesity and HDL cholesterol is usually low. Triglycerides and blood pressure are usually high. This syndrome often leads to coronary heart disease and diabetes. Primary treatment is to reduce obesity, lipid risk factors, glucose levels, blood pressure and increase physical activity.

- **GOUT** is a hereditary disease occurring mostly in males, characterized by a disturbance in purine metabolism and a high uric acid level in the blood. In its acute form, there are sudden attacks of severe pain in a joint, generally of the big toe, frequently following an exceptionally large protein and purine-rich meal, alcohol intake or stress.

  - Ketosis caused by some weight loss diets that are low in carbohydrate or those that require fasting for a period of time, may cause an attack. Repeated gouty attacks may result in deformity of joints.

➢ Medications are now used more frequently than a protein/purine-restricted diet, which avoids organ meats, meat extracts, shellfish and so forth. Medications commonly used include allopurinol (Zyloprim®) and colchicine which relieves pain but can impair absorption of vitamin B12.

- Individuals with **POLYCYSTIC OVARIAN SYNDROME (PCOS)** often have enlarged polycystic ovaries, insulin resistance and android obesity (caused by high levels of male hormones.) It affects a small percentage of women of childbearing age and is a leading cause of infertility. The cause may be genetic and/or environmental. Objectives for treatment are maintenance of a desirable body weight, weight loss, correction of dyslipidemias and maintenance of normal blood pressure and glucose tolerance.

  ➢ **Treatment:** Weight control and exercise plans are major aspects of the plan. Losses of small percentages of weight often reduce symptoms. Diet modification should include decreasing elevated blood glucose and lipid levels. Diets should contain about 30-40% fat because low fat, high CHO diets promote insulin secretion. Oral contraceptives, for regulation of the menstrual cycle, and oral hypoglycemic (Metformin) agents may be prescribed. Fertility medications are sometimes prescribed for women who want to become pregnant, to help normalize ovulation.

(7) Oncologic and hematologic conditions

Oncologic

- **CANCER** is a group of diseases in which malignant growths form. The treatments associated with it frequently place patients at nutritional risk. Current thinking is that many cancers can be prevented by positive nutrition practices.

- The American Cancer Society suggests that cancer risk will be reduced if one "achieves and maintains a healthy weight, is physically active on a regular basis and makes healthy food choices." Nutrition advice is at **www.cancer.org.**

- Diet suggestions include consuming a minimum of 5 servings of fruits and vegetables (including legumes) daily, especially those of high color, such as:
  ➢ Fruits and vegetables high in vitamin A: Apricots, cantaloupe, watermelon, carrots, spinach, mustard greens, turnip greens, collards, kale, broccoli, winter squash, sweet potatoes, mixed vegetables.
  ➢ Fruits and vegetables high in vitamin C: Oranges, orange juice, grapefruit, cantaloupe, vitamin C fortified fruit drinks and fruit juices, mangos, papayas, muskmelons, plantains, mustard greens, turnip greens, collards, kale, other deep-colored greens, broccoli, cauliflower, Brussels sprouts, sweet peppers.
  ➢ Cruciferous vegetables: Broccoli, cauliflower, Brussels sprouts, cabbage, turnips, collards, kale, mustard greens, turnip greens, kohlrabi, watercress, radishes.
  ➢ High-fiber vegetables: Dried peas and beans, corn.

- Other dietary suggestions include:
  ➢ Eating a minimum of 3 servings of whole grains daily such as: High-fiber cereal/bread: bran cereals, Shredded Wheat®, wheat germ, granola, whole wheat bread, rye crackers, Triscuits®, oatmeal.

- Reducing the amount of processed meats and red meat consumed.
- Avoiding charred foods especially meats.

- There is considerable evidence that rates of colon cancers are increased by diets low in fiber; rates of breast cancer by diets high in fat; and rates of mouth, throat and esophagus cancers are associated with high intakes of alcohol. Increasing carotenoids may protect against lung cancer. Fiber increases fecal bulk and decreases transit time, thus reducing bowel exposure to carcinogens and protecting against colon and rectal cancer. Fruits and vegetables that contain fiber also provide carotenoids and vitamin C, which are antioxidants that may reduce the risk of colon cancer. Foods rich in phytochemicals such as soy, grain and vegetable foods containing lignans may be associated with lower risk of breast, ovary and prostate cancers.

- Metabolic alterations may affect the nutritional status of cancer patients. Energy needs may increase, decrease, or remain normal depending upon the cancer type. CACHEXIA, or wasting of muscle, seen in cancer patients is not explained by an increased resting energy expenditure. Increased lipolysis and fatty acid oxidation results in the depletion of fat stores. Most cancer patients are in negative nitrogen balance with body protein being used preferentially by the tumor.

- Malnutrition is a serious problem for patients with many forms of cancer because appetite is often diminished from illness or treatment. Common nutrition problems associated with neoplastic disease include:

  - Anorexia with progressive weight loss and undernutrition.
  - Taste changes causing decreased or altered food intake.
  - Hypermetabolism.
  - Malabsorption associated with deficiency of pancreatic enzymes or bile salts.
  - Small bowel obstruction, bypass or blind loop syndrome.
  - Protein-losing enteropathy with various malignancies.
  - Hormonal abnormalities induced by tumors.
  - Anemia from chronic blood loss or bone marrow replacement.
  - Electrolyte and fluid imbalances.

- Treatment should be designed to achieve or maintain optimal nutritional status and to minimize the side effects secondary to therapy. Use whatever dietary strategies work to maximize food intake:

  - Offer small, frequent meals and snacks to maintain weight.
  - For chewing and swallowing problems, thick liquids or semisolid foods are better tolerated. Purees and thickeners may be used. For mouth ulcers, avoid highly spiced or acidic foods.
  - Nausea, vomiting, diarrhea caused by radiation or medication may be alleviated by medication. Use regular dietary methods to minimize nausea and diarrhea. Provide salted foods, if tolerated, to replace fluid losses.
  - For taste aversions and/or blunted taste, avoid offending foods or add spices and seasoning. Some cancer medications make foods taste metallic. Often cold or room temperature foods are preferred.
  - For weight loss and muscle wasting, increase protein and calories, encourage between-meal snacking; encourage eating when the patient most feels like it, usually

in the morning. Give whatever foods the patient will enjoy. Avoid dietary restrictions to promote appetite. Promote nutrient-dense bedtime feedings.

> Enteral formulas, high in protein and calories can improve the diet.
> For anorexia, provide foods preferred and well tolerated by the patient; use drugs to stimulate appetite. In some situations, favored foods prepared by family members are permitted even in the hospital. Release from liability forms may need to be signed if bringing in food is against hospital policy.
> Monitor carbohydrate intake if glucose intolerance develops.

- Some physicians and CAM practitioners advise vegan or raw diets to treat various types of cancer.

Hematologic conditions

- **ANEMIAS** can be defined as a deficiency in the size or number of red blood cells, or the amount of hemoglobin they contain. This can limit the exchange of carbon dioxide and oxygen between the blood and tissue cells. Many anemias are related to lack of nutrients but some are the result of medical conditions. The classification is based on cell size and hemoglobin content. The anemias that are caused by inadequate intake of iron, protein, vitamins, or some minerals are often called **NUTRITIONAL ANEMIAS.** Diagnosis of the specific type of anemia should be made before treatment because initiation of treatment for one type may mask the underlying anemia.

- **IRON DEFICIENCY ANEMIA** is a microcytic (smaller than normal red blood cells), hypochromic (pale color caused by deficiency of hemoglobin) anemia. While there are many possible causes, the most common are inadequate iron intake due to poor diet (e.g. vegetarian diet with inadequate intake of heme iron); a problem with absorption due to diarrhea, intestinal disease, partial or total gastrectomy or achlorhydria.

  > Drug interactions, excessive blood loss due to hemorrhage, bleeding ulcer and menstrual loss,are also common causes of iron deficiency anemia
  > During pregnancy and lactation, infancy and adolescence, when there is an increased blood volume, iron requirement is high.
  > Treatment is based on the cause of iron deficiency. The goal should be repletion of iron stores. A diet high in iron, including supplementation, if necessary should be accompanied by foods high in vitamin C (to help convert iron from food into the absorbable ferrous form), and/or supplementation of the vitamin.
  > It is also suggested that an individual with iron deficiency anemia avoid drinking large amounts of coffee or tea with meals because they both contain tannins, which interfere with iron absorption.

- **FOLIC ACID DEFICIENCY ANEMIA** is a hyperchromic (intense red color), macrocytic (larger than normal red blood cells), megaloblastic (large, immature, abnormal red blood cells in the bone marrow) anemia. Individuals with this type of anemia usually lose weight, are often anorexic, malnourished, have diarrhea and a smooth and sore red tongue. They also are lethargic, easily fatigued, have poor wound healing and cold extremities.

- Causes of folate deficiency include inadequate diet, alcoholism, pregnancy, intestinal malabsorption. Increased levels of folate are needed with burns, inflammatory diseases, hemolytic anemia, infection, hepatitis, cancers, pregnancy and lactation and major surgery.
- Current research suggests that there may be a genetic component to low folate levels and it may be linked to high levels of homocysteine.
- Differentiation must be made between folic acid deficiency anemia and vitamin B_{12} deficiency before treatment is initiated.
- The treatment goal is to replenish folic acid stores. The underlying cause of the deficiency should be treated, if possible accompanied by a diet high in folic acid, copper, iron, vitamin C and vitamin B_{12}. Food and Drug Administration regulations require folic acid supplementation of grains. Supplements of folic acid are also advised.

- **VITAMIN B_{12} DEFICIENCY ANEMIA** and **PERNICIOUS ANEMIA** are megaloblastic, macrocytic anemias. In pernicious anemia the body is unable to use vitamin B_{12} properly, possibly because of a lack of intrinsic factor. Current research suggests this may be caused by an autoimmune reaction and, in some people, it may have a genetic basis.

  - In rare situations, vitamin B_{12} deficiency is caused by poor intake, such as a vegan diet, in chronic alcoholism, faddism, or poverty, when the diet does not contain this vitamin.
  - Vitamin B_{12} is stored for a long time, so a deficiency in a previously well-nourished person may not be seen for five or more years.
  - In the elderly, there is diminished absorption. Individuals who have gastric disorders that cause inadequate secretion of intrinsic factor may also exhibit signs of vitamin B_{12} deficiency.
  - The goal of treatment is to cure the anemia and its cause, when possible.
  - In addition to vitamin B_{12} injections given daily for pernicious anemia, treatment includes a diet with a liberal use of proteins of high biological value and a soft bland diet, if the mouth is sore. The diet should be supplemented with iron, vitamin C, some other B vitamins and copper. Vitamin B_{12} deficiency can be treated with oral supplementation, in addition to a diet high in the vitamin.
  - A deficiency of either vitamin B_{12} or folic acid causes the circulating level of homocysteine to rise. Homocysteine has been associated with increased risk of cardiovascular disease, stroke and peripheral vascular disease, but recent research suggests this is not so. People with a genetic predisposition to low folic acid levels should be supplemented.

- **PROTEIN DEFICIENCY ANEMIA** is a macrocytic anemia (large, immature erythrocytes) associated with protein malnutrition. Usually multiple deficiencies are present. The treatment is a high protein, high calorie, nutrient-rich diet.

- **VITAMIN C DEFICIENCY ANEMIA** is a macrocytic anemia seen in severe vitamin C deficiency (**SCURVY**). Ascorbic acid (vitamin C) is needed to convert iron from the ferric to ferrous form for absorption, and to convert folic acid to the biologically active form - folinic acid. Vitamin C deficiency is seen more often in men than women, particularly in those who are homeless and those on marginal diets. The treatment is supplementation with ascorbic acid. Daily fruit and vegetable consumption should be increased.

(8) Organ system dysfunction

Gastrointestinal

- **GASTROESOPHAGEAL REFLUX DISEASE (GERD)** is caused by reflux of gastric fluid into the esophagus creating acid induced heartburn. It is caused by decreased lower esophageal sphincter pressure, irritation of esophageal mucosa by gastric acid, bile and pancreatic secretions, abnormal esophageal acid clearance or delayed gastric emptying. Treatment involves decreasing total fat intake and avoiding irritants such as chocolate, mint, alcohol, citrus juices, tomato products and coffee (including decaffeinated). Weight loss is recommended for overweight clients. Maintaining an upright posture during and several hours after eating can reduce the problem.

- **DUMPING SYNDROME**, also called **JEJUNAL HYPEROSMOLIC SYNDROME**, is a set of symptoms that sometimes occurs post-gastrectomy, particularly after a total gastrectomy and in some people after gastric bypass surgery. It results from alteration, ablation or bypass of pyloric sphincter. The food mass (especially simple carbohydrates) enters the jejunum and causes cramping, a full feeling, rapid pulse, weakness, sweating, dizziness, nausea, vomiting and diarrhea within one to two hours after a meal (late dumping). Early dumping occurs 10 to 15 minutes after consuming a meal, usually one high in carbohydrates. The goal is to slow the digestive process and maximize nutrient availability. Symptoms are caused by shifts in osmotic pressure, shifting the water from the blood into the intestines and release of intestinal hormones (serotonin, bradykinin, enteroglucagon, gastric inhibitory peptide, neurotensin.) About two hours later, when the carbohydrate is absorbed, there are often symptoms of mild hypoglycemia. The syndrome is likely to cause anxiety and weight loss.

  - **Treatment using food:** Five or six small meals daily; relatively high fat content to slow passage of food and help maintain weight; high protein content (meat, egg, cheese) to rebuild tissue and maintain weight; and relatively low carbohydrate content to prevent rapid passage of quickly absorbed foods. Typical diet includes no milk; no sugar, sweets or desserts; no alcohol or sweet carbonated beverages; liquids between meals only; no fluids for at least one hour before and after meals; relatively low fiber foods; and raw foods as tolerated. There is little evidence that eating or avoiding specific foods influences severity of disease or frequency of relapse or in any way induces a remission.

- **INFLAMMATORY BOWEL DISEASE (IBD)** includes ulcerative colitis and Crohn's disease. Malnutrition is common in IBD patients due to inadequate food intake, decreased absorption, excessive losses and increased requirements. Medications commonly used to treat IBD may interfere with nutrient metabolism (e.g., cholestyramine with fat-soluble vitamins, corticosteroids with calcium and sulfasalizine with folate).

  - **Treatment:** Maintain adequate protein and kcal intake. Monitor for possible vitamin/mineral deficiencies (vitamins A, B12, D, K, ascorbic acid, folate, iron, calcium, potassium, zinc). Use low fiber, low residue diet during and immediately after acute phases. Do not use low fiber, low residue diet long term. Total parenteral nutrition may be indicated for IBD patients, but is most effective with small bowel Crohn's disease. Anti-inflammatory drugs may be prescribed.

- > **Complications:** Fistula, bowel perforation, obstruction and abscess. Defined formula diets have been recommended for distal intestinal or colonic disease to facilitate bowel rest.

- **ULCERATIVE COLITIS** is a chronic inflammation of the mucosa of the large intestine, characterized by rectal bleeding, diarrhea, pain, anemia, fever, negative nitrogen balance, anorexia, dehydration and/or malnutrition. The etiology is not known, but immunological and emotional factors are implicated. Complications are toxic megacolon, fistula, hemorrhage, obstruction and growth retardation in children.

- **CROHN'S DISEASE (REGIONAL ENTERITIS, REGIONAL ILEITIS, and TRANSMURAL GRANULOMATOUS COLITIS)** is a chronic, progressive, inflammatory disorder that may involve any part of the intestine but primarily involves the distal ileum, colon and anorectal area. Symptoms include vomiting, anorexia, GI blood loss, fatigue, weight loss, pain, diarrhea, fever and anemia. Decreased growth rate is a complication in children with the disease. Unknown etiology but genetic, infectious, emotional and immunological factors are implicated.

- **CHRONIC PEPTIC ULCER DISEASE** results from repeated peptic ulcers, which are eroded lesions or excavated sores in the stomach or duodenum due to injury from digestive secretions.

  - > **Causes and contributing factors:** The main causes are heliobacter pylori bacteria, aspirin and other nonsteroidal anti-inflammatory agents, and stress such as from complications of severe burns or other hypermetabolic problems. High, prolonged doses of corticosteroids may increase the risk. Alcohol and smoking may exacerbate the ulcers, but do not seem to cause them.
  - > **Treatment:** Histamine H2 receptor blockers, proton pump inhibitors are used more often than antacids. Antimicrobial regimens are used to reduce the bacteria. Excessive and prolonged use of calcium antacids may induce hypercalcemia and development of kidney stones. The traditional bland diet does not decrease gastric acid secretion or promote rate of healing. Dietary treatment includes eating three or more well balanced meals per day; avoiding late night eating, which may promote acid production during sleeping hours; eliminating alcohol, salicylates and smoking; limiting caffeinated and decaffeinated beverages; and avoiding spices (black and red pepper) or other foods that cause repeated discomfort.

- **GASTRIC RESECTION** is the surgical removal of part or all of the stomach. Partial gastrectomy presents fewer nutritional problems than **TOTAL GASTRECTOMY**, in which the esophagus is joined to the jejunum (anastamosis). After a **VAGOTOMY** (cutting the vagus nerve) to reduce impulses carried by the vagus nerve, there is reduced acidity, gastric fullness and distention causing food fermentation, gas and diarrhea. Nutritional consequences are weight loss, dumping syndrome, diarrhea, malabsorption, anemia from deficiency of iron, B12, folate, metabolic bone disease and bezoar formation.

  - > **Treatment:** Initially after gastrectomy, for about two weeks, progressively increase the diet while restricting size of meals (small, frequent) and type of foods (mild, low in bulk). Limit volume and give beverages between feedings. Sometimes nutritional support must be used because patients have problems resuming adequate oral intake.

II. NUTRITION CARE FOR INDIVIDUALS AND GROUPS (50%)

If the patient is intolerant to intact nutrient formula, an elemental formula may be needed. Parenteral nutrition is primarily indicated for patients with gastric resection and/or small bowel resection due to intractable diarrhea and/or severe malabsorption.

- **GASTRIC BYPASS** is a surgical intervention for extreme obesity when weight is 100 or more pounds overweight and other dietary interventions have failed. Post-surgically small high protein meals are offered, with beverages between meals and supplementation of nutrients is required.

- **CELIAC DISEASE (GLUTEN-SENSITIVE ENTEROPATHY)** results from sensitivity to gliadin, a component of gluten, the proteins found in grains. Patients have damage to the villi of the intestinal mucosa causing a deficiency of enzyme for digesting gluten and must be on a lifelong gluten-restricted diet, free of the glutamine-bound fraction gliadin. Foods containing gluten that produce no ill effects in individuals with celiac disease are not restricted. The vegetable proteins found in rice, corn, potatoes, and beans, as well as protein found in fish and meat, are well tolerated. Buckwheat and millet have traditionally been restricted because of a lack of information, but current literature suggests they are safe for use. Recent research suggests that most adults with celiac disease can include a moderate amount of oats in a gluten-free diet. However, the commercially available oat flour may contain some wheat gluten or other restricted grains.

  - ➢ **Treatment:** Restrict wheat, rye, and barley and malt protein and their derivatives (e.g., hydrolyzed vegetable protein, soy sauce and malt from barley, malt seasonings, modified food starch.) Secondary lactose intolerance may be present, especially until healing takes place. Therefore, a low lactose or lactose-free diet may be indicated at the beginning of treatment. In severe cases, supplements of vitamins and minerals, especially fat-soluble vitamins, magnesium and calcium, may be indicated. Those on gluten-restricted diets must read food labels carefully to detect hidden sources of gluten on ingredient lists. When ingredients are questionable, it is advisable to check with the manufacturer to determine source of the ingredients. Cooking utensils may contain residue of restricted grains and cross-contamination must be avoided.
  - ➢ Gluten-free diets are increasing in popularity and recommended for weight-control, reduction of miscellaneous GI symptoms, etc. While this may not be medically necessary, it is a personal choice. As a result, many products are labeled and marketed as gluten-free, creating more dietary options for truly gluten intolerant people. There are also many books and references on gluten-free cooking. Specific lists and advice regarding gluten-free is in *Essentials of Nutrition for Chefs*, Culinary Nutrition Publishing, 2014, **www.nutritionforchefs.com** and many gluten-free cookbooks and guides.

- **CYSTIC FIBROSIS** is a disease that occurs primarily in children and extends into adulthood. It is characterized by a generalized dysfunction of the exocrine glands involving the pancreas, pulmonary system and, primarily, the biliary system.

  - ➢ **Symptoms:** Sweat contains large amounts of sodium chloride and to a lesser extent potassium.
  - ➢ **Treatment:** Give a high-protein, high-calorie diet with liberal amounts of fat and

sodium. Protein intakes should be 30-35% of an individual's total caloric requirement, and calories should be 150% of the RDA or 150kcal/kg for children and 200kcal/kg for infants. Give multivitamin with additional vitamins A, D, E and K, depending on nutrition status and drug/nutrient interactions. Other mineral supplementation (magnesium, zinc, calcium) may be needed. (Give multivitamin supplements, vitamin E, and vitamin K, in the first year of life.) 4-6g sodium chloride is needed to replace perspiration losses. Note: Former treatments included the use of a low-fat diet, which was found to be ineffective. The dosage of pancreatic enzymes is adjusted according to the fat/protein content of diet.

Cardiac

- **CORONARY HEART DISEASE (CHD)** is caused by the narrowing of coronary arteries and diminished blood flow because of atherosclerosis. Symptoms include **ANGINA** (chest pain) and heart attack, which can be fatal. The classic risk factors for CHD are high serum cholesterol, hypertension and smoking. It appears that reducing serum cholesterol levels, high levels of serum iron and maintaining appropriate body weight will reduce the risk of cardiovascular disease.

Risk status based on presence of CHD risk factors

- High risk is defined as having two or more CHD risk factors and leads to more vigorous intervention. Age (defined differently for men and women) is treated as a risk factor because rates of CHD are higher in the elderly than in the young, and higher in men than in premenstrual women. Obesity is not listed as a risk factor because it operates through other risk factors that are included (hypertension, hyperlipidemia, decreased HDL-cholesterol, and diabetes mellitus), but it should be considered a target for intervention. Physical inactivity is similarly not listed as a risk factor, but it, too, should be considered a target for intervention, and physical activity is recommended as desirable for everyone.

- Positive risk factors include:

  - Age: Male > 45 years and female > 55 years or premature menopause without estrogen replacement therapy.
  - Family history of premature CHD: Definite myocardial infarction or sudden death before 55 years of age in father or other male first-degree relative, or before 65 years of age in mother or other female first-degree relative.
  - Current cigarette smoking.
  - Confirmed hypertension: >140/90 mm Hg, or on antihypertension medication.
  - Low HDL cholesterol: < 40mg/dL
  - Diabetes mellitus: Risk is equal for men and women with diabetes.
  - Lifestyle: Sedentary and obesity.
  - High levels of homocysteine: Levels can be reduced by increasing intakes of vitamins B_6, B_{12}, riboflavin and folic acid by food or supplements. Recent research suggests that the link to high levels of homocysteine is not as strong as once thought.
  - Metabolic syndrome: The presence of abdominal obesity is more highly correlated with metabolic risk factors than is an elevated BMI.

- A negative risk factor is high HDL cholesterol (≥60mg/dL), which is considered to reduce risk of coronary heart disease. If the HDL cholesterol level is ≥60mg/dL, subtract one risk factor (because high HDL cholesterol levels decrease coronary heart disease risk).

Cholesterol

- **SERUM CHOLESTEROL** is composed of five types of lipoproteins: chylomicrons, intermediate density lipoproteins (IDL), very low density lipoproteins (VLDL), low density lipoproteins (LDL) and high density lipoproteins (HDL). High HDL is associated with decreased risk of coronary heart disease (CHD) and a high LDL increases CHD risk.

- **HDL CHOLESTEROL** is sometimes called the "good" form of cholesterol. It is part of the total cholesterol determination. Increasing the proportion of HDL cholesterol is protective and the amount (or ratio) of LDL to HDL cholesterol is an indicator of cardiovascular risk. Major causes of low HDL cholesterol include: cigarette smoking; obesity; lack of exercise and sedentary lifestyle; androgenic and related steroids, progestational agents and anabolic steroids; beta-adrenergic blocking agents; hypertriglyceridemia and genetic factors,such as primary hypoalphalipoproteinemia.

- Indicators for positive lipid profiles are total cholesterol less than 200mg/dL, LDL cholesterol less than 100mg/dL, HDL cholesterol greater than 40mg/dL and triglyceride less than 150mg/dL. Current research suggests HDL cholesterol at greater than 60mg/dL may be more protective against heart disease for women. Diet therapy is suggested for individuals with fewer than 2 risk factors and a LDL level greater than 160mg/dL. It should begin at lower LDL levels for those who have more than 2 risk factors.

- The **NATIONAL CHOLESTEROL EDUCATION PROGRAM OF THE NATIONAL INSTITUTES OF HEALTH** suggests trying the **TOTAL LIFE STYLE CHANGE DIET** (TLC), if LDL levels are above healthful levels. This diet includes:
  - ➤ <7% of total calories saturated fat
  - ➤ <200mg/day cholesterol
  - ➤ Increased soluble fiber (10-25g/day) and plant stanols/sterols (2g/day)
  - ➤ Weight management
  - ➤ Increased physical activity

- For each one percent reduction in serum cholesterol levels, there is a two percent reduction in risk of coronary heart disease.

- Medications such as bile acid sequestrants (cholestyramine), nicotinic acid and HMG CoA reductase inhibitors (statins, such as Pravacol® Mevacor ®, Lipitor ® and Crestor®) are the most common drugs used for treatment and are required for life. All of these have side effects, some nutritional, and patients should be carefully monitored.

- There is evidence that omega-3 fatty acids have a lipid lowering effect and decrease platelet aggregation. Omega-3 fatty acids are found in fish oils, and frequent consumption of fish is recommended. The benefit of fish oil capsules may be detrimental, as in large quantities they can inhibit blood coagulation and cause hemorrhages. The NCEP does not recommend fish oil supplements but supports eating seafood several times each week.

Some physicians suggest using flax seed oil in the diet, if the client is allergic to fish, or does not eat fish, for any reason.

- Physicians often prescribe low doses of aspirin to reduce the risk of heart attack. Taken in combination with fish oil capsules, severe bleeding may occur.

- There is also some evidence that antioxidants, particularly vitamin E, may affect the oxidation potential of LDL cholesterol. Diets high in tocopherol, and diets rich in flavonoids found in red wine and some fruits, appear to reduce cardiovascular risk.

ATP III LIPOPROTEIN LEVELS (mg/dL)

obtain after 9 – 12 hour fast

LDL Cholesterol

<100	Optimal
100-129	Near optimal/above optimal
130-159	Borderline high
160-189	High
≧190	Very high

Total Cholesterol

<200	Desirable
200-239	Borderline high
≥240	High

HDL Cholesterol

< 40	Low
40-59	The higher the better
>60 and higher	Considered protective against heart disease

Triglycerides:

<150	Desirable
159-199	Borderline
200 or >	High

Source: www.nhlbi.nih.gov

FOODS TO CHOOSE OR DECREASE for THERAPEUTIC LIFE STYLE CHANGE

Food Group	Choose	Decrease
Lean Meat, Poultry and Fish	Beef, pork, lamb—lean cuts well trimmed before cooking	Beef, pork, lamb—regular ground beef fatty cuts, spare ribs, organ meats
	Poultry without skin	Poultry with skin, fried chicken
	Fish, shellfish	Fried fish, fried shellfish
	Processed meat—prepared from lean meat, e.g., lean ham, lean frankfurters, lean meat with soy protein	Regular luncheon meat, e.g., bologna, salami, sausage, frankfurters
Dairy Products	Milk—skim, 1% fat (fluid, powdered, evaporated); buttermilk	Whole milk (fluid, evaporated, condensed) 2% fat milk (low-fat milk), imitation milk
	Yogurt - nonfat or low-fat yogurt or yogurt beverages	Whole milk yogurt, whole milk yogurt beverages
	Cheese - low-fat or reduced-fat natural or processed cheese	Regular cheeses (American, blue, Brie, Cheddar, Colby, Edam, Monterey Jack, whole-milk mozzarella, Parmesan, Swiss), cream cheese
	Frozen dairy dessert - ice milk, frozen yogurt (low -fat or nonfat)	Ice cream
	Low-fat coffee creamer, low-fat or nonfat sour cream	Cream, half & half, whipping cream, non-dairy creamer, whipped topping, sour cream
Fats and Oils	Unsaturated oils - safflower, sunflower, corn, soybean, cottonseed, canola, olive, peanut	Coconut oil, palm kernel oil, palm oil
	Margarine - made from un-saturated oils listed above, light or diet margarine, especially soft or liquid forms or those containing plant stanols, Enova® or other fat modified oils	Butter, lard, shortening, bacon fat, hard margarine
	Salad dressings - made with unsaturated oils listed above, or low-fat or fat-free	Dressings made with egg yolk, cheese, sour cream, whole milk
	Seeds and nuts - peanut butter, other nut butters	
	Cocoa powder	Milk chocolate, rich chocolates, candy bars

Breads and Cereals	Whole-grain - breads and rolls, English muffins, bagels, buns, corn or flour tortillas	Bread in which eggs, fat, and/or butter are a major ingredient; croissants, biscuits, sweet rolls, fruitbreads and muffins
	Cereals - oat, wheat, corn, multigrain	Most granolas and granola bars
	Whole-grain pastas	Pasta with cream or cheese sauce
	Brown rice and other whole-grains	White rice, refined grains
	Dry beans and peas, may be canned	
	Crackers, low fat - animal type, graham, soda crackers, breadsticks, melba toast	High-fat crackers, cookies, fried pita chips and other fried breads
	Homemade baked goods using unsaturated oil, skim or 1% milk, and egg substitute - quick breads, bran muffins, whole-grain pancakes and waffles	Commercial baked pastries, muffins, biscuits, waffles, pancakes
Soups	Reduced or low-fat and reduced-sodium varieties, e.g., chicken, or beef noodle, minestrone, tomato, vegetable, potato, reduced-fat soups made with skim milk or vegetable purees	Soups containing whole milk, cream, meat fat, poultry fat, or poultry skin
Fruits and Vegetables	Fresh, frozen, or canned, with little or no added fat, salt, sugar or sauce	Vegetables fried or prepared with butter, cheese or cream sauce Fruits canned in heavy syrup
	100% fruit juice, frozen fruit bars	Sweetened fruit beverages
	Frozen desserts - low-fat and nonfat yogurt, ice milk	Ice cream and frozen treats made with ice cream or whipped cream
Sweets and modified fat desserts	Cookies, cake, pie, pudding prepared with egg whites, egg substitute, skim milk or 1% milk, and unsaturated oil or margarine; gingersnaps; fig and other fruit bar cookies; fat-free cookies; angel food cake, whole-grain bars	High-fat and high-sugar pies, cakes, doughnuts, cookies, cream pies, sweet rolls, candies

- **HYPERTENSION (HTN)** is elevated blood pressure, a risk factor in the pathogenesis of cardiovascular disease, affecting about 20% of Americans. HTN is generally asymptomatic and is identified only when blood pressure is checked. Ninety percent of HTN is **ESSENTIAL HYPERTENSION** or **IDIOPATHIC HYPERTENSION** of unknown cause. Ten percent results from renal disease, tumor of the adrenal gland or brain lesions. HTN is positively correlated with obesity, psychological stress, and a high sodium intake, but all HTN is not responsive to sodium reduction. Ingesting the RDI/RDA levels for calcium and adequate potassium (based on a good sodium/potassium ratio in the diet (around 90mEq/day from high potassium foods) may protect against HTN. Caffeine may increase blood pressure by stimulating renin and catecholamines. Primary treatment for hypertension includes medication and weight loss, where indicated. Sodium may be restricted in some cases. Hypertension is diagnosed when there is systolic blood pressure of 140mm Hg or more and/or a diastolic pressure of 90mm Hg or more. Optimal levels are 120/80 or less.

> **Treatment:** Weight reduction if the patient is obese; exercise; relaxation therapy to decrease stress; blood pressure control; and if the patient is sodium sensitive, a low-sodium diet should be ordered; caffeine and alcohol consumption may be restricted.
> The **DASH DIET** (Dietary Approaches to Stop Hypertension) is widely used. This diet, the outcome of a research study, recommends foods low in total fat and saturated fat, high in fruits and vegetables and low or nonfat dairy products. DASH has a positive effect on prevention and control of HTN.
> Other dietary interventions are still in various stages of research and include recommendations for increased intakes of calcium and magnesium, potassium from increased intake of fruit and vegetable and fiber.
> Increased intakes of vitamins D, E and K may be appropriate. Aggressive drug and diet therapies are required for severe hypertension. Drug therapy includes diuretics, drugs acting on the sympathetic nervous system (beta-blockers), ACE inhibitors, vasodilators and others. The majority of these drugs have nutritional implications.

• **CONGESTIVE HEART FAILURE (CHF)** is characterized by decreased cardiac output, with impaired tissue perfusion and systemic and vascular congestion. Because CHF results in low renal perfusion, the glomerular filtration rate declines, thus decreasing the amount of sodium filtered. This activates the renin-angiotensin-aldosterone system of the kidneys, causing sodium and fluid retention.

> **Treatment:** Drug therapy, sodium-restricted diet and potassium replacement if necessary. Small frequent meals are usually better tolerated. Caffeine and fluid may be restricted.

• In an effort to reduce risk factors associated with heart attack and stroke, the American Heart Association (AHA) and the National Cholesterol Education Program (NCEP) have established guidelines for a safe and prudent diet that restricts total fat, saturated fat and cholesterol. The diet is especially important for clients with plasma cholesterol levels above 200mg/dL. The total cholesterol and type of lipoprotein and cholesterol influence risk.

Sodium restriction

The 2010 Dietary Guidelines for Americans make a major point of the general public reducing sodium intakes. The recommendation is to consume less than 2300mg sodium daily and that African Americans, those with hypertension, diabetes, chronic kidney disease and persons older than 51 consume less than 1500mg daily. This is a major challenge as typical intakes are over 3500mg daily and reduction to 1500 means omitting most processed foods, restaurant meals and significant dietary changes that are difficult to maintain for most people.

- **SODIUM-RESTRICTED DIETS** can be used in the management of essential hypertension, impaired liver function, cardiovascular disease, renal disease and renal or cardiac failure. Generally, most dietary sodium comes from processed foods. Many persons with hypertension are not responsive to decreases in dietary sodium intake and medications are required to control blood pressure.

- The aim of sodium restriction is to restore normal sodium balance to the body by promoting the loss of excess sodium from extracellular fluid components, thus reducing hypertension, edema and/or ascites. Sodium is the major cation of extracellular fluid. Normally, moderate sodium loads are excreted in urine. In certain pathologies, a breakdown in the body's normal homeostatic mechanism results in sodium and water retention in cells and an increased resistance to blood flow.

- Age modifies factors that determine renal handling of sodium: glomerular filtration rate, renal hemodynamics and responsiveness to the renin-angiotensin-aldosterone system.

- **ALDOSTERONE** is a sodium-conserving hormone that operates in the renin-angiotensin mechanism to conserve sodium in exchange for potassium causing resorption of water to maintain body fluids.

- **SALT (NaCl)** is 40% sodium and 60% chloride by weight. One teaspoon of table salt contains 2300mg sodium. **SALT SUBSTITUTES** generally replace the sodium with potassium and are intended to simulate the taste of salt (e.g., NuSalt®, No Salt®, Adolphs™, Morton™). Morton "Lite" salt is a potassium-sodium-chloride blend, yielding about 1100mg sodium per tsp. Kosher salt, because of larger flakes, has less weight and less sodium per teaspoon than table salt.

- **SODIUM CONTROLLED DIETS** include:

  ➤ **MILD SODIUM RESTRICTION:** 3g sodium (3000mg = 130mEq). Salt may be used lightly in cooking, but no additional salt is allowed after preparation. Foods in which salt is used as a preservative or a major flavoring agent are excluded, for example, pickles, olives, bacon, ham, chips and many other processed foods. Or omit table salt and use up to 1250mg in prepared foods.

  ➤ **MODERATE SODIUM RESTRICTION:** 2g sodium (2000mg = 87mEq). No salt is used in cooking, no salt is added to the food, and no salty foods are eaten. Canned and processed foods including salt are omitted. Regular bread is limited to four servings. Meat and milk are permitted in moderate portions. Most food must be prepared from scratch as most processed and prepared foods are too high in sodium.

  ➤ **STRICT SODIUM RESTRICTION:** 1g sodium (1000mg = 44mEq). Omit virtually all salt, and salt-containing foods. Use the diet for short term periods only or for tests.

  ➤ **SEVERE SODIUM RESTRICTION:** 0.5g sodium (500mg = 22mEq). This level is not recommended. It is too highly limited to be practical and is not needed anymore with available drug therapy.

Renal

- **ACUTE** or **CHRONIC GLOMERULONEPHRITIS** is an inflammatory process of the glomeruli of the kidney usually precipitated by a streptococcal infection. Symptoms include hematuria, proteinuria, edema, hypertension and renal insufficiency or failure.

  - ➤ **Treatment:** Controlled fluid intake equals fluid output. Provide sufficient kcal and control protein, sodium and/or K and phosphorus according to laboratory data and renal function. Vitamin D3, iron, calcium and multivitamin supplements may be recommended.

- **NEPHRITIS** is an inflammation of the kidney with diffuse, progressive, degenerative or proliferative lesions affecting the renal parenchyma, interstitial tissue and renal vascular system.

  - ➤ **Treatment:** Provide adequate calories. Use 70% high biologic value proteins to ensure positive nitrogen balance. Restrict protein, sodium or potassium when there is edema, hyperkalemia or uremia. Replace all lost fluids. Monitor phosphorus and vitamin A according to lab data and renal function. Use of fish oils may be beneficial.

- **UREMIA** is the toxic condition produced by the retention in blood of nitrogenous substances usually excreted by the kidneys. It is the terminal manifestation of renal failure. Symptoms include nausea, vomiting, weakness, anorexia, dizziness, convulsions and coma.

  - ➤ **Treatment:** Provide adequate calories and control protein, fluid, and electrolytes according to laboratory data and renal functioning.

- **NEPHROTIC SYNDROME** is a set of symptoms applied to renal disease characterized by marked edema, heavy albuminuria, proteinuria, hypercholesterolemia, increased coagulation and abnormal bone metabolism. As much as 30g of protein may be lost daily in urine. Vitamin D deficiency has been reported with nephrotic syndrome.

  - ➤ **Treatment:** Provide a diet containing sufficient protein and calories to maintain a positive nitrogen balance (0.8g protein/kg/day with 75% high biologic value, and approximately 35kcal/kg for adults and 100-150kcal/kg for children. Moderate sodium (3g) to reduce edema. Monitor closely for depletion of protein, potassium, vitamin D and other nutritional deficiencies (iron, zinc, vitamin C and folacin). Medical nutrition therapy for nephritis is controversial, with some research suggesting higher protein levels and stricter control of edema. Fluid restriction may not be warranted.

- When hyperlipoproteinemia (HLP) is associated with nephrotic syndrome, restrict intakes of fat, cholesterol, alcohol and concentrated sweets. Linoleic acid, omega-3 fatty acids and a vegetarian soy-based diet with additional amino acids may be useful.

- In **ACUTE RENAL FAILURE** nutritional priorities include:

  - ➤ Preserving body cell mass.
  - ➤ Providing sufficient energy to permit maintenance of vital functions.
  - ➤ Providing sufficient protein to replace amino acids lost from catabolism .

- Nitrogen balance is influenced by both calorie and protein intake. Treatment is usually based on the underlying cause of the failure. Optimum nitrogen balance is achieved with a caloric intake of 50-60kcal/kg of body weight. A minimum of 30-40kcal/kg dry weight is required for adults. Restoration of body weight in the malnourished child requires 1½-2 times normal energy requirements.

  - For children, protein should never be restricted below 1.0-2.0g of high biological value protein per kg of body weight.
  - Sodium levels vary according to fluid retention and hydration status.
  - Hyperkalemia may be acute due to release during catabolic processes
  - Protein needs in acute renal failure are often greatly increased by hypercatabolic states such as sepsis, hemorrhage, or open, draining wounds. Protein should not be severely restricted because (acute) temporary dialysis will remove products of a high protein intake.
  - Fluid and electrolyte intake should balance net output.

- **CHRONIC RENAL FAILURE** requires that protein intake be balanced with output to avoid inducing uremia or malnutrition. Hemodialysis or peritoneal dialysis may be required. Chronic renal failure occurs when the glomerular filtration rate (GFR) is less than 12ml/min/1.73 m2. A controlled protein, sodium and potassium diet is used to achieve and maintain adequate nutritional status in renal disorders. It is designed to lighten the work of a diseased kidney by reducing the urea, uric acid, creatinine and electrolytes that must be excreted. It also replaces substances (i.e., protein, sodium) that are lost in abnormal amounts because of impaired kidney function.

  - Treatment: Achievement of these goals requires regulation of protein intake; balance of fluid intake and output; adequate caloric intake; regulation of sodium, potassium and phosphorus intake; and supplementation with appropriate vitamins and minerals. The level of each restriction is not fixed, but is dependent on the patient's clinical and biochemical status at any particular time; therefore the diet must be adjusted often.

Diet in renal disorders

- The diet in renal disorders is based on a specialized list of foods that identify the amount of protein, sodium and potassium. Substitution is permitted within the list as long as the total protein, sodium, potassium, phosphorus and fluid intakes do not exceed the limits of the prescribed diet restriction. Protein of high biological value is preferred over other protein sources, especially in severe protein restrictions, and should supply three-fourths of the daily protein allowance. Essential amino acid supplements are tailored to meet the specific needs of these patients and are most beneficial for protein restrictions of less than 30g/day. For lower levels of protein intake, wheat starch products are used for baking. Low protein pasta and carbohydrate supplements provide extra calories. Fruits and vegetables, good sources of potassium, are restricted. To meet fluid restrictions, liquids are limited and all foods are well drained.

- Special renal exchange lists are used to plan appropriate intake of protein, calories, sodium and phosphorus. The diet should provide about 35kcal/kg/day or appropriate calories to maintain weight. Give 40-55% of calories from fat, and give protein in a quantity suitable to diet order or treatment.

  - **LOW PROTEIN DIET:** This diet provides 0.55-0.60g/kg/day with >0.35g/kg/day protein of high biologic value.
  - **VERY LOW PROTEIN DIET:** This diet provides about 0.28g/kg/day protein of any biologic value, supplemented with either a ketoacid and amino acid mixture or an essential amino acid mixture.
  - When patients undergo **HEMODIALYSIS,** the diet should provide 1.0-1.2g/kg/day protein with more than 50% of high biologic value. Because hemodialysis removes toxins and normalizes blood levels, the diet can be less restrictive than for patients with renal disease who are not dialyzed.
  - **CONTINUOUS AMBULATORY PERITONEAL DIALYSIS (CAPD):** For patients on CAPD, provide 1.2-1.5g/kg/day, with a minimum of 50% high biologic value protein.
  - Amounts of protein allowed for various types of dialysis may be based on **KINETIC MODELING,** which measures the urea removed during dialysis, over a set period of time. This is very individualized and specific protein requirements can be set for each patient.

- In chronic renal failure, nondialyzed patients are generally restricted to 1,000-3,000mg sodium unless the underlying disease is of the salt-losing type. Those on CAPD generally do not require sodium restriction unless there is poor blood pressure or fluid control.

- When urinary volume is adequate, a normal blood level of potassium is maintained. However, in renal insufficiency, potassium loads are not excreted in a normal manner. In end-stage renal disease, hyperkalemia can occur because cell metabolism releases potassium into the blood. If serum potassium is elevated and urine output limited, then potassium should be limited to 40-70mEq/day.

- Fluid tolerance must be ascertained prior to the start of renal failure fluid therapy, particularly in instances of oliguria. **OLIGURIA** is the diminished generation of urine (less than 500ml/24 hours). Fluid intake should balance output in the person with renal failure who is not being dialyzed. With dialysis, fluid is restricted to 750-1500ml/day, depending on weight gain allowed between treatments and frequency of treatments. If there is **ANURIA,** no urine output, fluid replacement is limited to 400-600ml/day to compensate for insensible water losses through respiration or perspiration.

- Diet influences the acidity or alkalinity of the urine. **ACID ASH DIETS** are high in meat, poultry and fish, peanuts, walnuts, whole grains, corn, lentils, cranberries, plums and prunes. **ALKALINE ASH DIETS** are high in milk and dairy products, almonds, beets, greens, spinach, fruits, except cranberries, plums and prunes.

Renal stones

  - **RENAL CALCULI** (nephrolithiasis) are kidney stones. The cause is generally unknown, but stones of concentrated urinary constituents are formed. Common types are calcium oxalate stones, struvite stones, uric acid stones and cystine stones. A low-calcium, high-animal-protein diet may precipitate stone formation.

- ➤ **Treatment:** Increase fluid intake to dilute urine. On the basis of stone type, control urine for acidity or alkalinity. Acid or alkaline ash diets may be used, but medication is more common.

- **CALCIUM OXALATE STONES** account for most kidney stones (calcium oxalate or calcium oxalate plus calcium phosphate).

  - ➤ **Causes:** May include alkali therapy or hard water; excess vitamin D causing withdrawal of calcium from bones; prolonged immobilization; hyperparathyroidism; renal tubular acidosis caused by abnormal ammonia formation or **IDIOPATHIC CALCIURIA** (excess calcium excretion with unknown cause); or a metabolic error handling oxalates. Some research suggests that overuse of vitamin C supplements increases risk of stone formation.
  - ➤ **Treatment:** A **HIGH CALCIUM DIET** including 800-1200mg/day of dietary sources of calcium from yogurt, milk, cheese, sardines, shellfish and calcium-rich vegetables, with limits on oxalate sources. **OXALATE** sources include fruits (berries, grapes, figs, rhubarb, tangerines); vegetables (beans, beets, celery, greens, okra, spinach, peppers, sweet potatoes, tomatoes); beverages (cocoa, tea, beer); nuts (almonds, cashews, peanuts, nut butters) and grains (wheat germ, soy products including tofu, grits).

- **STRUVITE STONES** are urinary stones made of a hard crystal of ammonium magnesium phosphate. These stones form when there are urinary tract infections. Dietary management has no significant role in managing this condition.

- **URIC ACID STONES** are caused by improper metabolism of purines, as with gout, or from tissue breakdown in catabolic diseases.

  - ➤ **Treatment:** Usually increased fluid intake with the same medications used for gout and, at acute phases. A **LOW PURINE DIET** in which meat, meat extracts, organ meats, shellfish, anchovies and sardines are restricted is sometimes used, but usually only foods very high in purines, such as those listed above, are restricted. The production of acid urine favors the body's retention of uric acid and stone formation. Alkalinzation of the urine (pH 6.0-6.5) through high alkaline ash diet and addition of citrate or bicarbonate increases uric acid excretion and is a cornerstone treatment for this condition.

- **CYSTINE STONES** are caused by a genetic defect in the ability to transport amino acids. These stones cause severe renal damage.

  - ➤ **Treatment**: Very high oral intakes of fluid, up to 4 liters per day, plus alkaline ash diet and/or D-penicillamine to alkalinize the urine and decrease protein intake.

Pulmonary

- Respiration is directly related to metabolic rate. As the metabolic rate increases, so does ventilatory drive. Patients with compromised ventilatory status may have decreased nutrient intake. Bronchodilators taken by **CHRONIC OBSTRUCTIVE PULMONARY DISEASE (COPD)** patients are gastric irritants and nearly 25% of COPD patients have peptic ulcers. Chronic sputum production alters the taste of food. Shortness of breath may hinder a patient's ability to prepare and eat food. Fluid retention may mask changes in body composition. Chronic illness may lead to depression, which results in decreased food intake. Caloric expenditure may be elevated in COPD patients due to infections or fevers and the increased work of breathing. Too much carbohydrate may raise CO_2 production to levels the respiratory system cannot handle.

- The ratio of carbon dioxide produced to oxygen consumed when carbohydrate, protein, and fat are metabolized is called the **RESPIRATORY QUOTIENT (RQ)**. The RQ for carbohydrate = 1.0, RQ for protein = 0.8, and RQ for fat = 0.7. In patients with respiratory disease, a diet lower in carbohydrate and higher in fat may be beneficial.

- Diet modifications for individuals with COPD are as follows:

  ➢ For oral feeding: Provide 50% of total calories as fat and restrict cholesterol and saturated fat as needed.
  ➢ For enteral tube feeding: Add a fat modular or some type of oil (corn, etc.) to a commercial feeding or give a commercial tube feeding formula that is designed to be high in fat (e.g., Traumucal® or Pulmocare®) that contains more than 50% of the nonprotein calories as fat. In addition, use a nutrient dense formula (2 kcal/ml) for patients who have a fluid restriction.
  ➢ For parenteral feeding: Provide 50% of nonprotein calories from a lipid source.

- **ACIDOSIS/ALKALOSIS** can be classified in two ways, **RESPIRATORY** from abnormal CO_2 excretion and **METABOLIC** from abnormal production, ingestion or excretion of hydrogen ion. The designation of acidosis or alkalosis refers to the pH alteration prior to medical correction.

- **METABOLIC ACIDOSIS** is characterized by decreased serum pH, CO_2, pCO_2.

  ➢ **Causes:** Ketosis of diabetes, starvation, or high-fat and low-carbohydrate diets; cellular hypoxia and lactic acidosis; decreased hydrogen ion excretion from renal disease; shock or cardiac failure; excess base loss from dehydration secondary to diarrhea or pancreatic or small bowel fistulas; intake of acidifying salts.
  ➢ **Respiratory:** Increased rate and depth of respirations.
  ➢ **Renal:** Decreased hydrogen ion excretion.
  ➢ **Treatment:** Correct bicarbonate level; combat hyperkalemia.

- **RESPIRATORY ACIDOSIS** is characterized by decreased serum pH; increased pCO_2.

  ➢ **Causes:** Hypoventilation, often because of asthma or COPD.
  ➢ **Compensation**: Increased bicarbonate resorption if caused by renal problems.
  ➢ **Treatment:** Depends on etiology.

- **METABOLIC ALKALOSIS** is characterized by increased HCO_3 and pH; decreased chlorine and potassium.

  ➢ **Causes:** Acid loss from vomiting or gastric suctioning; excess base intake from absorbable antacids, such as $NaHCO_3$; potassium depletion from diuretics; poor K intake.
  ➢ **Respiratory:** Small decrease in ventilation, renal bicarbonate, K excretion.
  ➢ **Treatment:** KCl, isotonic saline, stop causative agent.

- **RESPIRATORY ALKALOSIS** results in increased pH; decreased pCO_2, H_2CO_3.

  - ➢ **Causes:** Hyperventilation.
  - ➢ **Renal:** Bicarbonate excretion.
  - ➢ **Treatment**: Depends on etiology.

- **TUBERCULOSIS (TB)** is an infectious disease, caused by the bacillus, *Mycobacterium tuberculosis.* People who are immunocompromised are more susceptible to this disease, especially those who have AIDS. The bacterium invades the lungs and causes tissue wasting, exhaustion, productive cough, which sometimes produces bloody sputum and night sweats. TB can spread through the bloodstream, causing many other symptoms, including kidney damage and pain in the spine and bones.

  - ➢ **Treatment**: The diet should contain adequate calories (consider possible hypermetabolic state) and liberal amounts of protein, adequate calcium and vitamin D (RDA levels). Iron and vitamin C should be included in adequate amounts to assure hemoglobin formation and assure wound healing. The most common medication used is INH, which interacts with vitamin B_6. Therefore, vitamin B-complex should be adequate, especially vitamin B_6. Assure adequate fluids. Alcohol use should be minimized and supplemental vitamin A should be given if the body is not converting carotene properly.

Hepatic and pancreatic

- **CIRRHOSIS** is a chronic, progressive disease of the liver in which fibrous connective tissue replaces the functioning liver cells. It is often caused by excessive alcohol consumption. Enteral nutrition is indicated if there is inability to consume adequate nutrition to meet requirements with the presence of a functioning GI tract. Parenteral nutrition is indicated when there is gastrointestinal intolerance to feeding and there is uncontrollable GI bleeding.

  - ➢ **Treatment:** Use a liberal protein, high-kcal diet that is high in vitamins and moderate in fat. Give B-complex vitamins in active forms. Replacing long chain fats with medium chain triglycerides and supplementation with water miscible forms of fat-soluble vitamins are indicated if steatorrhea is present.

- **HEPATIC COMA** is a state of unconsciousness seen in people with advanced liver disease; it may be due to ammonia intoxication when the liver can no longer detoxify products of metabolism.

  - ➢ **Treatment:** Reduce protein and all nutrients requiring hepatic processing.

- **HEPATIC ENCEPHALOPATHY** may be due to ammonia intoxication, infection, acid/base imbalance, fluid and electrolyte imbalance, hypoxia, nitrogen overload, medications, GI bleeding or derangement of circulating amino acids.

  - ➢ **Treatment:** Reduce protein and nutrients requiring hepatic processing. Give lactulose (inhibits gastrointestinal absorption of ammonia and other toxic nitrogenous substances). Research suggests a positive effect of enriching formulas with branched chain amino acids for those patients who do not respond to lactulose therapy.

- **VIRAL HEPATITIS** is an inflammation of the liver most commonly caused by a viral infection (virus forms A, B, C). For form B, the treatment includes steroid therapy followed by injections of alpha interferon. In infectious hepatitis, type A, the virus is transmitted via the oral-fecal route through contaminated food and water. Hepatitis can also be passed by contaminated instruments or through sexual contact.

- **ALCOHOLIC HEPATITIS** is a serious pre-cirrhotic form of alcohol injury to the liver, affecting its structure and function. It is often seen with malnutrition.

  - ➤ **Symptoms:** Anorexia (loss of appetite) is very common; also seen are jaundice, malaise, weakness, diarrhea, fever, headache, and enlarged liver and spleen.
  - ➤ **Treatment:** Bed rest, adequate fluid, diet of small, frequent feedings that are high in protein, calories, vitamins and minerals to promote liver regeneration and glycogen synthesis, spare protein and prevent further liver damage.

- **PANCREATITIS** is an acute or chronic inflammation of the pancreas. It interferes with digestion because pancreatic enzymes may be unavailable.

  - ➤ **Treatment:** In the initial acute phase, all oral feeding should be withheld and hydration accomplished intravenously. Diet should progress, as tolerated to a low-fat, frequent small feeding diet using of medium chain triglyceride oil with pancreatic enzymes given as medication. Data suggest that nasojejunal or jejunostomy feedings decrease pancreatic secretion by bypassing cephalic and gastric phases of pancreatic stimulation and may be indicated if the patient is able to tolerate them. Parenteral nutrition is indicated for patients with severe protracted pancreatitis, dictating complete pancreatic rest. In severe states, it can be hypermetabolic and should be treated with the same type of regimen as any other hypermetabolic condition.

Neurological disorders

- **EPILEPSY**, a recurrent disorder of cerebral function, is characterized by sudden, brief attacks of altered consciousness, motor activity or sensory phenomena. Convulsive seizures are the most common form of attack. Sometimes a **KETOGENIC DIET** is used in certain forms of epilepsy in an attempt to modify the seizure pattern. This is a diet in which fat provides three to four times more calories than carbohydrate and protein combined to produce ketosis. Long term, a high-fat diet may lead to other medical problems. Medication is now used more frequently to control epilepsy than is diet.

  - ➤ For more traditional ketogenic diets, a condition of mild dehydration achieved through modest fluid restriction may be needed to achieve a desired level of circulating ketones.
  - ➤ Addition of medium chain triglyceride oil (MCT oil) is another approach used to achieve ketosis.
  - ➤ Medications used for epilepsy increase catabolism of vitamin D and supplements may be ordered. Folic acid supplements may interfere with the therapeutic affects of the medication and should be used with caution.

- **CEREBRAL VASCULAR ACCIDENT (CVA)**, commonly referred to as a **STROKE**, results when there is damage to the brain from a clot, rupture or vascular spasm. Once a stroke has occurred, assure adequate caloric, nutrition and fluid intakes with attention to any feeding difficulties such as motor skill deficits or swallowing disorders resulting from the stroke. The consistency and texture of foods may need to be modified and the patient checked for signs of aspiration. Limit intake of vitamin K-rich foods to one per day if patient is on anticoagulants.

- > **Risk factors:** Obesity, diabetes, hypertension, smoking and use of oral contraceptives.
- > **Treatment:** Primarily preventive, blood pressure control, dietary restriction of cholesterol, saturated fat and sodium, increased consumption of fruits, vegetables (potassium) and fish (omega-3 acids) and aspirin therapy.

- **ALZHEIMER'S DISEASE** is a common form of dementia characterized by a progressive loss of memory, speech, self-care behaviors, motor skills and cerebral function. Weight loss may be attributed to increased resting metabolic rate or energy output (e.g., constant pacing), or inadequate food intake because of losses in taste, forgetting to shop or eat, inability to cook or to swallow, etc. The diet offered should meet calorie and nutritional needs and provide for adequate fluid intake. Supervision is necessary to assure adequate and appropriate food intake.

  - > **Treatment**: Use nutrient-dense foods, frequent snacks and finger foods, nutritional supplements, verbal and sensory cues; frequent prompts and structured meal routines.

(9) Orthopedic/wounds

- **HIP FRACTURES** most commonly occur in elderly women from falls and other trauma. Risk factors include high alcohol intake, low intakes of calcium, old age, osteoporosis and bone cancer. Many traumas cause fractures of any bone at any age.

  - > **Treatment:** Hip fractures (and other fractures) are usually surgically repaired, so optimal nutrition is important for wound healing, prevention of infection and formation of new bone matrix. This is a hypermetabolic condition and nutrition needs increase as much as 25%. A high protein, high calorie diet, with adequate amounts of calcium, phosphorous, vitamin D and vitamin C is recommended. Fluid intake should be sufficient to assure excretion of excess calcium. Zinc supplementation may be necessary after surgery. If infection arises, calories must be increased. The patient should be mobilized as soon as possible to prevent calcium losses, kidney stones, pressure ulcers, urinary tract infections and blood clots.

- A **LONG BONE FRACTURE** is a hypermetabolic condition, sometimes increasing caloric needs by as much as 25%. It is often accompanied by shock, infection, bleeding and/or inadequate hydration.

  - > Treatment: After surgical repair, reduction of the fracture, a high protein, high calorie diet is recommended. Assure adequate amounts of vitamin C, calcium, phosphorus, vitamin D, zinc and vitamin A for bone and wound healing. Patient should be given exercises to prevent muscle atrophy in other limbs.

Wounds

- **WOUNDS** can be a serious problem especially in immunocompromised individuals. Burn wounds, pressure ulcers and other wounds that are exudative and or infected, require intensive nutrition therapy. Protein and calorie needs are increased and intake of vitamin A, vitamin C and zinc should be monitored carefully for adequacy.

c. Determine energy/nutrient needs specific to condition

- Energy and nutrient needs vary according to the medical condition and degree of pathology. Some conditions, such as cancer, may require alterations in energy, while others, such as COPD, need specific nutrient modifications. Still others, such as gout, have few energy and nutrient modifications. Nutritional intervention guidelines should be consulted when planning appropriate interventions regarding energy and specific nutrient intake adjustments.

WEIGHT MANAGEMENT - Added topic, not in CDR outline.

- The *2010 Dietary Guidelines for Americans* have 2 guidelines specific to weight management.
    - To maintain body weight in a healthy range, balance calories from foods and beverages with calories expended.
    - To prevent gradual weight gain over time, make small decreases in food and beverage calories and increase physical activity.

- There has been a marked increase in overweight/obesity in most developed countries in the world. It is also seen in urban areas of many developing nations where there is malnutrition found in the rural areas. The World Health Organization has called it a "global epidemic of obesity" and considers obesity to be one of the top ten causes of preventable death worldwide.

- Over the past 20 years, overweight and obesity have soared in the U.S. At present, about 2/3 of American adults are overweight or obese and 30% are obese according to the National Center for Health Statistics. Over half of Americans are trying to lose weight. Weight control is a focus of practice for dietitians in medical, community, counseling, food service and other settings. A growing percentage of children are now overweight or obese.

- The dietitian should determine the degree of overweight/obesity by calculating the BMI, measuring weight circumference, and checking for any of the life threatening side effects that often are seen in an overweight or obese person.

- Estimates of the prevalence of overweight and obesity are typically based on BMI. (See Domain II) Clinicians should be able to use good judgment in BMI interpretations to be sure that its accuracy, as an indicator of total body fat, is correct.

    - Examples of the indicators to question include the presence of edema, high amounts of muscles, muscle wasting and people who are short in stature.
    - Although the following circumstances do not influence validity of the BMI strongly, there may be variables with age, gender and ethnicity and differences in composition of lean tissue, sitting height and hydration status.

- The National Heart, Lung, Blood Institute (NHLBI), in their treatment guidelines advises that treatment of the overweight and obese person is a 2- step process: assessment to determine the degree of obesity and the absolute risk status and management that includes reduction of excess weight and maintenance of the lower body weight. NHLBI advises incorporating additional measures to control any associated risk factors.

- In addition to psychosocial and emotional consequences of obesity, there are many physiological consequences, such as hypertension, type 2 diabetes, gallstones, some types of cancer, osteoarthritis, non-alcoholic fatty liver disease, elevated serum LDL cholesterol and low serum HDL cholesterol.

- Losing weight requires motivation and a strong personal commitment to change behaviors. The NHLBI suggests that clinicians should consider the following issues when assessing an overweight/obese person's readiness for weight loss:

  1. Has the person sought weight loss on his or her own initiative?
  2. What events have led the person to seek weight loss now?
  3. What are the person's stress level and mood?
  4. Does the person have an eating disorder, in addition to obesity?
  5. Does the person understand the requirements of treatment and believe that he or she can fulfill them?
  6. How much weight does the person expect to lose? What other benefits does the person anticipate?
  7. Does the person understand that the program will cause weight to be lost gradually and that modest weight loss frequently improves health?
  8. Is there understanding that physical activity must be built into the program?

- As to the specifics of weight loss diet, a healthful diet should be designed that meets nutritional needs but with less calories than needed to maintain current weight. Generally, at least 1500 calories is necessary to maintain nutritional adequacy and provide enough food to avoid hunger. For almost all weight loss diets, physical activity is increased to burn calories and promote fitness and strength. Many types of diets work, and preferences vary, but an important factor is that the food plan is nutritionally adequate and can be sustained. Various counseling techniques are effective with individuals and groups.

- Where possible, obese children should be targeted early, and eating and activity patterns altered, because this may avoid physiological and psychological problems later in life There are many local and some federal weight loss programs that are targeting children and adolescents. Because many are relatively new, there are few research outcomes that have been published.

d. Determine specific feeding needs

(1) Oral

- **ORAL FEEDING** is providing nourishment by mouth. It is one form of enteral feeding and is the preferred feeding method when the patient is able to chew, swallow and digest food.

Routine house diets

- The **REGULAR DIET,** or **GENERAL DIET,** is also known as a **HOUSE DIET**. It is based on a general, palatable, varied diet and offers patients a selection of foods that provide adequate nutrients to repair, rebuild or maintain body tissue. House diets are designed to meet the RDI/RDA for nutrients. Modifications may be made to allow for individual food preferences and tolerances.

- The **SOFT DIET** is the step between the liquid and regular diet and appropriate for patients unable physically or psychologically to accept the regular diet. It provides tender foods, no raw fruits or vegetables, no coarse breads or cereals, and no gas forming or fried foods. Highly seasoned foods may be limited or omitted. When highly seasoned foods are also omitted, the diet is called a **BLAND DIET**.

- **BLENDERIZED LIQUID DIET** (sometimes called a **FULL LIQUID DIET**) is provided for patients unable to tolerate solid food because of illness or inability to chew or swallow. It may be used as a transition between a clear liquid and soft or regular diets. Frequent small feedings (6-8 per day) facilitate ingestion of adequate calories and protein. It may be necessary following oral surgery or mandibular (jaw) fracture, plastic surgery or radiation of the face and neck, for general surgery and for patients with esophageal strictures. A variety of foods including milk, plain frozen desserts, pasteurized eggs, custard, plain or flavored yogurt without fruit or nut pieces, strained cream soup or pureed thinned vegetables, pudding, fruit and vegetable juices, cereal gruels, broth, and milk and egg substitutes and blenderized thinned meat, poultry, fish etc. may be used. Often commercially prepared vitamin and mineral fortified liquids are used. The diet can provide 1,800-2,000kcal and 80g protein per day and, with careful planning, can be nutritionally adequate. Liberal use of milk and milk-based products makes the diet high in lactose and cholesterol. Reduce lactose by substituting hydrolyzed milk or lactose-free products, if indicated. Unless modified, the diet should not be used on a long-term basis for patients with hypercholesterolemia.

- **CLEAR LIQUID DIET** is highly restrictive with little nutritive value. It provides an oral source of fluids, a small amount of calories and electrolytes to prevent dehydration, and keeps colonic residue to a minimum. Fluid replacement and maintenance of the body's water balance become matters of prime concern when an acute illness produces a marked intolerance to food. The diet includes clear liquid food (fat-free broth, bouillon, tea, clear or strained fruit juices, carbonated beverages, popsicles and gelatin). Depending on the reason for restriction and hospital policy, coffee may or may not be given. Alcohol is excluded. This diet contains only about 500-600 calories, 5-10g of protein, 120-130g of carbohydrate, and almost no fat. It is nutritionally inadequate and should not be used for more than a few days.

(a) Composition/texture of foods

- Mechanical modifications (ground or pureed) can be used for patients with chewing or swallowing problems. If food intake or utilization is impaired in any way, alternate methods of feeding should be instituted. Oral feedings include a range of diets that may have modified nutritional content or textural consistency.

- Foods of appropriate composition and textures should be given that meet the client's individual medical needs.

- **DYSPHAGIA** is a disturbance in the transfer of food from the oral cavity to the stomach characterized by difficulty in swallowing foods and/or liquids which, if untreated, can lead to malnutrition. The cause of dysphagia can be Alzheimer's disease, various neurological diseases, head or neck cancer, structural lesions, motility disorders, pharmacological or medication induced, stroke or other diseases. Swallowing tests should be performed to determine how the patient tolerates different food and fluid textures and to avoid aspiration of food if swallowing is compromised.

- A **National Dysphagia Diet** is now the standard treatment. The diet provides foods that are modified in texture so that the patient can swallow. The treatment must be tailored to the individual's impairment and preferences, and foods offered should be chosen to reduce risk of choking or aspiration, in addition to sufficient fluid for adequate hydration.

- The National Dysphagia Diet consists of three levels and the level chosen is related to the results of the swallowing tests.

  - **Level 1:** Dysphagia Pureed consists of foods with "pudding-like" consistencies, which are very smooth and have no lumps. Liquids may have to be thickened.
  - **Level 2**: Dysphagia Mechanically Altered consists of foods that are moist, soft in texture and can easily be formed into a bolus. Liquids may have to be thickened, depending on recommended consistency. This is a transition from level one and the patient has to be able to chew.
  - **Level 3:** Advanced consists of textures that are nearly regular, except those that are very hard, crunchy or sticky. Foods should still be moist and should be cut into very small pieces. Beverage consistency is based on recommended level and patient must have a sufficient number of teeth to tolerate the consistency.

- Many companies have developed texture-modified foods for patients with dysphagia (e.g., thickened juices and powders to thicken pureed foods.) Correct positioning of the patient; sitting upright with a firmly supported body is important. The patient usually needs assistance to eat and careful observation is essential to avoid choking and/or aspiration pneumonia.

- A **High-Fiber Diet** is used in the prevention and treatment of gastrointestinal, cardiovascular and metabolic diseases including diverticular disease, cancer of the colon, constipation, irritable bowel disease, hypercholesterolemia, diabetes and Crohn's disease. The high-fiber diet is a general diet with emphasis on fiber-rich foods including vegetables, legumes, fruits, whole grain breads and cereals.

- **Fiber Restricted Diet** is used in acute phases of diverticulitis, inflammatory bowel disease (IBD), or infectious enterocolitis, when the bowel is markedly inflamed. Distension caused by bulky food and bowel movements may cause pain. The diet contains a minimum of fiber and connective tissue and is designed to prevent formation of an obstructing bolus of high fiber foods in patients with narrowed intestinal or esophageal lumen. Low fiber diets decrease the weight and bulk of the stool and lead to delayed intestinal transit. For a fiber restricted diet:

  - Avoid dry, fresh, and raw fruits except ripe banana. Limit fruits to canned fruit and juice without pulp.
  - Limit vegetables to juices without pulp and cooked, non-gassy, seedless vegetables such as asparagus tips, winter squash, green beans, spinach, carrots and beets.
  - Use white or refined grain bread and cereal products such as white rice, enriched pasta and white breads. Do not use whole-grain or bran products.
  - Avoid tough, fibrous meats. Use tender meat, poultry, fish and ground meats.
  - Avoid nuts, seeds, dried beans, peas and corn.

- A fiber-restricted diet is not synonymous with a **Low Residue Diet**. Colonic residue is increased by both high fiber foods and low-fiber foods such as milk, potatoes and prune juice, that increase stool weight that yield residue but are not fibrous.

➢ Fiber-restricted diets are contraindicated in healthy individuals and are associated with prolonged intestinal transit time and small, infrequent stools.

➢ Low-fiber diets containing large amounts of refined carbohydrates may be associated with diverticular disease. The reduced bulk of the diet may eventually result in narrowing of the colonic lumen by producing small compact stools that cause the colon to contract more tightly around the stool, thus decreasing the size of the lumen and increasing intraluminal pressures. These pressure increases may lead to herniation of the colonic muscle, leading to diverticulosis.

➢ Fiber-deficient diets have been linked to cancer of the colon in epidemiological data.

(b) Diet patterns/schedules; diagnostic test meals

- Diet patterns provide a guide for a patient's daily food intake. They are specific to the patient's nutritional needs, disease state, food tolerance and method of feeding. They help to individualize the diet pattern to meet the patient's needs. Three meals, three meals with a snack, or five to six small feedings are patterns commonly used. Further, the diet patterns should reflect the patient's food preferences, socioeconomic conditions and ability to store and prepare food. Finally, documentation should provide a communication tool for all members of the dietary department and healthcare team.

Preparation for diagnostic tests

- **FECAL FAT TEST** measures fecal fat for diagnosis of malabsorption or cystic fibrosis. The diet includes ingestion of 100g fat per day for three days prior to initiation of stool collection and three days of collection.

- **GLUCOSE TOLERANCE TEST (GTT)** is an oral test used to aid in diagnosis of diabetes mellitus.

  ➢ After initial blood sample is taken, the patient is given a standard dose of high carbohydrate liquid (75g), typically Glucola®, followed by postprandial blood tests to determine blood sugar levels for several hours after the test dose.

  ➢ In the past, a diet consisting of 300g carbohydrate was administered for three days prior to testing. The necessity of that diet has been questioned, especially for patients receiving an adequate diet of at least 150g carbohydrate.

- **MEAT-FREE TEST** is used to determine gastrointestinal bleeding. Meat, poultry and fish contain hemoglobin, myoglobin and enzymes that may give positive results for up to four days after ingestion. A meat free diet is eaten for several days and is followed by several days of stool samples to test for occult blood in stools. Some tests for occult blood also restrict other foods, such as beets, that may obscure test results.

- **CALCIUM TEST** is used to determine urinary calcium excretion in the diagnosis of hypercalciuria, which is detectable only at moderately high calcium intakes. A diet of 1,000mg of calcium is necessary, with 400mg of calcium likely to come from food sources, and 600mg derived from oral supplementation with calcium gluconate (an absorbable form of calcium).

- **SEROTONIN TEST** (5 HIAA or 5 hydroxyindoleacetic acid) is used to determine the metabolite of malignant tumors of the intestinal tract. The following foods should be eliminated from the diet at least 24 hours prior to the test: walnuts, bananas, plantains, avocado, tomato, red plums, purple plums, pineapple and pineapple juice and passion fruit.

- **VANILLYLMANDELIC ACID TEST (VMA TEST)** is a test of urine to diagnose a tumor, Pheochromocytoma, in cases of unexplained hypertension. In place of the screening test for urine VMA, urine metanephrines are measured. The procedure is not affected by dietary intake.

(c) Modified diet products and food supplements

- Real whole foods are the preferred method for meeting client nutrient needs. A variety of products, modified to meet medical needs and health promotion goals are available (egg substitutes, fat-free dairy products, unsalted products and fat-free dressings).

- **FOOD SUPPLEMENTS** are used for clients unable to meet their complete nutritional needs with regular solid food. Supplements include liquids and solids for specific medical purposes and ages, such as nutrient-dense liquid feedings, fortified pudding and fortified hard cookies.

(d) adaptive equipment

- Oral feedings require basic utensils (forks, plates, straws, etc.). Special equipment is available to accommodate handicapped individuals. Preserving and supporting self-feeding is to be encouraged to help patient(s) remain independent and functional. Feeding of fluids or nutrients by vein can be in addition to or replace oral feeding.

- Adaptive equipment, such as forks with formed special handles, plates with raised rims, cups with covers, etc. allow people with functional limitations to eat with less assistance.

(2) Enteral and parenteral nutrition

Enteral nutrition

- **ENTERAL FEEDING** is providing nourishment by mouth or by inserting a tube or catheter directly into the gastrointestinal (GI) tract. Enteral feeding includes feedings as oral supplements or by tube or catheter to meet individual requirements when oral intake is inadequate. For oral supplements, if the digestive system is functioning well, intact formulas can be given. If there are digestive or absorptive problems, then hydrolyzed formulas are given. In practice, the term enteral feeding usually refers to the delivery of nutrients by tube or catheter into the digestive tract when oral intake is inadequate. Enteral nutrition presents fewer risks to the patient than parenteral feeding.

- Use enteral feedings for:

  ➤ Neurological and psychiatric problems: Cerebrovascular accidents (CVA), trauma, neoplasms, severe depression, anorexia nervosa.
  ➤ Gastrointestinal problems: Neoplasm, inflammation, malabsorption, fistulas, pancreatitis, inflammatory bowel disease.
  ➤ Hypermetabolic states: Burns, HIV, AIDS, cystic fibrosis, comatose states, hyperemesis of pregnancy.
  ➤ Esophageal problems: Inflammation, trauma, neoplasm.

II. NUTRITION CARE FOR INDIVIDUALS AND GROUPS (50%)

- Dietitians generally plan enteral feedings, but nursing or nutrition support staff usually administer it. Dietitians should be aware of enteral feeding practices and procedures, but they do not usually insert or care for tubes and equipment for enteral or parenteral feeding unless they have received special training in nutrition support.

GUIDELINES FOR ENTERAL NUTRITION

Use enteral nutrition support by tube feeding in appropriate patients who are or will become malnourished and in whom oral feedings are inadequate to maintain nutritional status.

Initiate nutrition support in patients who have had inadequate oral intake for 7 to 14 days, or in patients where inadequate oral intake is expected over 7 to 14 days. Patients must have at least 2-3 feet of functional GI tract.

Gain access to the gastrointestinal tract in the most natural and least invasive manner, taking into account the gastrointestinal anatomy and function (effectiveness of gastric emptying, aspiration risk) and the anticipated duration of enteral nutrition.

Use the parenteral route only when the patient is at risk of malnutrition from not eating, a trial of enteral nutrition has failed, or severely diminished intestinal function due to underlying diseases or treatment is anticipated.

Evaluate potential candidates for home enteral tube feeding by a multi-disciplinary team of healthcare professionals.

Educate the home care patient and caregiver on the required procedures and potential complications before hospital discharge.

Tailor the nutrition program to meet lifestyle needs at home.

Purchase supplies and equipment in anticipation of the patient's hospital discharge; arrange for supportive care at home if needed.

Trained healthcare professionals knowledgeable of the potential infectious, mechanical, and metabolic risks of tube feeding should monitor patients during enteral nutrition support.

Parenteral nutrition

- **PARENTERAL FEEDING** systems use catheters to provide nutrients directly into the bloodstream, intravenously. They are used only for patients who cannot tolerate oral feeding or GI tube feedings.
- Forms include Partial Parenteral Nutrition (PPN); Total Parenteral Nutrition (TPN); and Cyclic Total Parenteral Nutrition.

(a) Formulas and calculations

Enteral formulas

- There are a variety of enteral feeding products on the market. Some are for oral supplementation and contain intact nutrients. These are either milk-based or lactose-free and the lactose-free formulas commonly contain 1.0-1.2 calories per milliliter. Some formulas (e.g., Ensure®) are directly marketed as meal replacements or supplemental feedings for seniors and others.
- Enteral formulas are indicated for use in patients who have a functioning gastrointestinal tract and are unable to tolerate food with sufficient nutritional content.

ENTERAL FORMULAS

Type	Copyrighted or Trademarked Products
Blenderized	Complete, homemade (care must be taken to avoid avidin or biotin problems and salmonella risks; if eggs are used, the pasteurized liquid form is recommended.) These are not recommended because of danger of contamination and concern about nutritive value.
Disease-specific	Hepatic Aid II, Pulmocare, Traumacal, Advera for the immunocompromised, Magnacal Renal,
Extra calories	Ensure Plus, Boost Plus, Novasource 2.0, Resource Plus
Fiber added	Boost with Fiber, Ensure with Fiber, Fibersource, Replete with Fiber
High nitrogen	Ensure HN, Ensure Plus HN, Precision HN, Osmolite HN, Isocal HCN, Two Cal HN, Impact
Modular	Casec, Promix, Moducal, Polycose, Sympt-X, MCT oil
Peptide-based	Reabilin, Peptamen, Vital HN, Perative
Predigested/elemental	Travasorb HN, Travasorb STD, Vivonex TEN, Tolerex
Protein powders	ProPac, Casec, ProMod
Special purpose	Travasorb, Criticare HN, Impact
Standard	Ensure, Osmolite, Isocal, Isosource, Boost

- Some formulas contain extra calories (for those on restricted fluid intake); some contain additional nitrogen (15% of calories as protein) and/or fiber. Predigested elemental tube feedings containing hydrolyzed macronutrients, are designed for use in a partially functioning digestive tract. They are hyperosmolar, and often low in fat (<10%.) Modular feedings provide specific nutrient sources (carbohydrate, protein, fat, including MCT oil, vitamins and minerals) that can be added to liquid feedings. Condition-specific formulas designed for renal patients, AIDS patients, those with pulmonary or liver disorders and/or diabetes are also available.

Parenteral nutrition

COMPONENTS OF TPN SOLUTIONS

Dextrose: Adult TPN solutions are generally 5-70% dextrose monohydrate. The larger central vein can handle highly concentrated sugar. A maximum of 10% dextrose can be infused into a peripheral vein. Maximum rates of CHO administration should be no greater than 5mg/kg/min to avoid hyperglycemia, pulmonary and hepatic abnormalities. 1 gram of anhydrous dextrose yields 3.4 calories.

Amino acids: Essential and non-essential crystalline amino acids are given to promote positive nitrogen balance. The type of amino acid product and its concentration is chosen on the basis of the disease state. The concentration of amino acids in these solutions ranges from 3.5 -20%. Generally 15-20% of daily caloric intake should come from protein. 1 gram of protein yields 4 calories.

Lipids: Lipid emulsions provide essential fatty acids and are a concentrated fuel source. Provision of a minimum of 10% of kcal from lipids is usual. Fat is isotonic and does not contribute to the osmolarity of the solution. Fat emulsions provide lipids as an aqueous suspension of soybean or safflower oil with egg yolk phospholipid as the emulsifier and with glycerol added to provide osmolarity. Maximum fat dosage should not exceed 2g/kg/day. The usual dose is 30% of non-protein kcals as fat.

A 10% fat emulsion yields 1.1kcal/cc or 550kcal/500 cc bottle. A 20% fat emulsion yields 2kcal/cc or 1000kcal/500 cc bottle.
The maximum TPN lipid for adults is 2.0g/kg body weight.

Electrolytes, vitamins, minerals: Vitamins, minerals and electrolytes are administered to maintain normal body function. Individual needs are based on laboratory data and other measures. Commercial balanced vitamin/mineral products are available to add to TPN formulations. A standard trace elements solution is provided routinely. These doses aim for maintenance, not repletion. Vitamin K and iron are not included in the parenteral infusion, but special formulations may be required in some cases. Typical fluid volume for TPN is 1½ -3 liters. Maximum volume of fluid for TPN rarely exceeds 3 liters.

- Fluids may include any nutrient needed by the body if provided in a form suitable for blood transport. Depending on how the solution is administered (orally or by tube or intravenously) appropriate sources of carbohydrate, protein, fat, vitamins and minerals can be selected.

- **NORMAL SALINE SOLUTION (NS)** is water with added salts and is used to replace fluids intravenously. Sodium chloride solution is 0.9%.

- **DEXTROSE SOLUTIONS**, sometimes called glucose solutions, range from a 5% solution (D₅W) of dextrose in water (often used in peripheral parenteral nutrition [PPN] support of fluids and electrolytes after surgery or to maintain hydration) up to 70% dextrose solutions available for total parenteral nutrition (TPN). Dextrose solutions given intravenously do not provide the standard 4 kcal/g of carbohydrate. These solutions are anhydrous, and provide 3.4 kcal/g. D₅W is the only solution within the range of normal body osmolarity (275-295 mmol/kg). Other solutions are hypertonic.

Enteral calculations

- Choice of formula is based on specific patient needs. Nutrients are calculated using the same methods with which a regular diet is calculated. Calorie, protein, carbohydrate, fat water and vitamin/mineral needs are used to choose a specific product. Tube placement is a deciding factor for formula choice. Once the formula is chosen, the number of feedings, volume and frequency can be determined.

Water content

- Most formulas contain 70-85% water. Provide additional water to meet the patient's fluid needs as appropriate. Also, increase fluid as tolerated for fluid loss secondary to fever, increased urine output, diarrhea, draining wounds, ostomy output, environmental temperature, vomiting, increased fiber intake or fistulas. Include fluid provided via oral intake, fluids and intravenous fluids in calculating fluid requirements.

Calorie-nutrient concentration

- Calorie and nutrient concentration affects the volume needed to meet nutritional requirements. In choosing a formula, it is important to determine if the RDI/RDA for vitamins and minerals can be met with the calculated volume. Formulas contain between 0.5kcal and 2kcal per milliliter and can be used as appropriate in the following situations:

  ➢ 0.5kcal/ml to meet increased fluid requirements.
  ➢ 1kcal/ml for standard formulas and transitional feeding.
  ➢ 1.5-2kcal/ml when there are volume limitations.

CALCULATING ENTERAL FEEDINGS

To establish the volume of the enteral feeding, the following steps are used.

1. Meet daily fluid requirements: Remember that formulas have solute and solvent. Free water needs to be calculated. Consult product literature for percentage of free water.

> **For example:**
> 1000 cc isotonic enteral feeding yields approximately 830 cc free water. Additional water can be given between feedings. **Adults:** 30-60 cc free water per kg/day **Children:** 100 cc/kg/day for the first 10kg
> > 1000 + 50 cc per each additional kg for 10-20kg
> > 1500ml + 20ml/kg over 20kg

2. Determine total volume per day continuous feeding:

> **For example:**
> Formula to run at 75 cc/hr: 75 cc/hr x 24 hr = 1800 cc or 1.8 liters total intermittent feeding
> **For example:**
> Formula to be given in a volume of 400 cc, 5 times per day 400 cc x 5 per day = 2000 cc or 2 liters total

3. Determine caloric content: Multiply the volume (cc) by the calories/cc of the formula.

> **For example,** 1800 cc x 1.06 kcal/cc = 1908 total kcal

4. Determine protein content: Multiply the total volume in liters by protein/liter of the formula.

> **For example,** 1.8 liter x 37g protein/liter = 67g protein

5. Determine actual calories and protein: Multiply the calories and protein per liter by the strength* of the formula:
¼ strength = 0.25
½ strength = 0.50
¾ strength = 0.75
1/3 strength = 0.33
2/3 strength = 0.67
full strength = 1.00

> **For example:**
> 1908kcal x 0.50 (½ strength) = 954kcal 67g PRO x 0.50 (½ strength) = 33.5g PRO

*Note: Dilution of formula is no longer recommended as start-up procedure—but dilution may be necessary to increase flow of high viscosity formulas and remains an option if total fluid requirements can be met by other methods.

II. NUTRITION CARE FOR INDIVIDUALS AND GROUPS (50%)

Parenteral calculations

- Once caloric needs of the patient are established, protein goals should be calculated. The remainder of the energy requirement is derived from carbohydrate and fat. Vitamin, mineral electrolyte and fluid requirements have to be added to the prescription.

- To calculate calories of IV fluids:

$$D_5W = 5\% \text{ of } 1,000 \text{ ml or } 50g \text{ of dextrose/liter}$$
$$50g \times 3.4 \text{ kcal} = 170 \text{kcal/liter}$$

- Amino acids provide 4 calories per gram, and for 1 liter of 7% amino acid solution, there are 280 k/cal.

$$7g/1000 \text{ ml} = 70g/\text{liter}$$
$$70 \times 4 \text{ kcal} = 280 \text{kcal/liter}$$

- Protein and carbohydrate calories are added to yield total calories of glucose plus amino acid solution.

- One liter of a typical TPN solution contains a final concentration of 25% dextrose and 3.5% amino acids, plus vitamins, minerals and electrolytes. Often 3 liters of solution are given daily; providing 3,000kcal and 105g protein, plus added vitamins and electrolytes. Because TPN is often used for prolonged periods, trace element deficiencies can occur, so trace elements should be monitored and added to solutions for long-term TPN.

- Other potential additions to TPN solutions include:

  ➢ Albumin is used to increase serum albumin levels.
  ➢ Insulin is used to regulate blood sugar levels. (Only Human Regular [U-100] insulin may be added to a total nutrient mixture. Insulin therapy may be provided subcutaneously, constantly infused, or added to the parenteral solution, which is more effective than adding insulin to normal saline.
  ➢ Heparin is used to reduce chance of blood clots forming and obstructing the catheter

(b) Routes, techniques, equipment

ENTERAL TUBE FEEDING

NASOENTERIC FEEDING

NASOGASTRIC: Tube from the nose to the stomach, usually short-term, 3-4 weeks.

NASODUODENAL/ NASOJEJUNAL: Tube from the nose through the pylorus into the duodenum or jejunum; used for short term nutritional support, usually 3-4 weeks in patients at high risk for aspiration, esophageal reflux, delayed gastric emptying, persistent nausea, vomiting.

NONSURGICAL PERCUTANEOUS ENDOSCOPIC GASTROSTOMY (PEG) Placement of the tube directly into the stomach through the abdominal wall, performed under local anesthetic using an endoscope. This is technically not a surgical procedure and is used for patients who require a tube for more than 4 weeks. It is a short procedure with minimal wound complications and once the site is healed the tube can be replaced with a low-profile device that allows more freedom of movement and ease in showering.

SURGICALLY INSERTED ENTERAL FEEDING TUBES

GASTROSTOMY: Placement of tube into the stomach; variety of techniques used; available in different sizes and tube flexibility; used when mouth and esophagus must be bypassed.

JEJUNOSTOMY: Short-term small bowel access methods. Can be needle catheter placement, direct tube placement, or creation of a jejunal stoma that can be intermittently catheterized. Usually used post-operatively with gastric decompression.

ENTERAL TUBE FEEDING

METHODS OF ADMINISTRATION

Continuous drip feedings may be given chilled. Other feedings should be given at room temperature to improve tolerance.

CONTINUOUS DRIP: Use of an infusion pump is required. Tube feedings are administered at a constant, steady rate over a 18-or 24-hour period. Method appropriate for patients who do not tolerate large volume infusions; such as those with compromised GI function due to disease, surgery, chemotherapy or radiation.

INTERMITTENT DRIP: Tube feedings are infused at specific intervals throughout the day. The volume of the desired feeding is divided into equal portions and given four or six times per day. The feedings are usually given by pump or gravity drip over a 20-minute or 1-hour time period. This method allows the patient to be free from equipment during rehabilitation activities. It may also be used for night feedings at the maximum tolerated rate. Should not be used for those with risk for pulmonary aspiration.

BOLUS FEEDING: For patients who are clinically stable with functional stomach. Refers to rapid delivery of 60 ml of feeding into the GI tract by syringe. If bloating or abdominal discomfort develops, it is suggested that the patient be encouraged to wait 10-15 minutes before ingesting the remainder of the allocated portion Those with normal gastric function are usually able to tolerate about 500 ml of formula at each feeding. This method is most like the normal eating process and 3-4 of these feedings can provide nutritional requirements for most people.

FEEDING TUBE SIZES

Soft, pliable tubes of polyurethane or silicone come in many lengths and diameters. Some have weighted tips. The smallest tube that the feeding will flow through is the best.

Generally, tube sizes are 5-12 "French." Sizes 5-6 are often used for protein hydrolysates; 7-10 for protein isolates; 8-12 for intact proteins. Smaller tubes can be used with infusion pumps.

Since proteins are the largest molecules given by tube, the type of protein influences tube size. The size of the feeding tube and drip chamber and the availability of pumps affect the choice of solution that can be successfully administered. Blenderized feedings and those containing soy polysaccharide fiber usually require pumps for infusion through smaller bore tubes, to avoid clogging tubes due to higher viscosity.

ENTERAL FEEDING PRACTICES

Safety:
Use closed feeding containers to reduce the risk of contamination by airborne organisms.
Change extension-tubing administration set and bag daily.
Never add a new supply of formula to old formula.
Refrigerate unused prepared formula immediately.
Do not allow feeding solutions to hang at room temperature longer than 8 hours.

Preventing Aspiration:
Check tube placement prior to administration of feeding.
Elevate head and shoulders at least 30 to 45 degrees.
Keep tubes patent (with opening clear and unblocked for fluid flow).
Irrigate tubes with a 20-30 ml of warm water every four hours during continuous feedings and before and after intermittent feedings and medication administration.
In case of clogging, irrigate tube with a syringe of warm water.

Monitoring:

Daily
Monitor for drug-nutrient interactions.
Confirm tube position, drip rate, and vital signs.
Check for edema.
Monitor for hydration and fluid intake and output.
Check gastric residuals frequently when feedings are started, if appropriate.
Hold feedings if residual volumes are more than 200 ml on two successive assessments.

Weekly
Record weight at least 3x per week, measure intake and output, stool output and consistency, and urinary excretion; check electrolytes, blood urea nitrogen, blood glucose until stabilized.
Check serum electrolytes, BUN, creatinine (2-3x/wk) nitrogen balance, if appropriate; reevaluate nutrition indicators to adjust nutrient composition, based on periodic chemistry values, blood counts and other measures.

Medications:
Medications added to tube feedings can alter absorption of both nutrients in the feeding and the drug itself.
Medications should not routinely be added to the tube.
Tube should be flushed after each medication to prevent clogging.
Some medications (e.g., antibiotics, H_2 antagonists) may cause diarrhea.
Dilantin should be given separate from tube feedings to prevent absorption problems.

Parenteral

- **PERIPHERAL PARENTERAL NUTRITION** (PPN) is also called **PERIPHERAL VEIN NUTRITION.** Parenteral fluid is infused through the vein, typically on the arm. It may augment an enteral nutrition program or may be used short term if a person takes nothing by mouth but is not hypermetabolic. Nutrient solutions not exceeding 800-900 mOsm/kg can be infused through a regular peripheral catheter that is place into a vein in good condition.

- **TOTAL PARENTERAL NUTRITION (TPN)** is a method of meeting all nutritional needs via feeding through a central vein, usually the superior vena cava. TPN is not indicated if other feeding methods can be used, if the need will be less than five days, or if aggressive nutritional support is not required or requested by the patient or his or her family. TPN is recommended for nourishment with the following medical problems:

  - An inability to absorb nutrients via the GI tract due to massive small bowel re-section.
  - Diseases of the small intestine.
  - Radiation enteritis.
  - Severe diarrhea or intractable vomiting.
  - High-dose chemotherapy, radiation and bone marrow transplants.
  - Patients with moderate to severe pancreatitis.
  - Severe malnutrition and a non-functional GI tract.
  - Severely catabolic patients with or without malnutrition.
  - When the GI tract is not usable within five to seven days.
  - Patients experiencing major surgery, moderate traumatic stress.
  - Inflammatory bowel disease or obstructions.

- **CYCLIC TOTAL PARENTERAL NUTRITION** is intermittent infusion of TPN solution. It may be used to create an infusion-free period to allow other activities or to prepare for home parenteral nutrition. Often the solution is given for 8-12 consecutive hours followed by a 12-16 hour period of no infusion. This should not be used if fluid or glucose intolerance is detected.

(c) Complications

METABOLIC COMPLICATIONS ASSOCIATED WITH PARENTERAL NUTRITION (PN)				
Complication	**Possible Etiology**	**Symptoms**	**Treatment**	**Prevention**
Hyperkalemia	Not common; trauma-induced catabolism; renal dysfunction; rapid potassium administration in presence of normal renal function; metabolic acidosis	Diarrhea, tachycardia, cardiac arrest, oliguria, paresthesia	Adjust potassium intake depending on protein and non-protein calories	Monitor serum levels for trends; assess for drug-nutrient interactions, especially potassium-sparing diuretics
Hypokalemia	Inadequate potassium; increased potassium losses	Nausea, vomiting, confusion, arrhythmias, cardiac arrest,	Increase PN potassium or provide intravenously	Give potassium daily if needed. Check for

METABOLIC COMPLICATIONS ASSOCIATED WITH PARENTERAL NUTRITION (PN)				
Complication	Possible Etiology	Symptoms	Treatment	Prevention
	(diarrhea, diuretics, intestinal fistulas); protein anabolism; potassium wasting drugs; alkaloids	respiratory depression		drug-nutrient interactions
Hypernatremia	Inadequate free water administration; excessive sodium intake; excessive water losses (fever, burns, hyperventilation)	Thirst, decreased skin turgor, mild irritability in some cases, elevated serum sodium, BUN and hematocrit	Decrease sodium intake; replenish fluids	Avoid excess sodium intake; monitor fluid status; monitor urine sodium
Hyponatremia	Excessive fluid administration or free water intake; nephritis and/or adrenal insufficiency; dilutional states (congestive heart failure, SIADH, cirrhosis of the liver with ascites)	Confusion, hypotension, irritability, restlessness, cold clammy skin, seizures, oliguria	Restrict fluid intake Increase sodium intake as dictated by clinical status	Avoid overhydration; provide 60 to 100mEq/dL unless contraindicated by cardiac, renal, or fluid status; monitor urine sodium; use concentrated solutions of nutrients
Hypoglycemia	Abrupt discontinuation of PN;insulin overdose	Weakness, sweating, palpitations, lethargy, shallow respirations		Taper PN solution; with abrupt discontinuation of TPN; hang 10% dextrose at the same rate as TPN to prevent rebound hypoglycemia
Hyperglycemia	Large doses of glucose started too quickly; stress, infection, pancreatitis, liver or renal failure; steroids; history of diabetes, obesity	Glucose levels above 200mg/dL, frequent urination, increased thirst, HHNK	Add insulin in small amounts to formula or in those who are severely resistant; give insulin drip; terminate PN if HHNK occurs	Give higher percentages of fat in formula; limit total daily CHO to ~3g/kg/min to those at risk and 5.0 for other adults

II. NUTRITION CARE FOR INDIVIDUALS AND GROUPS (50%)

METABOLIC COMPLICATIONS ASSOCIATED WITH PARENTERAL NUTRITION (PN)

Complication	Possible Etiology	Symptoms	Treatment	Prevention
Hypertriglyceridemia	Lipid provision exceeds ability to clear lipids from bloodstream (>4 mg/kg/min); sepsis, multi-system organ failure, pathologic hyperlipidemia, lipoid nephrosis; medication usage alters fat metabolism (i.e. Cyclosporin)	Serum triglyceride level 300 to 350 mg/dL 6 hr past lipid initiation; elevated levels in previously stable patients (ie. sepsis)	Decrease lipid volume administered; lengthen infusion time; simultaneously infuse glucose	Assess for preexisting history of hyperlipidemia before initiation of PN; use 20% lipid emulsion
Hypercalcemia	Renal insufficiency, some malignancies; such as breast cancer, bone cancer, excess vitamin D; prolonged immobilization, stress	Depression, lethargy; HTN; nausea, vomiting, constipation	Reduce or remove from PN solution	Encourage weight-bearing activity; monitor vitamin D intake
Hypocalcemia	Decreased vitamin D intake; hypo-albuminemia; hypo-magnesemia; hypo-tension; some drugs; citrate binding of calcium due to excessive blood transfusions	Parasthesia, tetany, irritability, ventricular arrythmias	Calcium supplementation	Provide sufficient calcium; monitor for trends
Hypermagnesemia	Renal insufficiency; excessive magnesium administration	With very high serum levels: hypotension, arrhythmias	Decrease magnesium intake	Monitor serum levels for trends
Hypomagnesemia	Excessive GI loss, renal loss due to renal dysfunction, or certain drug, active tissue synthesis	Apathy, muscle weakness, tetany, convulsions; nausea, vomiting; hypokalemia; hypocalcemia	Magnesium supplementation	Monitor serum levels for trends
Hyperphosphatemia	Excess phosphate administration or renal insufficiency	Not well described	Reduce or delete phosphorus from solution	Use 20% lipid solution

METABOLIC COMPLICATIONS ASSOCIATED WITH PARENTERAL NUTRITION (PN)

Complication	Possible Etiology	Symptoms	Treatment	Prevention
Hypo-phosphatemia	Nitrogen and glucose-rich solutions cause rapid shift of phosphorus into intercellular space; aluminum-containing medications	Irritability, confusion; parasthesia, muscle weakness; hypoventilation; anorexia nausea; vomiting	Give malnourished patients up to 40-50 mEq/L	Advance feeding slowly and monitor electrolytes
Prerenal azotemia	Dehydration; excess protein; inadequate nonprotein calorie intake with mobilization of own protein stores	Elevated serum BUN	Increase fluid intake; decrease protein level	Monitor serum BUN
Overfeeding	Excess carbohydrate or protein administration	Excess CHO; CO_2 retention, cardiac tamponade, liver dysfunction; excess PRO; elevated BUN, excess nitrogen excretion, elevated BUN/Cr ratio	Decrease CHO/PRO as needed	Avoid excess CHO/PRO in feeding
Cholestasis	Precise etiology unknown; theories include sepsis, GI pathology (shortbowel syndrome), IBD, ileal resection);lack of enteral stimulation; increased production of bile acid toxic to the liver	Increases in alkaline phosphotase, elevation of bilirubin and AST(SGOT)	Restrict daily CHO load to <5mg/kg/min; avoid over-feeding and minimize enteral stimulation	Use GI tract as early as possible
Gastrointestinal atrophy	Atrophy of villi; colonic hypoplasia	Decreased gastric function; impaired GI immunity and gut bacterial translocation in research; relevance to humans not yet determined; glutamine may be relevant	Transition to enteral feedings as quickly as possible	Keep patient NPO for short time as possible; increase to complex oral/enteral feeding as fast as possible

- **REFEEDING SYNDROME** is a complication that can occur during aggressive feeding after a long nutritionally compromised status. It is seen in nutrition support when too many calories are ingested too soon. It can be life threatening and must be treated promptly. Metabolic abnormalities such as hypophosphatemia, hypokalemia and hypomagnesemia are commonly seen. Fluid retention is due to increased insulin concentration. Sudden expansion of the extracellular fluid leads to cardiac decompensation in nutritionally compromised individuals. Administration of dextrose can cause significant hyperglycemia that may result in osmotic diuresis and dehydration. When any feeding is initiated in nutritionally compromised patients, close monitoring of serum phosphate, magnesium, potassium and glucose is necessary. Refeeding syndrome can also occur when treating marasmus.

Department policies and procedures

- Delivery of enteral and parenteral nutrition must follow the steps outlined in institutional policies and procedures. Policies may identify the clinical conditions that indicate the need for metabolic support and should designate the service or position responsible for implementing the procedures. Nutrition support policies and procedures are frequently team written. The dietitian should be familiar with the nutrition support policy, the role of the dietitian as well as roles of other team members.

- Procedures should outline the sequence of events from baseline assessment, to ordering, administration and monitoring. Metabolic support issues are under constant research, surveillance and evaluation. Therefore, policies and procedures about nutrition and metabolic support must be updated frequently. The AND dietetic practice group, Dietitians in Nutrition Support, provides useful information for updating policies and procedures.

(3) Complementary care/herbal therapy

- **ALTERNATIVE MEDICINE** is a term used to describe practices used in place of conventional medical treatments. These practices incorporate spiritual, metaphysical or religious underpinnings, non-European medical traditions or newly developed approaches to healing. There are almost 500 such systems. The term "alternative medicine" carries an inherent point of view. What in the west (1 billion people) is considered "alternative" medicine is for the rest of the world (>4 billion people) considered "traditional" medicine, i.e., Chinese medicine and Ayurveda. In this manual, the term "alternative medicine" should be taken to mean "alternative, from a Western viewpoint".

- Alternative medical systems include:

  - Ayurveda
  - Chiropractic
  - Herbalism
  - Homeopathy
  - Naturopathic Medicine
  - Osteopathy
  - Traditional Chinese Medicine
  - Unani

- **COMPLEMENTARY MEDICINE** describes alternative medicine used in conjunction with conventional medicine. Common complementary care methods include acupuncture, chiropractic, hypnotherapy, massage therapy, yoga, meditation, visualization and prayer. The AND has a Nutrition in Complementary Care Dietetic Practice Group, with members who are interested in the role of alternative therapies and dietary supplements in health and disease. For more information, their website is: **www.complementarynutrition.org**.

- The term, "complementary and alternative medicine" is an umbrella term for both branches. The U.S National Center for Complementary and Alternative Medicine (NCCAM), previously established as the Office of Alternative Medicine, defines **COMPLEMENTARY AND ALTERNATIVE MEDICINE** (CAM) as "a group of diverse medical and healthcare systems, practices and products that are not presently considered to be part of conventional medicine". A study by Ernst, published in 2003, estimated that about half the populations of developed countries use CAM. Their website is: **www.nccam.nih.gov**.

- NCCAM defines **INTEGRATIVE MEDICINE** as "[combining] mainstream medical therapies and CAM therapies for which there is some high-quality scientific evidence of safety and effectiveness." Andrew T. Weill, MD states that "integrative medicine is not synonymous with complementary and alternative medicine (CAM). It has a far larger meaning and mission in that it calls for restoration of the focus of medicine on health and healing and emphasizes the centrality of the patient-physician relationship." All CAM practitioners, however, are not physicians.

- Proponents of evidence-based medicine regard the distinction between conventional and alternative medicine as moot, preferring "good medicine" (with provable efficacy) and "bad medicine" (without it). "Bad medicine" is any treatment where the efficacy and safety of the product or treatment has not been verified through peer-reviewed, double blind placebo controlled studies, regarded as the "gold standard" for determining the efficacy. It is thus possible for a method to change categories in either direction, based on increased knowledge of its effectiveness or lack thereof.

- NCCAM classifies CAM into 5 categories. Some examples of each are described.

Alternative medical systems

- **AYURVEDA** is used in the Indian subcontinent. Much training in ayurvedic medicine is done in the province of Kerala. The word "ayurveda " roughly translates as the "science of life". Ayurveda deals with healthy living, along with therapeutic measures that relate to physical, mental, social and spiritual harmony. Ayurveda is one of the few traditional systems of medicine involving surgery. As a result of strong regulations in medical practice in Europe and America, the most commonly practiced Ayurvedic treatments in the west are massage and dietary and herbal advice.

  - Ayurveda operates on the precept that various materials of vegetable, animal and mineral origin have some medical value. The medicinal properties of these materials have been documented by practitioners and have been used for centuries to cure illness and/or help maintain good health. Ayurvedic medications are made from herbs or mixtures of herbs, either alone or in combination with minerals, metals and other ingredients of animal origin. The metals, animals and minerals are purified before being used for medicinal purposes.

- **CHIROPRACTIC** is a complementary and alternative healthcare profession that focuses on diagnosing, treating and preventing mechanical disorders of the musculoskeletal system, their effects on the nervous system and on general health. Chiropractic's premise is that spinal joint misalignments, which chiropractors call "vertebral subluxations", can interfere with the nervous system and result in diminished health.

  ➤ Some licensed chiropractors, with the degree of Doctor of Chiropractic (DC), specialize in treating lower back problems or sports injuries, or combine chiropractic with manipulation of the extremities, physiotherapy modalities, nutrition or exercises to increase spinal strength or improve overall health, as part of a holistic treatment approach. Chiropractors are not trained nor licensed to prescribe drugs. Many recommend essential oils, or homeopathic (non-prescription) medicines. Depending on the country or state in which the chiropractic school is located, some train in minor surgery. When indicated, the doctor of chiropractic consults with, co-manages or refers to other healthcare providers.

- **HERBALISM,** also known as **HERBAL THERAPY,** is the oldest healthcare known to mankind. Herb therapy is the use of herbs for therapy or medicinal purposes. Derived from plants, herbs are used for their medicine, aroma and spice in herbal therapy. Herb plants produce and comprise a myriad of chemical substances that interact with our bodies. Herbal therapy allows natural plants and herbs to empower organs and tissues to regain normal functionality.

  ➤ Currently, over 4 billion people or 80% of the world population use herbal therapy for some form of healthcare. Ayurvedic practitioners, homeopathic practitioners, naturopathic practitioners, traditional Oriental practitioners and Native American Indians commonly use herbal therapy. Common illness or conditions that herbal therapy can benefit are some digestive problems, sinusitis and irritable bowel syndrome. Other conditions like arthritis, post-cancer treatment, fertility issues, menopause, PMS, colds and even flu may be helped with herbal therapy. Herbal therapy can be in many forms; essential oils, creams, pills, patches, etc.

- **HOMEOPATHY** is based on the "Principle of Similars" and rests on the premise of treating sick persons with extremely diluted agents that in undiluted doses are deemed to produce similar symptoms in a healthy individual. Its adherents and practitioners assert that the therapeutic potency of a remedy can be increased by serial dilution of the drug, either with water or alcohol and then shaken by ten hard strikes against an elastic body (succussion). Homeopathy is more popular in Europe and India than in the U.S., where it is subject to tighter regulations. Stricter European regulations have recently been passed to limit this popular practice, especially in France and Belgium.

- **NATUROPATHIC MEDICINE (**also known as **NATUROPATHY)** is a medical philosophy and practice that seeks to improve health and treat disease by assisting the body's innate capacity to recover from illness and injury. Naturopathic practice includes different modalities such as manual therapy, homeopathy, hydrotherapy, herbalism, acupuncture, counseling, environmental medicine, aromatherapy, whole foods, and so on. Practitioners tend to emphasize a holistic approach to patient care. Although naturopathy originated in the United States, today it is practiced in many countries, where it is subject to different standards of regulation and levels of acceptance.

- Naturopathic practitioners prefer not to use invasive surgery or most synthetic drugs. They prefer "natural" remedies such as relatively unprocessed or whole medications like herbs and foods. Licensed physicians from accredited naturopathic medical schools are trained to use diagnostic tests, for example, imaging and blood tests before deciding on a full course of treatment. Naturopathic practitioners also employ the use of prescription medication and surgery, and when necessary, refer patients to medical practitioners. Naturopathic physicians (ND) are not medical doctors and must have a specific license in some states.

- **OSTEOPATHY** is a theory of disease and method of cure founded on the assumption that deformation of some part of the skeleton and consequent interference with the adjacent nerves and blood vessels are the cause of most diseases. Practitioners of osteopathy, called osteopaths (or osteopathic physicians in the U.S.) have a holistic approach. Osteopathic philosophy requires addressing the whole person in diagnosis, prevention and treatment of illness, disease and injury, using manual and physical therapies.

  - With its origins in the late 1880s, osteopathy was initially a variant of the contemporary Western medical approach and became integrated with mainstream medicine in 1969. Osteopathic physicians are licensed in the U.S. as DO and, in most states, have the same privileges as MDs. Outside the U.S., osteopathy is considered a complementary or alternative therapy and is limited largely to musculoskeletal conditions.

- **TRADITIONAL CHINESE MEDICINE (TCM)** is a range of traditional medical practices used in China that developed over several thousand years. These practices include herbal medicine, acupuncture, cupping and massage. TCM says processes of the human body are interrelated and constantly interact with the environment. Therefore the practitioner looks for signs of disharmony in the external and internal environment of a person in order to understand, treat and prevent illness and disease. TCM theory is based on a number of philosophical frameworks including the Theory of Yin-yang, the Five Elements, the human body Meridian system, Zang Fu theory and others. TCM developed as a form of non-invasive therapeutic intervention (also described as folk medicine or traditional medicine) rooted in ancient belief systems, including traditional religious concepts. Chinese medical practitioners before the 19th century relied on observation and trial and error which incorporated certain mystical concepts. Like their Western counterparts, doctors of TCM had a limited understanding of infection, which predated the discovery of bacteria, viruses (germ theory of disease) and an understanding of cellular structures and organic chemistry. Instead they relied mainly on observation and description on the nature of infections for creating remedies. Based on theories formulated through three millennia of observation and practical experience, a system of procedure was formed to guide a TCM practitioner in courses of treatment and diagnosis. Accupunture and cupping are also used in TCM.

  - Unlike other forms of traditional medicine which have largely become extinct, traditional Chinese medicine continues as a distinct branch of modern medical practice, and within China, it is an important part of the public healthcare system. In recent decades there has been an effort to integrate the discoveries made by traditional Chinese medicine with the discoveries made by workers in the Western medical traditions. The basic belief is that optimal health results from living harmoniously. The practitioner may give different herbal preparations to patients with the same type of infection because the symptoms reported may suggest a different type of imbalance indicated by observation, hearing and smell, asking questions and reading the pulse.

- **UNANI MEDICINE** has found favor in Asia especially India. In India, Unani practitioners can practice as qualified doctors, as the Indian government approves their practice. Unani medicine is very close to Ayurveda. Both are based on theory of the presence of the elements (in Unani, they are considered to be fire, water, earth and air) in the human body. According to followers of Unani medicine, these elements are present in different fluids and their balance leads to health and their imbalance leads to illness. While Unani was influenced by Islam, Ayurveda is associated with Vedic Hinduism.

  ➢ The base used in Unani medicine is often honey. Honey is considered by some to have healing properties and hence is used in food and medicines practiced in the Islamic world. Real pearls and metal are also used in the making of Unani medicine based on the kind of ailment to be healed. Unani medicine is also called as Graeco-Arabic medicine.

Mind-body intervention

- **AROMATHERAPY** is the use of volatile liquid plant materials, known as essential oils, and other aromatic compounds from plants to affect someone's mood or health. The main branches of aromatherapy include:

  ➢ Home aromatherapy (self treatment, perfume and cosmetic use).
  ➢ Clinical aromatherapy (as part of pharmacology and pharmacotherapy).
  ➢ Aromachology (the psychology of odors and their effects on the mind).

- **MEDITATION** describes a variety of practices. It usually involves turning our attention inward to the mind itself. Meditation is often a component of Eastern religions, originating in Vedic Hinduism. It has also become mainstream in Western culture. It encompasses a wide variety of spiritual practices which emphasize mental activity or quiescence. Meditation can also be used for personal development, such as the exercises of Hatha yoga. Many practice meditation in order to achieve internal peace, while others do it in order to become healthier and friendlier.

- **YOGA,** when used as a form of alternative medicine, is a combination of breathing exercises, physical postures and meditation, practiced for over 5,000 years. Yoga is considered a mind-body intervention used to reduce the health effects of generalized stress while increasing flexibility and body strength.

- Prayer and visualization are also frequently used as mind-body interventions to aid healing.

Biologically-based therapies

- **ACUPUNCTURE** is a technique of inserting and manipulating needles into "acupuncture points" on the body. According to acupunctural teachings, this will restore health and well-being, and is particularly good at treating pain. The delineation of these points is standardized by the World Health Organization. Acupuncture is thought to have originated in China and is most commonly associated with Traditional Chinese Medicine. Other types of acupuncture (Japanese, Korean and classical Chinese acupuncture) are practiced and taught throughout the world. In the U.S., acupuncture is provided by a variety of healthcare providers. Practitioners who specialize are usually licensed acupuncturists, L.Ac. Each state has its own laws and requirements.

- Whether acupuncture is efficacious or acts as a placebo, has been the subject of muchongoing scientific research. Scientists have conducted reviews of existing clinical trials according to the protocols of evidence-based medicine; some have found efficacy for headache, low back pain , headache, nausea, but for most conditions have concluded that there is insufficient evidence to determine whether or not acupuncture is effective. The World Health Organization (WHO), the National Center for Complementary and Alternative Medicine (NCCAM) of the National Institute of Health (NIH), the American Medical Association (AMA) and various government reports have also studied and commented on the efficacy of acupuncture. There is general agreement that acupuncture is safe when administered by well-trained practitioners and that further research is warranted.

Manipulative and body-based methods

- **MASSAGE** is the practice of applying structured pressure, tension, motion or vibration, manually or with mechanical aids, to the soft tissues of the body, including muscles, connective tissue, tendons, ligaments, joints and lymphatic vessels to achieve a beneficial response. A form of therapy, massage can be applied to parts of the body or successively to the whole body, to heal injury, relieve psychological stress, manage pain and improve circulation. Where massage is used for its physical and psychological benefits, it may be termed **THERAPEUTIC MASSAGE** or **MANIPULATIVE THERAPY**.

- **REFLEXOLOGY**, also called **ZONE THERAPY**, is the practice of stimulating points on the feet, hands and ears, to benefit some other part of the body or to improve general health. The most common form is foot reflexology. Practitioners believe that the foot can be divided into many reflex zones corresponding to all parts of the body, so that applying pressure to a person's foot will stimulate another part of the body to heal itself.
  - ➤ In reflexology, it is believed that there is a "vital energy" that is circulating between organs of the human body that penetrates into every living cell. Whenever this energy is blocked, the zone of blockage will be affected, and the reflex zones can indicate the blockage of energy in different organs. Therefore, if someone has a problem in a particular organ, a reflexologist will press on the corresponding reflex zone or zones and the person will experience pain. This pain is said to originate from the deposition of crystals in the reflex zone and, with massage, these crystalline structures can be broken down and the pain relieved. Simultaneously, the pressure applied to the reflex zones by the reflexologist is claimed to pass through the nerves to release energy blockages.

Energy therapy

- **ENERGY THERAPY** is a collection of techniques and therapies that are often classed as alternative medicine. Energy psychology focuses on the interrelationship of emotion, behavior, psychopathology and health through the electrical activity of the nervous system, acupuncture meridians, chakras, biofields and morphogenetic fields.
  - ➢ Though there are varying approaches, energy therapies are typically based on the premise that on a fundamental level, everything in the universe is made of energy. From this perspective, human beings are also fundamentally energy. Around the world, from ancient times to modern day, techniques have developed which focus on healing at this energy level. While many energy therapies make no claim of scientific verification, there are many who benefit from energy healings.

- Energy psychology includes many techniques aimed at healing emotional distress such as trauma, phobias and anxiety; cognitive distress, such as limiting beliefs; physical distress, such as head injury, heart rhythm asynchrony, neurological imbalances, biochemical imbalances and structural imbalances; and spiritual distress, such as existential issues, fears and limiting spiritual beliefs. Although the procedures are different, practitioners assert that they all deal with the body's energy system, be it meridians, chakras, auras, spirits or some other medium.

- **REIKI** is a form of spiritual healing and spiritual practice proposed for the treatment of physical, emotional, mental and spiritual diseases. Mikao Usui developed Reiki in early 20th century Japan, where he claimed to receive the ability of "healing without energy depletion" after three weeks of fasting and meditating on Mount Kurama. Practitioners use a technique similar to the laying on of hands, in which they claim to be channels for energy ("Ki" or "Qi") guided by a universal spirit or spiritual nature ("Rei"), flowing through their palms to heal a person wherever they may need healing. Some forms of Reiki are massage; others pass hands over a clothed body; still other Reiki healing is done through meditations. Since Reiki requires spiritual faith and so little is known about it scientifically, it is considered controversial by some people. There is little evidence-based research that Reiki works by any means other than suggestion or the placebo effect, though some theorists have described a scientific basis for calling Reiki an energy medicine.

- **THERAPEUTIC TOUCH (TT)** is a mostly secular variant of faith healing, started by Dolores Krieger in the early 1970s. The TT practitioner moves his or her hands over the patient's body, specifically the affected area, without actually touching the patient. The claim is that this allows the practitioner to direct the flow of chi (or Qi), allowing the patient to heal. It is based on the belief that humans, or all living things, have an energy field or aura extending beyond the surface of the body that can be manipulated by the therapist. Many nurses and hospice workers are trained in therapeutic touch. However, under scientific testing, no definitive evidence has been found establishing either the existence of Qi, or these energy fields. Additionally, no double blind clinical trials have established that TT is more effective at healing patients than placebo.

(e) Implementing care plans

(1) Nutrition therapy for specific nutrition-related conditions

- The **DIET MANUAL** is a book that describes the components of each diet prescribed and provided at the healthcare institution. It must be adopted by the medical staff; it guides healthcare staff responsible for translating a diet prescription into nutritionally adequate meals. A diet manual clarifies for all personnel what food the institution will provide to fulfill each diet prescription and provides guidance to those writing diet prescriptions. Many small institutions adopt diet manuals produced by larger institutions or professional associations.

(2) Basis for quality practice (evidence-based guidelines, standardized process (NCP), regulatory and patient safety issues)

- All implementation should be carried out by the registered dietitian using evidence-based guidelines and the NCP, within the Scope of Practice, while maintaining ethical standards.

- Quality practice, as outlined by the Institute of Medicine:
  - ➢ Follows a consistent process and model based on practice knowledge, evidence, research and science
  - ➢ Exists within an individuals's scope of practice, state licensure scope of practice, regulations and standards
  - ➢ Guides for self-evaluation and used by regulatory agencies to determine competency for credentialed dietetics practitioners
  - ➢ Aims for compensated, equitable and reimbursable services
  - ➢ Evaluates and measures patien/client outcomes through data sources
  - ➢ Enables lifelong learning with career ladder through credentialing, certification and advanced practice standards.

- A comprehensive scope of practice resource including 2012 Scope of Practice in Nutrtion Care and Standards of Professional Performance for RD's and DTR's is the the June 2012 Supplement of the Journal.

- For current information on quality management visit and websites www.eatright.org/quality, www.eatright.org/qualityresources, www.eatright.org/sop

Regulatory and patient safety issues

- The **JOINT COMMISSION FOR ACCREDITATION OF HEALTHCARE ORGANIZATIONS (JCAHO)** provides an accrediting service to healthcare facilities. Standards and performance measures have been developed to provide this service. JCAHO standards are recognized as defining a national consensus on quality healthcare that reflects changing practices and delivery trends in the healthcare industry. Healthcare organizations apply for JCAHO accreditation because they obtain an objective evaluation of the organization's performance. In addition, the accreditation process allows facilities to focus their quality improvement efforts, enhance professional recruitment, expedite third-party payment, fulfill licensure requirements in most states and meet certain Medicare certification requirements, favorably influence managed care contract decisions, and provide a method for staff education. JCAHO standards focus on outcomes of nutrition care.

> ➢ As of 2006, JCAHO standards require "all entries in medical records be dated and authenticated, and a method established to identify the authors of entries."
> ➢ The entry must include the full name of the author and certification(s). Student entries should include the full name and student or intern after the name. All student entries must be countersigned by a certified practitioner.

- **MEDICARE** was established in 1965 to cover the medical care of people 65 and older and was expanded in 1972 to include the severely disabled and people with end-stage renal disease. Medicare, which is managed by the Health-care Financing Organization, has two parts. Part A is the hospital insurance that is provided automatically to beneficiaries. Participating healthcare organizations must meet the Medicare Conditions of Participation. These conditions are considered met if the facility is accredited by JCAHO. Part B is the supplemental coverage that is optional for persons covered under Part A. Medicare Part D is the Drug Plan that began on January 1, 2006.

- The exact services that are covered by Medicare are delineated in Medicare regulations. Dietitians should be familiar with the regulations specific to their service or specialty to facilitate cost effectiveness for the patient, facility, and healthcare personnel. The policy for covering the costs of medical nutrition therapy has not been consistent. In settings other than those accredited by Medicare or JCAHO, dietitians, in order to receive reimbursement, must be certified individually by Medicare. Prescribed medical nutritional products are reimbursed in inpatient settings. Currently, in the outpatient setting, dietitian's services are a reimbursable expense for diabetes and non-dialysis renal disease. Expanding Medicare coverage for other dietetic services is a high priority for the dietetics profession. Key to obtaining this coverage is the demonstration of cost effectiveness of dietetic services through outcomes research.

- Nationally available health insurance with a variety of health promotion and disease prevention services, known as the Patient Protection and Affordable Care Act (PPACA), commonly called the Affordable Care Act (ACA), was signed into law in 2010.

- The dietetics practitioner must be sure that while implementing plans, safety issues such as ability to swallow, food/medication interactions, feeding positioning, food allergies and any other nutrition/food related items that might have an impact on the patient's safety are addressed.

(3) Counseling

- Depending upon the patient's ability and disease state, counseling should begin as soon as there are orders for a maintenance diet. Family and/or caregivers should be involved as they can reinforce counseling and often prepare food eaten by the patient. (See Domain I for counseling techniques.)

(4) Communication and documentation

- Communication in the implementation phase involves many people. This includes primarily the patient/client and family or significant others, in addition to other healthcare providers.

- Communication with other healthcare providers is an important part of documentation in medical records.

  - ➢ The notes should be well-organized and the language used should be understood by all medical personnel who use the document.
  - ➢ Universally accepted abbreviations may be used. However, if the abbreviations are internal to the dietetics profession, use may cause misunderstanding for other healthcare providers.

Documentation

- Documentation is a continuous process.

- Documentation in the medical record during the implementation phase provides among other issues, a review of quality of care. Notes recording progress, participants in care decisions and changes in patient care direction should be carefully noted.

- New laws require all physicians and healthcare facilities to document electronically.

(5) Discharge planning and disease management

- During the implementation portion of NCP, if there is a determination of positive progress with the nutrition intervention(s) and other aspects of patient care, discharge planning should begin.

- When a client is discharged to his or her home, written diet instructions should be given for reference and reinforcement, or referral to a community health agency or a private nutrition practitioner should be made.

- Nutrition support programs may be contacted in advance and arrangements made for home-delivered meals. It is essential for the dietitian to collaborate with other members of the healthcare team, including the physician, nurse, pharmacist and social worker to ensure that the patient's feeding-related needs, equipment and supplies will be arranged for prior to discharge.

- In certain instances, the dietitian and other members of the healthcare team may need to interface with home care and nursing agencies to process certification of medical necessity and treatment authorization request forms and to negotiate with the insurance company to arrange payment for nutritional therapies at home.

- When a patient is discharged to a hospital or other nursing facility, the discharge summary can be a source of dietary information on nutrition status, explaining the degree of and the resident's response to nutrition intervention. This information can save the admitting facility time and prevent it from trying approaches that were previously unsuccessful. The nutrition discharge summary also can highlight a problem such as weight loss that might not be readily apparent to the admitting facility.

II. NUTRITION CARE FOR INDIVIDUALS AND GROUPS (50%)

- A discharge care plan is developed in accordance with facility protocol and is a part of the individual's medical record. The discharge care plan should be reviewed regularly to assure that all approaches to improve or maintain the client's state of health are effective.

3. Implementation and promotion of national dietary guidance for populations (e.g., MyPlate, *Dietary Guidelines for Americans, etc.*)

    a. Legislation and policy development

- **MYPLATE** is a graphic representation of the food recommendations that are included in *Dietary Guidelines for Americans*, published by the USDA and the DHHS. It replaced MyPyramid in 2011 as basic dietary guidance. MyPlate translates RDA/DRI and *Dietary Guidelines for Americans* information into the kinds and amounts of foods to eat each day.

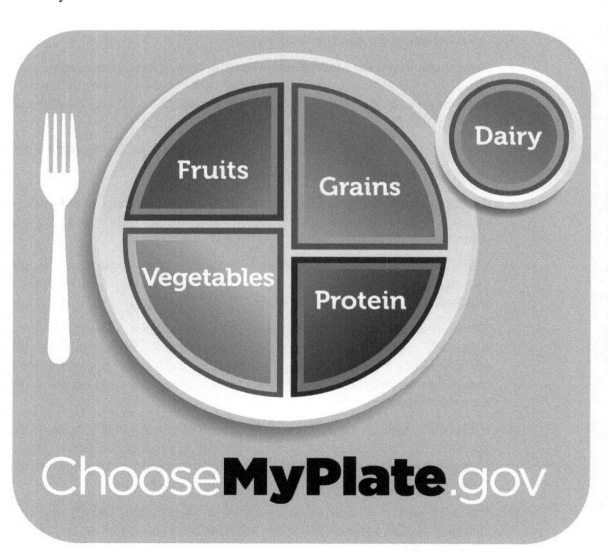

- Most health organizations endorse the *Dietary Guidelines for Americans*, but some, such as the American Cancer Society, have their own guidelines that are congruent with *Dietary Guidelines for Americans,* but specific to the prevention or treatment of a disease. Over the past 25 years, other U.S. government agencies have issued different forms of *Dietary Guidelines for Americans*. While some are very specific, such as the National Heart, Lung, and Blood Institute (NHLBI) whose guidelines contain recommended intakes of saturated, monounsaturated and polyunsaturated fat, others are general in nature. There are also ethnic and age-related graphics developed by various organizations and practitioners.

- Many countries have food guidance systems, with various graphics. MyPlate was released in 2011, after much consumer research, to arrive at the graphic that the largest portion of the adult population in the United States would understand. The website provides many resources for professionals and consumers and information in several languages is being developed.

- The website: **www.ChooseMyPlate.gov** "features practical information and tips to help Americans build healthier diets". Some selected messages are meant to help consumers focus on key behaviors.

Selected messages include the following:
  - ➤ **Enjoy your food, but eat less.**
  - ➤ **Avoid oversized portions.**
  - ➤ **Make half your plate fruits and vegetables.**
  - ➤ **Switch to fat-free or low-fat (1%) milk.**
  - ➤ **Make at least half your grains whole grains.**
  - ➤ **Compare sodium in foods like soup, bread, and frozen meals—and choose foods with lower numbers.**
  - ➤ **Drink water instead of sugary drinks.**

Dietary Guidelines for Americans

- *DIETARY GUIDELINES FOR AMERICANS* are dietary recommendations for healthy Americans age 2 years and over about food choices that promote health specifically with respect to prevention or delay of chronic diseases.

- The key recommendations for the general population contained in the 2010 *Dietary Guidelines for Americans* are:

  - ➤ **Make half your plate fruits and vegetables**. Eat red, orange and dark-green vegetables, such as tomatoes, sweet potatoes and broccoli, in main and side dishes. Eat fruit, vegetables or unsalted nuts as snacks—they are nature's original fast foods.
  - ➤ **Switch to skim or 1% milk**. They have the same amount of calcium and other essential nutrients as whole milk, but less fat and calories.
  - ➤ **Make at least half your grains whole.** Choose 100% whole-grain cereals, breads, crackers, rice and pasta. Check the ingredients list on the food package to find whole-grain foods.
  - ➤ **Vary your protein choices.** Twice a week, make seafood the protein on your plate. Eat beans, which are a natural source of fiber and protein.

> ➤ **Cut back on foods high in solid fats, added sugars and salt**. Many people eat foods with too much solid fat, added sugar and salt (sodium). Added sugars and fats load foods with extra calories you don't need. Too much sodium may increase your blood pressure.
> ➤ **Eat the right amount of calories for you.** Everyone has a personal calorie limit. Staying within yours can help you get to or maintain a healthy weight. Avoid oversized portions. Use a smaller plate, bowl and glass. Stop eating when you are satisfied, not full. Order a smaller portion or share when eating out. If you drink alcoholic beverages, do so sensibly—limit to 1 drink for women or 2 drinks for men daily.
> ➤ **Use food labels to help you make better choices.**
> ➤ **Be physically active your way.** Pick activities that you like and start by doing what you can, at least 10 minutes at a time. Every bit adds up and the health benefits increase as you spend more time being active.

Surgeon General's Report on Nutrition and Health

- The *SURGEON GENERAL'S REPORT ON NUTRITION AND HEALTH, Healthy People* published in1979, subtitled, *Promoting Health—Preventing Disease: Objectives for the Nation,* set an agenda for health promotion and prevention of chronic disease with a group of health objectives that, it was hoped, would be accomplished by 1990. The next report was published in 1988 gave information regarding dietary practices and health status was included along with specific health recommendations and the scientific basis for them and raised discussion about health policy decisions for prevention purposes. The *Healthy People* reports with goals for the following ten years were an outcome of the original Surgeon General's Reports.

Healthy People 2020

HEALTHY PEOPLE 2020 is a comprehensive set of health objectives for the nation to achieve by 2020. The objectives were created by scientists from both within and outside of the government. It is set forth by the Office of Disease Prevention and Health Promotion of the United States Department of Health and Human Services and identifies a wide range of public health priorities and specific measurable and evidence-based objectives. The "Overarching Goals" are to attain high quality, longer lives free of preventable disease, disability, injury and premature death, achieve health equity, eliminate disparities, improve the health of all groups, create social and physical environments that promote good health for all, promote quality of life, healthy development and healthy behaviors across all life stages. There are 18 Nutrition and Weight Status Objectives. **(www.healthypeople.gov)**

Five-a-day

- The **FIVE-A-DAY NUTRITION EDUCATION PROGRAM** was developed when researchers found that there was a link between increased consumption of fruits and vegetables and decreased incidence of certain types of cancer. Five-A-Day was initiated by the National Cancer Institute (NCI), a unit of the National Institutes of Health (NIH), and funded by a joint partnership of NCI and the Produce for Better Health Foundation. The program's goal is to increase consumption of fruits and vegetables to five or more servings per day in the expectation that the incidence of cancer will decrease. There are media, retail, community and research components to promote the message.

National groups and programs

- The **NATIONAL HEART, LUNG AND BLOOD INSTITUTE (NHLBI)** is a unit of the federally supported National Institutes of Health (NIH), a division of the United States Department of Health and Human Services (DHHS). The NHLBI conducts and supports research in diseases of the heart, blood vessels, lung, blood and blood resources and sleep disorders. It also has administrative responsibility for the NIH Woman's Health Initiative. NHLBI conducts educational activities and develops and distributes educational material for health professionals and the public, which are funded through NIH. (**www.nhlbi.nih.gov**) NHLBI has suggested the Dietary Approaches to Stop Hypertension (DASH) diet as an option within the *Dietary Guidelines for Americans* that meets the criteria for prevention of diseases specific to their research and education focus.

- The **NATIONAL CHOLESTEROL EDUCATION PROGRAM (NCEP)** is a program of NHLBI. It began in 1985 and its mission is "to contribute to the reduction of illness and death from coronary heart disease, by reducing the percent of Americans with high blood cholesterol." (**www.nhlbi.nih.gov/aboutncep**)

- The **NATIONAL CANCER INSTITUTE** (NCI) is also a unit of the NIH. It was established in 1937 and is the US government's principal agency for cancer research and training. It coordinates the National Cancer Program and conducts research relating to cause, diagnosis, prevention, treatment and control of cancer. Education and training programs are also part of its mission and are funded through NIH for cancer related prevention.

- The **AMERICAN CANCER SOCIETY** is a voluntary health organization that provides community education and funds research on cancer. (**www.cancer.org**) The American Cancer Society has established general dietary and lifestyle guidelines for cancer prevention and lists some specific guidelines for individual types of cancer. The general guidelines are:

  - Eat a variety of healthful foods, with an emphasis on plant sources.
  - Eat five or more servings of vegetables and fruits each day.
  - Choose whole grains in preference to processed (refined) grains and sugars.
  - Limit consumption of red meats, especially those high in fat and processed.
  - Choose foods that help maintain a healthful weight.
  - Adopt a physically active lifestyle.
  - Maintain a healthful weight throughout life.
  - If you drink alcoholic beverages, limit consumption.

- The **AMERICAN HEART ASSOCIATION** is a voluntary organization that promotes a heart-healthy diet, has a public education program and supports heart disease research. (**www.americanheart.org**) The American Heart Association Eating Plan for Healthy Americans is:

  - Eat a variety of fruits and vegetables. Choose 5 or more servings per day.
  - Eat a variety of grain products, including whole grains.
  - Include fat-free and low fat milk products, fish, legumes (beans), skinless poultry and lean meats.
  - Choose fats with 2g or less saturated fat per tablespoon, such as liquid and tub margarines, canola and olive oil.

➤ Balance the number of calories you eat with the number you use every day. (To find that number, multiply the number of pounds you weigh now by 15 calories. This represents the average number of calories used in one day if you're moderately active. If you get very little exercise, multiply your weight by 13 calories instead of 15. Less active people burn fewer calories.)

➤ Maintain a level of physical activity that keeps you fit and matches the number of calories you eat. Walk or do other activities for at least 30 minutes on most days. To lose weight, do enough activity to use up more calories than you eat every day.

➤ Limit your intake of foods high in calories or low in nutrition, including foods like soft drinks and candy that have a lot of sugars.

➤ Limit foods high in saturated fat, trans fat and/or cholesterol, such as full-fat milk products, fatty meats, tropical oils, partially hydrogenated vegetable oils and egg yolks. Instead choose foods low in saturated fat, trans fat and cholesterol from the first four points above.

➤ Eat less than 6g of salt (sodium chloride) per day (2,400mg of sodium.)

➤ Have no more than one alcoholic drink per day if you're a woman and no more than two if you're a man. "One drink means it has no more than ½ ounce of pure alcohol." Examples of one drink are 12 oz. of beer, 4 oz. of wine, 1-1/2 oz. of 80 proof spirits or 1 oz. of 100-proof spirits.

- The **NUTRITION SCREENING INITIATIVE** is a national joint effort of The American Academy of Family Physicians, Academy of Nutrition and Dietetics, National Council on Aging, Inc., and other organizations established in 1989, to screen older Americans for signs of poor nutritional status and promote interventions that will enhance their quality of life and health. Screening forms and procedures are available.

- There are many other national groups, some federally funded and some privately funded, that have nutrition initiatives for the public.

a. Legislation and policy development

- Becoming involved in legislation and public policy issues, especially regarding nutrition matters is the responsibility of every dietetics professional.

- New legislation usually is introduced because of a perceived problem with an issue under the control of federal, state or local government. Anyone can call the problem to the attention of a legislator or the legislator's staff to request action that will help the problem.

- The action can be in the form of new legislation or more explicit guidelines for the public. In order to have those who can help hear about the problem, one has to be an advocate. AND members have been advocates for providing healthful school lunches, senior feeding programs, compensation for medical nutrition therapy and other issues.

- It is important for dietitians to understand the legislative process, be aware of current issues, know who their legislators are, and convince them of the importance of the issue to their constituents.

- To refresh understanding of the legislative process and how you can work within it go to the AND website (**www.eatright.org**) click on Advocacy and read the online booklet: *ANDAdvocacy Guide—Effective Nutrition and Health Policy Begins with You.* Members of and can also subscribe to the online newsletter, *On the Pulse,* to keep abreast of national legislative information regarding nutrition and dietetics practice.

- There are many ways dietitians can become involved in influencing legislation and public policy at the national and state level. Dietitians can also act as nutrition policy advisors to legislators and/or testify at hearings, regarding matters of importance in setting nutrition policy throughout the United States.

- **LICENSURE** is a state policy that provides consumers an assurance that a professional is competent to provide certain services and is used to exclude the non-licensed practitioner from providing those services for a fee. AND's Washington office has played an important role in getting either licensure or other credentialing for dietitians at the state level. Licensing statutes make it illegal to practice dietetics without first obtaining a license from the state. Statutory certification limits the use of particular titles to persons meeting predetermined requirements, but persons not certified can still practice dietetics with a different title. Registration is the least restrictive form of state regulation. It prohibits use of the title "Registered Dietitian" or other job titles by persons not meeting state-mandated qualifications. However, unregistered persons may practice the profession using nutrition-related titles that are not protected by licensure.

b. State and community resources and nutrition-related programs

(1) Block grants to states

➤ The federal government has many community programs that are administered by state or local governments. One way the government supports these initiatives is by awarding a **BLOCK GRANT** of money to the administering government for broad purposes. The receiving agency can use the money where they can use it best, as long as it meets the criteria for the basic grant. There are five federal block grant areas: Maternal and child health; Community services; Social services; Preventive health and health services and; Primary care.

(2) Federal and state funded food and nutrition programs

This information is described earlier in this Domain.

(3) Community interventions

- As defined in Domain II, a **COMMUNITY** is a group of individuals who can be defined by location, function, shared interest or social cohesion. Various researchers believe that these defined communities can act together as a vehicle for behavioral change. Issues such as weight loss, decreasing fat consumption, lowering blood pressure, blood glucose and cholesterol control, have met with mixed results. Access to health professionals, reinforcement of specific health messages and the general environment has produced some positive results.

- Communities are often informal groups with no one in charge. Actions are based on consensus. The community itself seems to make the individual stronger by tapping the strengths of each member. Flexibility is built into each program and change strategies are based on each group's needs.

STEPS Grants

- **STEPS TO A HEALTHIER US GRANT** was a program established in 2004, by the Centers for Disease Control (CDC) through the US Department of Health and Human Services (DHHS). A total of $35.7 million dollars was awarded 22 grants, covering 40 communities throughout the country to support the health initiative. Topics included in the grant are diabetes, asthma, overweight and obesity. They also address risk factors such as physical activity, poor nutrition and tobacco use. Agreements were for five years, with a goal to "help Americans live longer and healthier lives."

  > ➤ The program targeted rural communities, low income and minority populations, immigrants, youth, senior citizens, uninsured and underinsured people and other high-risk populations. Partners in the programs included Departments of Health and Education, school districts, healthcare providers and other diverse organizations. Programs in schools, workplace and healthcare settings used interventions such as walking programs, media campaigns, smoking cessation programs, increasing healthy food choices in schools and health education training to involve the community members.

4. Development programs and services

a. Identification and attainment of funding

- New programs or services are established because of a need that has been identified within the community. The need is usually identified by conducting a community needs assessment or by other research done in the area.

- Proper planning requires that the goals and objectives of the program must be established so sources of funding can be identified. Some money may be available from the agency or business that is planning the program. Other revenue sources, such as "in kind" donations or small amounts of cash, might be available from the local community. Depending on the topic of the program, grants may be available from governmental or private sources.

b. Resource allocation and budget development

- Tentative budgets should be developed before any funding is requested. The outside grantor will want to know the purpose and expected outcome of the intervention before they will give any resources. This will also help to separate the specific needs of the proposed programs, so those with limited resources can choose the part of the plan or program they might want to support.

c. Provision of food and nutrition services to groups

- High-risk groups include people who have serious and often incurable illnesses; those who are very poor and/or are unemployed; who are unable to communicate because they cannot speak or hear; those who do not speak English or the language of instruction. Some may be lacking education or have a literacy problem. There may be a large number of people in the community who have poor housing or are homeless. There may be many who have no health insurance. Some, especially the elderly, may be isolated due to infirmity. Most of these people are food insecure.

- Community agencies should periodically assess the community to see the kind of services that are needed and try to provide them in the best way possible. Sometimes trained non-professionals or community volunteers can provide basic services that would allow the professionals to manage programs and work with those at highest risk.

- Involve members of the community in working with the agency so it has access to those who most need service. Try to set the agency's hours of operation to accommodate the working members of the community.

- The goal of all of these efforts should be client self-sufficiency, wherever possible.

TOPIC D - MONITORING and EVALUATION

- Nutrition monitoring and evaluation is the fourth step of the Nutrition Care Process.

- Monitoring should be scheduled and reviewed at specific intervals.

- Evaluation measures current information with previous status, progress towards goals and success or failure to meet goals and objectives.

1. Monitoring progress and updating previous care

a. Monitoring responses to nutrition care

- **MONITORING** is the portion that looks at outcomes that have been measured and recorded at pre-planned intervals. If performed correctly, they measure the responses to nutrition care and the degree to which the patient/client goals have been met.

b. Comparing outcomes to nutrition interventions

- An **OUTCOME** is a measured result of a healthcare process, system or episode of care. Outcomes are monitored to conduct risk-benefit analyses (comparison of morbidity, mortality and quality of life preceding a specific treatment to morbidity, mortality and quality of life resulting from the treatment), cost-benefit analyses (monetary benefits of treatment relative to monetary costs of treatment) and cost-effectiveness analysis (ability to achieve desired outcome relative to achievement costs).

- When evaluations of nutrition interventions are compared with outcomes, consideration should be given to the individual for whom the therapy was prescribed, in addition to collection of aggregate numbers, because the individual may not be able to fulfill the potential of the therapy for other than clinical reasons.

- Outcome measures must be objective, reproducible, transferable to other sites, quantitative, clinically relevant, easy to measure and able to be assessed over a period of time. Monitoring outcomes allows for an assessment of the usefulness of nutrition practices and interventions. This assessment should go beyond statistical significance; the clinical significance of outcomes research results must be considered in the evaluation of nutrition therapies.

- Clinicians, healthcare organizations, healthcare policy makers and third-party payers use data obtained from monitoring outcomes. Outcome research helps to identify the best treatment options, thereby making patients the ultimate beneficiaries.

2. Measuring outcome indicators using evidence-based guides for practice

- Evidence-based guides are very important tools to use for practice because the information is validated through well-documented research. However, critical thinking skills need to be used if change has not occurred. Additional or new interventions may be necessary to reduce barriers to success.

a. Explaining variance

- Dietitians must know statistical methods to evaluate variance.

- The ability to think critically helps one to ask informed questions regarding issues that arise and cannot be answered with mainstream information. The critical thinker will ask why an outcome was not as expected and seek the answer if the reason for the variance is unclear.

b. Using reference standards

- Reference standards are usually the result of previously conducted and validated research, and standards should be used to compare outcomes with results of earlier research.

c. Selecting indicators

- After goals are established, indicators are selected to measure information regarding specific goals. The indicators should be standardized measures that have been validated. An example of an indicator might be repeat attendance, scores on tests, weight loss or other measurable factors that contribute to attaining goals.

3. Evaluating outcomes

a. Direct nutrition outcomes

- Current findings should be compared with previous status, intervention goals and/or reference standards to see if changes have occurred from the nutrition interventions.

- Outcomes for nutrition monitoring and evaluation are organized into 4 categories: 1) Nutrition-Related Behavioral and Environmental Outcomes; 2) Food and Nutrient Intake Outcomes; 3) Nutrition-Related Signs and Symptoms Outcomes and; 4) Nutrition-Related Patient/Client Outcomes.

- The dietitian must monitor the patient/client progress in all of these areas to see if the nutrition intervention has been implemented and provide evidence that the intervention is or is not changing the behavior or status. An evaluation and comparison of the current findings with the previous status, intervention goals and/or reference status should be done to see if there are positive or negative changes.

b. Clinical and health status outcomes

- In addition to evaluating direct nutrition outcomes, it is important to evaluate other clinical and health status for changes; i.e., improved lab values.If the outcome is negative, it may mean that the condition of the patient has deteriorated, or expected behavioral changes did not take place, then the clinical and nutrition care portion of the evaluation should be reevaluated.

c. Patient-centered outcomes

- When patients/clients are involved in goal setting, they will "buy into" therapies more easily and positive outcomes will most often result, thereby improving customer satisfaction.

d. Healthcare utilization outcomes

- Using fewer resources to achieve goals is a positive utilization outcome.

- Standardized formats are designed to be cost-efficient. All agencies that deal with health costs in any way, are seeking methods to reduce the cost of healthcare. In addition to positive nutrition outcomes, utilization costs are measurable and cost-effective.

4. Relationship with outcomes measurement systems and quality improvement

- Performance outcomes can be measured in looking at outcomes of planned care. If outcomes are not positive, performance of the healthcare professional can be measured and quality improvement can be implemented.

5. Determining continuation of care

a. Continuing and updating care

- As long as the patient/client is able to work with dietitians and other healthcare professionals, care should be a continuing process.

- Once goals are reached and sustained, healthcare professionals should be available to update care as necessary if conditions change.

b. Discontinuing care

- Care should be discontinued when goals are attained and sustained, is no longer effective for patient comfort, or if the patient/client and family do not want to continue care.

6. Documentation

- Much documentation is electronic to increase readbility, clarity and ease of information sharing among the healthcare team.

- Appropriate charting techniques include all relevant information including plans for care and follow-up, including evaluation mechanisms.

- All medical personnel should respect confidentiality of the patient/client and should not identify or discuss the person in any public place or with anyone who is not immediate family or involved in that person's care.

- The **PROBLEM-ORIENTED MEDICAL RECORD (POMR)** is an organized system of data analysis and client care planning used in documentation of medical records in many hospitals and healthcare settings. A POMR includes the following:

  - ➢ **Database:** The database includes admission or registration data, such as name, age, sex, race, referral source and brief medical and social histories. Results of laboratory tests, X-rays and physical examinations, diagnosis, surgery or treatment, consultations and diet history will be noted. Medications, records of vital signs, temperature, height and weight, including changes in weight, and physician orders will also be recorded.

- ➢ **Problem list:** Established problems, temporary problems, allergies, sensitivity or intolerance problems and drug or dietary problems are delineated, found on the database.
- ➢ **Plans:** Each problem is addressed and a plan is formulated to include therapy and education.
- ➢ **Continuing care record:** The record is a current problem list that can be updated, changed or resolved. Continuing care progress is recorded.

- **SUBJECTIVE OBJECTIVE ASSESSMENT PLAN (SOAP)** format is used to record POMR information:

  - ➢ **Subjective**: Data are collected from the client, family or caregiver. Data reflect perceptions of the client's condition or problems.
  - ➢ **Objective:** Information comes from laboratory tests or X-rays, nutritional analysis, physical findings and performance tests. Currently much of this information is "charted by exception" meaning that only the information that is not within normal limits is recorded.
  - ➢ **Assessment:** The professional interprets the subjective and objective information relative to the client's nutritional status using the Problems, Etiology and Signs (PES) format for assessing problems.
  - ➢ **Plan:** The plan is the action to be taken to resolve identified nutritional problems. The plan may be diagnostic, therapeutic or educational and should contain an evaluation component.

- To reflect the Nutrition Care Process the **ASSESSMENT, DIAGNOSIS, INTERVENTION, MONITORING AND EVALUATION (ADIME)** format has been established. This is considered to be a more precise way of charting - restricting the information to only the most relevant information, with the nutrition diagnosis as the focus.

- **Assessment:** The Assessment portion looks similar to the third step of the SOAP note. It might include significant medical and family history, medical diagnoses, important and relevant data compared with a standard, etc.

  - ➢ **Diagnosis:** The PES Statement should be in this portion of the note.
  - ➢ **Intervention:** Plans for treatment and goals; client involvement, expected results.
  - ➢ **Monitoring and Evaluation:** Progress or lack of progress and reasons; changes in patient/client condition, future plans.

- Documentation is necessary for determining the effectiveness of program or treatment and for cost-benefit or cost-effectiveness analysis. Documentation includes:

  - ➢ Recording the process and outcome of intervention in the medical record or the client file.
  - ➢ Documenting progress toward achievement of program or treatment objectives by changes in biochemical parameters, anthropometric measures and food patterns.
  - ➢ Recording the process and outcome of training or counseling.
  - ➢ Documenting changes in behaviors by frequency of clinic visits, observation of food choices and frequency of referrals to other healthcare professionals to dietitians.
  - ➢ Documentation should be done usng standard nomenclature and abbreviations so that the medical team can easily read and interpret charting.

SELECTED ABBREVIATIONS USED IN MEDICAL CHARTING

a	before	H&H	hemoglobin and hematocrit
a.c.	before meals	Hb	hemoglobin
ad lib	as desired	Hct	hematocrit
A/G	albumin/globulin ratio	Hgb	hemoglobin
AI	adequate intake	HS	at bedtime
ASHD	arteriosclerotic heart disease	Ht	height
aq	water	HTN	hypertension
a&w	alive and well	hx	history
bid	twice daily	ICU	intensive care unit
bm	bowel movement	IDDM	insulin dependent diabetes mellitus (type 1)
BMR	basal metabolic rate	IM	intramuscular
BP	blood pressure	I&O	intake and output
BPH	benign prostatic hypertrophy	IV	intravenous
BS	bowel sounds	Kcal	kilocalories (food calories)
BUN	blood urea nitrogen	kg	kilogram
c	cups	L	liter
c	with	lb	pound
Ca++	calcium	LBW	low body weight
CA	cancer	LBM	lean body mass
CBC	complete blood count	LI	large intestine
CC	chief complaint	LMD	local medical doctor
CHD	coronary heart disease	MI	myocardial infarction
CHF	congestive heart failure	Mg	magnesium
CHO	carbohydrate	mg	milligram
chol	cholesterol	NG	nasogastric
CNS	central nervous system	NPO	nothing by mouth
COPD	chronic obstructive pulmonary disease	NIDDM	non insulin dependent diabetes (type 2)
CPN	central parenteral nutrition	NR	not remarkable
CPR	cardiopulmonary resuscitation	N&V	nausea and vomiting
CRF	chronic renal failure	O2	oxygen
CSF	cerebrospinal fluid	OB	obstetrics
C.T.	clotting time	OHA	oral hypoglycemic agent
CVA	cardiovascular accident	OJ	orange juice
DAT	diet as tolerated	para	pregnancy
D/C	discontinue	PC	present complaint
D&C	dilatation and curettage	PCM	protein-calorie malnourishment
def.	deficiency	PEM	protein energy malnourishment
DM	diabetes mellitus	PI	present illness
DOB	date of birth	po	by mouth or postoperative
D5W	5% dextrose and water	pm	whenever necessary
dx	diagnosis	PT	physical therapy
ECG	electrocardiogram	PTA	prior to admission

SELECTED ABBREVIATIONS USED IN MEDICAL CHARTING

EEG	electroencephalogram	PZI	protamine zinc insulin
EKG	electrocardiogram	q	every
ENT	ear, nose, and throat	qd	every day
excl	exclude	qh	every hour
FBS	fasting blood sugar	qid	four times a day
GBD	gallbladder disease	qod	every other day
gest	gestation	RBC	red blood cells
GI	gastrointestinal	R/O	rule out
gt	a drop	RQ	respiratory quotient
GTT	glucose tolerance test	Rx	prescription
GYN	gynecology	s	without
SCA	sickle cell anemia	TC	total cholesterol
SOB	shortness of breath	TF	tube feeding
SOBOE	shortness of breath on exertion	tid	three times a day
stat	at once	TPN	total parenteral nutrition
sub	substitute	UTI	urinary tract infection
Sx	symptom	VS	vital signs
t	teaspoon	WBC	white blood count
T	tablespoon	WNL	within normal limits
T&A	tonsillectomy & adenoidectomy	wt	weight
TB	tuberculosis		

Domain III - Management of Food and Nutrition Programs and Services

Domain III = 21% of the test.

TOPIC A - FUNCTIONS OF MANAGEMENT

1. Functions
   a. Planning
      (1) Short and long range
      (2) Strategic and operational
      (3) Policies and procedures
      (4) Disaster planning
   b. Organizing
      (1) Work scheduling
      (2) Structure/design, department/unit
      (3) Workload, simplification, productivity and FTE requirements
      (4) Establishing priorities
      (5) Tasks/activities and action plans
      (6) Resources
   c. Directing
      (1) Coordination
      (2) Delegation
      (3) Communication
      (4) Motivation strategies
      (5) Leadership styles, skills, techniques
      (6) Management approaches
   d. Controlling
   e. Evaluating
2. Characteristics
   a. Skills
      (1) Technical
      (2) Human/managing diverse work force
      (3) Conceptual
   b. Roles
      (1) Informational
      (2) Conflict resolution
      (3) Problem solving
      (4) Decision making
      (5) Other
   c. Traits
      (1) Interpersonal communications
      (2) Use of authority, influence and power
      (3) Ethical practice

3. Professional standards of practice
    a. *Standards of Practice in Nutrition Care*
    b. *Standards of Professional Performance*
    c. Legislative process

TOPIC B - HUMAN RESOURCES

1. Recruitment and selection
    a. Laws and regulations
    b. Job analysis, specifications, descriptions
    c. Performance standards
    d. Candidate recruitment
    e. Candidate screening
    f. Candidate interviewing
2. Employment process and procedures
    a. Personnel information
        (1) Records
        (2) Confidentiality
    b. Unions/contracts
    c. Disciplinary action
    d. Grievances
    e. Performance evaluation
    f. Retention strategies
    g. Compensation

TOPIC C- FINANCIAL MANAGEMENT

1. Budget development/resource allocation for food and nutrition programs and services
    a. Budget procedures
    b. Types
        (1) Operational
        (2) Capital
    c. Methods
        (1) Incremental
        (2) Performance
        (3) Zero-based
        (4) Flexible
        (5) Fixed
    d. Components
        (1) Direct expenses
        (2) Indirect expenses
        (3) Capital expenses
        (4) Profit margin
        (5) Revenue
    e. Resources allocation
        (1) Financial and materials
        (2) Cost control decisions

      (3) **Factors affecting available resources**

2. Financial monitoring, evaluation, and control
    a. Accounting procedures
      (1) **Cash/credit procedures**
    b. Financial statements
      (1) **Profit and loss statements**
    c. Value analysis

TOPIC D- MARKETING and PUBLIC RELATIONS

1. Marketing analysis
    a. Process
      (1) **Identification of target market**
      (2) **Determination of needs/wants**
      (3) **Marketing mix**
      (4) **Customer satisfaction**
      (5) **Documentation and evaluation**
2. Pricing
    a. Strategies
      (1) **Breakeven**
      (2) **Revenue-generating**
      (3) **Loss leader**
    b. Rationale
3. Public relations
    a. Media relations
    b. Social networking
    c. Campaign development

TOPIC E - QUALITY IMPROVEMENT

1. Regulatory guidelines (e.g., federal, local, TJC)
2. Process, implementation. evaluation
    a. Cost/benefit analysis
    b. Productivity studies
3. Outcomes management systems
4. Vendor performance and evaluation

TOPIC A - FUNCTIONS OF MANAGEMENT

1. Functions

a. Planning

- Typical planning questions include: Why must it be done? What action is necessary to do it? Where and when will it take place? Who will do it? How will it get done? What will be the cost?

- Mission statements are vital to successful organizations, projects, departments and individuals within organizations. The **MISSION STATEMENT** is a philosophy or creed, the "reason for being." Each organization and each individual has a unique mission. For maximum effectiveness, everyone involved in an organization should participate in formulating the mission statement for that organization. If all members "buy into" the mission, they are more likely to feel personally responsible for working to achieve its end. In addition, a mission gives everyone a sense of shared values and personal security. The mission statement remains relatively stable, though plans change constantly.

- **VALUES** are beliefs about the way things should be. Values are reflected in actions. Values are not necessarily good or positive; for example, racists share common values.

- **PRINCIPLES** are guidelines for human conduct that have enduring, permanent value, for example, honesty, fairness, integrity, quality, service and respect for others. **PRINCIPLE-CENTERED VALUES** are values based on moral principles.

- **NEEDS ASSESSMENT** gathers data (from research, surveys, focus groups, interviews, etc.) to shape strategies for accomplishing the mission.

- An enterprise can operate efficiently if the organization's goals and aims and the needs of individual employees are kept in balance. An example would be an organization that provides a day care facility for employees to meet both worker and parental needs. The day care program would reduce absenteeism and promote job satisfaction.

(1) Short and long range

- **SHORT RANGE PLANS** are generally one year in duration.

- **LONG-RANGE PLANS** generally are for 3-5 years or more.

(2) Strategic and operational

- **STRATEGIC PLANNING** is an interrelated process that identifies internal and external forces related to the mission and values of the organization. Key stakeholders (management, staff, etc.) evaluate the identified opportunities and threats, and a plan evolves. The plan clearly sets forth the vision or mission, goals and objectives, and strategies to attain the objectives. **OPERATIONAL PLANNING,** including budgets and staffing patterns, should focus on attainment of the objectives of the strategic plan. Functions and services that are not important to the plan should be discontinued. All levels of management, from line supervisors up, are involved in strategic planning.

- The top level of planning focuses on company-wide objectives, top management's view of its mission and how best to allocate resources. This level generally sets forth the strategies to meet the objectives. The second level of planning develops more detail about each department's contribution to the strategic plan. Often this level develops tactics, action plans or annual plans.

Approaches to planning

- **INDEPENDENT PLANNING:** Only one person is involved, usually the boss, chair or department head. Independent planning allows more flexibility to make quick changes, but it takes a considerable amount of time of the individual responsible for it. Another disadvantage is that ideas are those of only one person and others may not be committed to the plan because they did not participate in its development.

- **ASSOCIATIVE PLANNING:** The leader and others are involved, each contributing ideas to planning before or during the process. Additional input is the advantage. The disadvantage is that it slows down the decision-making process.

- **PARTICIPATIVE PLANNING:** A general outline of the plan is provided and employees fill in the details. The advantage is that employees have input and develop allegiance the success of the plan. The disadvantage is that employees might not agree or might delay the process.

- **REMOVED PLANNING:** Employees make a complete plan and submit it to the manager for approval. The advantage is more cooperation, since employees become involved, minor details that the manager does not see can be handled. The disadvantages are that employees do not have as many resources as managers, that the employee plans might not be realistic and reasonable and that management and employees can have conflicting goals and priorities.

(3) Policies and procedures

- **POLICIES** are general guidelines for decision-making. A policy sets boundaries around decisions. Policies channel organizational thinking so it is consistent with organizational objectives. Examples include specified areas where employees may smoke, dress codes and grievance procedures. Policies should be recorded in a policy manual that is periodically revised and readily available to all employees. All employees (or volunteers) should know about all policies that they are to follow so they can do their jobs in accordance with established policy.

- **PROCEDURES** specify in chronological order the steps necessary to achieve an objective or carry out a policy. Examples include maintaining patient records, organizing the patient Cardex/file, receiving and acknowledging diet orders and diet changes, carrying out nutritional assessments, menu marking, editing and recording in the medical record.

(4) Disaster planning

- Every food service organization should have a disaster plan that covers employee responsibility in a disaster. The plan should include having ample amounts of non-perishable foods, water and supplies on hand. Disaster plans are to be reviewed periodically and supplies and water refreshed. Disaster plans should include evacuation of the facilities in case of fire, flood or water damage, electrical failure, etc.

b. Organizing

(1) Work scheduling

- **TIME MANAGEMENT** is a way of establishing priorities on the basis of importance and urgency. Effective management requires time for urgent matters, including problem solving (crisis management), and for giving attention to important matters, such as relationship building, planning, training and recreation. The goal of time management is efficiency without undue stress.

- Good time management includes clearly defined goals and objectives; i.e., daily work plans, establishing priorities, setting deadlines, well-trained support staff, limited interruptions, effective meetings, control of stress, few errors and mistakes, reasonable span of responsibility and control, and a balance between what is important and what is urgent.

- **SCHEDULING** is the time frame and time sequence for the performance of a specified work activity; for example, work hours of 6 am to 2 pm or 9 am to 5 pm.

  - An **IRREGULAR SCHEDULE** is one in which an employee begins work at different times, depending on the day; such as Monday at 7 am; Tuesday at 10 am.
  - In a **SPLIT SHIFT** schedule, the employee is not scheduled for 8 consecutive hours; for example, serve lunch and dinner with a 2-hour break between 4-hour shifts.

(2) Structure/design, department/unit

- A **FORMAL ORGANIZATIONAL STRUCTURE** uses a framework established by top management to describe the relationships of people. The structure indicates who supervises whom, who reports to whom, who makes decisions, and who holds the power.

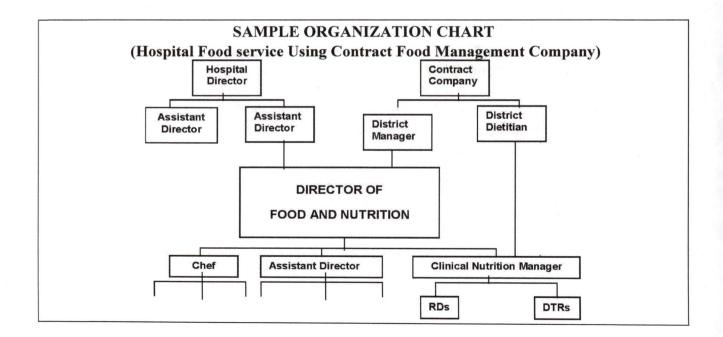

SAMPLE ORGANIZATION CHART
(Hospital Food service Using Contract Food Management Company)

- An **INFORMAL ORGANIZATIONAL STRUCTURE** is a network of personal and social relationships that arise spontaneously as people work together. This is the way relationships actually work. Managers must recognize that informal groups exist within all formal structures. By reinforcing informal groups and creating a sense of togetherness, a manager can maximize achievement of company objectives.

- In many organization charts, the solid lines indicate channels of authority, with those who have the most authority at the top of the chart. Advisory or staff lines of responsibility and communication are shown with dotted lines.

- **LINE PERSONNEL** give and receive orders along the chain of command from the head of the company to the lowest level. Each person is directly accountable to the person above. **STAFF PERSONNEL** are outside this chain of command although they may have their own chain of command within their distinct departments. They aid and support line personnel. Examples of staff personnel include legal advisors or human resource department employees.

- **FORMAL AUTHORITY** that derives from a person's status or rank is based on (1) the right to take action and, (2) the power to enforce compliance with policies and procedures. In all organizations, people are conscious of levels of authority called "top," "middle" and "first-line" management. Each level is endowed with a certain degree of authority.

- The guidelines in an **INFORMAL AUTHORITY** structure are loose and considered social. Informal authority patterns provide additional channels of communication through the "grapevine" and give groups stability and necessary social values. Informal leaders are key influencers of group behavior. Informal authority may be based on personality, leadership, charisma, status, relationships or other personal qualities.

(3) Workload, simplification, productivity, and FTE requirements

- Management is responsible for deciding how and to whom the resources of the organization will be allocated and how management time will be spent.

- Staffing needs are determined by the number of employees in a work area required to meet a demand for services, based on a forecast of consumer/client/patient needs and wants. Staffing is the basis of an organization's recruitment, selection and training process. Staffing deals with personnel rather than equipment needs.

- **MEASUREMENT-ENGINEERING APPROACH** to staffing measures the work content of tasks, establishes standard times to complete tasks and specifies the number of employees needed to complete the tasks.

- **PRODUCTIVITY** is determined by the relationship between output of goods and services (O) and input of resources (I), expressed in ratio form as O:I. The higher the numerical value of this ratio, the greater the productivity.

  - Factors influencing productivity include literacy and technical training, research and development, energy costs, facilities and equipment, family structure, use of alcohol and drugs, worker attitudes and motivation, cost of government regulations, legal and/or liability costs, inflation.

> **THEORY Z PRODUCTIVITY** is a theory of management prevalent in Japan that has resulted in remarkable productivity. It emphasizes workers and management planning and working together to enhance mutual goals.

- A **FULL-TIME EQUIVALENT (FTE)** is equal to 40 hours per week or 2,080 hours per year (or whatever the designated full-time is at that place of business.) FTE is a term used to compare the management of regular, full-time workers to the management of part-time or short-hour workers. It is customarily used to count the number of employees who work for an organizational unit.

  - One full-time relief worker can cover the schedule of 2.5 FTE. (See Example 2.)

    Example 1:
    25 employees x 40 hours/week = 1000 hours
    12 employees x 20 hours/week = 240 hours
    6 employees x 10 hours/week = 60 hours
    TOTAL HOURS = 1300 hours/week

    1300 hours divided by 40 = 32.5 FTEs
    The department has 43 employees, but only 32.5 FTEs.

    Example 2:
    Each full-time employee works 5 days per week and has 2 days off. A full-time relief worker works 5 days per week and has two days off. The relief worker can cover the work of employee A for her 2 days off, employee B for her 2 days off and employee C for one of her 2 days off.

  > The workload documents the number of staff needed to accomplish objectives.

Environmental factors

- Working conditions, such as comfortable temperatures, appropriate noise levels, lighting, ventilation and safety factors (e.g., handling of toxic chemicals), contribute to output and employee morale. Poor environmental conditions lead to increased absenteeism, increased health risks to employees and increased costs to the organization.

Turnover

- **TURNOVER** is the percentage of employees replaced each year for any reason. Each industry has expected turnover rates. The turnover rate for fast-food establishments and college cafeterias is higher than for nursing home food service operations. Each institution maintains records of annual turnover rates for particular departments. A turnover rate of less than 10% is generally acceptable for hospital food and nutrition services.

  Turnover rate = <u>Total employee terminations* x 100 </u>
          Average work force for a specific period
            (*voluntary and involuntary)

- Excessive turnover is expensive to an organization and reflects management problems, unless the work force is expanding due to growth.

- Steps to reduce turnover include:
  - Clearly conveying goals, objectives and philosophies.
  - Documenting and communicating policies and procedures.
  - Hiring based on job descriptions and specifications.
  - Training and supervising effectively.
  - Evaluating job performance regularly.
  - Providing reasonable salaries and benefits.
  - Ensuring a safe and sanitary working environment.
  - Recognizing employee achievement.
  - Establishing and enforcing a grievance policy.
  - Encouraging participation in meetings.
  - Keeping records on reasons for reprimands, resignations or firings.
  - Evaluating reports and providing feedback.

- The following costs are associated with turnover:
  - **BREAK-IN COST** are those incurred because of a new employee's reduced performance while learning a job.
  - **LOST PRODUCTION COST** comes from running with low or reduced staff when people leave and have not yet been replaced. Overtime, at a higher hourly rate, may be necessary for remaining employees.
  - **TAXES** are a cost associated with turnover. The employer pays Federal Unemployment Tax (FUTA) Index(see TAXES in Index p.341). on the first $9,000 earned by an employee in a given year. If an employee collects unemployment, the unemployment insurance tax rate increases, resulting in costs to both employer and employees.
  - **BOOKKEEPING COSTS** are incurred to complete necessary paperwork when employees are hired or terminated.

- Reports that show absenteeism, complaints related to an employee's tasks, or departmental statistical data can be used to evaluate performance and take corrective actions that may reduce turnover.

(4) Establishing priorities

- One important managerial function is establishing priorities. Managers of most healthcare food service organization work with limited funds. Priorities, based on both the organizational mission statement and long and short-term goals should be set and placed into the budget as finances permit.

- Sometimes, the priorities are so urgent that funds must be made available immediately. Other priorities do not necessarily have a fiscal component and can be accomplished faster.

(5) Tasks/activities and action plans

- **TASKS** are activities that implement the process of planning. Tasks might include assessing resources, identifying components of a project, assigning activities to personnel, and so on. Tasks and activities define what must be done, and by whom, to achieve objectives.

- **ACTION PLANS** are specific projects or programs designed to achieve the organizational goals developed by units. Action plans identify activities, outcomes, budget, staff needed and so forth. In some organizations, action plans must contain a mechanism for evaluation or cost-benefit determination.

6) Resources

- The manager decides how resources of all kinds will be allocated. Some funds will come from the organization itself, and if more funds are necessary to accomplish priorities and long and short-term goals, the manager should identify income sources within the department to facilitate the process.

- Other resources to be allocated include staff, materials, equipment and food.

c. Directing

- **DIRECTING** includes motivating, educating, guiding and communicating with employees. It is also called **SUPERVISING.**

- The **SPAN OF CONTROL** is the number of people one person supervises. A reasonable span of control is necessary for the supervisor to have time to monitor and evaluate activities and personnel properly. The span can be quite large if many people are doing similar tasks, for example, tray line workers. A smaller span of control is more appropriate if professionals are working in a technical area; i.e., a clinical dietitian supervising diet technicians.

(1) Coordination

- **COORDINATION** means synchronizing all departments and/or activities so that the organization's objectives are met with an efficient work flow.

(2) Delegation

- **DELEGATION** is the transfer of responsibility and authority for making decisions within the organizational structure.

- ✱Guidelines for delegating work are:
  - ➢ Delegate to those capable of accomplishing the assigned task.
  - ➢ Give the appropriate power and authority to act.
  - ➢ Provide sufficient facts to accomplish the task.
  - ➢ Provide training when necessary.
  - ➢ Provide necessary equipment, supplies and technology.
  - ➢ Add responsibility gradually.
  - ➢ Be available as a resource.
  - ➢ Tolerate some mistakes; be supportive.

(3) Communication

- **COMMUNICATION** is transmitting information from a sender to a receiver who must receive and interpret the information. People perceive and interpret information through individual filters of backgrounds, needs, emotions, values and experiences. They tend to trust or mistrust messages depending on the source. The biggest issue in communication is miscommunication, which happens with both oral and written messages. The manager is generally responsible for communication within a unit and to other units.

- Important communications should be in writing so that everyone receives the same message. All formal communications (e.g., employee evaluations) should be written to provide documentation.

- Effective oral communications require a respect for privacy, eye contact, speaking the same language on the same level and feedback that the communication has been received.

- Patterns of communication, within an organization, include the following:

  - ➤ **CIRCLE COMMUNICATIONS** are those in which each person can send messages to colleagues (peers, superiors, subordinates) openly and freely. Circle communication may sometimes be inefficient, but participants are generally happier and more motivated than in a more autocratic system. Quality assurance systems depend on circle communications.
  - ➤ **STAR COMMUNICATIONS** channel all messages through one individual who is in a leadership position (e.g., department heads who report to the same manager but have little direct contact with one another). Decision-making may be faster and more consistent because decisions are made by the leader. Members of a star communications system often send more messages, have more checkpoints, and take more responsibility for locating and correcting problems. This may be because they know the leader is aware of their actions and responses.

- With the popularity of e-mail, much of the communication in the workplace is electronic.

- Employers often have policies about use of e-mail, can track e-mail usage and content, and limit use of e-mail to business purposes. Inappropriate use of e-mail at work, including personal non-business communications during work hours, can be the cause for disciplinary, legal action or termination.

(4) Motivation strategies

- **MOTIVATION** is that which causes, channels and sustains human behavior. Motivation is the internal force that urges an individual to want or to act. A manager's leadership strengths include the ability to motivate subordinates to increase their performance and satisfaction. **ROLE PERCEPTION** is the understanding of the aspects of behavior that are necessary to achieve excellent performance. **PERFORMANCE LEVEL** is often described as the interplay between motivation, ability and role perception. *— good interview thought*

ABRAHAM MASLOW'S HIERARCHY OF HUMAN NEEDS is based on the premise that human needs depend on what one already has, and only unsatisfied needs influence behavior. Maslow lists five levels of universal needs to explain human behavior:

MASLOW'S HIERARCHY OF NEEDS

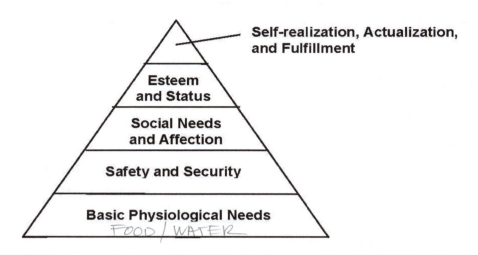

- Self-realization, Actualization, and Fulfillment
- Esteem and Status
- Social Needs and Affection
- Safety and Security
- Basic Physiological Needs *FOOD / WATER*

- For each need to become activated as a motivating factor, the need immediately preceding it must be fulfilled. Maslow believes that the way to stimulate motivation is to determine which of a person's wants is most unsatisfied and work to satisfy that need. For example, school lunch (physiological need to satisfy hunger) precedes learning how eating a variety of foods can keep you healthy (self-realization)—a hungry child does not care about a well-balanced diet.

meeting pt where they are at.

- **MCCLELLAND** found that people with a high need for achievement have the following characteristics of interest to managers:

  ➢ They like to take responsibility for solving problems.
  ➢ They tend to set moderately difficult goals for themselves and take calculated risks.
  ➢ They place great importance on concrete feedback on how well they are doing.

- **HERZBERG'S THEORY OF MOTIVATIONAL FACTORS** says that job satisfaction and motivation come from giving workers increasingly greater responsibility, autonomy and feedback on job performance. Key concepts are ability for growth in the job, keeping abreast of the organization, recognition of achievement and participation in group meetings.

- **HERZBERG'S MAINTENANCE (HYGIENE) FACTORS** is a two-factor theory that states that workers are more likely to be satisfied with marginal hygiene factors, such as pay, benefits, fair administrative policies and good working conditions if motivational factors, such as achievement, recognition and promotion opportunities are high. However, good hygiene factors help prevent reduced worker performance (work slow down) and reduce stress-related illness and absenteeism. These factors are necessary but not sufficient for employee motivation.

(5) Leadership styles, skills, techniques

- **LEADERSHIP** is the ability to accomplish organizational objectives by inspiring and influencing others through interpersonal relationships between the leader and those led.

- Effective leadership skills include the ability to get the job done through human interaction, integrity, character, empathy and objectivity. A leader presents facts, reviews alternatives to problems and continuously assesses and reviews needs.

- Personal traits of a successful leader include intelligence, dependability, objectivity, abundant energy, self-discipline, total commitment to goals of the organization, talent for swift, "cool" action when "the heat is on," desire to study and remain updated, involvement in outside social, political and civic activities, ability to spread enthusiasm, consistency in action, ability to control anger, ability to act with purpose, persuasive skills and good communication skills. A leader is able to talk and write clearly and forcefully, is self-assured, perceptive, creative and able to empathize, has confidence, is well adjusted; listens well; and believes in his or her ability to effectively handle most situations.

- Leadership styles vary. Effective leaders are dynamic and flexible and can adapt their style to meet varied situations.

  - **AUTOCRATIC** leaders make decisions and announce them to subordinates. The autocratic leader is "the boss."
  - **CONSULTATIVE DIPLOMATIC** leaders make decisions and then sell actions to subordinates.
  - **PARTICIPATIVE** leaders identify purpose, problems, and a tentative plan of action, but invite input from subordinates before making the final decision. Japanese management often uses this style.
  - **DEMOCRATIC** leaders ask subordinates to make decisions within limits defined by the manager.
  - **LAISSEZ-FAIRE** leadership is based on the economic doctrine that government should not interfere in commerce. In the same manner, the manager/leader is a figurehead who does not interfere with the decision-making process, but does set limits. This style of leadership is seldom found in healthcare organizations. It is more common in academic settings; i.e., rotating chairperson of a department.

- **QUALITY CIRCLES** are a participative management form started in Japan in 1962. In the quality circle, eight to ten employees from a work area meet regularly with a leader to solve problems related to quality, productivity, cost, safety, morale, housekeeping, working environment and so forth. Participants are taught problem-solving techniques. With good leadership and coaching, quality circles can improve communication between line workers and management, improve attitudes and behaviors, develop leadership and supervisory skills and generally result in measurable savings on projects. This style of leadership requires support and empowerment from management to implement recommendations.

• OHARI'S WINDOW is a management-style inventory developed by Luft and Ingham to help determine work and communication styles, as well as "fit" in a specific job situation. Individuals and their peers are asked to choose from a variety of adjectives which describe the individual's personality. These are then mapped into the following concepts:

> PUBLIC SELF is apparent to most people (color of eyes, height, sex).
> BLIND SELF needs feedback; others are aware, but individual is not aware (e.g., unconscious gestures like fingering hair, constant blinking).
> PRIVATE SELF involves self-perception. Trust is an issue; others are unaware, but individual is aware (eating behavior, birthplace, color preference).
> UNKNOWN or POTENTIAL SELF is still learning; requires future developments, such as the next job. Using this framework, the size of each compartment fluctuates depending on behavior observed by others. When more is known and shared and less is unknown by others, there is more opportunity for feedback for self-knowledge.

• The BLAKE-MOUTON MANAGERIAL GRID is used to help managers determine whether their values and feelings are task or people-oriented. On a Blake-Mouton grid, the vertical axis rates concern for people; the horizontal axis rates concern for production and structure. Both are nine point scales. Ratings high in consideration for both people and production indicate a team approach to leadership. Those high in consideration for people and low on production suggest a social or "country club" approach. Scores high in production and low on people indicate a task oriented leadership style. Those low both in production and people are identified as an "impoverished" leadership style..

(6) Management approaches

Classical/traditional approaches

• FREDERICK TAYLOR (1856-1915) was an engineer who took the scientific approach to management. Major concepts of SCIENTIFIC MANAGEMENT include:

> Emphasizing expertise and efficiency.
> Identifying the one right way to do a task.
> Matching the worker to the task.
> Educating and training the worker.
> Motivating with dollars.
> Formal management education. (Taylor was the first to advocate training).

• HENRY FAYOL (1841-1925), a mining engineer, organized management by function and grouping of activities (e.g., production, sales, finance) in France at about the same time as Taylor. Major contributions of MANAGEMENT BY FUNCTION include:

> Developing the principles of management - planning, organizing, leading, coordinating and controlling.
> Creating line and staff organizational chart.
> Emphasizing chain of command and formal authority.
> Advocating a narrow span of control.

- Taylor studied the individual in terms of time and motion; Fayol concentrated on major functions. Both took a passive view of the individual (simply a cog in the wheel) and advocated economic rewards for the worker.

Behavioral approaches

- The behavioral approach to management looks at the social and psychological nature of workers, the workplace as a social system, group dynamics, the impact of the small work group and leadership styles. Leaders in the behavioral management movement include the following:

  - **MARY PARKER FOLLET** (1868-1933) was the transitional agent from the classical approach to the behavioral or human relations approach. She was people-oriented and believed that where people work together, conflict would exist and that managers need to be able to resolve these issues.

  - **ELTON MAYO** (1880-1949) integrated behavioral sciences of psychology and sociology into management theory. Employee participation was emphasized and the needs of the employee stressed. Self-direction and self-control are common in this type of management. He believed that power centers are the interpersonal relationships in the working unit and that the leader facilitates the goals of the organization and the workers. Mayo based his theories on studies conducted at Western Electric's Hawthorne plant near Chicago. The **HAWTHORNE EFFECT** is the positive influence a change in the work environment has to increase employee output.

  - **DOUGLAS MCGREGOR** (1960) described two basic management attitudes toward employee behavior: Theory X and Theory Y.

    - **THEORY X** corresponds closely to the classical management theory where managers exert direct control over their employees. Theory X assumes that work is inherently distasteful to most people and that workers are not ambitious, do not want responsibility, and have little creativity. Managers who believe in Theory X are usually strict because they expect the worst from their employees, which may result in their employees acting or performing poorly.
    - **THEORY Y** parallels the human relations model that holds that workers accept responsibility and are self-motivated. Theory Y assumes that work is natural and enjoyable, and that workers are motivated, creative and want control of their work situation. Believers in Theory Y promote employee growth and development.
    - In practice, managers must adapt their style to the nature of workers and situations. No single approach will achieve the same results with all employees.

  - **RENSIS LIKERT** developed the theory of **PARTICIPATIVE MANAGEMENT** which states that management that encourages and rewards employee participation will result in higher productivity. Likert emphasized the multiple groups that exist within any given organization, encouraged decision making by group consensus and coined the term "linking pins" to identify those individuals who belong to and thus link more than one group.

384

- **THEORY Z**, proposed by **WILLIAM OUCHI** (1981) suggests that the key to Japan's economic success is management expertise and personnel policies. Theory Z emphasizes planning, decision-making by general agreement, and loyalty between workers and employers. Workers' loyalty is enhanced by guaranteed lifetime employment, evaluation and promotion, non-specialized careers and collective decision-making.

Management by Objectives

- **MANAGEMENT BY OBJECTIVES (MBO)** originated by **PETER DRUCKER**, involves setting specific, measurable goals with each employee and then periodically reviewing the progress made. MBO usually is a comprehensive, organization-wide program involving professional and managerial personnel.

  ➢ Benefits of MBO are that it improves commitment and motivation, directs work activity toward organizational goals, forces and aids in planning and control and assists in problem identification.

  ➢ Potential problems of MBO are setting unclear or immeasurable objectives, spending excessive amounts of time setting objectives, evaluating progress and the focus on achieving a goal hindering the actual quality of work.

Systems approach

- The **SYSTEMS APPROACH** (1970s) to management views the organization as a unified system of interrelated parts operating as a part of the larger, external environment. Systems theory says the activity of any part of the organization affects the activity of every other part. To mesh one department with the whole organization, a manager must work with other employees, other departments and representatives of other groups. The systems approach calls attention to the dynamic and interrelated nature of an organization and management tasks. Key terminology of the systems approach includes the following:

  ➢ **SUBSYSTEMS**: Parts that make up the whole.
  ➢ **SYNERGY**: The whole is greater than the sum of its parts.
  ➢ **OPEN SYSTEM**: The system interacts with its environment.
  ➢ **CLOSED SYSTEM**: The system does not interact with its environment (e.g., prison).
  ➢ **FLOW**: A system has flows of information, material and energy. These enter the system from the environment as **INPUTS** (raw materials), undergo transformation processes within the system and exit the system as **OUTPUTS** (goods and services).

Contingency approach

- The **CONTINGENCY APPROACH** (1960s) holds that there is no one best way to manage in every situation but that managers must find different ways to fit different situations. There are two inputs to increased productivity; the individual and the nature of the situation. The answer to the question, "What do I do?" is "It depends." The manager needs to diagnose the problem as it presents itself.

- **NETWORK ANALYSIS** helps the manager plan and control a project with many interdependent and sequential activities. Examples of network analysis include the following:

  ➢ **PROGRAM EVALUATION AND REVIEW TECHNIQUE (PERT)** uses a network analysis diagram to coordinate complex production processes. A **PERT CHART** aids a manager in organizing the production sequence, spotting possible scheduling difficulties, estimating completion time and controlling the entire production process. Using PERT technique, the manager needs to list all the activities required in the project, arrange the activities sequentially and estimate the time to accomplish each activity.

➤ The **CRITICAL PATH** is the sequence of events to complete a task. The activities along the critical path are those with time limits of greatest importance. A delay in any activity along the critical path will result in a delay of the whole production process. Computers usually generate this information. **CRITICAL PATH ANALYSIS** refers to identification of the longest set of adjoining activities from the start to the end of the network. The critical path analysis helps the manager to identify and plan all activities; coordinate planning, performance and control tasks; facilitate scheduling; and establish responsibilities and goals.

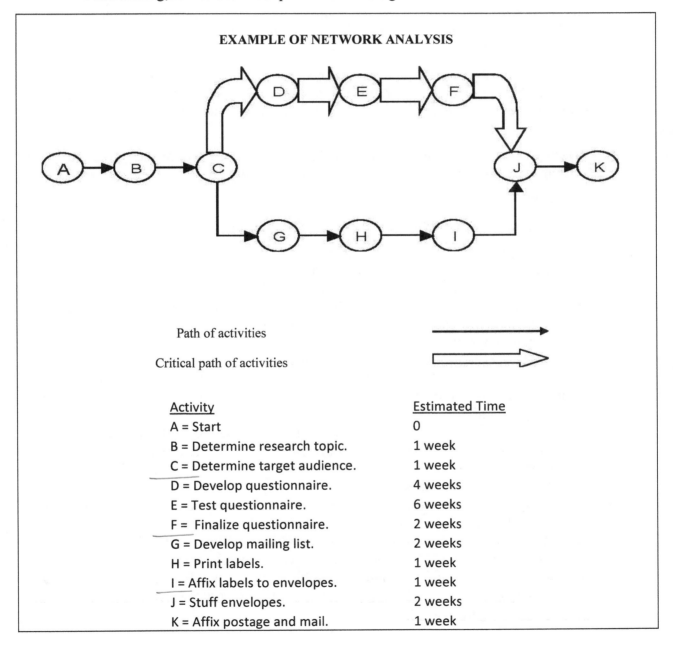

EXAMPLE OF NETWORK ANALYSIS

Path of activities

Critical path of activities

Activity	Estimated Time
A = Start	0
B = Determine research topic.	1 week
C = Determine target audience.	1 week
D = Develop questionnaire.	4 weeks
E = Test questionnaire.	6 weeks
F = Finalize questionnaire.	2 weeks
G = Develop mailing list.	2 weeks
H = Print labels.	1 week
I = Affix labels to envelopes.	1 week
J = Stuff envelopes.	2 weeks
K = Affix postage and mail.	1 week

d. Controlling

- The controlling function of management measures output, quality of product or service, supplies and labor costs and efficient use of employee time. Control prevents present and future deviations from plans and stimulates employees to keep on course. Directives should be put in terms of guidance rather than commands.

- Standards measure both quantity and quality of performance in specific, meaningful terms that enable managers to detect deviations from plans and take corrective actions. **QUANTITATIVE STANDARDS** include production figures, sales figures, labor hours, bacterial counts, temperatures, etc. **QUALITATIVE STANDARDS** include the number of rejects, complaints and returns.

- **STEERING CONTROLS** are reliable indicators that detect deviations that will influence results. Steering controls act as early warning indicators, allowing managers to take corrective actions. Examples include temperature of prepared food, bacteria count of product, monthly financial statementS, and suppliers delivering materials that do not meet specifications.

- **YES/NO CONTROLS** mandate specific aspect(s) that must be approved or conditions that must be met before an operation can continue. They are most often used where safety is a factor; for example, inspection for safety and sanitation of food transport vehicles.

- **POST-ACTION CONTROLS** measure results of a completed action; such as the number of participants in the program the last time it was offered.

e. Evaluating

- When conducting an evaluation interview, the evaluator should:

  - Select appropriate time and private place for interview.
  - Recognize that evaluations are stressful and emotion-laden.
  - Emphasize strengths on which to build rather than weaknesses to overcome.
  - Suggest appropriate actions rather than focusing on traits that are hard to change.
  - Point out opportunities for growth in the position.
  - Evaluate progress in relation to potential.
  - Treat a failure or mistake as an opportunity to learn.
  - Emphasize problem-solving. Determine the cause of problems (lack of training, inefficient system or equipment, personal problem) and assist with removing barriers when possible.
  - Discuss and identify several specific goals that can be accomplished within a reasonable period of time. The next evaluation uses the identified goals to assess performance.
  - Document goals and timelines.

- Monitoring must be a continuous process in order to correct defects and take advantage of opportunities. Managers cannot wait until all results are in to begin to evaluate performance. **CONTINUOUS IMPROVEMENT (CI) (**sometimes called **CONTINUOUS QUALITY IMPROVEMENT (CQI)** encourages each employee to monitor and report, without fear of reprimand, any potential problems that may affect intended goals and outcomes. In healthcare, CQI focuses on improving the processes of healthcare services to meet the needs of patients.

- Deviations from standards must be analyzed to determine corrective action or to take advantage of unexpected opportunities. Statistically significant variations are the basis of quality-assurance programs.

- A well-designed control system usually includes feedback of information to those performing the activity. The individuals whose actions are being monitored are usually in the best position to take corrective action because they are closest to the activity that needs correction.

- Care must be taken to assess whether the problem occurred because of the worker, the system or the equipment. Whenever possible, corrections should become "institutionalized" so they are not repeated elsewhere in the organization.

- Some institutions routinely assign the corrective action to the individual who made the error or caused the problem. Corrective actions should be noted on evaluation forms and plans should be developed to improve performance. Firing employees who err generally places the responsibility for correction on others.

2. Characteristics

a. Skills

(1) Technical

- TECHNICAL SKILLS include knowledge of and ability to use the processes, practices, techniques or tools of a specialty area. The relative importance of these skills depends on the level of management. Some technical skills (such as use of food service equipment) are more important at the lower levels of management, whereas conceptual skills are more important in top management. Computer skills are valued at all levels but top management can access support staff for some technical services.

(2) Human/managing diverse workforce

- HUMAN SKILLS include the ability to interact with other people successfully and the ability to understand, work with and relate to individuals and groups to get the work done.

- Diversity as a concept focuses on a broader set of qualities than just race and gender. In the context of the workplace, valuing diversity means creating a workplace that respects and includes differences, recognizing the unique contributions that individuals with many types of differences can make, and creating a work environment that maximizes the potential of all employees.

- Benefits of diversity in the workplace include:
  - ➤ Boosting employee morale.
  - ➤ Increasing employee productivity by utilizing talents.
  - ➤ Creating a work environment that allows all employees to reach their full potential.
  - ➤ Providing multiple options for dealing with workplace diversity.
  - ➤ Reducing complaints and grievances.
  - ➤ Acquiring multiple perspectives on problem solving.

(3) Conceptual

- **CONCEPTUAL SKILLS** include the ability to view the organization as a whole and to see how the parts of the organization relate to and depend upon one another, including the ability to integrate and coordinate the parts of an organization and its processes and systems.

  Management at all levels needs a combination of conceptual, human and technical skills in order to be effective. First-line management needs proportionately more technical skills in order to directly supervise employees. Middle management uses primarily human and communication skills. Top management focuses on planning and other functions that require relatively equal amounts of conceptual and human skills. Top management needs few technical skills. For example, first line management in a hospital food service operation must know scoop sizes to monitor portion control on the tray line, but the hospital administrator need not have these skills.

b. Roles

(1) Informational

- This role includes monitoring information, disseminating information from upper management to subordinates and keeping upper management informed. The role is one of a spokesperson and communicator. This role often requires writing and computer skills.

(2) Conflict resolution

- A manager must act as a mediator to resolve disputes that can be disruptive and lower morale and productivity. Conflicts should be resolved as quickly as possible and involve only the parties involved to limit extending the conflict.

(3) Problem-solving

- Managers have to make rational choices among alternatives. Problem-solving is a link between the five management functions - planning, organizing, staffing, directing and controlling. Managers have to deal with difficult problems and sometimes have to make unpopular decisions, such as closing a facility or reducing employee count.

- Steps in problem solving:
  - ➢ Step 1: Define the problem.
  - ➢ Step 2: Identify the limiting or critical factors.
  - ➢ Step 3: Develop possible alternatives.
  - ➢ Step 4: Analyze the alternatives.
  - ➢ Step 5: Select the best alternative.
  - ➢ Step 6: Implement the solution.
  - ➢ Step 7: Evaluate the outcome.

(4) Decision-making

- **HENRY MINTZBERG** (1975) defined management in terms of an organized set of behaviors including interpersonal, informational and decisional roles.

- **INTERPERSONAL ROLES** - The manager acts as a figurehead, leader or liaison. Figurehead roles are ceremonial, such as attending company dinners or signing proclamations. <u>Leadership roles</u> involve motivation and service on committees, both internal and external. <u>Liaison roles</u> involve gathering and sharing of information, establishing and maintaining contacts and effective communications

- The <u>three</u> **INFORMATIONAL ROLES** of managers are: 1) <u>Monitor - researching, receiving and collecting information relevant to the work to be done;</u> 2) <u>Disseminator - sharing information within the organization;</u> 3) <u>Spokesperson - sharing information outside of the organization.</u>

- There are <u>four</u> **DECISIONAL ROLES** of all managers: (1) <u>the entrepreneur initiates change to improve the situation;</u> (2) <u>the disturbance handler responds to situations beyond his or her control;</u> (3) <u>the resource allocator decides on the use of resources and screens all important decisions;</u> and (4) <u>the negotiator is usually the manager who has the information and authority to negotiate.</u>

  [handwritten: 1. entrepreneur   3. resource allocator]
  [handwritten: 2. disturbance handler   4. negotiator]

  (5) Other

- An organization's mission, history, traditions, goals and objectives including the style of the present top management, determines the manner and expectations for managers. The organization's expectations are reflected in its <u>policies</u>, operating <u>procedures</u>, <u>controls</u> and customs. Supporting charities or community activities is a strategy for building awareness and recognition for organizations and businesses.

c. Traits *[handwritten: p.360 - measures output, quality of product/service, supplies/labor cost & emp. time efficiency]*   *[handwritten: P.347: general guidelines for decision making / steps to achieve an objective or carry out = policy]*

  (1) Interpersonal communications

- Management effectiveness depends on how well an individual's traits match the requirements of a specific situation. Different traits such as aggressiveness, creativity and an outgoing or shy personality lend themselves to different leadership and/or management styles. Each person brings to the job a unique way of looking at things, a personal frame of reference that influences whatever is seen or heard. Current business practice values and supports diversity to achieve maximum potential from the workforce. Listening, particularly non-evaluative listening, promotes understanding the other person's point of view and is essential in the communication process. Other factors that influence interpersonal communications include differences in status, bias (racial, ethnic, gender, age) and education or training.

  (2) Use of authority, influence and power

- **AUTHORITY** is the right to make decisions that commit resources or give orders. Authority comes with the position, that is, from placement within the management hierarchy.

- Power and influence come from both management and workers. **POWER** is the capacity to act, and the strength and ability to accomplish something and to make choices and decisions. Power enables a person to influence or induce compliance from others. Power and influence can emanate from the position (job, rank) and from personal actions (behavior, personality). Some individuals are very influential within groups because of age, seniority or demonstrated personal characteristics that have earned the respect of the group.

- Good managers have, and respect, both kinds of power – that which comes from position as well as that which comes from behavior of personality. Specific types of power include the following:

  - ➢ **COERCIVE POWER:** Ability to punish or withhold benefits.
  - ➢ **REFERENT POWER:** Power from imitation or identification with an individual in power (e.g., the son of a business owner).
  - ➢ **EXPERT POWER:** Power from knowledge or expertise.
  - ➢ **REWARD POWER:** Power to reward through promotion, compensation, job assignment, office location, etc.

- Groups of workers, especially when informal leaders or unions are involved, have considerable influence and power within most organizations. Worker power can be expressed positively or negatively in increasing or decreasing personal and group productivity.

(3) Ethical practice — Three governing documents: ① Code of ethics ② SOP ③ SOPP

- All professionals should abide by a code of ethics for their profession. The Academy of Nutrition and Dietetics has established a *Code of Ethics for the Profession of Dietetics.* All parts of the *Code* pertain to all dietitians. . (See *AND/CDR Code of Ethics for the Profession of Dietetics,* JADA, August 2009, pp. 1461-67.)

- The **CODE of ETHICS** reflects values and ethical principles, setting forth commitments and obligations to the public, clients, the professors, colleagues and other professionals.

- Managers who make purchase decisions should be careful not to obligate themselves by accepting gifts or favors. Violations of the *Code of Ethics* can lead to removal of one's RD credential or exclusion from membership in AND.

- Managers must have the ability to build relationships and use persuasion and compromise to promote organizational goals and goodwill within the company and in dealing with customers, clients, contractors, government officials and others. The reputation for integrity requires consistent ethical practices.

3. **Professional standards of practice**

   a. **Standards of practice (SOP)**

   - **2012 STANDARDS OF PRACTICE IN NUTRITION CARE** are in the June supplement of the Journal.

   - Many AND dietetic practice groups have developed standards of practice for their particular areas of specialization.

   b. **Standards of professional performance**

   - The Academy of Nutrition and Dietetics (AND) has developed **STANDARDS OF PROFESSIONAL PERFORMANCE (SOPP)** for both RD's and DTR's, which describe minimum expectations for competent levels of practice and responsibilities for accountability. These are not rules or requirements of practice but rather they guide the practice and performance of nutrition professionals. They are supposed to be used as outcomes upon which the practitioner's performance is assessed and evaluated validly and reliably.

- As the SOP are specific to activities related to patient/client care in acute and long-term care, public health, community, extended care, and ambulatory care settings, they are formatted according to the four steps of the Nutrition Care Process. The SOPP are focused on professional behavior in all practice settings and cover six domains: 1) provision of services; 2) application of research; 3) communication and application of knowledge; 4) use and management of resources; 5) quality in practice; and, 6) competence and accountability.

- These two documents, along with the *Code of Ethics*, guide professional dietetics practice and can be used to effectively assess performance. (For more information see **www.eatright.org**).

c. Legislative process

- Dietetic professionals should understand the legislative process in any way that will help the nutritional health of their patients/clients and the well being of their employees.

- Dietitians can be advocates by communicating with legislators on the national, state or local level through visits to the legislators' offices, writing to them by e-mail, regular mail, or by calling their offices. Clients who have had successful experiences with dietitians can be encouraged to write to their legislators or testify at hearings on behalf of the dietetics profession. Legislators and/or their aides can be invited to visit the dietitian's work place to see what the dietitian does. Some dietitians become expert witnesses and some serve on campaign committees, donating their time and money.

- Legislators propose bills addressing situations where they or staff or friends have had personal problems or that have been called to their attention by constituents. Laws passed by legislative bodies are usually very broad in scope and are not specific. Once a law is passed, the departments to which they have been assigned write the specific regulations. At the federal level, all regulations must be published in the *Federal Register*, and the public is given a specific amount of time to answer the regulations, usually 90 days. AND's Washington office submits comments on some legislation and regulations on behalf of the Academy but individual dietetics professionals should take the time to comment on regulations regarding food and nutrition legislation as well.

TOPIC B - HUMAN RESOURCES

1. Recruitment and selection

- **RECRUITING** is the process of seeking a well-qualified individual for a position. Many companies have a personnel department or human resources department to assist in recruiting. Recruitment may be internal, external or both. Internal recruitment has many positive advantages, especially because the employee is familiar with the organization and its culture, thus training time may be significantly reduced. In some instances, internal recruitment alone may be illegal. External recruiting can be done through an employment agency, a school placement service, advertisements and/or announcements placed on a bulletin board at the facility. Posting jobs internally encourages current employees to apply for different or more challenging jobs. Online recruitment is a very popular method of seeking the most qualified applicants for a position. Applicants can post resumés to online resumé databases, which can be searched by human resources personnel to find suitable matches, or a company can post job availability on their website, Internet classified ads or chat rooms.

a. Laws and regulations

- For income tax purposes, an **EMPLOYER** is an individual, trust, corporation, partnership, estate, joint-stock company, association, group, pool, joint venture, group or entity that employs one or more employees. In general, an **EMPLOYEE** is an individual who performs services that are subject to the will and control of an employer regarding what must be done and how it must be done. Neither the number of employees, nor the length of time in which they work (i.e., part-time or full-time), method of payment, nor their age is material. It does not matter whether the employee is referred to as a partner, agent or temporary worker. For employees, an employer must withhold income and payroll taxes, contribute to the employer's portion of Social Security taxes (FICA) and pay unemployment and workers' compensation insurance.

- For income tax purposes, an **INDEPENDENT CONTRACTOR** is defined as one who is subject to another's control or direction merely for the result to be accomplished and not the means and methods for accomplishing the result. Payments to independent contractors are not subject to withholding taxes. Health insurance and other benefits need not be provided. An independent contractor needs to carry his or her own health and liability insurance and worker's compensation. The Internal Revenue Service (IRS) has a list of factors that determines the amount of control the recipient of services has over an individual who performs work. The importance of each factor is determined on a case-by-case basis. Those who engage the services of independent contractors or classify themselves as such (i.e., weight control counselors, freelance health writers) should seek professional advice from a tax expert.

- The **SOCIAL SECURITY ACT** of 1935 and its amendments encompass a variety of programs that include old age, survivors, disability, health insurance, unemployment compensation, public assistance, health and welfare.

  ➢ The original act provided payments to retired employees, age 65 and older.
  ➢ It was amended in 1956 to lower eligibility age of women to 62.
  ➢ It was amended in 1961 to lower eligibility age of men to 62.
  ➢ It was amended in 1983 to increase retirement age from 65 to 66 by the year 2009 and to age 67 by 2027 for full benefits. One can choose to receive benefits as early as 62 but monthly benefits are permanently reduced by 20-30% for early payments.

- The **OLD AGE, SURVIVORS AND DISABILITY INSURANCE** (OASDI) gives old age benefits after retirement in monthly payments for the rest of the beneficiary's life. Benefits are provided to survivors and disabled children whose disability occurred before age 18. Employers and employees share equally in the cost of programs. Deductions from paychecks are taken from each paycheck in an amount specified by the federal government. The employer must match the amount.

- The **SUPPLEMENTARY SECURITY INCOME ACT** of 1972 (SSI) supports individuals with limited income and assets and who are 65 years or older, blind or disabled..

- The **MEDICARE ACT** of 1965 pays for most hospital and medical care for individuals age 65 and over. Part A covers hospitalization, and Part B covers doctors and some other out patient services. Part B is optional and must be paid for separately. Registered Dietitians can be reimbursed for nutrition care services for diabetes and non-dialysis renal disease through Part B. Registered Dietitians must apply to Medicare in order to be providers of MNT. See and website, **www.eatright.org** for further information. Another optional Medicare program is the Drug Plan (Part D), which started on January 1, 2006.

- **UNEMPLOYMENT INSURANCE** includes both federal (Federal Unemployment Tax [FUTA]) and state programs. To be eligible for unemployment pay, an individual must be able and available for work. An individual is not eligible if he or she quits a job without good cause, is discharged because of misconduct, is involved in a labor dispute causing a work stoppage, or if he or she refuses to take suitable employment.

- **WORKERS' COMPENSATION** is a state-regulated program that originated in 1908 to cover medical costs for injuries incurred on the job. Workers' compensation must be secured by insurance obtained and paid for by the employer or the individual who operates as an independent contractor, if required by those with whom they do business. Workers must prove they were injured on the job and the extent of their injuries in order to be compensated.

- The **NATIONAL LABOR RELATIONS ACT (NLRA)** of 1935, also called the **WAGNER ACT**, established the National Labor Relations Board to enforce provisions of this law. This act is pro-labor in its intent because workers had been exploited in the past. It established the right of workers to organize and join labor unions, to choose representation, to bargain collectively, and, in most cases, to strike. It prohibits management from interfering with employees joining a union and from discriminating against those who do.

- The **FAIR LABOR STANDARDS ACT (FLSA)** of 1938 helped reduce poverty, create purchasing power and establish a Federal minimum wage. Maximum hours, equal pay, overtime pay, record keeping, employee meals and meals credit, tip regulations, uniform and uniform maintenance, and child labor provisions covering the majority of American workers are also included in this Act. It has been amended many times for the purpose of raising the minimum wage. The act is enforced by the U.S. Department of Labor.

- The **TAFT-HARTLEY ACT** of 1947 also known as The **LABOR MANAGEMENT RELATIONS ACT** is pro-management. It amended the Wagner Act, although most provisions of the Wagner Act were left in place. It outlaws **CLOSED SHOPS** that require union membership before hiring. It permitted **UNION SHOPS** in which a person must join the union within a specified time after being hired. Provisions are aimed at limiting unions by: (1) prohibiting union unfair labor practices, (2) stating the rights of employees as union members, (3) stating rights of employers, and (4) allowing the president of the United States to temporarily stop national strikes for up to 80 days. The law was extended in 1974 to include private nonprofit hospitals and nursing homes. Requirements are that unions representing workers in these healthcare facilities give 90 days notice (30 days more than other industries) before terminating a labor agreement. Labor disputes in healthcare facilities must automatically be submitted to mediation conducted by the Federal Mediation and Conciliation Service or a similar state agency to avoid strikes that would close essential services.

- The **LABOR-MANAGEMENT REPORTING AND DISCLOSURE ACT** of 1959 (Landrum-Griffin Act) is a second amendment to the Wagner Act. It protects union members from misconduct by the union, for example, misuse of pension funds.

- The **EQUAL PAY AMENDMENT** of 1963 amended the Fair Labor Standards Act. It requires equal pay for women doing the same work as men. This act is enforced by the Equal Employment Opportunity Commission (EEOC.)

- The **CIVIL RIGHTS ACT** of 1964 states, "No person in the United States shall, on the basis of race, color or national origin, be excluded from participating in, be denied the benefits of, or be subjected to, any program or activity receiving federal financial assistance."

- **TITLE VII OF THE CIVIL RIGHTS ACT** of 1964, as amended by the **1972 EQUAL EMPLOYMENT OPPORTUNITY ACT**, forbids employers, employment agencies and labor unions from using race, sex, color, religion or national origin as a basis for making employment decisions, except where possession of a particular characteristic is a bona fide occupational qualification. Seniority or merit systems are acceptable as long as they do not discriminate. This law applies to all firms with more than 25 employees. The Equal Employment Opportunity Commission (EEOC) was created by Title VII to investigate complaints. The law was further amended in 1974, to include sexual harassment by an employer. In 1978, the **PREGNANCY DISCRIMINATION ACT** was passed. This broadened the definition of sexual discrimination to include pregnancy, childbirth or related medical conditions.

- The **AGE DISCRIMINATION IN EMPLOYMENT ACT** of 1967 prohibits discriminatory employment practices, based on age, for persons between the ages of 40 and 69. It was amended in 1978 to extend coverage age to 70, and again in 1986, to prohibit employers from requiring retirement at any age.

- The **OCCUPATIONAL SAFETY AND HEALTH ACT** of 1970, sets standards to ensure every working man and woman in the nation safe and healthful working conditions. It is enforced by the Occupational Health and Safety Administration (OSHA), an agency within the Department of Labor. The act requires occupational illnesses and occupational injuries to be reported by employers with 11 or more employees.

- The **JOB TRAINING PARTNERSHIP ACT** of 1983 replaced the earlier Comprehensive Employment and Training Act (CETA). This act provides funds to state and federal agencies to train and find employment for those in the community who are hard to employ. For example, some Women, Infant and Children (WIC) programs hire outreach workers under this act.

- The **IMMIGRATION REFORM AND CONTROL ACT** of 1986 (IRCA) discourages illegal immigration by requiring employers to hire only persons who may legally work in the United States. Legal workers include citizens and nationals of the United States and aliens authorized to work. The law was amended in 1990 to provide that no individual be discriminated against because of national origin or citizenship in hiring, firing, recruiting or referring. Form I-9 must be completed for every employee hired after November 6, 1986, and must be kept on file for three years after termination. The U.S. Department of Justice, Immigration and Naturalization Service (INS) issues the form. The form is completed when the employee begins work. Within three business days, the employer must review the employee's documents. The employee must present one original document that establishes identity (e.g., U.S. passport, certificate of naturalization, U.S. driver's license, ID card with photo or current refugee travel document). In addition, the employee must provide one original document that establishes employment eligibility (e.g., U.S. Social Security card, original birth certificate, Native American tribal document or current employment authorization document issued by the INS).

- The **AMERICANS WITH DISABILITIES ACT** (ADA) was enacted by Congress in July 1990. It is important civil rights legislation protecting people with disabilities from discrimination and promoting equal access to opportunities in the workplace. The Americans with Disabilities Act defines an individual with a disability as a person with a physical or mental impairment that substantially limits one or more major life activities. The individual must have a record of such impairment or be regarded as having impairment. Examples of disabilities include; mental retardation, mental illness, paralysis, visual impairment, loss of limbs, cancer, AIDS, learning disabilities, recovered alcoholics or drug addicts who no longer use alcohol or drugs, individuals with controlled high blood pressure and individuals with disfigurements.

  - The Act applies to government at all levels, private employers, employment agencies and labor unionswith over 15 employees.
  - Employers are required to provide *reasonable accommodation* for *qualified individuals* with disabilities, unless doing so would cause great financial hardship. Appropriate actions include making facilities readily accessible, modifying work schedules and providing qualified readers or interpreters.
  - Under the Act, people with disabilities are entitled to full and equal goods, services, facilities, privileges and accommodations. Public transit vehicles must be adapted to be accessible to those with disabilities.
  - Telephone companies must provide special services (TDD) for individuals with hearing and speech disabilities as of July 26, 1993.
  - New public facilities designed and constructed for first occupancy after January 26, 1993 must be handicapped accessible. Redesign of some facilities may be eligible for tax credits. Design or redesign may include installation of ramps, removal of steps, wider aisles and doorways, worktables of altered height, Braille buttons on elevators, handrails and so forth.

- The **FAMILY MEDICAL LEAVE ACT (FMLA)** of 1993, covers all private employees, state employees, and federal employees who work for an employer with 50 or more employees within 75 miles of a given workplace. The act entitles all eligible employees a maximum of 12 weeks leave during any 12-month period. An eligible employee is an individual who has worked for the employer a minimum of 12 months and 1,250 hours in the past year. Health insurance must be continued at the same level it was when the employee was working. The employee must be allowed to return to the same job or a job with equivalent status and pay, under most conditions. The leave can be unpaid or accrued paid leave may be used, for the following:

  - Birth of a child.
  - Placement (by the state) of a child for adoption or foster care.
  - Caring for a spouse, child, or parent with a serious health condition (inpatient care in hospital, hospice, residential medical facility, or continuing care by an MD or DO.)

b. Job analysis, specifications and descriptions

- A **JOB ANALYSIS** indicates all aspects of the job activities of the individuals who will be hired to achieve the goals of the organization. It includes the work to be done, the type of person who should be hired to do it and its relationship to other jobs. An uninvolved individual usually does the job analysis. From the job analysis, the job specification and job description are created

- A **JOB SPECIFICATION** sets minimum qualifications needed to perform the job. It typically includes payroll title, department, supervisor, job summary, education, experience, skills, physical and personal requirements, references, hours and wages and promotional opportunities.

- A **JOB DESCRIPTION** also called **POSITION DESCRIPTION** should be available for every position in a department. It is used as the basis for preparing job evaluations, recruitment procedures, training requirements and performance appraisals. It includes job titles, job code, location, job summary, performance requirements (responsibilities, knowledge, skills, equipment used, standard of production expected), supervision, relation to other jobs and qualifications (experience, education).

- **STAFFING PATTERNS** are established by management to determine the appropriate number of employees presently employed and the number needed for future employment.

Types or categories of employees

- **FULL-TIME EMPLOYEE** is one who is expected to work the number of hours each week that the employer designates as "full time." The usual number of hours designated as full time is 40, but in some instances, 35 or 37.5 hours per week is considered full-time. An employer can expect to pay a full-time worker who works 40 hours a week for 2,080 hours of work in a year. Full-time workers probably do not actually work 2,080 hours however, because they are usually entitled to some paid time off such as for vacation, holidays, sick or personal leave.

- **FULL-TIME EQUIVALENT EMPLOYEE (FTE)** A full-time equivalent is the ratio of the total number of paid hours during a specific time period. The employee who is full-time is paid as one FTE. Part-time employees are considered fractions of one FTE. If full-time employees work 40 hours per week and a part-time employee works 20 hours per week, the employee would be considered as 0.5 FTEs.

- **PART-TIME EMPLOYEE** works a pre-determined number of hours a week, but that number is less than what is considered to be full-time (e.g., 24 hours per week). They may work more hours than this, but they are guaranteed only the pre-determined work hours.

- **SHORT HOUR EMPLOYEE** is defined as one who has a pre-determined number of hours to work per week, but that number is less than half-time, or less than 20 hours per week. These workers are typically not entitled to benefits such as health insurance or retirement, and are used to help organizations save on labor costs.

- **CASUAL EMPLOYEE** is a worker who is not guaranteed a set number of hours each week but who may be scheduled to work as needed. These employees are sometimes referred to as "on call" workers because they may be called in to work on short notice to meet a particular need. However, the term "casual" is a better term since these employees are often scheduled in advance, such as when they cover for another employee who is going on vacation.

- **JOB SHARING** occurs when two or more individuals work in tandem to perform a full-time job. The workload may be divided in any number of ways to meet the situation and the people involved. A benefit of this arrangement includes the fact that there are two people who bring their individual ideas, talents and skills to the job. It can also provide the benefit of a flexible schedule for the employee. Disadvantages are that there can be a lack of continuity and decreased productivity and communication problems can occur about who is responsible for tasks and when they are to be done.

- **PROBATIONARY EMPLOYEE** is one who is newly hired into a position. For a set period of time, typically 60 to 90 days, the worker is learning a job and getting acquainted with the work environment. During the probation period, the employer can terminate the worker "without cause" if it appears the worker cannot learn the tasks required or demonstrates behavior that is problematic. Employees who work beyond the probationary period cannot usually be fired unless there is cause.

- **TEMPORARY WORKERS** may be needed for a specific job or project, to cover leave of absence or when there is a short-term need for extra employees. They may or may not be placed on the payroll of the employer. Temporary workers who are not on the employer's payroll may be hired through a temporary employment agency. All types of workers from unskilled to professional staff may be hired in this way. Workers are employed and paid by the agency. The employer, in turn, pays the agency for the use of these workers.

- **CONTRACT EMPLOYEE** is one who is hired to do a job that is finite in nature. The work is frequently contracted out as a one-time job. A contract employee may be hired from a temporary or contract agency, or the worker may be hired as an independent or freelance consultant. The contract employee may be paid a fee for the project or may be paid at an hourly rate.

- Both temporary and contract employees may be grouped together under the term **CONTINGENT WORKER.** This term differentiates these workers from career employees. Contingent workers know that their positions are not permanent, whereas career employees expect to have a job as long as their work performance is acceptable. Contingent workers do not get any health benefits, paid vacation days or sick leave.

c. Performance standards

- Performance standards and indicators are used to plan workload and to evaluate the performance for an individual, a group of workers or a department. Standards are an important element in the continuous improvement process of a quality assurance program.

- **MEASURED STANDARDS** define the quantitative content of work tasks, establish the standard time it takes to perform such tasks and determine the number of employees required to accomplish the work to be done. The standards are recorded in written form. The measurement process is complex, time consuming and applicable only to conditions at the time of measurement. Measured standards are not always feasible. Measurement is easier in production- oriented departments, such as medical records and housekeeping.

- **STANDARD METHODOLOGIES** are descriptions of a typical workload and times to accomplish components. In some hospitals, computer-based data processing systems perform the calculations and produce desired managerial information based on the workload needs of the department.

- **CONSTANT WORKLOAD** includes activities that are not directly associated with departmental output or that must be performed regardless of volume, such as maintaining the facilities.

- **VARIABLE WORKLOAD** is directly related to production, such as number of admissions, examinations and laboratory tests.

d. Candidate recruitment

- **DIVERSITY** refers to human qualities that are different from our own and those of groups to which we belong; but that are manifested in other individuals and groups. Dimensions of diversity include, but are not limited to: age, ethnicity, gender, physical abilities/qualities, race, sexual orientation, educational background, geographic location, income, marital status, military experience, parental status, religious beliefs, work experience and job classification.

- Diversity is a goal and the work force should generally reflect the population of the community it serves in all its dimensions. Training to promote diversity promotes an atmosphere of inclusion and respect. Affirmative action and other laws require that workplaces do not discriminate in hiring, promotion or other practices. Sensitivity is needed to assure that all workers are treated respectfully. One should not assume that others have the same values, customs or beliefs. The need to participate in religious observances of those of varied ethnic and religious traditions should be accommodated. Many religions have specific food laws and holiday traditions that must be respected for patients, clients, staff and others.

e. Candidate screening

- **SCREENING** is choosing the best potential candidates for a job from among those who inquire about the position. Someone often does screening other than the person(s) who will make the final employee selection.

- **HIRING** is making a formal offer of a job. Hiring is accomplished through applications, interviews, and an optional review examination and physical examination. Before hiring, management needs to examine a candidate's ability to be trained, desire to learn, willingness to cooperate, ability to accept criticism, work effectiveness and skill level.

- References should always be checked before hiring. Inadequate reference checking is one of major causes of high turnover, theft and white-collar crime.

- Before hiring, potential employees should be informed if drug testing and/or a physical examination are required for employment. That way a prospective employee can decline, without taking a drug test. A physical examination cannot be required before a position is offered.

f. Candidate interviewing

- To prepare for the interview, the interviewee should be provided with the job description to ensure familiarity with requirements of the job. The interviewer should schedule a face-to-face meeting with each candidate to assess their abilities, their aptitude for the job, their potential for contributing value to the organization, and their willingness to work the times necessary for the job. Because food service and healthcare is a 7-day a week job, many employees must work weekends and holidays. This requirement should be made clear early in the interview process to avoid wasting time of both parties.

- The interview process consists of several steps:
  - (1) Pre-interview—The interview should be relevant. Review the job description, secure a quiet setting for the interview, review applications, provide a position description to the applicant and schedule the interview.
  - (2) Opening the interview—Review roles and responsibilities of the position, functions of the agency and allow the applicant to pose questions to clarify the position. It is at this point that the interviewer must attempt to establish rapport with the applicant.
  - (3) Questioning the applicant.

- The structure of the interview should be determined before the appointment. A **STRUCTURED INTERVIEW** consists of a series of carefully planned questions that the interviewer asks of each job applicant. The interviewer does not deviate from the list.

  - The advantages to this type of interview are that the interviewer optimizes his/her ability to compare candidates and maximizes the amount of consistent documentation acquired for each candidate. The latter relates to Equal Employment Opportunity since it becomes more difficult for a rejected candidate to claim discrimination.
  - The disadvantage is that the interviewer cannot react to a candidate's responses.
  - The **UNSTRUCTURED INTERVIEW** requires the least amount of preparation. While the interviewer should have a complete understanding of the job requirements, only general questions need to be formulated before the interview takes place.
  - The advantage is that there can be responses to answers and additional questions can be formulated.
  - This type of interview takes more time, which can be a disadvantage, especially if there is a large applicant pool.
  - A mixture of the two types of interview, the **SEMI-STRUCTURED INTERVIEW**, may offer a good alternative.
  - (4) Closing the interview—Inform applicant how notification will occur, confirm address, e-mail address, and telephone number (home or cell), obtain references and answer questions from applicant. Specific job duties and responsibilities, work hours and conditions, opportunities for advancement, department and facility organization should be provided to the interviewee.
  - (5) Post-interview—Review the selection criteria, rank applicants, check references on top choices. Notify all applicants interviewed prior to announcing the selection.

- By law, questions cannot be asked about national origin, religion, marital status or age, physical or mental disability, sexual orientation, transportation, children, height or weight, type of discharge from the military, credit history or reference or arrest record. Citizenship status may not be asked unless you decide to hire the person. Be careful that the questions you ask are job related. Acquired immune deficiency syndrome (AIDS) testing is a recurring issue. There is an emerging legal view that AIDS is a handicap and therefore cannot be considered a negative factor in hiring. Acceptable interview questions fall into general, technical and situational categories:

  - General: "Why do you want this job?" "In what areas do you excel?"
  - Technical: "What software programs are you familiar with?" "What enteral or parenteral products have you used?" "What special training programs have you taken?"

> ➤ Situational (to evaluate interpersonal skills and management potential): "How would you deal with a subordinate who repeatedly does not complete required documentation about patients?"

- The interview and selection process should conform to ethical standards assuring privacy and confidentiality as well as legal requirements.

- Pre-employment testing may be valuable in the selection of the best candidate. Tests, such as skill tests, intelligence tests, personality tests, integrity tests may be required as long as they are relevant to the position. In clinical areas, a model case study may be given to the prospective employee to complete before leaving on the day of the interview.

2. Employment process and procedures

Orientation and training

- All new employees should be offered a well-planned **ORIENTATION PROGRAM.** This familiarizes and acquaints a new employee to the organization, the department, and the job responsibilities. A good orientation program will save time because the employee will understand the responsibilities of the job in a timely fashion, and learn proper ways to carry out the requirements of the position.

- **TRAINING PROGRAMS** differ from orientation programs in that training programs should teach or improve skills and concepts. A primary objective of training is to keep skills at a good level or to improve performance to acceptable levels. Training programs should also be established for employees you think may have the potential to be promoted. Re-training may be necessary for current employees who are not performing at a high enough level or if the job or equipment has changed since initial employment.

a. Personnel information

(1) Records

- **EMPLOYMENT RECORDS** are written information concerning a specific employee (e.g., name, address, spouse, children, educational background, former employment, hiring date, job assigned, wage rate, absences with reason, adjustments in work and wages, performance appraisal reports, promotions, demotions, transfers and information concerning insurance and health benefits). Records form a basis for employee merit ratings, salary adjustments and documentation for termination or disciplinary action.

- Organizations have policies about how to handle employee information, including job descriptions, performance reviews, disciplinary actions and so forth.

- A **PERSONNEL FILE** includes a description of an employee's job as it relates to the mission and purpose of the company. Documentation related to hiring, contracts, tax information and performance evaluation are in this file. Specific written documentation of actions that are particularly noteworthy (e.g., letters of commendation, awards) or negative (complaints, safety problems, high absentee rate) should be filed and used in the employee's performance appraisal. Federal laws give individuals the right to review the items in their personnel files.

- The Immigration Reform and Control Act requires employers to complete an I-9 form verifying workers identity and eligibility to work in the United States. This form should be in the employee's records.

- It is important that written records be kept to document what the employee has been told, what agreements have been made and any other information. After a performance appraisal, both employee and supervisor should sign a copy of the appraisal and the agreed upon goals. One copy goes to the employee, and one copy goes in the employee's personnel file. If an employee is given an ultimatum (e.g., reduce patient tray errors, attend an alcohol treatment program, learn new computer system) to meet within a set period of time or be terminated, the supervisor should have a letter acknowledging understanding of the conditions signed by both the employee and a witness.

(2) Confidentiality

- The **PRIVACY ACT** OF 1974 gives individuals the right to review their records in any private business that contracts with a federal agency.

- All employee records should be maintained as confidential records with access limited to personnel contributing to or maintaining the records.

- When giving information on a former employee, managers should be careful not to violate confidentiality. The **EQUAL EMPLOYMENT OPPORTUNITY ACT** and the **FAIR CREDIT REPORTING ACT** allow a rejected applicant access to the background information that was part of the recruitment process. Some organizations have policies to release only information that the individual was employed on particular dates and to provide no additional information. This verifies employment but avoids giving reasons for separation.

b. Unions/contracts

- A **LABOR UNION** is a legally sanctioned, formally organized association of workers united to represent their collective views on wages, hours and working conditions.

  - ➢ Principles of unions are: strength through unity; equal pay for equal work; employment practices based on seniority (i.e., promotion, raises, layoffs).
  - ➢ Rights and responsibilities of unions are to: protect the welfare and well-being of workers; raise living standards; establish job rights and security; use strength of numbers to get fair wages and working conditions; bargain for employees; set standard wages and procedures; adjust grievances; help employees find work; influence government on behalf of employees.
  - ➢ Union member rights and responsibilities are to: take part in union affairs; attend meetings; vote in union elections; discuss wages and conditions of contracts; enjoy union benefits; receive death burial benefits; receive union publications; pay dues.

- **COLLECTIVE BARGAINING** is negotiation between representatives of management and employees (union) about conditions of employment, wages and hours, leading to an agreement (contract) between employees and management. Arenas in which bargaining takes place include single unit (department), company-wide, industry-wide and coalitions.

- Bargaining strategies include the following: *"Labor-management relations"*

  - ➢ **GOOD-FAITH ATTITUDE** is the cornerstone of effective labor-management relations. Both parties communicate and negotiate. Proposals are met with counter-proposals and both parties make reasonable efforts to reach agreement.
  - ➢ **MILITANT ATTITUDE** is based on conflict; this is called the "blue sky" approach because the initial demands by both parties are excessive.

> **HORSE-TRADING ATTITUDE** involves trading one demand for another, based on strength; for example, increased health benefits may be offered in exchange for limits on accrued vacation time.
> **DEFEATIST ATTITUDE** is prevalent among smaller, inexperienced management teams who fear unions and agree to the demands of a dominating union or to small unionized groups who fear plant closings.
> **ACCEPTANCE ATTITUDE** is considered to be realistic, quiet and passive.

- **MEDIATION** involves a neutral mediator agreed upon by both parties who takes part in negotiations. Parties are not obligated to accept recommendations made by the mediator. Often parties reach an impasse and their dispute remains unsettled.

- **ARBITRATION** is the most definitive type of third-party intervention. The appointed arbitrator usually has power to determine and dictate the settlement terms, guaranteeing a solution to an impasse. In **BINDING ARBITRATION**, both parties are required to accept the arbitrator's decision. In **NON-BINDING ARBITRATION**, they are not.

- Unions are active in companies through the following:
  > **UNION SHOP:** Any employee may be hired but must join the union after hiring. The union represents the workers in bargaining as the bargaining agent. In certain states, union shops are illegal.
  > **OPEN SHOP:** Employees are not required to join the union. This is also called a **NON-UNION SHOP.** Those who do not join the union do not pay dues.
  > **CLOSED SHOP:** Employees must join the union before they are hired. This was outlawed in 1947.
  > **AGENCY SHOP:** Any bargaining unit employee who is not a union member must pay a service fee to the union for its representation on the assumption that union efforts benefit all employees.

- Management's best strategy in dealing with a union is to prepare for negotiations and to be realistic and flexible. Generally, the Human Resources Department represents management and strives to avoid confrontations with unions by providing fair compensation and working conditions. Benefits given to unions are seldom rescinded and become cumulative over the years. Legal actions of management include:

  > **LOCKOUT** in which management locks the doors, thus preventing union employees from entering. The lockout is rarely used because it often generates negative publicity toward management in the community.
  > **PLANT CLOSING** is when management sells the facility and moves rather than surrender to demands of labor. The threat of closing and subsequent job loss often leads to compromises.
  > **INJUNCTION** is a court order prohibiting either party from performing an unjust, inequitable or injurious act. For example, there may be an injunction to keep a facility open because it provides power or needed services to a community.
  > **STRIKEBREAKERS** are non-union workers who perform jobs until striking workers come to terms with management. They are called "scabs" by union members.
  > **MANAGEMENT-RUN OPERATIONS** occur when supervisory, technical or clerical personnel run equipment or perform functions when the regular personnel walk off the job.

- ➢ Hiring **LOBBYISTS** is when persons are employed to influence state and federal legislators to sponsor or vote for or against laws that further particular interests (either union or management.)

- Illegal actions of management include:

  - ➢ **BLACKLIST:** A list of pro-union workers is circulated and employment opportunities are denied to them.
  - ➢ **YELLOW-DOG CONTRACT:** Employees sign an agreement with management that they will not join a union.

- Labor strategies include the following:

  - ➢ **STRIKE:** Temporary work stoppage to protest working conditions.
  - ➢ **PICKET:** Employees publicly air complaints against the employer by staging a demonstration outside the building, usually with signs that discourage patrons from entering.
  - ➢ **BOYCOTT:** Refusal to do business with a given party or buy services until demands are met. Labor may also place ads in newspapers asking potential patrons to boycott a business that is unfair to labor.

c. Disciplinary action

- The purpose of employee discipline is to try to help employees improve the quality and/or quantity of their work and to help decrease/eliminate abusive, disruptive or unsafe practices.

- If the disciplinary process is effective, fellow employees will have an improved work environment.

- Each organization should have its own clear written policies and procedures regarding disciplinary action but there are some general guidelines.

  - ➢ The first formal step in the disciplinary process is a verbal warning in the privacy of the manager's office where the employee and manager discuss the problem and possible solutions from both points of view. The meeting is documented, but the report is not usually placed in the employee's file. If improvement is shown in a pre-specified time, the report is not usually filed, but if there is no improvement, then the report is placed into the employee's personnel file. If there is not sufficient improvement, a written warning should be followed with suspension, and depending on the nature of the problem, termination.

  - ➢ Generally, the manager should not be confrontational, but should point out the problems seen in the employee's work. If this is a probationary employee, a time limit should be set for employee improvement, suspension or possible termination. Written comments should be shown to the employee. After the conference the manager and employee should both sign the report so there is a written record to place in the employee's file.

d. Grievances

- A **GRIEVANCE** is a circumstance regarded as a justifiable cause for protest on the part of an employee. Grievances are usually settled on an informal basis. If employees are unionized, the contract includes formal grievance procedures, including presentation of the grievance in writing and guidelines for handling disputes. Usually, the first attempt to settle disputes is at the supervisory level rather than higher management levels.

- All employees should be aware of the codes of conduct for employees. Procedures for disciplinary action should describe authorized penalties and mechanisms for employee appeal.

- Employees should feel comfortable going to managers or supervisors with grievances regarding real or perceived mistreatment on the part of a supervisor or a co-worker. Departments should have a written process for dealing with these issues and workers should be made aware of the steps to be taken.

- State and federal law prohibits harassment of employees because of their sex. Both males and females can be victims of sexual harassment. This should be further spelled out in company policy. Employers can be held legally liable for sexual harassment that occurs in the work place. Examples of **SEXUAL HARASSMENT** include:

  ➢ Verbal or physical abuse of a sexual nature, including graphic comments about a person's body, sexually degrading words and display of sexually explicit objects or pictures.
  ➢ Overt or subtle pressures or requests for sexual favors.
  ➢ Unnecessary or inappropriate touching.
  ➢ Suggestions or a threat that imply that an employee's work status and/or career advancement is contingent upon sexual toleration or acquiescence to sexual advance.
  ➢ Unwelcome sexual advances or conduct that creates an intimidating, hostile or offensive working environment.

- Sexual harassment is included as a form of sex discrimination, prohibited by Title VII of the Civil Rights Act of 1964. Government guidelines suggest that employers have clear policy statements discouraging harassment, procedures for reporting incidents, employees designated to receive complaints, defined actions for violators, management support for policies and protection from reprisal for those initiating harassment complaints.

- An individual who views another's conduct as inappropriate (e.g., sexual comments, touching or threats) may make an allegation of sexual harassment. Accused individuals will be held accountable, even if the conduct was not intended to be offensive. Employers or individuals found to be engaging in harassment are subject to warning, disciplinary action or termination. All allegations should be investigated promptly, handled confidentially and documented thoroughly.

- If one becomes aware of an incident of sexual harassment, he or she should report it to the authorized individual, but not discuss the issue with the alleged offender or anyone else. If the case or issue is discussed with anyone other than those who legally need to know, there is risk of a personal lawsuit for defamation of character.

- The **EQUAL EMPLOYMENT OPPORTUNITY COMMISSION (EEOC)** is the agency of the federal government responsible for enforcing laws prohibiting employment discrimination. In addition, the Civil Rights of 1991 allows up to $300,000 punitive and compensatory damages.

Employee counseling and assistance programs

- Counseling may be verbal or written communication between an employee and a supervisor regarding work habits, or it may be counseling provided by or through the personnel or human resource department (e.g., alcoholism, child care, retirement.) Employee counseling is important in the quality assurance program because it helps employees do their jobs correctly and supports them in times of need.

- Employee assistance programs help employees with personal problems that can potentially affect job performance such as substance abuse, mental health problems, AIDS or family problems. These programs benefit companies because employees who have these problems, cannot perform at peak levels, use more sick time and are more likely to have accidents at work. This lowers the overall productivity of the organization. Employee assistance programs can be in-house or contracted out.

e. Performance evaluation

- The **ANNUAL REVIEW,** also called **PERFORMANCE REVIEW**, is a regularly scheduled evaluation of pre-determined goals, objectives and performance of tasks. Usually annual reviews are tied to salary increases, promotions, bonuses or benefits. A manager may do the review alone or it may be done separately by the employee and the manager, who then compare the ratings. The type of appraisal is determined in part, by the type and level of job (e.g., clerical, production, professional).

- Every employee should know what is expected and how he or she is performing on the job. A performance appraisal serves to document proficiencies and strengths, and to identify areas in which improvement is desired. Statements should be made in a positive and constructive way.

- The written performance appraisal generally states the employee's name, job title, department, current pay rate, new rate and dates of review period.

- Often there is a rating scale (1-10) ranging from unsatisfactory performance to exceptional or outstanding performance in specified aspects of the job.

- Categories for evaluation may include job knowledge, work quality and quantity, dependability, attitude and compatibility, initiative and adherence to safe practices and established policies and procedures. Each category should provide space for explanation as well as a number rating.

- A plan for improvement that sets performance goals to be attained during the next review period is included.

- The performance appraisal should be signed by the evaluator and reviewed by the employee. After review, the employee signs it. The employee's signature says that the employee has seen the appraisal. If the employee does not agree with the appraisal, the employee may write a rebuttal. A copy of the original appraisal and rebuttal are filed in the personnel record and a copy must be given to the employee. A performance appraisal report can become a legal document if there is a lawsuit.

- In a profit center, performance is measured by the numerical difference between the revenues and expenditures for which the manager of the organizational unit is responsible. Higher performance scores, often with financial rewards, are given to individuals or groups that exceed revenue projections.

- The **RATING SCALE METHOD** examines each trait or characteristic of a job (e.g., knowledge of work, initiative, application, quality, volume) and rates it on a scale, based on performance standards defined by the rater. Some forms leave room for remarks to help explain the rating.

- **BEHAVIORALLY ANCHORED RATING SCALES (BARS)** define specific behaviors at different points on the scale. This helps raters define where an individual fits on the scale.

- With the **ESSAY METHOD**, the evaluator writes a statement describing the employee's strengths, weaknesses and unique qualities.

- **SELF-ASSESSMENT** shifts the emphasis from manager appraisal to self-analysis by the employee and from focus on past performance to focus on the future (goal setting). The management by objectives (MBO) system uses this type of self-assessment for evaluation.

- A **GLOBAL RATING** is a single rating of overall job performance. A global rating (a grade or single score) provides little information that will help an employee identify specific areas for improvement or set personal goals that will motivate better performance unless the global rating is a composite score of several factors. The global rating may be the basis for a salary adjustment.

f. Retention strategies

- Employee retention is vital to the health and success of an organization. If your best employees leave after a short period of time, the money and time spent on training is lost. If many people leave, there is probably a serious problem. Employees need to be satisfied by clearly knowing what is expected at all times. Expectations that change from day to day cause employee stress because the person does not feel secure. If change has to be made, employees should know the new expectations. The quality of supervision is key to their security.

- The employee should feel secure about expressing concerns, to suggest innovations and provide feedback. Perception of fairness, such as promotions, raises and general treatment also provide a secure environment.

- Use of employees' talents, uniqueness, special skills, experience even if outside of the job description helps to make a comfortable environment in which to work.

- Employees need to feel appreciated. Thanking them for doing a good job, awards and recognition for good work, even if not monetary, are important to a comfortable and happy work environment.

g. Compensation

- **COMPENSATION** is the rate of pay given to employees for performance of work or provision of services. The definition may also include benefits received, such as health and vacation.

- **SALARY** is annual, monthly or weekly income to employees holding positions with regular schedules. Usually salaries are subject to federal and state income tax and Social Security tax withholding. Frequently, salaries also have deductions for health insurance, life insurance and investment plans.

- **WAGES** are compensation paid to workers with irregular hours based on the number of hours they work. Wages are also subject to withholding and may or may not have associated benefits packages.

- The Fair Labor Standards Act, which governs minimum wages, distinguishes between **EXEMPT** and **NON-EXEMPT EMPLOYEES.** Exempt employees are not subject to minimum wage requirements and are not paid for overtime. This category includes anyone employed in an executive, administrative or professional capacity. Non-exempt employees must be paid minimum wage and are paid for hours worked, including overtime.

- Upon discharge, **SEVERANCE** may be paid to an employee. No employment laws specify that severance must be paid or govern the amount, if any, to be paid. Sometimes, severance is given on the condition that the employee sign a contract that he will not compete with the employer or approach former clients.

- Employees may apply for unemployment benefits following discharge for performance related issues and/or a reduction in force. Employees discharged for wrongdoing, such as stealing, are not eligible for unemployment payments. State and federal laws govern eligibility for unemployment compensation.

TOPIC C - FINANCIAL MANAGEMENT

1. Budget development/resource allocation for food and nutrition programs and services

- A **BUDGET** is a financial plan used to plan and evaluate the results of future actions. The budget indicates how and at what rate money is to be spent. This allows expenditures to be regulated over a period of time (usually one year). Budgets provide systematic financial bookkeeping to account for funds in a continuous, verifiable and accurate manner. A budget is developed to conform to policies of an organization. Budgeting usually begins with a forecast of revenue from sales of products or services, such as cafeteria meals or nutrition counseling. Estimates are made of expenses, costs, collections, and payments reflecting anticipated sources of revenue and expense.

- Benefits of a budget include: forcing management to consider future directions and developments; providing review of previous expenditures as a basis for justifying future requests; giving standards for comparison against actual transactions; anticipating and planning for changes in costs from inflation; cost of-living raises, etc.; setting spending limits; providing goals for revenues and profits; and providing continuity in the event of management change.

- Potential problems with budgets include: ignoring rigid budgets; budget preparation and budget meetings that take personnel away from other activities; undesirable competition between departments; missing current opportunities that may not be in approved plans; emergencies; or failure of capital equipment requiring unbudgeted expenditures. Changes beyond the control of the budget makers may alter budget assumptions and make it appear that management planned poorly.

a. Budget procedures

- Good planning and monitoring are the keys to cost control. It is easier and less disruptive to operations to keep costs down than to reduce costs. Budget development must reflect the high priority placed on items and services that promote attaining organizational goals and/or the strategic plan.

- Budget development includes consideration of:
  - ➢ Expenditures of the preceding period (past fiscal year).
  - ➢ Budget of the present period (this fiscal year).
  - ➢ Changes in the present budget period (this first quarter).
  - ➢ Actual income and expenditures to date (e.g., to July 3, 2013).
  - ➢ Object of expenditures (items in current budget).
  - ➢ Budget requests for the next period (e.g., $5,000 for computer equipment).
  - ➢ Comparison between present and anticipated budgets (e.g., evaluation of current and subsequent fiscal year).

- The 4 phases of a budget cycle are:

  1. Budget Preparation: Compilation and discussions about departmental requests, evaluation of potential revenues and expenses. The administrator, director of finance and/or officers adjust line items. Usually a **BALANCED BUDGET** (revenues = expenses) is submitted for approval by top management.
  2. Justification: Process of review, revision and approval by those responsible for authorizing or granting funds.
  3. Execution of Budget: Translation of the budgeted expenditures into operational programs. Monitoring and adjusting revenues and expenses within set time frames (e.g., quarterly).
  4. Review and Evaluation: Before an audit, programs and budgeted items are evaluated for compliance with budget policies and if expenditures and income were within budgeted amounts. Books are prepared for an external audit, usually annually.

b. Types

(1) Operational

- **OPERATIONAL BUDGETS** provide a basis for control, planning and coordination. This budget shows the overall structure of the operation and enables staff to visualize its place in it. It includes revenue and expenditures such as sales, supplies, services, small equipment, food and labor.

- A **REVENUE BUDGET** includes estimated income from sales or services. It can also include other sources such as grants, endowments, property and investments. It is considered part of an operational budget.

- **CASH FLOW BUDGETS** are detailed estimates of anticipated cash receipts and disbursements throughout the budget period, usually by the month. It includes cash-on-hand, accounts payable, accounts receivable, the cost of credit and cash flow. It assists management in coordinating cash inflow and outflow and in synchronizing cash resources with need. Seasonal effects on cash positions thus become apparent, and the availability of cash for taking advantage of discounts is identified. Historical records and dates of current income-generating events or services or dates of major expenditures influence the cash flow budget.

(2) Capital

- A **CAPITAL BUDGET** is a budget plan for improvements, expansions and replacements in buildings, major equipment and land. These major capital investments may be for purposes of expanding or improving facilities and may be prorated over several budget periods/years.

- A **MASTER BUDGET** is a composite of the operational, capital, budgeted balance sheet, and cash flow budgets and includes a projection of profit or break-even. Various ratios should be computed to determine if the appropriate relationships of expenditures to revenues has been projected. Depending on the type of budget, there are published industry standards that indicate typical percentages for food, administrative costs, salary, number of personnel, etc.

c. Methods

(1) Incremental

- An **INCREMENTAL BUDGET** is based on the existing budget, with a fixed percentage added to each category to cover inflation or projecting change for the following year based on expected changes. An incremental budget may also be variable in that actual dollars allocated will vary in proportion to the work done. *+Variable or Fixed*

(2) Performance

- A **PERFORMANCE BUDGET** gives priority and additional funding to functions that exceed income generation projections, that have high productivity or that meet other performance-related variables.

(3) Zero-based

- A **ZERO-BASED BUDGET (ZBB)** is newly created each year without extensions of current activity costs. Managers must justify all requests for funds and reevaluate activities each year. Zero-based budgets do contain some fixed costs (rent, utilities) that are used as a starting point in budget preparation. A zero-based budget may be fixed or variable. *+Variable or Fixed*

(4) Flexible

- A **VARIABLE BUDGET** or **FLEXIBLE BUDGET** can be applied to both incremental and zero-based budgets. Expenses are projected, based on variable amounts of production, volume or revenues. It is more flexible than the fixed budget when income increases or decreases.

(5) Fixed

- **FIXED BUDGETS** are used to compare actual financial performance with expected performance. They are characterized by firm projections that are set for the whole budget cycle. Fixed budgets assume that business will be stable for the entire budget cycle. The advantages are that managers can be provided with financial performance goals that can be measured in each accounting period, but they are not flexible enough to react to important changes. Both incremental and zero-based budgets can be fixed.

d. Components

(1) Direct expenses

- **DIRECT COSTS** or **DIRECT EXPENSES** are costs that can be identified with specific products, departments or activities (e.g., food costs in food service departments).

- The direct cost of labor and wage incentive programs are part of the total cost of labor (salaries and benefits) which can be computed as a percentage of the total budget.

- **PRODUCTIVITY** is a measure of quantifiable output per full-time equivalent (FTE). Examples include the number of meals per labor hour and its effect on bottom line (profit or loss) or the number of counseling appointments per week.

(2) Indirect expenses

- **INDIRECT COSTS** or **INDIRECT EXPENSES** are based on expenses that cannot be identified with specific products, departments or activities (e.g., taxes, insurance). Overhead costs are often not scrutinized as carefully as direct costs. Some indirect costs can be changes in service providers or operating procedures altered (e.g., changing insurance carriers, using energy conservation techniques).

- **FIXED COSTS** are costs required by an operator to exist and do not vary with sales. Fixed costs include insurance, rent and property tax.

(3) Capital expenses

- **CAPITAL INVESTMENTS** have a longer life than the operating period (e.g., property, physical plant, equipment). Capital expenditures are often in a separate capital budget for accounting purposes to distinguish items on which depreciation occurs.

(4) Profit margin

- The **PROFIT MARGIN** is a measure of operating profitability. The profit margin may be expressed in a percentage. To determine the cost of an item or service, a specific percentage of profit should be built into the price.

$$\% \text{ PROFIT MARGIN} = \frac{\$ \text{ Net Profit}}{\$ \text{ Sales}}$$

- **PROFITABILITY RATIOS** measure the ability of an organization to generate profit in relation to sales or the investment in assets. Profit (net income) is the monetary amount of income after all expenses have been deducted from income or revenue. Return on equity and return on assets are profitability ratios. Return on equity measures adequacy of profit in relation to owner's investment. Return on assets measures management's ability to generate a return on corporate assets.

$$\text{RETURN ON EQUITY} = \frac{\text{Net Profit}}{\text{Equity}}$$

$$\text{RETURN ON ASSETS} = \frac{\text{Net Profit}}{\text{Total Assets}}$$

- Most food service operations generate some level of net income whether for profit or not-for-profit. In not-for-profit operations, net income is applied to provide additional services. In for-profit operations, net income is distributed as profits to shareholders and owners.

(5) Revenue

- **REVENUE** is the total income generated from sales, services, property, grants, fund-raising, investments, etc.

e. Resources allocation

(1) Financial and materials

- Analyses will determine what changes in equipment and facilities will promote long-term cost savings. Increased productivity must be evaluated when examining new and existing equipment and facilities.

- **SUNK COSTS** are those that have already occurred because of previous decisions that cannot be altered; such as equipment and supplies already purchased.

- **DIFFERENTIAL COSTS** are estimated future costs or costs that differ among alternative courses of action, for example, purchase of a steamer vs. microwave oven.

(2) Cost control decisions   *or repair vs. replace*

- Purchase specifications and negotiated contracts fix costs for particular materials, labor, equipment and facilities for a given period of time. Specifications ensure that quality and quantity will not be compromised even if the supplier's costs go up.

- A **JOB CONTROL CLAUSE** in a union contract can inhibit management's right to bring down operating cost by changing standards, methods or making improvements.

- **OPPORTUNITY COSTS** are cost control mechanisms that use the preferred option for decision-making. Opportunities may be available for only a short time because of a consumer concern or government action. Opportunity costs evaluate how much cost is incurred, or potential profit is lost, if an opportunity is missed. For example, choosing to spend time on one project means that time is not available for another project that may produce more revenue or benefits.

- **DISCRETIONARY COSTS** do not have to be incurred immediately. They are costs that can be incurred at any time or not at all, for example, new advertising.

Cost control strategies/procedures

- Cost control strategies are generally short-term drives to reduce cost by having everyone increase production or decrease expenses. Hiring freezes, early retirement, limiting raises to cost-of-living adjustments and increasing responsibility or productivity expectations are common cost-control strategies. A quality control program that encourages everyone to "do it right the first time" is one of the most effective cost-control systems. Cost controls evaluate cost within a time period. Knowing where the money goes will not bring it back, but will help control costs in the future.

- Common cost-control formulas are:

$$\text{COST PER MEAL} = \frac{\text{Total cost}}{\text{Number of meals prepared}}$$

$$\text{MEALS PER LABOR HOUR} = \frac{\text{Total number of meals served}}{\text{Total labor hours to produce meals}}$$

$$\text{MEALS PER FTE} = \frac{\text{Total number of meals served}}{\text{Total FTE to produce meals}}$$

$$\text{LABOR MINUTES PER MEAL} = \frac{\text{Total labor minutes to produce meals}}{\text{Total number of meals served}}$$

Food service industry records typically used

- Inventory controls
  - ➤ Requisition or storeroom issue records
  - ➤ Perpetual inventory
  - ➤ Physical inventory
- Other Records
  - ➤ Food production and service records: Menus; Standardized recipes; Portion control standards
  - ➤ Production schedule and leftovers report
  - ➤ Menu tally
  - ➤ Dining room/patient room records
  - ➤ Census reports: Number of meals served Count of regular and special meals
  - ➤ Income/expense records: Cash sales register reports Guest checks Cash disbursement records for expenses
  - ➤ Storage and storeroom records: Log of items and people entering and leaving storerooms
- Record of expenses
  - ➤ Personnel records (related to cost control): Time card/payroll records Work schedules Benefits records
  - ➤ Purchasing and receiving records: Purchase orders Invoices Receiving records Purchase records Summary of purchases record

(3) Factors affecting available resources

- **DIAGNOSIS-RELATED GROUPS (DRGs)** were created by the Social Security Reform Amendment in 1983, now Public Law 98-21. Originally for inpatient services to Medicare patients, it is now used for most third-party payment for hospitalized patients. The DRG system identified 467 categories of treatment and set a standard fee or **PROSPECTIVE PAYMENT SYSTEM (PPS)** for each treatment, regardless of length of hospital stay. Upon discharge, a case is assigned to a DRG. DRG designation is determined by:

  - ➤ Principal diagnosis, which may include up to four co-morbidities or complications. A **CO-MORBIDITY** is a pre-existing condition. A **COMPLICATION** is a condition that arises during the hospital stay.
  - ➤ Principal procedure, which may include up to two secondary procedures.

- Patient's age.
- Patient's sex.
- Discharge status, for example, released from the hospital, died in the hospital, transferred to a hospital or unit not covered by PPS.

- Healthcare entities not covered by DRGs include psychiatric units, rehabilitation hospitals, childrens' hospitals, long-term care hospitals and substance abuse treatment centers. Special adjustments regarding payments fall into two categories; extended length of stay (**DAY OUTLIERS**) and excessive cost (**COST OUTLIERS**) of specific products or services.

- Nutritional support is included in the prospective payments. To keep costs down, the nutrition services staff must correctly identify patient needs and use supplies, such as parenteral nutrition, efficiently. Nutrition intervention is cost-effective when it reduces the length of hospital stay, complications or severity of illness.

- Other factors affecting available resources include:
  - Unexpected reduction in revenues, forcing cutbacks in budgeted programs.
  - Cuts in government funding or slow payment by insurers.
  - Loss of staff or facilities, including mergers.
  - Priority spending in other areas of the operation.
  - Changes in management and/or insurance contracts.

2. Financial: monitoring, evaluation and control

- **CURRENT ASSETS** are cash, accounts receivable, marketable securities and inventory expected to be turned into cash, sold or exchanged (usually within one year).

- **FIXED ASSETS** are the monetary value of equipment, land, buildings, patents and other items used to produce goods and services.

- **LIABILITIES** are the amount (debt) owed by a business to an outside entity, payable in money (e.g., bank loan, outstanding bills and payroll). Long-term liabilities include mortgages, bonds and other debts that are being paid off gradually.

- **CAPITAL** or **OWNER'S EQUITY** is the owner's share of assets or the amount the owner has invested in the organization. It may also be shareholders' equity or stockholders' equity.

- Ownership may be one of several kinds:

  - **PROPRIETORSHIP:** Is a business owned by a single individual.
  - **PARTNERSHIP:** A business owned by two or more people.
  - **CORPORATION:** A business incorporated under the law of a state with ownership held by stockholder. In a not-for-profit corporation, members may be the owners. Some not-for profit organizations that meet certain legal conditions have a 501 c (3) tax status and may accept charitable contributions.
  - A **SUBCHAPTER S CORPORATION** is an IRS designation for a corporation with 75 or fewer shareholders that can be taxed as if it were a partnership.
  - A **LIMITED LIABILITY COMPANY (LLC)** is a hybrid business that allows pass-through income and limits liability of shareholders. It is more flexible than a

corporation and often has a sole or very few owners.

a. Accounting procedures

- **ACCOUNTING** is a specialized part of a management information system. It is an organized approach to gathering, recording, analyzing, summarizing and interpreting financial data to determine financial condition.

- Standard methods of accounting and presentation of financial statements, termed **UNIFORM SYSTEMS OF ACCOUNTS**, have been established in specific industries, including certain segments of the hospitality services industry. These uniform systems of accounts within a particular industry provide for the uniform classification, organization and presentation of revenues, expenses, assets, liabilities and equity. They include a standardized format for financial statements, which permits comparability of financial data within an industry. Financial statements can be prepared using computer spreadsheets or customized software programs.

(1) Cash/credit procedures

- Institutions and businesses that handle cash must have specific written policies and procedures for handling cash and processing payments, such as checks or credit card purchases. Policies should state who is authorized to handle cash, how and where cash is held, how often deposits must be made and security procedures.

Cash security

- As few employees as possible should handle cash and payments. Each employee should be responsible for cash gathered during a set time period. Register receipts should equal cash in the drawer. Cash should be deposited in a secure place (bank or safe) to minimize opportunities for theft.

- Credit card sales should be verified at set amounts. Even small purchases should be processed within the time limit set by financial policy.

b. Financial statements

- **FINANCIAL STATEMENTS** are documents that show, in dollars, the flow of goods and services to, within, and from an organization. Financial statements provide a means for controlling or determining **LIQUIDITY**, the ability to convert assets into cash to meet current expenses, **GENERAL FINANCIAL CONDITION**, the long-term balance between debt and equity and **PROFITABILITY**, the ability to earn profits over a period of time.

- Basic financial statements include the operating statement, balance sheet, income statement and statement of changes in financial position.

- The **BALANCE SHEET** is a statement of financial condition that shows the financial position of the enterprise at a particular time, including the economic resources (assets), economic obligations (liabilities) and the residual claims of owners (owner's equity).

Total Assets = Total Liabilities + Owner's Equity

- The **OPERATING STATEMENT** compares the actual fiscal performance to the planned budget.

- The **INCOME STATEMENT** is the financial report that presents the net income or profit of an organization for the accounting period. It provides information about the revenues and expenses that resulted in net income or loss.

- The **STATEMENT OF CHANGES IN FINANCIAL POSITION** provides information about the source and use of funds.

- An **ANNUAL REPORT** is a document in which businesses or organizations summarize their financial condition and key policy changes once a year.

- The **STATEMENT OF CASH FLOW** reports the amount of cash flow from an organization's operating, investing and financing activities. Primary cash receipts and cash payments from each of these activities are shown. Cash flow needs to be generated in adequate amounts and at the right time to keep the organization financially sound. Cash flows vary at peak times of income or expense. The statement of cash flow links the balance sheet and the income statements and is presented for each period. The statement helps users of financial statements to assess the ability of the organization to meet its financial obligations.

- Monthly financial statements provide a status report of expenses and income-to date (actual) in relation to budget projections. Based on these figures, the manager can determine whether corrective adjustments are warranted.

- A budget may be changed during the fiscal year if projected income does not materialize (e.g., research grant proposals are rejected or there is a major unplanned expense.) Programs and services must be reevaluated based on actual fiscal resources. Corrective adjustments are usually made quarterly with particular attention during the last quarter of the budget year.

(1) Profit-and-loss statements

- The **PROFIT-AND-LOSS STATEMENT** is also known as the **INCOME STATEMENT**, lists revenues, expenses, gains and losses for a given period. Net income (or loss) for the period is the bottom line.

c. Value analysis

- Value is the result of the relationship between the price paid for an item and the item's utility in the function it fills. **VALUE ANALYSIS** is the systematic investigation of all components of an existing product or service with the goal of eliminating unnecessary costs without interfering with the effectiveness of the service or product. Value analysis in food service includes monitoring of:

  ➤ Food costs- menu, menu pricing, purchasing, storage and storeroom control, food production, portion size and waste.
  ➤ Labor costs- type and extent of services offered, hours of service, number of employees and cost per category of employee.
  ➤ Operating and other expenses- maintenance and repair, laundry and linen, supplies and utility costs.

TOPIC D - MARKETING and PUBLIC RELATIONS

1. Marketing analysis

The fundamental steps to marketing analysis are determining the objectives, selecting a target market, analyzing the needs and preferences of potential consumers and studying the competition.

MARKETING DIETETICS: A PLANNING MODEL

Step 1: Identify the target market and product line. Consider the dietitian's unique skill and strengths in relation to what is needed or wanted by potential clients or customers. Narrow the product or service to a manageable level.

Step 2: Conduct market research. Why has no one thought of it before? Conduct SWOT Analysis. SWOT is an acronym for strengths, weaknesses, opportunities, threats. A SWOT analysis is conducted by a group of individuals who are knowledgeable about a situation.

Step 3: Set measurable and realistic goals. Identify checkpoints and levels of success that warrant continuation and/or expansion.

Step 4: Determine strategies. These strategies should be based on an analysis of the environment, relating the organization to the market, the competition and financial, technical, socioeconomic and political factors.

Step 5: Develop action plans and assign responsibility. Determine what tasks are required to accomplish the strategic plan, what timing is appropriate and who is responsible for each task.

Step 6: Establish a financial reporting system.

Step 7: Measure and evaluate results. Set a timetable for review. The review includes both financial review and an evaluation of the extent to which the operation has met its stated goals and objectives.

Step 8: Enlist organizational commitment. Develop a strategy for selling the project to key decision makers within the organization.

---

a. Process

(1) Identification of target market

- The **TARGET MARKET** (audience) is the group of potential clients or customers with the authority and ability to purchase or take advantage of a particular product or service that satisfies their shared demand.

- There are two major market types:
    1. **CONSUMER MARKETS** - Individuals buy products or services for personal use.
    2. **INDUSTRIAL MARKETS** - Business, government agencies or other institutions buy products to use in operations or in making other products.

- **MARKET SEGMENTATION** is the division of the total market into groups with similar characteristics or interests (e.g., oat bran cereal eaters, males over age 65). Markets that are segmented can be reached with messages of specific importance to them.

- **SOCIAL MARKETING** describes application of commercial marketing principles to the advancement of a social cause, idea or behavior. It seeks to increase acceptability of a social idea or cause. This is used most often in public health, such as campaigns to reduce smoking, increase vegetable consumption, etc.

(2) Determination of needs/wants

- Through the use of market research, information is obtained on those needs and characteristics necessary to segment the market. Markets can be segmented based on:
  - ➢ Family income, geographic location, race.
  - ➢ Behavior patterns.
  - ➢ Physical characteristics (age, sex, health).
  - ➢ Psychological traits.
  - ➢ Opinions of goods on the market.
  - ➢ Degree of competition from other products.

- Quality assurance establishes programs and services based on the identified needs of the customer or client, rather than on the supplier's estimation of what is wanted or needed.

(3) Marketing mix

- A good **MARKETING MIX** is an effective meshing of product, program or service, price, promotion and distribution strategies to achieve success. These strategies change, depending on the product's life-cycle stage. For example, different strategies are needed to launch new community programs than to support existing ones.

(4) Customer satisfaction

- As institutions become more competitive for customers, one method of differentiation is customer satisfaction. More emphasis is being placed on evaluation/feedback given by the customers in order for the establishment to give customers the products/services they wish, within reason. Customer satisfaction is becoming one of the most important measures of a food service's rank placement and market share. Comment cards, evaluation forms and Internet surveys following service are tools to get direct feedback from customers. Unsigned, anonymous feedback is often more honest and more useful, than asking customers who may be uncomfortable giving a negative response.

- Filling a unique market niche results in a competitive advantage. It can be achieved by offering a unique service, a faster service or one of greater quality or lower price. This differentiates an organization from its competition. In food service, an example would be providing delicious, heart-healthy food choices. Analysis of sales, demand, pricing and promotion to the target audience also creates a competitive edge. Follow-ups and after sales services add to the competitive advantage.

(5) Documentation and evaluation

- Documentation and evaluation should be built into any marketing program from the outset. Documentation and evaluation measures include:
  - ➢ Financial data.
  - ➢ Evaluation forms to gather feedback from clients or participants.
  - ➢ Surveys.
  - ➢ Studies to measure effectiveness (e.g., increased nutrition knowledge, attitude and

compliance scores (pre-test/post-test), dietary intake records, changes in blood pressure or serum cholesterol).

2. Pricing

a) Strategies

- **PRODUCT STRATEGIES** include labels, packaging, trademarks, new product development, guarantees, finding new uses and new users.

- **SERVICE STRATEGIES** include convenience, individual attention, assistance with forms/applications, transportation and guaranteed satisfaction.

- **PLACEMENT STRATEGY** uses systems and channels to place the product or service into consumers' hands, maximizing speed and ease while minimizing cost. Some products or services are best advertised in local newspapers, community bulletin boards, upscale magazines, websites, social media, etc., based on intended customers.

- Considerations in food pricing include the following:

  - ➢ Consumers want value, a good product for the price.
  - ➢ Low cost menu items can have a proportionately higher markup to offset items that must be priced lower than the standard markup.
  - ➢ Menu items priced too high decrease sales and increase operating costs.
  - ➢ Sales volume is increased through customer satisfaction, based on taste, market research, promotions and good service.
  - ➢ Effective record keeping on sales mix, food and labor costs, costs for supplies, and overhead are necessary for proper pricing.
  - ➢ Factors such as a competitor's pricing, supermarket food prices, and consumer demand affect pricing.
  - ➢ Pricing is always important but especially when fast food or other options are convenient to potential patrons.

- **PRICING STRATEGIES** include meeting the competition's price, pricing above the competition (to promote perceptions of quality) and pricing under the competition (to promote cost advantage).

- **COST-BASED PRICING** is calculated as total costs divided by estimated attendance or units sold.

(1) Break-even

- **BREAK-EVEN ANALYSIS** seeks to identify a level of production to cover all fixed and variable costs of production in the short term. Profit at the break-even level of output is zero.

- The **BREAK-EVEN POINT** is the point at which an operation is making no profit but incurring no loss, where total revenue is equal to total expenses. The following is the break-even equation:

$$BEP = \frac{\text{Fixed Cost}}{1 - (\text{Variable Cost/Sales})}$$

Example: The following data are available for ABC cafeteria:

    Fixed cost = $ 38,000

    Variable cost = $ 75,000

    Sales = $180,000

Substituting the figures in the formula, the break-even point for ABC cafeteria is calculated as shown below:

$$\text{BEP} = \frac{\$38,000}{1 - (\$75000/\$180,000)} = \frac{\$38,000}{1 - .42} = \frac{\$38,000}{.58} = \$65,517.24 \text{ revenue.}$$

(2) Revenue-generating

- Most food service organizations must generate revenue to offset the costs of their operations. Some are established as not-for-profit, but others are for-profit. Each organization must decide how to price the items they sell in order to generate income. Some healthcare organizations generate revenue in cafeterias or coffee shops, while others have catering operations or special services, such as meals for the family or special meals on the birth of a baby.

Methods

- The **DEMAND ORIENTED METHOD** is based on what customers perceive the cost to be and are willing to pay. This is often used for a new or trendy item. Close control and monitoring of sales are required to justify the pricing. For example, coffee, nachos and popcorn have low raw food costs, but consumers may expect, and may be willing, to pay more than standard markup. This additional profit can offset other items that may be sold at less markup because their raw food cost is high.

- The **FOOD COST PERCENTAGE** is the ratio of the cost of food over the revenue received from selling the food.

- A 40% **RAW FOOD COST** in relation to sales is a general rule-of-thumb for the total menu.

- To calculate raw food costs for each recipe ingredient, multiply the quantity (as purchased [AP] weight or measure) by the ingredient unit price.

    Example:

3 #10 cans tomatoes x $2.50/can	=	7.50
5 lb carrots x $.62/lb.	=	3.10
2 lb onions x $.68/lb.	=	1.36
3 lb navy beans x $.78/lb.	=	2.34
Total raw food cost =		**$14.30**

- To calculate **RAW FOOD COST PER SERVING**, divide the total raw food cost for all ingredients by the number of servings.

> **Example:** $14.30/(25 servings) = $.572
> **Raw food cost per serving is $0.57**

Markup

- **MARKUP** is determined by dividing the desired percentage of food income spent on raw food costs (e.g., 40%) into 100 (representing total sales). The resulting figure is the **MARKUP FACTOR**. The markup factor is usually set to include overhead, labor, utilities, equipment etc.

> **Example:**   100/40 (percent of sales for food) = 2.5
> **The markup factor is 2.5.**

- To figure the **SELLING PRICE**, a food manager must also calculate "hidden costs" (e.g., staples, salt, pepper, condiments) and losses that occur during preparation, cooking and serving. Many managers add 10% (or some other standardized percentage) to raw food costs before figuring the markup factor.

> **Example:**
>
> | | |
> |---|---:|
> | Raw food costs | $0.86 |
> | Hidden costs (10% of raw food costs) | +0.09 |
> | | $0.95 |
> | Markup factor (x 2.5) | x 2.5 |
> | **Realistic selling price** | **$2.375** |

> **Rounded to the next reasonable menu price: $2.50.**

- The **PRIME COST METHOD** was initiated by **HARRY POPE** to reflect labor costs directly. Some high priced items, like steak and lobster, require relatively little labor time to prepare, whereas stew, is labor intensive. Prime costing spreads the cost of food service evenly among customers.

> **Example:**
>
> | | |
> |---|---:|
> | Raw food costs | $0.86 |
> | Hidden costs | 0.09 |
> | Labor (60 minutes @ $4 y 25 portions) | +0.16 |
> | | $1.11 |
> | Markup factor (x 1.5)* | x 1.5 |
> | **Realistic selling price** | **$1.665** |

> Rounded to the next reasonable menu price: $1.75.
> (*The markup is lower because labor costs are added separately.)

(3) Loss leader

- A **LOSS LEADER** is selling of an item at a sale price that is lower than the actual cost of the item. This is meant to bring consumers to the store, in the expectation that they will purchase other items not on sale. It is a type of promotional pricing.

b. Rationale

- **PRICING ADJUSTMENTS** include discounts for employees or free and reduced prices for participants in the National School Lunch Program.

- **OPTIONS PRICING** allows for increases in pricing as customers add options to the basic product, such as àla carte pricing. It can be used in clinical services when a nutritional assessment is offered with or without a computerized dietary analysis.

- **PRODUCT LINE PRICING** offers a range of prices for a variety of products offered. A restaurant may offer table service and self-service, with similar products priced differently, depending on the type of service.

3. Public relations

- **PUBLIC RELATIONS** is the relationship that is developed between the public and an organization, business or individual. Effective communications are needed to get your message across, sell your product or idea. Maintaining excellent public relations is a key to success in any field.

a. Media relations

- While paid advertisements can be effective tools for establishing and maintaining a public presence, utilizing the media (television, newspapers, radio, Internet) can be at times a more effective (and cost effective) way of sharing your message.

- In dealing with media it is important that you be proactive and reach out to them. Press releases, press kits and media kits are all ways to reach out to media to generate interest around a particular issue, story or product.

- Typically, news outlets are deadline oriented, so there may be limited time to research answers. Professionals should stay up to date with current research and information in their field and/or specialty so that they are always ready to respond in a coherent and timely manner to media requests for information.

- Messages released through the media should be concise and understandable. Short, easy to understand messages that drive home key points are much more effective than complicated explanations. During interviews, poise and confidence is key, and this can be developed through practice and experience.

- Messages sent out through the media should be relevant to the public at large. Pointing out what is new, novel or different about your product or idea will help consumers buy into your message. Generally, consumers are most interested in things that will affect their "heart" (family, pets), "health" or "pocketbook."

- After any media interview, it is important to follow-up, provide any further resources needed to complete the story, maintain rapport and thank the contact for interest in the story.

b. **Social networking**

- Social networking allows for a more informal method of communicating with the public. Methods of social networking can include:

  ➢ **BLOGS/VLOGS** - Online web "diaries" where entries are published in chronological order. Blogs can be general in nature and include a variety of discussions or focus on a specific topic. Vlogs are similar except that they are in video format.

  ➢ **PODCASTS** - Streamable or downloadable audio files of information. Some podcasts are rebroadcasts of existing radio shows and some are solely released as podcasts. Vodcasts are similar except that they also include video in addition to audio content.

  ➢ **SOCIAL NETWORKING SITES** (examples are Facebook/LinkedIn) - Online sites that allow individuals and groups to interact, exchange information and publicize events, etc. Facebook is a more social site whereas LinkedIn is focused on professional networking.

c. **Campaign development**

- To develop an effective campaign, it is important not only to communicate your message but also that your message is:

  ➢ Relevant to your audience.
  ➢ Understandable- clear and concise, not overly wordy or complicated.
  ➢ Doable, affordable and manageable for your intended audience.
  ➢ Meaningful to your intended audience.

- **PROMOTIONAL STRATEGY** consists of developing a blend of advertising, personal selling, sales promotion and publicity to meet sales or revenue objectives.

- Successful promotions share the following qualities:

  ➢ They are at a reading level appropriate to the target audience. They use consumer language, for example, "eat," not "consume"; "foods," not "nutrients".
  ➢ They are as brief as possible.
  ➢ They are positive. They use active verbs in their written or spoken messages.
  ➢ They use attractive, interesting visuals to support the message.
  ➢ They use appropriate distribution channels to reach the target audience. For example, most working women cannot be reached through daytime television. Notices that go out with bills, newsletters or bulletin boards in grocery stores are more effective.
  ➢ They may include a sample of the product or service, for example; such as a free evaluation, an open house or a tasting of the product.
  ➢ They may use spokespersons that are known and respected by the target audience.

TOPIC E - QUALITY IMPROVEMENT

1. Regulatory guidelines (e.g., federal, local, TJC)

- Quality assurance needs the commitment of every employee to do the best possible job under the constraints of the system. Management should make every effort to provide systems that allow workers to do quality work. Regulatory guidelines provide comprehensive quality guidelines for systems, products and services.

- A regulatory system implemented with an inspection program will facilitate early disclosure of defects and non-conformities. The sooner these discrepancies are discovered and corrections are made, the more the organization can save. For example, a guideline allows for collection of X menus per hour. If fewer menus are collected per hour, the process must be improved and staff costs and time reduced.

- **HAZARD ANALYSIS CRITICAL CONTROL POINT (HACCP)** is the systematic analysis of all process steps in food service subsystems starting with food products from suppliers to consumption of food by consumers to ensure that food is safe for consumption.

- The National Restaurant Association Education Foundation developed **SERVSAFE**, a risk management series program that includes serving safe food, responsible alcohol service and employee and customer safety. Many managers in healthcare and school food service have been trained using SERVSAFE. For more information on HACCP and food safety procedures, go to the National Restaurant Association website: **www.nraef.org.**

Federal regulations

- The **OMNIBUS BUDGET RECONCILIATION ACT (OBRA)** of 1987, and its amendments, address nursing home reforms. The law mandates individualized resident assessments and a team planning process to support resident autonomy and independence. Facilities must meet OBRA guidelines if they are Medicare or Medicaid certified.

- Dietitians are required to determine the resident's nutritional status by assessing weight, height, hematological and biochemical values, to observe the resident for clinical and physical signs of malnutrition and to take appropriate action.

- Dietitians must provide a balanced diet that is responsive to the needs of each resident, determine the adequacy of nutritional intake and initiate appropriate responses for each resident when necessary. For example, residents with pressure sores are to have diets that replenish protein, vitamin C, calories and perhaps other nutrients. Residents who must be tube fed are to be given the amount and strength of the feeding recommended by the manufacturer to meet the RDA for protein, calories, minerals and vitamins. The dietitian is to document performance of the nutritional outcome demonstrated by the resident.

Voluntary regulations

- **The Joint Commission -** Founded in 1951, is an independent and non-profit organization whose mission is to continuously improve healthcare for the public, in collaboration with other stakeholders, by evaluating healthcare organizations and inspiring them to excel in providing safe and effective care of the highest quality and value. (See The Joint Commission website **www.jointcommission.org.**)

> ➢ The Joint Commission develops standards for quality and safety in the delivery of healthcare, evaluates organization performance based on these standards and makes recommendations for improvements so that healthcare providers can continually assess and improve how they administer care. The standards are set in areas such as patient rights, patient treatment, medication safety and infection control. In order to earn The Joint Commission's Gold Seal of Approval™, an organization must undergo an on-site survey by a Joint Commission survey team at least every three years. (Laboratories must be surveyed every two years.) Such objective audits result in a variety of benefits for the healthcare organization, patients, employees and the community including:
> ➢ Enhanced quality, patient safety and confidence in delivery care , treatment and services.
> ➢ Structured framework for program delivery and management resulting in improved, consistent patient care.
> ➢ A competitive edge in the marketplace along with facilitation of marketing, contracting and reimbursement.
> ➢ Improved risk management and risk reduction and possible lowered insurance costs.
> ➢ Education on good practices to improve business operations and enhanced staff education
> ➢ Enhanced loyalty and cohesiveness of clinical teams and a "culture of excellence" across the organization.

- Healthcare organizations that undergo Joint Commission evaluations can obtain either accreditation for the entire healthcare organization (hospital, long-term care facility, medical office, etc.) and/or certification for a particular program or service within a facility or community (i.e., diabetes education program in a hospital).

- **Accreditation** programs include those specific to:
  - ➢ Ambulatory care facilities.
  - ➢ Behavioral health organizations.
  - ➢ Critical access hospitals (small and rural hospitals that meet certain conditions of the Centers for Medicare & Medicaid Services).
  - ➢ Home care services (including in-home personal care or support, home medical equipment, hospice, etc.).
  - ➢ Hospitals (including general, children's long-term acute, psychiatric, rehabilitation and surgical specialty hospitals).
  - ➢ Laboratory services.
  - ➢ Long-term care
  - ➢ Office-based surgery

- **Certification** programs are:
  - ➢ The Disease-Specific Care Certification Program, which is designed to evaluate clinical programs specific for treatment of chronic disease or conditions (diabetes, heart disease, asthma) across the continuum of care.
  - ➢ The Healthcare Staffing Services Certification Program, which focuses o the ability of a health staffing firm's ability to provide qualified and competent services.

- Some states have licensure or certification of dietitians or dietitian/nutritionists, usually with the intent to protect the public.

2. Process, implementation, evaluation

- A **QUALITY ASSURANCE (QA)** program or **QUALITY IMPROVEMENT (QI)** program is a planned, systematic program that includes all actions necessary to provide adequate confidence that the product or service will satisfy given needs. Quality assurance provides some degree of confidence that products/services will be fit for use, reliable, consistent and reasonably priced. Quality assurance should be continuous andongoing to correct and improve products and processes. Quality assurance is a process that monitors and evaluates the quality and appropriateness of patient care.

- Evaluate care by identifying problems and looking for trends. A problem is present when a deficiency in care is serious, repeated or widespread. An "opportunity for improvement" is present when a level of quality is acceptable but, given the resources available, could be improved. Sometimes a composite score meets the threshold but incidences not meeting criteria can be traced to the actions of one or more staff members.

- **TOTAL QUALITY MANAGEMENT (TQM)** is a management theory to improve quality based on involving the total organization, using statistical quality control, seeking to raise workers' performance and continuously reevaluating performance to plan further interventions.

- **TOTAL QUALITY MANAGEMENT (TQM)** and the **QUALITY IMPROVEMENT PROCESS (QIP)** began during World War II when statisticians W. Edwards Deming, Joseph Juran, and W.A. Shewhart pioneered new methods of quality management that were applied to wartime industries. After the war, Deming's philosophy was the basis of Japan's extraordinary manufacturing success. Since the 1980s, increasing numbers of U.S. organizations have employed Deming's original "14 Points" in developing quality assurance programs. A modified version of the TQM process has 8 stages:

  1. Identify the project. Select problems or opportunities for improvement.
  2. Assess the current situation by examining statistical data. Evaluate the present process in detail. Analyze clients' needs and expectations through focus groups, surveys and interviews.
  3. Analyze the cause of the problem. Carefully separate the symptoms from the cause. Ask "why" to get to the root of the problem.
  4. Develop solutions by brainstorming, risk-benefit analysis and consideration of barriers to change. Consider doing a pilot project. Evaluate and improve the pilot project before instituting widespread change.
  5. Implement the improved pilot project. Make changes until it is stable and predictable and then, institute the full process.
  6. Standardize the improvement. Standardization transfers what one person or project team learns to a system that becomes part of the organizational routine.
  7. Relate the improvement to future plans. Did other projects arise as you dealt with this one? Apply what has been learned to other activities.
  8. Continue to monitor and evaluate and make modifications as necessary.

Indicators

- Expected standards and criteria to be met that apply to each area of service or production should be written. Criteria should be written in behavioral terms to express a single action or consequence of a single action. Behavioral criteria are written to evaluate whether nutritional intervention has altered the client's nutritional status or actions.

Criteria

- In designing a control system, managers must decide on the types and number of measurements to be used, what the standards will be, the frequency of measurement and the direction that feedback will take. In the field of nutrition, standards must be developed for nutritional assessment and nutrition intervention in order to demonstrate outcomes of services.

- **CRITERIA** are predetermined elements or standards against which quality of care or service can be compared. These criteria are developed from professional judgments based on current accepted research. Criteria should be stated in behavioral terms and should be measurable and achievable.

- Steps to develop quality assurance criteria are:
  1. Select target population.
  2. Select specific condition(s) or problems.
  3. Write criteria (process or outcome) including critical time, expected level of performance and exceptions.
  4. Reference criteria from the literature.
  5. Verify criteria to be sure they apply.
  6. Validate criteria by a field test.
  7. Revise as necessary.

Measure performance

- Measurement is an ongoing and repeated process with frequency dependent on the type of activity being measured. Accuracy of anthropometric measurements in a preschool clinic may be continuously monitored in a healthcare setting, whereas a progress report on long-term expansion objectives of several clinics may be requested by top management only once or twice per year. The time between measurements should not be unduly long.

Compare performance to criteria

- Performance should be analyzed to determine if the established criteria have been met or if problems exist in any criterion. Criteria may be changed if unforeseen problems cause alteration of the original design.

Plan corrective action

- Corrective action should be taken if performance falls short of standards or there is a negative response to actions or programs. Corrective action may change one or more activities of the organization's operations, or it may involve a change in the standards originally established.

Integration

- Quality control integrates quality standards acceptable to the client or customer with cost containment policies of the supplier. Quality control means providing maximum quality for the resources used. For example, group diet instruction may be adequate and acceptable and also less costly than individual instruction.

Collection of data and monitoring

- An effective quality improvement plan begins with commitment and involvement of top management. Employees get involved through quality circles, improvement process teams and department improvement teams. The whole process, not just the final product or service, is constantly monitored for quality. Every employee, not just a QA officer, is responsible for and involved with continuous improvement of systems, products and services. This approach differs markedly from training employees only to do as told. Quality assurance asks employees what, when, where and why systems and procedures should be changed and implements these actions as appropriate.

  - Assign personnel in each department for QA activities (indicators, data collection, etc.).
  - Describe the scope of care and type of patients served.
  - Identify the important aspects of care delivered. Those activities with the greatest impact on patient care should be the focus. Give priority to aspects of care for which there is large volume, high risk or high probability of problems. The JCAHO has specific QA standards for food and dietetic services that are a basis for evaluation. The standards are usually built into the institution's standards to prepare for JCAHO audits.
  - Identify the quality indicators. Indicators should be **R**elevant, **U**nderstandable, **M**easurable, **B**ehavioral and **A**chievable (RUMBA) index. Indicators can be resources, processes, clinical events, complications or outcomes.
  - Establish a threshold for evaluation. This threshold will be a pre-established level. For example, 90% of all patients on clear liquid diets will be advanced to other diets within 48 hours.
  - Collect and organize the data. Data sources include patient records, department logs and screening tools. Determine who will collect the data, when it will be collected and what sample will be used.

- Both quality and productivity must be measured to determine whether goals have been met. You can only control or manage what you can measure. Measurements are obtained from complaints, returns, reworks, inventories, surveys, data sheets, performance records, plate waste, weight loss of patients, serum cholesterol values or other measures.

Evaluation of effectiveness

- Effectiveness, according to Deming, is based on the degree of variation between the intended goal of a product or service and its actual performance. The service user's (not provider's) expectation and appraisal are measured and evaluated.

- For examples of evaluation problems and solutions, see **www.jcaho.org.**

- A 100% performance standard is unreachable for most situations, so thresholds for evaluation have been introduced. **THRESHOLDS** designate a point (lower limit) at which collected data require further investigation. Thresholds of 100% are set for **SENTINEL EVENTS** in which even one error is unacceptable. For example, serving food that causes an extreme reaction in a patient with a known allergy or intolerance is a sentinel event. Sentinel events are ones to guard against because error causes severe illness, injury or death.

- The **COMPLIANCE RATE** is a percentage established for each item monitored. For example, a threshold level of 70% is set for inpatient meal acceptability. If your survey reveals that the actual acceptability rate was 92% in January, your facility is in compliance with that item.

Implementation of corrective action

- Take actions to solve the problems. Develop a plan of corrective action, identifying who or what is expected to change. Look for the cause. It may be lack of knowledge, system defect or deficient behavior or performance.

- Correct by giving further education and training, supplying reference sources, changing policies and procedures, redistributing staff, altering use of equipment and supplies, correcting communication problems or counseling or transferring staff.

- Assess the corrective action and document improvement. Communicate relevant information to the hospital-wide QA program coordinator.

Report

- Like monitoring, documenting and reporting results according to established procedures, is an ongoing process and required for quality assurance, program funding and legal reasons.

a. Cost benefit analysis (CBA)

- **COST BENEFIT ANALYSIS** is conducted to determine if alternative actions will produce better financial or operational results. Cost/benefit analysis can be done prospectively or retrospectively. For example, record keeping in a nursing home is still done by hand. The food service director wants to computerize recipes, menus, purchasing and receiving forms, budgets and equipment repair records. She anticipates the need to hire an extra person to enter data, maintain the records and train current personnel on basic computer use. The savings should offset the increased personnel costs and personnel training time. A cost/benefit analysis will determine if the change will be beneficial before any action is taken.

- Cost benefit analysis provides an evaluation whether or not a particular project (intervention, program, etc.,) is worth completing or whether one project is more worthwhile than others. This is done by comparing the total costs of the project with the total benefits, all delineated in financial terms. Translation of costs and benefits into strictly financial terms can be difficult. (Placing a monetary value on certain things, such as the cost of a human life when evaluating the efficacy of drug, or the cost of a facility's reputation after a food-borne illness outbreak, has many ramifications).

- Another consideration in CBA is the "time value of money". Since the value of money changes over time, it is important that the true costs and benefits are reflected over the course of a project in the same terms. This is usually done by adjusting future costs into current or "present value" using a discount rate.

- **COST EFFECTIVENESS** is an analytic tool in which costs and effects of a program, and at least one alternative, are calculated and presented in a ratio of incremental costs to incremental effects. Effects are health outcomes; such as cases of a disease prevention, years of life gained or quality adjusted life years rather than monetary measures as in cost/benefit analysis.

b. Productivity studies

- **PRODUCTIVITY** is measured as the ratio of input to output. Increased productivity promotes increased profit. Operations analysis provides information that increases productivity.

- **WORK SIMPLIFICATION** is the process of finding easier, more efficient ways to handle tasks so that operations, time and motions can be reduced; thus increasing production and decreasing costs.

- **WORK SAMPLING** is a tool for fact-finding. Periodic work checks are cheaper than a continuous study. Work sampling is also known as **RANDOM RATIO DELAY SAMPLING** and **OCCURRENCE SAMPLING.** In this method there is intermittent observation of the worker engaged in various work-related activities.

- **TOTAL EFFICIENCY UNITS** are measures of quantity of work performed per unit of time; such as per hour.

- **PATHWAY CHARTS** (Flow Diagrams) are scale drawings of the path of a worker, measuring time and distance. Saving steps and actions saves time and money, especially if a task is repeated many times. **OPERATION CHARTS** document efficient movement of hands based on transport and action.

- **PROCESS CHARTS** are graphic presentations of work motions designed to improve the efficiency of the method. They track motions in a vertical column, using only a few symbols. The method was devised by **FRANK AND LILLIAN GILBRETH.**

- **MICROMOTION STUDIES** use photographs of motions taken at fractions of a second. The Gilbreth's formulated the idea. **CHRONOCYCLEGRAPHS** are photographic records of work patterns made by tying lights to hands. These records can be used to identify and reduce motions that are unnecessary.

3. Outcomes management systems

- An outcomes management system evaluates the effectiveness and efficiency of an operation. For dietetics that can be in the clinical setting, the community setting or in department operations.

- In 2004, President George W. Bush set a goal to establish an electronic health record for all Americans by 2014. This had been anongoing effort, first suggested by the Institute of Medicine because of patient safety and privacy. The electronic record will also be more efficient and, it is believed, save many errors on patient charts.

- Insurance companies want to use the data to see if the procedures and consultations they are paying for have positive outcomes.

- Financial officers also want the systems in place to see if there are positive outcomes for department operations.

4. Vendor performance and evaluation

- The ability of a vendor to supply an organization with necessary equipment and supplies can make or break that organization. For this reason an appropriate vendor evaluation program is imperative. Vendors should be regularly and formally evaluated as to whether or not they are meeting (or can meet) the needs of the organization.

- Vendor evaluations should include examination of the following criteria:
  - ➢ Product line- availability of items; quality, packaging, size and amounts
  - ➢ Delivery- schedule, reliability, methods and promptness, honesty
  - ➢ Sales personnel0- professionalism, knowledge, promptness, honesty
  - ➢ Accounting- correct, timely with both billing invoices and refunds
  - ➢ Company- stability, reputation, location, size, capacity, labor/trade relations
  - ➢ Facilities- cleanliness and reliability of storage facilities, trucks and related equipment

- Vendors should not be evaluated on the basis of one order/delivery but rather at regular intervals. This should be done with the use of a standard evaluation form that should be completed to formally evaluate all vendors. Results of such evaluations should be shared with vendors so that they can make changes, adjustments and be told the reasons for the termination of services.

Domain IV - FOOD SERVICE SYSTEMS

Domain IV = 17% of the test.

TOPIC A -MENU DEVELOPMENT

1. Types of menus

   a. Patient/resident
   > (1) Select/non-select
   > (2) Restaurant
   > (3) Room service

   b. Commercial

   c. Non-commercial

2. Menu development

   a. Master menu
   > (1) Concepts
   > (2) Development

   b. Guidelines and parameters
   > (1) Aesthetics
   > (2) Nutritional adequacy
   > (3) Cost
   > (4) Regulations

   c. Modifications
   > (1) Diet/disease states
   > (2) Substitutions
   > (3) Nutritional adequacy
   > (4) Allergies and food sensitivities

   d. Clients
   > (1) Age/life cycle stage
   > (2) Cultural/religious influence
   > (3) Vegetarian
   > (4) Satisfaction measurement
   >> (a) Customer evaluation
   >> (b) Sales data

   e. Operational influences
   > (1) Equipment
   > (2) Labor
   > (3) Budget

   f. External influences
   > (1) Trends
   > (2) Seasonal
   > (3) Disaster
   > (4) Product availability

TOPIC B - PROCUREMENT, PRODUCTION, DISTRIBUTION, and SERVICE

1. Procurement, receiving, and inventory management
    a. Procurement principles, concepts and methods
        (1) Bidding
        (2) Specification development
        (3) Group purchasing/prime vendor
        (4) Ethics
    b. Procurement decisions
        (1) Product selection/yield
        (2) Product packaging
        (3) Cost analysis
    c. Receiving and storage
        (1) Equipment and methods
        (2) Records
        (3) Security
    d. Inventory management
        (1) Control procedures - par levels, rotation, minimum/maximum
        (2) Issuing procedures

2. Principles of quantity food preparation and processing
    a. Cooking methods
    b. Equipment
    c. Preservation and packaging methods
    d. Modified diets

3. Food production control procedures
    a. Standardized recipes
    b. Ingredient control
    c. Portion control and yield analysis
    d. Forecasting production
    e. Production scheduling

4. Production systems
    a. Conventional
    b. Commissary
    c. Ready prepared
    d. Assembly serve
    e. Cook-chill
    f. Display cooking

5. Distribution and service
    a. Type of service systems

        (1) Centralized
        (2) Decentralized

    b. Equipment/packaging

IV. FOODSERVICE SYSTEMS (17%)

TOPIC C – SANITATION AND SAFETY

1. Sanitation and food safety
    a. Principles
        (1) Contamination and spoilage
        (2) Factors affecting bacterial growth
        (3) Signs and symptoms of food-borne illness
    b. Sanitation practices and infection control
        (1) Personal hygiene
        (2) Food and equipment
        (3) Food storage
        (4) Temperature control
        (5) Food hling techniques
    c. Regulations (government and other agencies)
    d. Food safety
        (1)Time and temperature control
        (2) Additives
        (3) Documentation and record keeping
        (4) HACCP
        (5) Recalls
        (6) Operational emergencies
        (7) Bioterrorism

2. Safety
    a. Employee safety
        (1) Universal precautions
        (2) Equipment use and maintenance
        (3) Personal work habits
    b. Safety practices
        (1) Environmental conditions
        (2) Regulations
        (3) Fire safety
        (4) Accident prevention
    c. Safety documentation and record keeping

TOPIC D – EQUIPMENT AND FACILITY PLANNING

1. Facility layout
    a. Equipment and layout planning
        (1) Menu
        (2) Service system
        (3) Safety and sanitation
        (4) Privacy/accessibility
        (5) Codes and standards
        (6) Fiscal aspects

IV. FOODSERVICE SYSTEMS (17%)

b. Planning team
  (1) Composition
  (2) Roles
  (3) Responsibilities

2. Equipment specifications and selection

TOPIC E - SUSTAINABILITY

1. Food and water
2. Non-food
  a. Supplies
  b. Equipment
3. Waste management
  a. Storage
  b. Reduction
  c. Disposal

TOPIC A - MENU DEVELOPMENT

- The menu is the primary way in which a food service operation communicates with its customer.

- The menu determines all aspects of production and service. Planning menus well is key to any successful food service operation.

- The menu is not only a price sheet, it is a selling and public relations device.

- The menu card should be designed and worded to appeal to the client, to stimulate sales and to influence choices. The menu should be easy to read, easy to handle, and spotlessly clean.

- Menus in healthcare settings should reinforce nutrition education parameters of the facility and provide a variety of healthy, tasty foods appropriate to the population served.

- Menu items should be clearly described, usually with the primary food in the description

- Menu items should use plural forms only when more than one unit is used. ("Scrambled eggs" contain more than one egg.)

- Menu items must be served as described. ("Vanilla Pudding with Whipped Cream" should be served with whipped cream, not whipped topping.)

- Patient menus should be easy to read and mark. Hospitals use a variety of scanning and other devices to tabulate menu items for patient trays. The menus determine food and staffing needs.

1. Types of menus

a. Patient/resident

- Facilities that provide all foods consumed by patients, residents, clients, etc., must provide food that meets total nutritional needs of the population served.

- Generally, cycle menus are longer for resident populations to avoid boredom and reduce repetition than they would be for populations with short stays in a facility.

- When different people (staff, visitors) eat in the facility, and have other options and meals elsewhere, it is appropriate to serve healthful meals, but three meals do not have to meet total daily needs.

(1) Select/non-select

- **SELECT MENUS** allow for food choices to be made by the patient/resident hours or days before the meal is served. Menus are distributed to patients and then collected by staff. This menu option allows for the control of amounts of various foods to be purchased and prepared as well as reduces waste and cost per meal. In medical facilities, different menus are written to provide acceptable options for those with medical issues and modified diets.

- **NON-SELECT MENUS** are predetermined menus that give the customer no menu choices. Variety is limited to items most likely to be consumed. Prior to writing menus, the dietetics professional should establish cost and nutrient parameters, define the target group, include cultural food preferences, check production feasibility, evaluate cost and nutrient content and establish menu guidelines (i.e., each lunch entrée will include 3 ounces of protein-rich food.)

(2) Restaurant

- Many hospitals and extended care facilities offer on-site restaurant-style food services for patients, residents, employees and others. These run the gamut of quick service to white tablecloth operations and can be a profit center.

- Restaurants and other food service operations offer a **FIXED MENU**, which is the same basic menu offered every day. "Daily specials" may be included. It is commonly known as **RESTAURANT-STYLE**, but is currently being used in healthcare settings, especially those with cook-chill, cook-freeze or assembly-serve systems. Fixed menus include popular items that are always available.

(3) Room service

- Some hospitals offer room service and individually prepared meals for patients and guests. Others have special units with this service at additional cost.

- **HOST/HOSTESS MENUS** are being used in many healthcare facilities for both public relations and cost purposes. A host/hostess is assigned to a specific floor and breakfast and sometimes lunch is chosen from a **SPOKEN MENU** and prepared on the floor.

- Regardless of the type of menu, menus planned by dietetics professionals should meet the energy and nutrient needs of the population served. *Dietary Guidelines for Americans* and DRI/RDAs are planning documents. Menus should meet the nutritional needs of the population, especially if the meals served are the only source of nutrients; as in residence halls, camps, correctional facilities, extended care facilities or hospitals.

b. Commercial

- **RESTAURANT MENUS** and menus for commercial establishments are printed selective menus that give customers a range of available foods allowing them to choose what they wish to eat. Menus should be planned to provide desired, frequently chosen items and a variety of special items selected to appeal to the population served.

  - ➤ **TABLE D' HÔTE** is a complete meal offered at fixed price. Customers are often offered a selection from each course. It is also called **PRIX FIXE MENU.**
  - ➤ **DU JOUR MENU** or menu of the day, is planned and written one day at a time. It offers flexibility and can be planned to use leftover food, seasonal foods, food bargains or food market specials.
  - ➤ **À LA CARTE MENU** includes items or groups of items priced separately and chosen by the customer.

- Menus are usually printed, but some facilities use menu boards or spoken menus. Often restaurants present daily specials as spoken items. In cafeterias, consumers self-select food items. The cafeteria line may be straight or arranged in a scatter or hollow-square configuration. The hollow-square accommodates more people and minimizes back-ups. Many cafeterias now feature a number of stations serving different types of food (i.e., soups and sandwiches, salads, baked potatoes with toppings and Mexican foods.) Some food service operations offer carryout foods. Employee cafeterias may be subsidized to give employees quality food at low prices and operated by an outside food service contractor. Contracts for services are negotiated and reviewed on a regular basis.

- **VENDING** is a total self-service system that does not require food service employee staffing. Food selection is limited by size, perishability and packaging. The decision of what selections to offer in machines is a menu planning issue. Customers may use microwave ovens to heat or finish foods that are purchased from vending machines.

- Mechanical dispensing of food, beverages and sundries offers convenience in areas where volume is not sufficient to justify a full-service facility. Vending may be available when the full food service is not open, for example, to outpatients in emergency rooms or in university dormitories.

- There is a large profit potential in vending. Vending may be self-operated or contracted to a vending company. Self-operating units assume full responsibility for stocking, currency collection and banking, security, maintenance and refunds. The vending contract should be awarded on bid basis, focusing on service levels, availability of preferred menu items, projected sales volume and commission to be paid to the host facility. Commissions are typically 25-30% of sales.

- Menu items in a coffee shop, restaurant, cafeteria or fast-food establishment are often posted, as are daily specials. Information should be logically organized and should include price. Menus and signs should be neatly printed and immaculately clean. Menu labeling of calories and the availability of additional nutrition information is now required for chain restaurants and some other food service venues.

- **CATERING** is the provision of food, and possibly service and equipment, for a predetermined group or set of functions. It is done by both commercial and non-commercial food service operations. Unlike other businesses, the client base changes continuously. The customer has more direct input about menu design and cost than in most other situations. A food service department typically negotiates special parties and conference meals as additional catered events. Services may be made available to outside groups (i.e., congregate dining programs or Meals-on-Wheels). Catered events may be a major source of additional revenue to a non-commercial food service operation, such as a hospital.

- Catering has the following characteristics:

  - The client sets the menu and cost parameters.
  - It may be on-site or off-site; may require provision of all service equipment and tableware; may require wait staff; and may involve coordinating other services (i.e., audiovisual equipment, security, flowers and musicians).
  - Catering frequently requires special licenses or permits, especially if alcohol is served. For not-for-profit organizations offering catering services, corporate tax-exempt status may be compromised by providing outside catering activities.
  - A contract should be written to include the specifics of the engagement, including scope of services provided, menu, number of staff, number of people to be served, use of outside facilities, insurance, trash removal, cleaning, method of payment and responsibility for obtaining permits.
  - Catering contracts may or may not include equipment rental, table lines, decorations or other items needed for the event.
  - Pricing will be influenced by the type of services provided and competition in the particular market. Pricing must cover all direct and indirect costs as well as contribution to profit.

c. Non-commercial

- Non-commercial food service operations include healthcare, school food service, correctional facilities, colleges and universities and the military.

- School food service must meet specific governmental guidelines as to type and amount of food groups served that meet the needs of school-aged children.

- Colleges and universities generally offer several meal plans and students can choose meal plans that provide some or all meals. Often school foodservice must compete with off-site food operations and plan menus that are particularly appealing to students. Typically fast-casual, comfort and ethnic foods are offered.

- For the military:
  - ➤ Appropriate feeding plans are based on where the personnel are based and availability of safe supplies, water, facilities and personnel for meal preparation.
  - ➤ In addition to the previously mentioned types of service, troops in the field have a variety of meals including **TRANSPORTABLE READY-TO-EAT MEALS** for when soldiers are not on the base. These include vegetarian and meals to meet the religious needs of individual soldiers.
  - ➤ There are special cold weather rations available to support nutrition needs in the colder climates.
  - ➤ There is also the **UNITIZED GROUP RATION (UGR),** which is basically an entire meal that is prepared by submerging a sealed food tray in water or by adding hot water to reconstitute the product.

2. Menu development

a. Master menu

(1) Concepts

- Menus are usually developed in a ten-step process. Every menu should be evaluated for variety, balance, nutritional value and cost.

  1. Distribute dinner and lunch entrées over the cycle, varying category (meat, poultry, fish, etc.) and preparation method, including sauces, if any.
  2. Select starchy items, if required, to accompany entrées or indicate that it has been deliberately eliminated (i.e., entrée of beef stew made with potatoes does not require additional starch).
  3. Select vegetables, considering color, texture and shape.
  4. Select salads, varying types, and dressings.
  5. Select desserts, varying types.
  6. Select soup and/or appetizers, if any.
  7. Select breads.
  8. Select breakfast entrées.
  9. Select breakfast cereal and breads.
  10. Select fruits/juices.

- Use fresh fruits and vegetables that are in season whenever possible. In peak season, produce is at maximum flavor and is generally less expensive.

- A variety of hot and chilled beverages should be offered with each meal.

- In **CYCLE MENUS** different items are offered daily for each meal. Menus are planned for a set period of time (weekly, biweekly, monthly and/or seasonally), after which the cycle is repeated. It is often used in institutional settings, based on the client length of stay. In long term care facilities and schools, the cycle should be longer than in hospitals with rapid client turnover. Most food service operations use a cycle menu. The goals of the cycle menu are:

  - ➢ To reduce time spent on menu planning.
  - ➢ To increase control over production.
  - ➢ To achieve efficiencies through increased familiarity with production and menus.
  - ➢ To reduce costs as a result of more accurate knowledge of inventory requirements over time.
  - ➢ To minimize staff training time that would be required by introducing new menu items often.

- The length of the cycle depends on the facility. In a hospital, where a typical patient stay is five days or less, a seven-day cycle is often used. For hospital cafeterias or for long-term stays, such as in a nursing home or for home-delivered meals, a cycle menu is typically four weeks.

- The beginning and end of a cycle menu must fit together with no repetition.

- Cycle menus are planned to take into consideration seasonal variations. Often there is a fall, winter, spring and summer cycle menu each repeated 2-3 times to take advantage of produce plentiful during that season. The summer cycle might include more salads; in the winter cycle more hearty stews and soup.

- Special holiday meals may be inserted on appropriate days as substitutes for the cycle offerings.

- **SINGLE USE MENUS** are planned for a specific day, holiday or event. This type of menu is frequently used in catering, where there are specific requests.

(2) Development

- The menu is the primary control system in food service. It dictates all of the other components of the food service system, what resources are required and how they are used to create the final product. The primary goal of a food service operation is to serve food that appeals to and meets the needs the consumer (nutritional, financial, etc.) while reflecting the mission, goals and objectives of the operation itself. This should be kept in mind while planning the menu. The menu-driven concept controls the entire organization and menu planning should be approached as a team effort including individuals with knowledge and skills in (but not limited to) nutrition, procurement, food preparation, facility management and hiring and training employees. Customers may be asked for menu suggestions.

- Factors that determine the final menu and recipes include time, nutrition needs of clients, staff skills, clientele demographics, season, geographic location, food costs, equipment and budget/profit goals.

b. Guidelines and parameters

(1) Aesthetics

- Visual appeal affects appetite and perception of food quality as much as taste and smell. Variations of color, temperature, shape and size increases meal appeal. Simple garnishes heighten interest. Texture can also add variety to a menu. Try to balance crisp, firm and soft foods. Provide both bold and mildly flavored foods to appeal to individual tastes.

- Avoid planning a menu that combines too many starchy foods, sauces, mixed foods (casseroles), fruits and vegetables of the same type or fried foods. Do not repeat food items too frequently. Hot and cold food items offered at the same meal provide temperature variety.

- Plating is key to eye appeal. Generally an odd number of foods on a platter is more visually appealing than an even number. Garnishes and sauces should complement the food and provide added color, texture and flavor.

(2) Nutritional adequacy

- Meals must meet the total energy and nutrient needs if the food service provides all meals for an individual, such as in a nursing home or correctional facility. When one meal a day is provided, it should supply at least 1/3 of the daily nutrients for the population served. Follow a meal pattern to ensure provision of recommended numbers of servings from the MyPlate Guidelines (**www.choosemyplate.gov**). Develop menus to meet the specific needs of individuals served, (i.e., those on modified diets). Menu items and complete meals may be evaluated for nutritional adequacy, using computer programs and should meet the DRI of the population served.

- Generally, menus should include foods from each food group at each meal. Low-fat milk should be offered as a beverage to meet the dairy group recommended servings although many adults will choose another beverage.

- Meals offered should generally meet recommendations of *Dietary Guidelines for Americans.* While some offerings can be high in calories, there should be a variety of healthful offerings so that the diner can select a meal that is appropriate and moderate in calories.

(3) Cost

- Menu pricing is influenced by labor, competition, customers and atmosphere and location as well as food costs.

- **FOOD COSTS** are the total expenditures for ingredients and edible products. The cost is obtained by determining the cost of ingredients, using purchasing specifications, quantity, weight, portion size and number of portions. Food in the food service budget is one of the most readily controlled costs and is subject to the greatest fluctuation. Menu planning, portion control and pricing strategies affect control of food costs.

Food cost terminology

- **AS PURCHASED (AP) WEIGHT** is the total amount of product purchased, including bones, fat, unusable portions and inedible outer layers.

- **EDIBLE PORTION (EP)** is the net amount of product obtained after processing, preparation and cooking. The ready-to-eat amount is, for example, the weight of chicken without bones.

- **PORTION SIZE** is the amount of food served to a customer as a single portion. This weight may include some inedible portion, i.e. chicken bones, grapefruit peel. It may be stated in ounces, cups or count, such as ½ grapefruit or 2 cookies.

- **WASTE** is the amount of food lost during processing, cooking or portioning. The percentage of waste equals the waste (loss) weight divided by the AP weight of the product.

  % Waste = Waste ÷ AP weight

- **FOOD COST PERCENTAGE** is a control mechanism that can be applied to total operation, a day, a meal or even a recipe.

  Food Cost % = Dollars raw food costs x 100
  Dollars food sales

  Examples:
  For operation: $\underline{\$400,000}$ x 100 = 36% which is the Food Cost %
  $\$1,110,00$

  For recipe: $\underline{\$0.25}$ x 100 = 33%, which is the Food Cost %
  $\$0.75$

- **YIELD** is the usable product remaining after processing, cooking and portioning. The **PERCENTAGE OF YIELD** equals the net weight of usable product divided by the AP weight.

  Yield % = Yield ÷ AP Weight

- Yield is the reciprocal of percentage waste.

  100% AP Weight = Waste % + Yield %

- **PORTION FACTOR** is the actual number of servings per pound of any food product.

  Portion Factor = 16 oz. ÷ Portion Size

- **PORTION DIVIDER** is obtained by multiplying the portion factor by the percentage yield of a food product.

  Portion Divider = Yield % x Portion Factor

Example:

The menu offers roast beef. A decision must be made as to whether to purchase raw round of beef at $4.00 per pound (75% yield) or precooked beef round at $6.25 per pound (95% yield). The menu requires 200 4 oz. servings. The manager must determine how much to buy, portion costs and whether it is more economical to purchase the raw or precooked product.

1. Determine the portion factor: 16 oz. ÷ 4 oz. = 4 which is the portion factor
2. Determine portion divider: Raw beef: 0.75 x 4 = 3.0; Pre-cooked beef: 0.95 x 4 = 3.8.
3. Determine the amount to buy: Number of servings ÷ portion divider = AP weight

Raw beef: 200 ÷ 3.0 = 66.60 x $4.00 = $266.40
   Precooked beef: 200 ÷ 3.8 = 52.63 x $6.25 = $328.94
The raw beef will cost less even though more pounds will be needed.

- Sometimes menu item prices are adjusted because a $5.95 selling price may be more acceptable to customers than a $6.15 selling price. Other times, items may have a higher than calculated selling price (i.e. coffee or popcorn) because customers expect to pay a higher price even though the actual food cost is low. These higher than normal factored prices may offset items with higher food costs.

(4) Regulations

- In governmentally mandated food programs, such as school breakfast and lunch and senior citizen feeding programs, there are specific regulations that require certain levels of nutrients to be offered or served and certain types of food (i.e., milk) that must be provided.

- Some school districts have additional regulations that limit or ban soft drinks or other empty calorie items from being served or available in dispensing machines.

- **TRUTH IN MENU** guidelines require that:

  ➢ Brand name, if used, must be represented accurately.
  ➢ Dietary and nutritional information must be accurate and supported with statistical data. Anything marked 'low-fat' must meet that nutritional claim.
  ➢ Presentation of food must be accurate. "Fresh fish" must not have been frozen.
  ➢ Location of ingredients must be accurate. Vermont maple syrup or Dover sole must come from these locations.
  ➢ Quality or grade must be accurate. Prime sirloin on a menu may not be choice grade beef.
  ➢ Proper cooking techniques must be stated. Broiled chicken may not be baked.
  ➢ Pictures must be accurate. If pie on the menu is shown à la mode, the item must be served topped with ice cream.
  ➢ Description of food products must be accurate. If an entrée is to be served with wild mushrooms, that entrée must have wild, not white regular mushrooms. If jumbo shrimp is listed, it may not have medium sized shrimp. "Homemade" anything must not be a commercial product. It must be made from raw ingredients on the premises.

Menu labeling

- While a number of states and local governments have proposed and/or passed a variety of menu labeling regulations in recent years, in March of 2010, Section 4205 of the Patient Protection and Affordable Healthcare Act (HR 3590) provided menu labeling regulations at a federal level.

- The regulations stipulate that restaurants or similar retail food establishments with 20 or more locations, doing business under the same name and offering for sale substantially the same menu items, must post calorie information of menu items that are offered for at least 60 days throughout the calendar year. Calorie content is to be displayed clearly and prominently on all menus and menu boards including drive through menus and food display tags. Calories for variable menu items, such as combination meals, would be displayed in ranges. An example of a combination meal could be a choice of sandwich, side dish and beverage.

- A succinct statement concerning suggested daily caloric intake is to be posted prominently on menus and menu boards to help the public understand the significance of the calorie information provided on menus and menu boards.

- A notice that additional nutrition information for menu items is available upon request must be displayed. Additional information for calories from fat, total fat, saturated fat, cholesterol, trans fat, sodium, total carbohydrates, sugars, dietary fiber and protein must be made available when requested.

- State and local governments are not able to impose any different or additional nutrition labeling requirements for food sold in restaurants and similar retail food establishments covered by the Federal requirements but can establish nutrition labeling requirements for establishments not covered by the new law or regulations (those with less than 20 locations and/or those not defined as a restaurant, i.e. bowling alleys, etc.).

- HR 3590 also includes similar legislation for vending machines so that nutritional information for foods is either visible on individual packages while it is still in the machine or provided nearby to (in the same line of vision) of the food items in the machine.

- The intent of such legislation is to provide consumers with tools and resources to make informed and healthful food choices. However, it is not yet clear what impact menu labeling will have on purchasing decisions and/or nutritional intake of consumers. Dietetics professionals have a role in helping consumers interpret and use the information provided.

c. Modifications

(1) Diet/disease states

- Foods served in hospitals and healthcare facilities must meet the special health needs of patients or residents. Because many people on modified diets go to restaurants or other commercial establishments, healthful options should be available on the menu, or upon request. The most common dietary requests are for low-fat and low-sugar options. There are increasing requests for gluten-free, reduced-calorie and reduced-sodium options.

- Many people have food allergies. Managers and wait staff should be aware of common allergens and be able to respond to questions from customers about ingredients used in food preparation.

- Dietary modifications for therapeutic diets and medical nutrition therapy are described in Domain II.

(2) Substitutions

- Clientele, market, market cost, season, availability, food preferences, regulations and health needs of client affect substitutions and number of choices in menus and menu items. Substitutions may be made for the soup, salad or entrée of the day in many healthcare units. Often standard substitutes, such as broiled fish or a peanut butter and jelly sandwich, are routinely available but not listed on the menu.

Substitutions and food preferences

- Quality food services offer enough variety and choices to allow individuals to choose preferred foods. Even in limited-menu operations, there should be substitutions available upon request. Generally, items like peanut butter and jelly, cereal with milk, soup, salads, pudding and simple cooked items (broiled or baked chicken) are available as food substitutes when offered food is disliked by the patient/client.

- When individuals are ill or stressed, appetite disturbances are common and personal "comfort" foods are preferred. As it is important to maintain nutrient intake and hydration, flexibility is needed. Selective menus should be used when possible to promote choosing foods more likely to be eaten. Hospital policies determine if family members may bring in favored foods (especially for terminally ill patients).

COMMON FOOD SUBSTITUTES

Food Group	Use	Instead of
Milk and dairy products:		
	Low-fat or skim milk	Whole milk
	Low-fat cheeses	Whole-milk and full-fat cheeses
	Low-fat yogurt; reduced-fat sour cream	Whole-milk yogurt; sour cream
	Ice milk, frozen yogurt	Ice cream
	Whole milk or fat-free half and half	Cream
Vegetables, including starchy vegetables:	Baked or low fat chips	French fries, potato chips
	Unsalted vegetable juices	Highly salted vegetable juices
	Steamed, roasted, grilled, stir-fried or raw vegetables	Fried vegetables or vegetables in cream sauce
Fruits:	Fresh, frozen, dried, juice pack	Fruits in heavy syrup
	Unsweetened fruit juices	Highly sweetened fruit juices and fruit drinks

---

Breads, starches and cereals:	Whole grain cereals	Highly sweetened cereals with refined grains
	Whole grain, reduced-fat or low fat chips or crackers	Regular snack chips or crackers
	English muffins, bagels, tortillas	Doughnuts, biscuits, croissants, sweet rolls
Meats or substitutes:	Lean meats, fish, shellfish, poultry	Fried or fatty meats, fish or poultry with skin
	Reduced-fat cheeses (such as part-skim Mozzarella cheese); fat-free cheeses	High-fat cheeses (such as brie, Cheddar and processed cheeses)
	Soybeans, tofu, dry beans and peas	Nuts, peanuts
	Egg whites, egg substitutes	Egg yolks (more than four per week)
Fats:	Corn, cottonseed, olive sesame, soybean, safflower, sunflower, peanut, canola oils	Butter, lard, bacon fat, meat fat and drippings
	Reduced-fat mayonnaise	Regular mayonnaise
	Reduced-calorie salad dressings	Regular mayonnaise
	Whipped margarine or butter	Coconut or palm oil as ingredients in packaged foods, hydrogenated vegetable Shortenings
	Reduced-fat salad dressing	Regular salad dressings
Soups:	Vegetable soups; broths; lightly salted soups with fat skimmed	Most commercially prepared soups and mixes
	Cream-styled soups (with low-fat milk)	Regular cream soups
	Reduced-sodium soups, stocks without salt	Salted, canned soups or high sodium dried mixes
Sweets and desserts:	Fruit and other desserts that have been sweetened lightly and/or contain only moderate fat	Desserts high in sugar and/or fats, such as candy, pastries rich cakes, pies, puddings
Beverages:	Water, mineral water, unsweetened or artificially sweetened soft drinks, juices	Highly sweetened beverages, including soft drinks
	Low-alcohol beer, wine	Alcoholic beverages in significant quantity
Miscellaneous:	Herbs, spices, flavorings, aromatics	Salt and salt/spice combinations

- If substitutions must be made because a listed menu item is not available, the customer/patient should be asked if the substitution is acceptable or if he/she would like to change the choice before the food is served.

IV. FOODSERVICE SYSTEMS (17%)

(3) Nutritional adequacy

- Menus should meet the specific needs of the dietary prescription, based on personal medical needs, age, food intolerance, need for modified texture, etc.

- Facilities that provide meals in non-therapeutic settings, such as university food services, may need to provide special foods/preparation for students who are gluten-intolerant, lactose-intolerant or have food allergies or other needs.

(4) Allergies and food sensitivities

- Patients with allergies and food sensitivities are now requesting information on food content and preparation methods that may affect their health. Common food allergens include milk, nuts, (especially peanuts), eggs, soy products, wheat, dairy and shellfish.

- Employees must be trained to answer questions about ingredients and preparation methods. Medical emergencies and possible lawsuits can result if incorrect answers are given or a food with an allergen is served to a person who declared a sensitivity or allergy to an ingredient. See Domain I – Food Allergies and Intolerances.

d. Clients

(1) Age/life cycle stage

- Nutritional needs vary through the life cycle. Menu selections should be planned so that the most likely combinations meet both physical and psychological needs. (For example, the vegetables offered most frequently in school lunches should be those children enjoy, such as corn and green beans, not Brussels sprouts or beets.) Physiologic needs will be met if RDI/RDA levels of nutrients needed by the population served are available but only if the food is eaten.

(2) Cultural and religious influence

- Menu choices should take into consideration age, sex, health, activity level, race, religion, ethnic preferences, regional preferences, peer group likes and dislikes, etc.

FOOD PATTERNS OF SELECTED CULTURAL GROUPS

Group	Characteristic Foods
African American	
Dairy:	Buttermilk, Cheddar cheese, American cheese, processed cheese
Fruit/vegetable:	Melon, greens, corn, potatoes, black-eyed peas
Grain:	Grits, biscuits, rice, cornbread, bread
Protein group:	Pork, chicken, macaroni and cheese, dried beans, organ meats, meat parts (tails, ears, etc.), fish (catfish, buffalo fish, perch), sandwich meats
Preparation methods:	Frying, boiling, addition of gravies
Beverages:	Carbonated beverages, fruit drinks, coffee
Italian/Mediterranean	
Dairy:	Ricotta, mozzarella, parmesan, gorgonzola cheeses, custards
Fruit/vegetable:	Figs, grapes, tangerines, tomatoes, olives, eggplant, artichoke, zucchini, roasted peppers
Grain:	Pasta, rice, polenta, Italian bread, breadsticks
Protein group:	Veal, chicken, sausages, seafood, including shellfish, legumes
Preparation methods:	Many combinations of foods and sauces; garlic, herbs; olive oil is primary fat
Beverages:	Wine and coffee
Puerto Rican	
Dairy:	Native white cheese, evaporated milk, custards, milk in coffee
Fruit/vegetable:	Starchy vegetables (viands) include yautia, malanga, plantain, yucca, sweet potato, squash; also green peppers, onions, lettuce, citrus fruits Including acerola; an excellent source of vitamin C
Grain:	French-type breads, rolls, rice
Protein group:	Chicken, beef, pork, variety meats, salted codfish, tuna, beans, legumes
Preparation methods:	Frying, soups, combinations with Sofrito, an orange colored sauce high in fat, achiote also used
Beverages:	Fruit juice, coffee, beer
Mexican	
Dairy:	Goat milk cheese, native cheeses, evaporated milk, flans (custards), milk in coffee drinks
Fruit/vegetable:	Prickly pears, bananas, peppers, corn, melons, oranges, tomatoes, avocados, potatoes, salsa, mango, cactus (nopales)
Grain:	Corn and flour tortillas, rice, macaroni, sweet rolls
Protein group:	Frijoles (beans), chicken, pork, ground beef, tripe, fish (including raw)
Preparation Methods:	Frying in lard; combination foods; chili peppers
Beverages:	Soft drinks, fruit drinks

IV. FOODSERVICE SYSTEMS (17%)

Southeast Asian

Dairy:	Not usually consumed: primary sources of calcium to replace milk: tofu, dark green vegetables, broth from bones cooked in acid solution, dried fish
Fruit/vegetable:	Stir-fried vegetables (Chinese, Filipinos); broccoli, mushrooms, pineapple, pickled vegetables (Japanese, Thai, Korean), sweet potatoes, beans
Grain:	Basis of meal; rice, thin noodles
Protein group:	Bite-sized pieces of raw fish (Japanese); dried seafood; pork, poultry
Preparation methods:	(Hmong, Chinese) Steaming, boiling, grilling, stir-frying; may have several entrées per meal, "family-style" bowls rather than individual portions; broth-based soups; use of soy and fish-based seasonings; lemon grass, chili pepper, green onion, basil, ginger, garlic, MSG; peanut or corn oil for frying (Chinese); lard for frying (Hmong); communal eating preferred
Beverages:	Coffee with sweetened condensed milk (Thai); strong coffee (Vietnamese); black or green tea (Chinese, Japanese, Korean); fermented beverages and juices (Chinese)

Middle-Eastern

Dairy:	Cow and goat milk, feta cheese, custards, yogurt
Fruit/vegetable:	Olives, figs, dates, persimmons, pomegranates, grapes, citrus, tomatoes, eggplant, avocado, mushrooms
Grain:	Rice, cracked wheat, (bulgur couscous), millet, white seeded breads, pita bread, sesame seeds
Protein group:	Lamb, poultry, some pork, salt-water fish, fish roe, white beans, squid, octopus, eggs, chickpeas, almonds
Preparation methods:	Roasting, grilling; olive oil, garlic, lemon and oregano commonly used
Beverages:	Coffee and wine

Native American

Dairy:	Not often consumed
Fruit/vegetable:	Soups and bean dishes; wild gathered vegetables, nuts and seeds, melons, beans, squash, potatoes, berries
Grain:	Fry bread; corn in all forms; flour tortillas
Protein group:	Sheep, goat, mutton, game, poultry; processed meats; Alaskan natives eat much meat and fish and few vegetables, pine nuts
Preparation methods:	Fried foods prepared with lard; roasting, boiling, baking, stews; food has many social and ceremonial religious customs
Beverages:	Tea, soda pop, fruit drinks

WORLD RELIGIONS AND FOOD PRACTICES

Type of religion	Practice or Restriction	Rationale
Protestants	Few food restrictions or fasting observations Moderation in eating, drinking and exercise is promoted	God made all animal and natural products for humans' enjoyment Gluttony and drunkenness are sins to be controlled
Roman Catholicism	Meat restricted on certain days Fasting practiced	Restrictions are consistent with specified days of the church year
Seventh-day Adventist	Pork prohibited and meat and fish avoided Vegetarian diet is encouraged Alcohol, coffee, and tea prohibited	Diet satisfies practice to "honor and glorify God"
Mormonism	Alcohol and beverages containing caffeine prohibited Moderation in all foods Fasting practiced	Caffeine is addictive and leads to poor physical and emotional health Fasting is the discipline of self-control and honoring to God
Eastern Orthodox Christianity	Restrictions on meat and fish Fasting selectively	Observance of Holy Days includes fasting and restrictions to increase spiritual progress
Judaism (Orthodox and Kosher)	All food inspected and marked as Kosher Pork and shellfish prohibited Meat and dairy at same meal prohibited Leavened food restricted during Passover Fasting practiced	Land animals that do not have cloven hooves and that do not chew their cud are forbidden as unclean (e.g., hare, pig, camel) Kosher process is based upon the Torah
Buddhism	Refrain from meat, vegetarian diet is desirable Moderation in all foods Fasting required of monks	Natural foods of the earth are considered most pure Monks avoid all solid food after noon
Hinduism	Beef prohibited All other meat and fish restricted or avoided Alcohol avoided Numerous fasting days	Cow is sacred and can't be eaten, but products of the "sacred" cow are pure and desirable Fasting promotes spiritual growth
Islam	Pork and certain birds prohibited Alcohol prohibited Coffee/tea/stimulants avoided Fasting from all food and drink during specific periods	Eating is for good health Failure to eat correctly minimizes spiritual awareness Fasting has a cleansing effect of evil elements

WORLD RELIGIONS AND FOOD PRACTICES		
Rastafari	Meat and fish restricted Vegetarian diets only, with salts, preservatives, and condiments prohibited Herbal drinks permitted; alcohol, coffee, and soft drinks prohibited Marijuana used extensively for religious and medicinal purposes	Pigs and shellfish are scavengers and are unclean Foods grown with chemicals are unnatural and prohibited Biblical texts support use of herbs (marijuana and other herbs)
Baha'i	All foods can be eaten except alcohol in any form	Belief that living simply and abstaining from alcohol and mind-altering drugs benefits spiritual development, reduces illness and has a good effect on character and conduct
Jainism	Ascetic practices Strict vegetarians Avoid onions and garlic Avoid honey, eggs, figs Avoid root vegetables Generally do not eat after dark	Desire for non-violence, to do no harm to any creature or environment Belief that onions and garlic increase sexual desire No root vegetable s because insects are killed in their harvest Belief that eating after sundown might kill minute organisms that emerge after dark
Sikism	Halal and Kosher meat forbidden Alcohol forbidden Simple, natural food preferred Some Sikhs do not eat beef or pork; others are vegetarian	Sikhs do not believe in ritual killing thus no halal or Kosher meat No alcohol or drugs promotes mental and physical fitness Whether a Sikh eats meat or is vegetarian depends on personal interpretation of the writings of Guru Granath Sahib Ji All food served in gurdwara (Sikh place of worship) is vegetarian

Chart from *Essentials of Nutrition for Chefs*, Culinary Nutrition Associates, 2013

(3) Vegetarian

- Within most populations there are some individuals who are vegetarians so vegetarian options should be available at every meal, either on the menu or upon request. Also any requests for avoidance of ingredients, for reasons of health, religion or preference, should be honored.

- Vegetarian diets can be healthy or unhealthy depending on food choices and methods of preparation. Many "heart healthy diets" are vegetarian or vegetarian with poultry, fish or shellfish. With any restricted diet, care should be taken to assure nutrient adequacy especially during periods of growth. Although vegetarians tend to have lower iron and protein intake, there is not a greater risk of iron deficiency than among non-vegetarians.

- A **VEGAN** or **STRICT VEGETARIAN** diet excludes all foods of animal origin (e.g., meat, poultry, fish, eggs, gelatin, dairy products) and relies heavily on grains, legumes, fruits and vegetables. Fats and sugars are used. Since plant proteins are incomplete, they must be complementary in order to assure all essential amino acids are consumed during the same day (not necessarily within the same meal). For example, a grain product will complement beans. This diet is deficient in B_{12}, which should be supplemented, and may be lacking in iron, zinc and calcium. In planning, provide plenty of non-animal food sources of iron, zinc and calcium.

- The **LACTO - VEGETARIAN** diet is as above but includes dairy products.

- The **LACTO - OVO -VEGETARIAN** diet is as above but includes dairy products and eggs.

- The traditional **ZEN MACROBIOTIC** diet is a nutritionally inadequate dietary regime composed of a series of 10 diets, each more restrictive than the one before. The ultimate diet is all grains. There are diets currently called macrobiotic, which are not as restrictive as the traditional and are mainly forms of vegetarian diets. The dietitian should check the contents of specific diets to see if they are nutritionally adequate. Some macrobiotic diets promoted as cancer cures or treatment may be dangerous if they are the traditional type, which are nutritionally inadequate and usually promote weight loss. Adherents may be advised to avoid traditional medical treatment in favor of alternative therapies.

- **RAW VEGAN** includes raw vegetables and fruits, nuts and nut pastes, grain and legume sprouts, seeds, plant oils, sea vegetables, herbs and fruit juices. Excludes all food of animal origin, and all food cooked above 118° F.

- **FLEXITARIAN** is a mostly vegetarian diet with occasional meat consumption , a "semi" or sometimes vegetarian often for health reasons or preferences but not based on religious beliefs.

- **PESCETARIAN** a mostly vegetarian diet that includes fish and shellfish but excludes mammals and birds.

(4) Satisfaction measurement

(a) Customer evaluation

- Customers expect competent and friendly service, consistency in the food served and a clean, comfortable environment.

- Customer evaluations may be obtained by survey, through observation of plate waste, informal customer comments, comment cards or formal or informal questionnaires. Survey statistics should help guide menu revisions and planning.

- Children's satisfaction may be rated using a **FACIAL HEDONIC SCALE** with various expressions of smiles or frowns.

- Ratings are established by surveys or by asking diners to rate which foods they prefer. Foods that are most popular should be included more frequently in the menu cycles to increase sales and satisfaction. If less popular foods are included in menu cycles, other options should be available at these meals. Suggestions from diners will generate new items to try on future menus. A representative (nursing home resident, student, consumer) advisory group may be appointed to help plan menus.

(b) Sales data

- Sales data monitor items served. A food service manager can examine up-to-the-minute information on sales via computer tracking and can evaluate the profit or contribution margin of each menu item. A low-popularity/low-contribution item should probably be removed from the menu if it cannot be improved. A low-popularity/high-contribution item with a consistent customer following might be retained. If an item is unpopular, determine if it is the preparation method, the recipe, including level and type of seasonings, the appearance or a competing menu item that minimizes sales. Do not take it off the menu without a fair trial.

e. Operational influences

(1) Equipment

- Evaluate equipment needed at each meal for each menu item to ensure that equipment availability and capacity is not exceeded. For example, if fruit cobbler is served in sauce dishes, other items using sauce dishes should not be served at the same meal if the number of sauce dishes is limited. For tray service, all items must fit on the tray.

- Plan menus that do not overtax cooking equipment. Avoid multiple roasted or fried menu items if there are limited ovens or deep-fat fryers.

(2) Labor

- Consider availability and skill of production and service personnel. Menus should balance the production workload from day to day. Avoid last-minute preparation that exceeds employee capabilities. Prepared frozen and partially prepared foods (like fresh precut vegetables) can reduce on-site labor. Costs of such items are usually higher, but may be justified based on available labor. For example, one could buy whole or shredded carrots to make carrot and raisin salad. Whole carrots will have a lower food cost, but labor costs to peel and shred whole carrots must be added to the whole carrot cost to arrive at comparable costs for the purchase of shredded carrots.

- Many facilities purchase ready-to-serve desserts, sauces, salad dressings, soups, breads, and entrées because they can get consistent quality with less need for labor and equipment. Decisions on scratch cooking vs. ready-to-serve are often based on availability, food quality and cost of labor.

(3) Budget

- The amount of money available that can be spent on food is based on anticipated sales or income from funding, which may also have to cover the cost of labor, equipment and other overhead expenses. In a healthcare facility or residential institution, a raw food cost allowance per person must be established and meals must balance out to this amount over a given period. For example, serving ground beef in a meat sauce for pasta one day offsets the higher cost of serving fresh fish another day.

f. External influences

(1) Trends

- Social, economic, political and environmental factors or conditions influence choices. A switch to biodegradable containers for carryout food service may be a sound decision if patrons are environmentally conscious. More vegetarian patrons may create demand for vegetable/soy-based entrées. Waste disposal facilities in the community and cost of waste removal may create need for more or less dishes and dishwashing equipment or more or less disposable products. Prevalence of at-risk individuals or populations with communicable diseases may require use of disposables or additional precautions.

(2) Seasonal

- Favorable climactic conditions may lead to an abundance of produce at lower costs while adverse conditions may create shortages and higher costs. Adjust menus accordingly by increasing the frequency of seasonally available produce.

- Summer menus usually have more salads, lighter entrées, more fresh fruits and vegetables and locally grown produce. Winter meals may have more hot foods and more soups, stews and casseroles. Well planned menus reflect the seasons by abundant use of seasonally available produce. While most foods are available year-round, the quality and flavor of produce in season is optimal and the cost far less than at other times of year. So, serve fresh peaches and tomatoes in the summer and fresh apples and hard-shelled squash in the fall.

(3) Disaster

- Food service operations must have disaster management plans to cover fire, flood, labor strikes (on premises or with delivery or supplier personnel), weather problems, electrical outages and other emergencies. Ample supplies of food; including non-perishable food, with manual can openers and bottled wate, should be available to provide food and water (plus juice or other liquid) for the population served, for a few hours and up to three days. Assume power outages and no refrigeration for many crises. Use perishables first before they spoil. As water supplies may be adversely affected and power outages may occur, disposables that do not require washing should also be stored for emergencies. The amount of food and water should be determined in the organization's crisis or disaster plan. Food, including water, should be checked for date codes regularly to assure adequate inventory for when disaster may strike.

(4) Product availability

- These days, most foods are available year round from somewhere, but costs escalate sharply for rare and out- of-season foods. Sometimes, a specific product will not be available or is too costly to obtain. Similar foods are usually substituted, with explanation to the diner, but menu development should consider the availability of unusual ingredients.

TOPIC B – PROCUREMENT, PRODUCTION, DISTRIBUTION and SERVICE

1. Procurement, receiving and inventory management

- The purposes of policies and procedures are to facilitate communication between the buyer and vendor; assure that products are purchased, delivered and paid for in a timely manner, and be certain that products are purchased and delivered in the desired quantity and quality.

a. Procurement principles, concepts and methods

(1) Bidding

- In ONE-STOP-SHOPPING, a full-line supplier provides most foods, except bread and dairy. The purchaser may receive a discount for large orders and may spend less time ordering and processing invoices. This method is not very flexible. Menus may have to be changed if the vendor does not have a particular item.

- In purchasing by the item, the purchaser buys from a specialized company (i.e., meat from a meat company, baked goods from a bakery). Advantages are that specialty companies often have top quality and "signature" items, and their salespersons are usually knowledgeable about products. Overhead costs may be lower than with large multi-product purveyors. Specialty companies may also be able to provide emergency deliveries. A disadvantage is that purchasing from a variety of specialty companies takes more time and paperwork than ordering from a full-line supplier.

- CONTRACT PURCHASING involves a binding agreement between the vendor and the purchaser. Oral contracts are not binding unless there is written confirmation within ten days or unless the goods have been received, stored and paid. A phone order can become a contract even though it is not in writing. It is best to have written contracts with terms agreed upon by both seller and buyer.

- BID REQUESTS invite potential suppliers to submit prices on specific items or specifications and should be issued 30-40 days before the scheduled due date. A purchase of a minimum of $500 per week is necessary to make the bid process worthwhile. The bid request may also ask for samples to be tested for quality. Quotations are usually required from two or more vendors. Bids are kept sealed until a formal time of opening. The opening should take place with an appropriate official present. If the facility is a public institution, bid opening may be open to the public.

- To maintain the integrity of the purchasing process, the person awarding bids or placing orders should not be in a position to sign receiving documents or authorize payments.

- Criteria for objective decisions in awarding bids requires consideration of the following:

  - Ability of the bidder to perform the contract and supply a quality product or service.
  - Ability of the bidder to provide the product or service in a timely manner.
  - Integrity and reputation of the bidder.
  - Bidder's previous performance.
  - Compliance with laws and with specifications of contracts and service.
  - Bidder's qualifications and licenses.
  - Bidder's financial resources.

IV. FOODSERVICE SYSTEMS (17%)

- When bids are solicited on an open or competitive basis, the contract is usually awarded to the lowest bidder who meets quality and service standards. If the award is not given to the lowest bidder, the reason for the decision should be fully stated and filed with documents related to the transaction. For example, a bidder may have a history of sending products that do not meet specifications or has a record of not meeting food safety or sanitation standards.

- The **PURCHASE ORDER** is a form that verifies quantity, quality and cost of an order. Purchase orders contain a purchase order number for tracking, name and address of purchaser, delivery destination, billing information and supplier; date of order, description of items being ordered, including quantity and quality, price, discount and general restrictions; and authorized purchaser's signature. Perishable or time-sensitive items may specify the time, date and required food temperature at delivery.

- **MONTHLY PRICE QUOTES** are obtained from vendors who agree to a fixed price for a given time. For produce, meat, eggs and poultry, the quote may be for one week, as prices vary more for these items than for staples, frozen food and non-food supplies. Within the food distribution system, food service operations and/or retail food stores can purchase foods three ways: 1) directly from food producers and processors through the processors' sales offices and branch warehouses; 2) from food wholesalers; 3) from food brokers and commissioned agents (middlemen).

(2) Specification development

- **SPECIFICATIONS (SPECS)** are a precise communication between the buyer and the seller describing the product to be purchased. Specifications include the following:

  ➢ Exact descriptions of each product are written to include factors such as; product, grade, form (i.e., fresh, frozen, precooked), degree of ripeness, size, thickness, count and product use. The specs may also contain other requirements such as geographic origin, brand name, packing medium and portion size.
  ➢ Product test procedures may also appear on the specs. For example, if the product is to be delivered at a refrigerated temperature, it can be tested with a thermometer on delivery. If meat is delivered in cut portions, it can be randomly weighed.
  ➢ General quality information about the desired product should be provided (i.e., "iceberg lettuce, heads to be green, firm, without spoilage, excessive dirt or damage. No more than 10 outer leaves, packed 24 heads to a case.")
  ➢ General specifications that accompany a contract include method of payment, billing procedure, terms and conditions, submission of samples for testing, what happens when either party fails to perform, rejection of products and delivery and receiving policies.
  ➢ Additional information necessary to clearly show quality expectations can also be included (i.e., bidding procedures, delivery and service requirements).
  ➢ All food shipped through interstate commerce must meet the requirements of one or more federal laws and regulations established by the FDA, the USDA, the National Marine and Fisheries Service and the U.S. Public Health Service.
  ➢ For facility planning, a set of written documents must be compiled by the architect to present to contractors for bidding. The documents include general conditions; scope of work; schedule of operations, with a timetable that includes possible late penalties; responsibility for installations and inspections; and specifications for all parts of work.

- ➤ Written equipment specifications may include the name of the equipment, the catalog and model number, material, construction, size, color, finish, quality, fittings, cost, type of power and heating source needed (pounds per square inch (psi) for steam; type and approximate BTU per cu. ft. for gas; and voltage, phase, AC, or DC and cycles if
- ➤ AC, and wattage for electricity), controls, performance requirements, dimensions, certification (by National Sanitation Foundation (NSF), Underwriter's Laboratory (UL), etc.), warranty, delivery requirements, installation and options, operating and maintainence instructions.

TYPICAL SPECIFICATIONS FOR FOODS BY CATEGORY

Category	Specifications can include:
Meats	Inspection, which is mandatory Grading Fat limitations Refrigeration requirements Tying, boning, packaging, etc. Portion size
Seafood	Type (fin or shellfish) Market form: fin-whole, eviscerated, fillets shell-alive, shucked Grade Processing Inspection, which is voluntary Temperature upon delivery
Poultry	Specific kind of poultry (chicken, duck, goose, turkey) Class (age) Grading Inspection, which is mandatory Style Refrigeration requirements; Size (weight ranges) Delivered on crushed ice or frozen
Fresh fruit and vegetables	Grade Variety Size Type of pack Count per container Geographic origin
Processed fruits and vegetables	Drained weight Packing medium (water or juice pack or type of syrup) Container size and type

---

- • **ORGANIC FOOD** is food that has been cultivated and processed in a more ecologically sustainable way.

  - ➤ The labeling requirements of the National Organic Program (NOP) apply to raw, fresh products and processed foods that contain organic ingredients. Except for food produced by small operations, foods must be certified by USDA accredited certifying agencies, to be labeled 100% Organic or Organic. Organic labeling is voluntary.

➤ Organic meat, poultry, eggs and dairy products come from animals that are given no antibiotics or growth hormones. Organic food is produced without the use of most conventional pesticides, petroleum-based fertilizers or sewage sludge-based fertilizers. Use of genetically engineered seed, ionizing radiation and artificial additives is not permitted.

➤ Products labeled **100% ORGANIC,** must contain (excluding water and salt) only organically produced ingredients. Products made with at least 95% organic ingredients (excluding water and salt) may be labeled as **ORGANIC.** Products that contain at least 70% organic ingredients can use the phrase "made with organic ingredients" on the principal display panel.

➤ The USDA seal and the seal or mark of the certifying agent(s) may appear on product packages and in advertising of any product that is labeled 100% Organic or Organic.

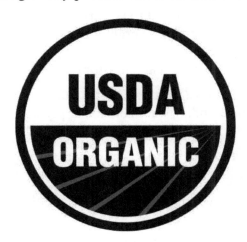

➤ The use of the terms" natural", "free-range", or "hormone-free" are still permitted, but are not interchangeable with organic.

- **SUSTAINABLE AGRICULTURE** promotes food production that protects the environment. Many chefs try to purchase products from local farms that use organic practices, even if their products are not 100% organic. Obtaining the official label as being organic is expensive and requires considerable legal documentation, many small farms that use sustainable practices grow food that could be labeled organic because it meets those standards do not have the time, desire or funds to go through the process.

- **CLEAN FOODS** is an emerging term for fresh ingredients and processed foods that are free of genetically modified organisms (GMO), have no preservatives or additives, and/or are organic. Culinarians have become involved in the clean food movement. This movement has led to the increased availability of heirloom varieties of fruits and vegetables, particularly in Whole Foods and similar market,s as well as farmers markets.

<u>**Vendor performance and evaluation**</u>

- Vendor performance requirements may be delineated by specifications for each food item to be purchased. If the food or supplies are not satisfactory, or are not delivered at the expected time, the buyer may negotiate a price adjustment or return the merchandise.

- Clearly, it is an advantage to deal with vendors who consistently provide quality food and deliver it at the right time. Food service institutions are disrupted by menu changes required by failure to deliver food that has been ordered or is of unacceptable quality at the time of delivery.

(3) Group purchasing/prime vendor

- **GROUP PURCHASING** is used by facilities with similar needs that join together to achieve the cost and service benefits of volume. Purchasing may be centralized (i.e., all hospitals in a particular chain) or may include decentralized individual facilities (i.e., healthcare facilities in a particular metropolitan area). Vendors are given preferential access to sell their products at the group-negotiated price to each facility.

Types of written contracts

- A **TYPE A CONTRACT (EXCLUSIVE)** is a written agreement to make purchases from only one purveyor for either a certain price or a period of time. For example, the purchaser may agree to purchase dairy products exclusively from one local dairy for six months and from another local dairy for the next six months.

- A **TYPE B CONTRACT (PARTIALLY EXCLUSIVE)** is a written agreement with one vendor, but if that vendor is not able to supply needs, the buyer is free to go to another vendor.

- A **TYPE C CONTRACT (OPEN)** is a written agreement in which the buyer can contract with any vendor and decisions are based on price only.

- A **DUAL A CONTRACT** is like an exclusive contract, except the buyer may purchase from two vendors and no others.

- With a **PRIMARY** or **PRIME VENDOR**, one vendor provides an institution with most (75% or more) of its supplies (excluding bread and dairy), but the institution maintains a back-up supplier. The facility can get good prices because of the volume being purchased from the primary supplier and the availability of other possible suppliers to fill the orders, which keeps the primary supplier cost and quality competitive.

Terms used in contracts

- **FREE-ON-BOARD (F.O.B.) AT SHIPPING** means that the buyer assumes responsibility as soon as the goods are loaded. **FREE ON BOARD (F.O.B.) AT DELIVERY** means the seller is responsible for goods until they reach the buyer. This determines who pays freight charges as well as who assumes liability if goods are lost or damaged in transit.

- **C.O.D.** means **CASH-ON-DELIVERY** (demand). It is used when credit is not established or previous bills are unpaid. Full payment is required at delivery.

(4) Ethics

- Good working relationships with vendors require adherence to ethical practices. The buyer should avoid being placed in a position of obligation to a particular vendor who could restrict the buyer's freedom to act in the future. A buyer should not accept personal gifts, anything with a significant cash value or favors from a vendor. Acceptance of small good-will items like calendars, samples or holiday cards does not compromise ethics. (See *and/CDR Code of Ethics for the Profession of Dietetics,* JADA, August 2009.)

IV. FOODSERVICE SYSTEMS (17%)

b. Procurement decisions

(1) Product selection/yield

- The form of food (i.e., canned, cubed, chopped) chosen is based on cost of product, labor, storage, equipment, intended use and other factors.

- Foods, like produce, are often available in fresh, frozen, peeled, cut, washed, chopped or other forms that reduce labor costs and increase yield by providing more edible product.

- Pre-preparation may reduce or increase raw food costs but may be balanced by reduced labor and equipment costs.

(2) Product packaging

- Disposable serviceware and packaging are convenient but require additional storage prior to use and create waste when disposed. Washing and reusing plates, glasses, etc. is preferable to reduce waste, but requires additional labor. Sensitivity to environmental impact of choices of serviceware, including reduction of foam and other non-biodegradable or recyclable materials, is essential.

- Food and food supplies are requisitioned at set order points to meet the food preparation plan, the cycle menu or other needs. This requires knowledge of time needed for preparation and of how long the item can be stored without sacrificing quality.

- Order points are based on storage capacity, perishability and turnover. Different case sizes are used for various food products, i.e., #10 cans come six to the case, 46-oz. soup concentrate and juice cans come twelve to the case and gallons usually come four to six to the case. Most food and supplies must be ordered in full cases.

(3) Cost analysis

- COST ANALYSIS is a procedure used to determine the total and unit costs of alternative strategies. Accurate cost information is necessary to plan and negotiate budgets, determine prices and to generate data for cost effectiveness analyses. Accounting records need to be examined in order to conduct an adequate cost analysis.

c. Receiving and storage

(1) Equipment and methods

Equipment

- Where possible, the receiving area should be within close proximity to the storage areas.

- Depending on the size of the facility and the frequency of delivery, a forklift might be necessary. Hand trucks and/or carts will be necessary to carry the merchandise to the storage areas. Box cutters, crate hammers, specifications and purchase orders should also be at the receiving site.

- Scales should be calibrated regularly. Thermometers to check food temperature on arrival should be available.

IV. FOODSERVICE SYSTEMS (17%)

- The receiving areas should have a defined schedule for cleaning and sanitation and should be inspected regularly.

Methods

- In **INVOICE RECEIVING,** also called **OPEN RECEIVING,** items delivered are checked against the purchase order or purchase record. The receiving clerk looks at the quantity, quality and price of the delivered product and compares it with the original purchase order (not the delivery invoice.)

- **BLIND RECEIVING** is more time consuming but more accurate. The receiving clerk uses a receiving record (either an invoice or a purchase order) that has the quantity order column blanked out. The clerk records the actual quantity of the product received. If there is a discrepancy between the amount ordered and the amount received, there is a delay in the discovery of the error.

- The temperature of food that is frozen or refrigerated should be taken immediately upon delivery. Containers of fresh produce should be opened and inspected for quality and absence of pest infestation. Items should be counted, measured or weighed. A chart showing average weight of perishable food items aids in checking in deliveries. If temperatures for produce, eggs, milk or other perishables are higher or lower than is safe, deliveries should be rejected. If acceptable, these foods should be put into refrigerators or freezers as soon as possible. Canned, dry goods and non-food items should then be inspected.

- Avoid potential food safety hazards by making sure foods are received at the proper temperatures. Reject shipments of food that do not meet the following temperature guidelines and retain the name and signature of the delivery driver on any rejected goods.

- Other guidelines for receiving include:
  - ➢ Post a chart showing average weight of perishable food items and the acceptable and unacceptable standards for receiving various food items.
  - ➢ Inspect the interior of delivery trucks for broken boxes, leaky packages, dented cans, raw products positioned near processed foods and fresh produce or dried spills on the floor.
  - ➢ Refuse food items delivered in dirty trucks and avoid delivery services that use them.
  - ➢ Check date codes.
  - ➢ Date and store all items promptly.
  - ➢ Schedule deliveries at off-peak service hours when there is trained staff to receive and store food items properly.
  - ➢ Reject any cans that are unlabeled, dented, leaking, bulging or show signs of rust at edges.
  - ➢ Save the identification tags for live mollusk and shellfish for 90 days after the last shellfish has been used.

Storage

- All storage areas must be kept clean and be large enough to provide adequate space to store food under proper conditions. Items should be stored using a **FIRST IN/FIRST OUT (FIFO)** method of rotation. The storage facilities should be accessible to both receiving and food preparation areas to reduce transit time and labor costs. It is preferable to have food storage on the same floor as food service. If that is not possible, the kitchen storage area should be large enough for a one or two day supply of food.

- Prepared foods should be labeled with name and date and should be sold, consumed, or discarded, as appropriate.

- Store food in durable, leak-proof, sealed or covered containers.

- Floors should be constructed of quarry tile, terrazzo or concrete that has been sealed to make an easily cleaned surface. Floors should be slip-resistant.

- A door width of 42 inches or more will allow easy movement of carts in or out of the storage and cooking areas.

- Lighting should be adequate to check inventory, food quality and for cleaning.

- Limiting access to all food storage areas to specific personnel, decreases loss due to theft. Vendors should not be permitted access to storage areas.

- Dry storage areas should be free of water or heating pipes, easy to clean and free of rodents and insects. Temperatures should be between 50°F and 70°F with 50% humidity. Cool storage areas should be at 40°F or lower and temperatures checked regularly.

- Food supplies must be kept separate from chemicals and supplies used for cleaning and sanitation. Pesticides and chemical cleaners should be stored in their original containers, with labels intact and within locked cabinets in an area separate from food.

- Quantity lots of bagged items, such as flour and sugar, should be cross-stacked on slatted platforms or racks at least six inches off the floor to allow for circulation. To avoid problems with rodents, covered plastic or stainless steel bins may be used for bagged items. Cartons of foods packed in glass jars should be kept closed because light tends to change colors and flavors. All opened boxes of food should be covered, labeled and dated.

- Dented or swollen cans and damaged items to be returned for credit should be segregated and clearly labeled.

- Bananas are kept in dry storage and are the only fresh produce that is never refrigerated. Tomatoes lose flavor when refrigerated. Whole tomatoes may be held at room temperature but should be refrigerated if cut.

- The storage area should contain a worktable near the entrance for unpacking supplies and assembling orders. Large and small scoops should be provided for each food container in use; such as bins of flour, sugar, cereals, etc. Scoops may not be stored in the bins. Scales for weighing large or small quantities should be available. Boxes may harbor pests and should be removed after unpacking food items.

- A regular schedule for the cleaning of floors, walls, shelving, vents, fans, etc, should be developed and maintained. Routine inspections should be made. Any violations of safety or sanitation standards should be corrected immediately.

- Heavy items should be stored on lower shelves. Dollies or carts should be available and employees instructed on proper lifting techniques to avoid back injuries.

- Supplies are to be stored on metal or high-impact plastic shelves at least 2 inches from wall and 6-12 inches from the floor. Shelves 16 inches deep will hold two rows of No. 10 cans or three rows of No. 2 or No. 2.5 cans. There should be at least an 18-inch clearance between the tops of supply items and sprinkler heads.

- Slatted shelves or wire shelving permits better air circulation and discourages pest infestation.

Refrigerator and freezer storage

- Cold storage is used for perishable foods to preserve nutritional value and sensory quality and to slow the growth of microorganisms. A few microorganisms can grow at refrigerator temperatures.

- Low-temperature storage may include large walk-in units (more common in large institutions) or smaller reach-in units that require less floor space and less capital investment. The trend is toward reach-in units, to accommodate a day's worth of perishables, located near work stations. This leaves the walk-in units for general and long-term storage.

- The refrigeration system may be divided into several units so that failure in one will not disrupt the operation. Because dairy items may absorb odors, they must be tightly sealed. Often they are stored in separate refrigerators.

Temperature and humidity

- Many outbreaks of food- illness are attributed directly or indirectly to improper refrigeration in a food service establishment. All potentially hazardous foods should be stored at 40°F or less in the refrigerator and 0°F in the freezer.

- Refrigeration equipment is frequently equipped with a recording thermometer mounted outside the unit. It continuously records the temperature of walk-in or reach-in, low-temperature storage equipment. If a refrigeration unit does not have a thermometer built into it, a bulb thermometer should be hung or mounted on a shelf inside the unit. An internal thermometer should be in place to verify the reading of the external thermometer.

- Thermometers should be placed in the warmest part of low temperature storage areas and should be checked at the start of each shift.

- Freezers should be kept at 0°F (-18°C) to maintain the quality of frozen foods. When freezers are at higher than desirable temperatures, the quality of products drops dramatically. For example, at 0°F, frozen spinach retains its quality for six months; at 10°F, for less than 3 months; at 20°F, for 3 weeks.

- A humidity range of 80-95% is recommended for most foods requiring refrigeration.

Storage and thawing

- Refrigerated and frozen foods should be stored and covered to reduce moisture loss, limit odor absorption and prevent damage from possible leakage or dripping. Meat and poultry defrosting in a refrigerator should be stored below cooked products so there is no dripping into other foods.

- Foods should be thawed in the refrigerator at 38° to 40°F. Usually this takes 12 to 24 hours. Once thawed, a product should be used immediately and not refrozen. Failure to thaw food properly (particularly chicken and ground beef) is a common source of food safety problems. Foods should never be thawed at room temperature. Some foods may be thawed under cool running water as a quick thaw method or in a microwave oven as part of a continuous cooking process.

- Ready-to-eat (RTE) or cooked items should be placed on the top shelves of reach-in or walk-in refrigerators.

- Frozen products should be stored in their original containers until preparation time. Thawing before preparation is needed for frozen fruit to be used in pies and for frozen eggs, poultry and meat.

- Prior to storage, hot cooked foods should be chilled quickly in an ice-water bath or using an ice paddle, then refrigerated in shallow containers to facilitate cooling. Divide large quantities into smaller containers. The center of the food should reach 70°F within two hours and 40°F within four hours. Roasts should be cut into pieces prior to refrigeration.

(2) Records

- An **INVOICE** is the delivery slip that comes from the purveyor giving price, quantity and form of payment. Once signed, it is a legal document that represents accepted inventory and money owed. The invoice should be checked against the purchase order, specifications, price quotations and other documents before payment is issued.

- The **RECEIVING CLERK** is usually one employee specially trained to receive foods and supplies. A receiving scale is used to check quantity. A receiving stamp documents when the order was received and by whom and verifies both quantity and quality. The receiving clerk should have a thermometer available and be trained to check for proper food temperatures before food is accepted.

(3) Security

- **INTERNAL SECURITY** is a system to prevent damage, pilferage and stealing of money, food, equipment or supplies by employees. It is also used to prevent sabotage and tampering with computers and computer files. Basic guidelines include the following:

  ➤ Implement and enforce well-defined policies and procedures to promote security. Employees should know that theft is cause for immediate termination and criminal prosecution.
  ➤ Keep food and other supplies in secured areas and limit access to authorized personnel only.
  ➤ Hire and train trustworthy employees.

> Conduct frequent inventories to reconcile stock issues, receipts and stock on hand to uncover pilferage problems early.
> Limit number of keys and accessibility to storage areas, walk-in cold storage and cash registers. Safe combinations should be available to as few personnel as practical for efficient operation of the food service department.

- **EXTERNAL SECURITY** secures the department and its resources from intrusion by outsiders. Basic guidelines include the following:

  > Doors to the outside should be locked, including doors to the receiving and loading docks.
  > Employees should display identification to enter.
  > Employees should immediately report any unusual activities or the presence of unauthorized individuals.
  > Most institutions have security guards and/or procedures to maintain security, including after-hours security, using a sign-in system. Some institutions have badges, identification cards, video monitoring or other security systems.

d. Inventory management

(1) Control procedures - par levels, rotation, minimum/maximum

- A **PAR STOCK SYSTEM** establishes the quantity needed for each item for menu preparation, allowing for special circumstances. Orders are placed at a fixed interval over a period of time and usage is monitored between order dates. Orders bring the item level back to the predetermined level.

- **INVENTORY ROTATION** requires that when new inventory is received, there should be enough room to store it behind similar products that are already on the shelves. Older items should always be in front to be used first.

- Minimize dangers of spoilage and decrease inventory costs by rotating inventory using the **FIFO (FIRST-IN/FIRST-OUT)** rule. Oldest inventory is used first. This requires dating of stored food and rotating inventory so new deliveries are used last rather than first.

- A **MINI-MAX (MINIMUM/MAXIMUM)SYSTEM** determines a minimum and maximum amount of stock to have on hand. Products are ordered when the minimum is reached, and only in quantities to bring stock up to the maximum level. The amount of product ordered remains the same, but the time of purchase will vary. To use the mini-max system, one must know:

  > **MAXIMUM LEVEL** is the number of units used during the order period plus safety level.
  > **MINIMUM LEVEL** is the point to reorder.
  > **SAFETY LEVEL** is minimum stock required to be on hand.
  > **USAGE RATE** is the amount of product used per day or per month.
  > **LEAD TIME** is time it takes to receive an item after placing order.

Labor cost

- Labor costs generally constitute 50-60% of food service expenses. Because of the increase in labor costs, many operations are using more partially prepared items, precooked meats and prepared salads to reduce or stabilize labor costs.

- Factors influencing labor cost include:
  - The wage rate in the local area.
  - The availability of particular skills.
  - The negotiated contract for wages, benefits and conditions of work.
  - The type of service, extent of services offered and hours of service. (A hospital food service is open seven days per week all year, so labor costs will be higher than for an operation open five days per week.)
  - The menu pattern and the form in which food is purchased. (A static menu that offers the same foods every day will be less difficult for labor than a cycle menu that changes; foods purchased partially prepared require less labor time.)
  - The physical plant, including the size and arrangement of units, the equipment and its arrangement.
  - The personnel policies and productivity. (Average productivity for the food service industry is 50%.)
  - Training costs related to turnover.

- The time that is required to complete a task and the base pay rate represent the two major factors contributing to labor costs.

  Example: An employee with a base pay rate of $12.21 (salary and fringe benefits) takes 3 hours to complete 100 salads for lunch. The labor costs for salad preparation would be $12.21 x 3 =$36.63 ÷ 100 salads = $.366 labor cost per salad.

- **LABOR COST PERCENTAGE** is the percent of meal cost attributable to labor costs:

  Labor Cost % = Cost of Labor ÷ Meal Cost x 100

  Example:
  A hospital serves 1520 patient and non-patient meals per day. The daily meal cost totals $5,350. The total labor cost per day is $2,160. Using the formula:
  Labor cost % = ($2,160 ÷ $5,350) x 100 = 40%.

- **INVENTORY TURNOVER RATIO** is one of the most widely used activity ratios. It shows the number of times the inventory is used up and replenished during a period. A high ratio indicates that a limited inventory is being maintained by a food service operation, and a low ratio indicates that larger amounts of money are tied up in inventories. Inventory turnover ratio is calculated as follows:

  Inventory Turnover Ratio = Cost of Goods Sold ÷ Average Inventory Value

Example:

$10,000 (Costs of goods sold) ÷ $1,500 (Average inventory value) = 6.67

This means that total inventory turns over 6.67 times a month. This is an average. Some foods (i.e., milk) turn over far more often, whereas it will take much longer to use up the pepper.

- **PHYSICAL INVENTORY** is the actual count of items on the shelf at a specific time using a standard recording form. Results of a physical inventory may be used to determine food costs for the preceding month.

- **PERPETUAL INVENTORY** is a continuously monitored record of stock on hand. Products coming into the facility are added to the balance on hand. The perpetual inventory form reflects food items, quantity on hand, quantity used, price of foods bought and used and current value of that item. A perpetual inventory should be verified monthly with a physical inventory. Reasons for discrepancies should be identified. Products taken from inventory are subtracted from the amounts on hand:

Food on Hand = Beginning Inventory + Food Purchased

Food Used = Food on Hand - Final Inventory

- **ABC METHOD OF INVENTORY CONTROL** classifies products according to their value:

  - **A-CLASS ITEMS** are the most expensive. Control and security are tightest and inventory is kept at a minimum (i.e., wines, lobster, meat). Total A-class accounts for approximately 70% of food costs.
  - **B-CLASS ITEMS** are of lesser value (i.e., canned apricots). The total B-class accounts for approximately 20% of total food costs.
  - **C-CLASS ITEMS** have the lowest dollar value (i.e., rice).

- The cost of food used may be found by adding the cost of purchases to the beginning inventory cost. That yields the cost of food available. Subtracting the cost of the ending inventory yields the cost of foods used.

(2) Issuing procedures

- Using a requisition form to remove food items from storage areas reduces pilferage and documents unnecessary waste. The **REQUISITION FORM** should contain date, item issued, weight or quantity, price and authorization signature. The form should be completed in duplicate or triplicate for record keeping and security reasons.

- In some operations, ingredients needed for specific recipes for the day are weighed, measured and assembled in advance in a central controlled-access area usually called the ingredient room. Some pre-preparation may also be done there (i.e., peeling, chopping, thawing, breading). When ready, ingredients are packaged and labeled. Advantages of an ingredient room are increased production control, improved security, consistent quality control and efficient use of equipment. Personnel must be able to read, write, follow directions exactly and must be trained to perform accurate measuring.

2. Principles of quantity food preparation and processing

a. Cooking methods

- **HEAT** is created by agitating molecules in a substance. The degree of agitation and the number of molecules in motion determine the heat produced. Cold is the absence of molecular movement.

- **ENDOTHERMIC** methods are chemical reactions that absorb heat.

- **EXOTHERMIC** methods are chemical reactions that release heat.

- **MOIST COOKING** techniques include boiling, blanching, parboiling, simmering, poaching and steaming.

- **DRY COOKING** techniques include baking, roasting, sautéing, stir-frying, pan-frying, deep-frying, grilling and broiling.

- **COMBINATION COOKING** techniques include braising and stewing wherein the food is cooked by dry and then by moist heat.

Methods of heat transfer

- In **CONDUCTION**, kinetic energy is transmitted from molecule to molecule. A source of heat is applied to the food product. This causes the molecules to vibrate and strike against each other. Molecules with greater energy give up some of their energy to the molecules with less energy. This action continues until the molecules farthest from the original source of heat have received some of the heat energy. Different materials conduct heat at different rates: water, fat and metals are good conductors, whereas air and glass are not. Conduction is a slow method of heat transfer.

- In **CONVECTION**, currents of air, water or fat carry heat or cold. When a gas or liquid is heated, it becomes less dense, causing it to rise. The cold gas or liquid will flow downward to the heat source. The circular flow of convection currents keeps the temperature somewhat uniform throughout the medium. Currents of hot air, hot fat or hot water circulate rapidly to the object being heated, and energy passes from the hot medium (air, fat or water) to the object by conduction.

  - Convection currents heat more rapidly than conduction alone.
  - Convection is involved in cooking food in a saucepan of water and in deep fat frying. A convection oven uses a fan to circulate air around the object being heated. This causes the heat to be transferred more quickly, so the food cooks in a shorter amount of time.

  - **RADIATION** transfers energy from a source to the food by waves. Only the surface is heated by the waves; they cannot penetrate below it. The rest of the food is heated by conduction. Dull, black and/or rough surfaces absorb radiant energy better than smooth and/or white surfaces.

  - **INFRARED RADIATION** applies a heat source to the side of the food. Broilers, toasters and hold lamps are examples of infrared radiant cooking.

- Water molecules in food are affected by **MICROWAVE RADIATION** which is energy production through friction in an enclosed space. Waterless materials will not heat in a microwave oven. That is the reason plastic or paper containers are used in a microwave oven. However, microwave containers may become hot to the touch through conduction. Use only microwave-safe containers and wraps in microwave ovens because other containers may melt, release toxic substances or damage the microwave. No metal can be used in microwave ovens.

Boiling point

- The **BOILING POINT** of a liquid is the temperature at which the vapor pressure of the liquid becomes greater than the **ATMOSPHERIC PRESSURE**, the opposing pressure (air) that is exerted against it. At the boiling point, bubbles form, float to the top of the liquid and vaporize. Atmospheric pressure is measured with a barometer and is also called **BAROMETRIC PRESSURE**.

- Factors affecting the boiling point include:
  - The boiling point of a liquid varies with altitude. Atmospheric pressure is lower at high altitudes and higher at low altitudes.
  - At sea level, water boils at 100° C (212°F). The boiling point drops 1° C or 1.8°F for each 960 feet above sea level.
  - The low boiling point of water at high altitudes alters many cooking operations so that modification of methods, leavening and altering the ratio of liquid to solids are necessary for use in mountainous areas. Longer cooking times are expected at higher altitudes.
  - The creation of a partial vacuum will artificially lower the boiling point of water. Similarly, an increase in air or steam pressure may raise the boiling point of water.
  - Substances in boiling solutions do not go off in steam. They decrease the vapor pressure of the water in which they are dissolved and will increase the boiling point.
  - The larger the number of solute particles in the solution, the less the escape of vapor and the higher the temperature necessary to produce boiling.

Dispersions

- A **DISPERSION** is a solution composed of particles throughout another substance. Types of common dispersions include:
  - **SOLUTIONS** are homogeneous mixtures of different substances such as molecules (sugar), and/or ions (salt). A solution usually includes water. The molecules are usually small, and higher temperatures increase solubility (i.e., sugar-sweetened lemonade or tea).
  - **COLLOIDAL DISPERSIONS** hold larger size molecules in solution. The molecules are too large for a true solution and too small to settle out. Proteins form colloidal solutions (i.e., gelatin in hot water, protein in milk and in egg white).
  - **EMULSIONS** are combinations of two immiscible liquids. This may include oil in water or water in oil (i.e., mayonnaise).
  - **SUSPENSIONS** contain particles too large or complex to dissolve or form colloidal dispersions (i.e., cornstarch in water).

- Other terms relating to dispersions:

  - A **SOL** is solid-in-liquid, a colloidal dispersion in the liquid state (i.e., gelatin before chilling).
  - A **GEL** is a liquid-in-solid dispersion, when a sol assumes a rigid form (i.e., cooled gelatin).
  - **FOAM** is a gas-in-liquid dispersion (i.e., whipped topping).
  - **SYNERESIS** is when liquid seeps from a gel (i.e., meringue topping on a pie).
  - **HOMOGENIZATION** is a process stabilizing emulsions by finely dividing one substance and dispersing it throughout another (i.e., homogenized milk).

- Heat, cold, enzymes, acids, alkali or stirring foods during processing or preparation may change the dispersion so that the particles are more finely divided and dispersed or more aggregated. Changes in the extent of dispersion may markedly alter the properties of a food product; such as the separation of oil from peanut butter or salad dressing.

- **BOUND WATER** in solution cannot be extracted from a food product (such as in bread). **FREE WATER** can be extracted from food with pressure (such as in grapes.)

FOOD ACCEPTABILITY

Qualitative (subjective) evaluation

- Observing plate waste and conducting consumer surveys will provide information about food acceptance. Foods offered but not chosen and foods yielding high plate waste should be reevaluated for quality and acceptability.

Sensory aspects of meals

- **APPEARANCE** refers to the size, shape, wholeness, gloss, transparency, color, attractiveness and consistency of individual foods and of the total meal.

- **FLAVOR** is determined by tastes perceived by tastebuds (sweet, salty, sour, bitter and umami), aroma, texture and temperature and by the strength of flavoring materials. Herbs, spices and flavoring extracts affect flavors and food acceptability to individuals. Method of preparation, as in grilling or frying, imparts specific "mouthfeel" that contributes to flavor.

- **AROMA**, the odor or fragrance of food, is a primary component of flavor. Aroma creates anticipation of flavor and can stimulate salivation and appetite. Heat intensifies aroma (i.e., baking bread, burning coffee). Aroma is a major factor in what most people consider as the taste of food.

- **TEXTURE** refers to the hand and "mouthfeel" of firmness, softness, juiciness, crunchiness, crispness and chewiness and the fibrous and crystalline qualities of the food.

Qualitative (sensory) tests

- **HEDONIC SCALES** measure the extent of the like or dislike of sensory characteristics of food. Hedonic scales are used to measure sweetness, sourness, brownness, acceptance, etc.

Discrimination tests

> **PAIRED COMPARISON** compares only two samples at one time. A judge is given the samples and asked to indicate how they differ. This testing is valuable for controlling and maintaining the quality of a product.

> **TRIANGLE TESTS** present judges with three samples, two of which are identical. The judge must decide which two are alike. This method is useful when only small differences exist between samples.

> **DUO-TRIO TESTS** present judges with one identified sample first (control). The judge then receives two coded samples (one is the same as the identified sample) and must determine which of the two coded samples is like the control sample. There is a 50% chance of guessing the correct answer with this method, so the paired comparison and triangle tests may be more valuable.

Descriptive tests

> In **RANKING**, trained judges rank samples according to the intensity of the characteristic being evaluated. This is useful for evaluating samples on a single quality characteristic (i.e., saltiness, crispness).

> **SCORING** involves giving a product a score on a scale, such as 1-5 or 1-10, for a given characteristic. Much information about the product can be accumulated because both qualitative and quantitative data can be collected. This type of testing requires trained judges and well-established standards.

> **FLAVOR PROFILES** involve a specially-trained panel working together to produce a written record of the aroma and flavor of the product. Aroma and flavor are examined separately and tabulated according to individually detected components or character, intensity of each, order of appearance and aftertaste.

Quantitative (objective) evaluation

- Quantitative measures use instruments and test procedures to measure food qualities.

- **IMITATIVE TESTS** measure food properties the way humans perceive them.

- **NON-IMITATIVE TESTS** measure the chemical of the physical properties of food.

INSTRUMENTS AND TESTS FOR OBJECTIVE TESTING

Instrument	Test
Colorimeter or Spectrophotometer	Measures color of food and clarity of liquid
Viscometer (Bostwick Consistometer)	Measures viscosity of foods
pH Meter	Measures tartness (acidity) of foods Measures hydrogen-ion concentration
Refractometer	Measures the sugar concentration of syrup Measures the soluble solids in juice
Microscope	Examines the microscopic structure of foods
Shortometer (Lee-Kramer Shear Press)	Measures product firmness and crispness
Textureometer	Tests the texture of food products
Penetrometer (Bloom Gelometer)	Measures product tenderness or gel strength
Line Spread Test	Determines product viscosity and consistency
Shear Value	Tests meat tenderness

---

b. Equipment

The choice of equipment needed depends on type of operation and menu items (i.e., convenience products, quantity, variety and preparation times). Operations that reheat or finish food require microwave ovens and other heating equipment, but not the full range of equipment required for preparation of food from basic ingredients that is necessary for conventional food preparation operations.

EQUIPMENT FOR CONVENTIONAL FOOD PREPARATION

Receiving
Scale, thermometer, storage, refrigerator at medium/low temperature, refrigerator for thawing

Bake Shop
Scale, mixer (vertical cutter/mixer), divider, rounder, dough roller, proofer, retarder, doughnut machine and fryer, oven, steam kettle, hood, refrigerator at medium/low temperature, blast freezer

Beverages
Ice maker with plastic or metal scoops, coffee makers, espresso/cappuccino makers, tea-making equipment, blender

Meat Preparation
Scale, meat saw, cutting boards, thermometer, chopper, grinder, tenderizer, patty machine, slicer

Meat/Fry Cooking
Scale, mixer, steam kettle, braising pan or kettle, oven, range, griddle, grill, broiler/charbroiler, fryer/pressure fryer, hood, thermometer

Vegetable Preparation
Peeler, pulper/disposer, vertical cutter/mixer, food cutter, cutting boards, vegetable slicer, dicer, slicer

Vegetable Cooking
Low-pressure steamer, high-pressure steam cooker, steam-jacketed kettle, oven, range, hood

Salad Preparation
Food cutter, vertical cutter/mixer, cutting boards, pulper/disposer, mixer, dicer, vegetable slicer

Plating
Refrigerator for holding, food warmer, bain marie, roll warmer, infrared lamp

Serving
Steam table, sandwich counter, slicer, salad station, dessert station, coffee urn, ice machine, beverage dispenser, self-leveling dispenser

Ware Washing
Dish machine, conveyor, pulper/disposer, booster, burnisher, blower-dryer, condensor

Pot Washing
Pot-washing machine, pulper/disposer

Sanitation/waste removal
Can washer/crusher, bottle crusher, steam-cleaning, pulper/disposer, incinerator, baler, compactor

---

Note: Less equipment is needed for convenience operations. Convenience equipment usually includes microwave ovens.

OVENS

Type of oven	Benefits	Constraints
Conventional ovens	Versatile and good for baking, roasting, and braising. Electric or gas.	Reliable but larger than other ovens.
Microwave ovens	Food cooks very rapidly. "On-demand" feeding can be accommodated.	Foods are easily overcooked and may reheat unevenly.
Convection ovens	Oven cavities can accommodate 12-30 meals at a time, making them more efficient than the microwave system.	About 30% faster than a conventional oven, but not as fast as a microwave. Excessive cooking losses or thickened surface layer develops on surface of some food.
Infrared ovens (Flash Bake Ovens)	Cooks faster than conventional ovens. Accommodates 16-24 meals at a time, resulting in greater efficiency, compared to a microwave system. Needs no preheating or venting.	Energy consumption is relatively high. Soups must be handled separately. Dishes and covers become very hot. Foods may burn or stick to heated dishes.

c. Preservation and packaging methods

- Refrigeration and freezing are among the most common methods of food preservation.

- **CHEMICAL PRESERVATIVES** are used to extend shelf life of some minimally-processed foods. Preservatives must not impair or mask product wholesomeness.

- **BLANCHING** is done by exposure to boiling water, steam or hot air for 1-3 minutes to inactivate enzymes, remove air from tissues and destroy contaminating microorganisms. Foods are usually blanched before canning, freezing or dehydration.

- **STERILIZATION** during canning destroys microorganisms that are of public health concern or that might cause spoilage under normal storage conditions. Canned, low-acid foods must be heated to destroy Clostridium botulinum (230-275°F for 12-325 minutes, depending on container type and size). Treatment of high-acid foods is less severe, because acid inhibits growth of C. botulinum (212-220°F for 5-280 minutes).

- **ULTRA-HIGH TEMPERATURE (UHT) PASTEURIZATION/STERILIZATION** is a process that extends the shelf life of food through pasteurization at very high temperatures for short periods. This process reduces microbial count with minimal quality deterioration. If the UHT product is aseptically packaged (packaging free of microorganisms), the product can be stored at room temperatures until it is opened, then stored at refrigerator temperature. UHT products that have not been aseptically packaged must be stored at 40°F or lower. Some UHT foods are whipping cream, coffee creamer and lactose-reduced milk. Aseptic packaging is used for fruit juice (boxes), soymilk, rice milk, soup and tomatoes. Containers must be air tight to be shelf stable.

- **DEHYDRATION** is the reduction of water in foods (i.e., dried fruits and vegetables).

- **CONTROLLED ATMOSPHERE (also called MODIFIED ATMOSPHERE)** is used for foods sealed in a "retort pouch." This vacuum-packed, hypobaric storage is achieved through reduced O^2 and CO^2. Packaging using controlled atmospheres requires special permits and extra handling procedures with regard to time, temperature and refrigeration to prevent growth of anaerobic bacteria and their toxins.

- *SOUS VIDE*, meaning "under vacuum", is a technology invented in France, in which individual portions of food are vacuum-packed, cooked at low temperatures for long time, then chilled and immediately frozen. Flavors are preserved, creating excellent palatability with minimal shrinkage (possibly as low as 2%). *Sous vide* foods are reheated in hot, not boiling, water to preserve texture and other food properties. Though expensive and not widely used in the US, the primary concern with this technology is the creation of an anaerobic environment conducive to the growth of Clostridium botulinum and its toxins. Extreme care in production and storage of foods at refrigerator or freezer temperatures is essential.

- **REFRIGERATED EXTENDED SHELF LIFE** is provided for fresh salads and cut fruit by packing produce in a package filled with an inert gas.

- **FERMENTATION** preserves by adding microbial cultures that promote controlled bacterial growth (i.e., aged cheese, soy sauce, sauerkraut, summer sausage, yogurt, sourdough bread, beer and wine).

- **FOOD IRRADIATION** is a technology that can reduce or destroy foodborne pathogens and extend food shelf life. The food, after processing, carries no residual radioactivity. Irradiation has been proven safe; it does not make the food radioactive. Because temperatures are relatively low during processing, the texture, color, flavor and nutrients are retained. Irradiation of meat and poultry products is viewed as a significant step to reducing the increasing number of food-borne illnesses each year related to those products. FDA regulates food irradiation processes. Some eggs in shell are irradiated to destroy potential salmonella. These eggs are safe to eat either poached or raw in recipes. Spices are often irradiated (especially when imported) because they can carry insects or insect eggs.

  - A **GRAY (GY)** is a unit of measurement of absorbed radiation equivalent to one joule of energy absorbed per kilogram of irradiated matter. 1,000 Gray (Gy) = 1kiloGray (kGy).
  - Low doses (< 1kGy) are used to kill or sterilize insects in grain and disrupt cell components to inactivate bacteria and parasites in meat and poultry. Low doses also delay ripening of fruit (strawberries) and inhibit sprouting of vegetables such as onions, garlic and potatoes.
  - Moderate (1 – 10kGy) doses actually sterilize foods. This dosage is seldom used, except to sterilize foods that may be useful in hospitals for surgical and immune-compromised patients.

➤ Currently whole foods, with the exception of imported spices, must be labeled with a **RADURA** symbol if they have been irradiated.

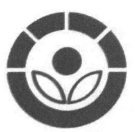

Radura symbol

- There is concern about the extent to which paper/plastic/styrofoam packaging products contribute to waste and whether that waste is biodegradable. Use of disposables must be evaluated on a cost/ benefit basis. Paper is biodegradable, but is a potential safety hazard when used for hot carry-out beverages. Some styrofoam is biodegradable and contributes less actual volume to landfills than paper. Styrofoam can be collected and recycled, if there is a reliable recycler available. Styrofoam disposed of via a slurry system will raise the fat content of a facilities waste stream. This is closely monitored by many municipal wastewater treatment agencies, and total fat limits may be mandated.

d. Modified diets

- Modified diets are described in detail in Domain II. Foods for special diets may be modified in content or form and are tailored to the physiologic needs of individuals with medical conditions.

3. Food production control procedures

a. Standardized recipes

- **STANDARDIZED RECIPES** specify amounts and proportions of ingredients, methods for combining ingredients and other preparation procedures, number of portions produced and portion size. Standardized recipes enable food to taste and look as it should, regardless of the preparer. The results yield a known quantity and quality of the product. Standardized recipes also help control preparation time, quality, quantity and costs and simplify purchasing because the quantities and forms of food needed are standardized.

- With increasing frequency, recipes are being adpted to meet HACCP guidelines. Criteria, such as time and temperature requirements and procedures to avoid contamination, cross-contamination and other hazards, are being written into recipes. Recipes that meet HACCP guidelines provide the final cooking temperature and the temperature at which the food must be held.

- To develop a standardized recipe, begin by analyzing proportions to see whether they are balanced (i.e., ratio of sugar to flour in a cake). Ingredients should be listed in order of use, generally with larger amounts listed first and dry ingredients before liquid ingredients.

- Directions in a recipe must be clear, in the right sequence and easy to follow. Ingredients must be listed accurately in the order of use.

- A standardized recipe includes product name, yield, portion size, ingredient quantity, preparation procedures, equipment, cooking temperature, cooking time.

- In many recipes, ingredients are quantified by volume measure (cups, quarts, etc.), but baking recipes usually list ingredients by weight for more accuracy.

STANDARDIZED RECIPE FORMAT
RECIPE: PASTA PIZZA

Portions: 96

Pans: 3

Pan Size: 12 x 20 x 2½

Cooking Temperature: 350°F (177°C)

Cooking Time: 20-25 minutes

Portion Size: 8 x 4 inches
Portion Utensil: Spatula

Total Recipe Cost:_____

Cost per Portion:_____

Date Calculated:_____

Ingredients	Amount	Procedure
Ground beef	4 lbs.	1. Sauté ground beef and sausage until cooked
Pork sausage, bulk	2 lbs.	
Spaghetti, thin	4 ½ lbs.	2. Drain excess fat.
Salt	3 Tbs.	3. Rinse meat in colander.
Vegetable oil	2 Tbs.	4. Cook spaghetti in boiling salted water in steam-jacketed kettle.
Tomato sauce	1 #10 can	5. Add oil to water to prevent boiling over.
Oregano, dry	3 Tbs.	
Sweet basil, dry, crushed	3 Tbs.	
Mozzarella cheese, grated	8 lbs.	6. Drain spaghetti.
Onions, chopped	2 cups	7. Put spaghetti in pans.
Green peppers, chopped	2 cups	8. Pour equal amount of sauce over spaghetti in each pan.
Mushrooms, drained	3 1-lb. cans	9. Spread cooked meat over sauce.
Ripe olives, sliced	3 cups	10. Sprinkle oregano and basil over meat.
		11. Sprinkle cheese over oregano and basil.
		12. Top with chopped onions, green peppers, mushrooms and ripe olives,
		13. Bake to a minimum internal temperature of 165°F for 15 seconds.

- To test a standardized recipe, all ingredients must be carefully weighed and measured, production time noted, condition at each stage described, yield measured, serving size defined and serving instructions noted. To accurately determine nutrient content, measure and subtract the weight of any part not included in the portion served (i.e., drained or trimmed fat, bones, cooking liquid, fruit peel). The whole recipe should then be critiqued, changed as necessary and re-tested two to three times (average). Periodic evaluation of standardized recipes ensures continued quality.

Modifying a standard recipe using an adjustment factor

- Standardized recipes can be modified by using an **ADJUSTMENT FACTOR** TO change portion calculations.

  - If you are reducing a recipe, the adjustment factor will be less than 1.0. If you are increasing a recipe, the adjustment factor will be more than 1.0
  - In order to compute your adjustment factor, divide the new yield by the original yield. Use this adjustment factor to revise your recipe by multiplying the ingredient amount in the original recipe by the adjustment factor.

  Example 1:
  The recipe you have yields 100 portions and your desired yield is 225 portions. Divide 225 by 100. Your adjustment factor is 2.25. If your original recipe calls for 3 teaspoons of salt, and your adjustment factor is 2.25, you would multiply 3 teaspoons by 2.25. The amount of salt in your revised recipe would be 6.75 teaspoons of salt.

  Example 2:
  If you want to make the yield of a recipe smaller, you would again take the desired yield and divide it by the original. The yield of the original recipe is 75 and you would like to serve 35 people. Divide 35 by 75 and your adjustment factor is 0.47. If your original recipe calls for 3 teaspoons of salt, and your adjustment factor is 0.47, you would multiply 3 teaspoons by 0.47. The amount of salt in your revised recipe is now 1.41 teaspoons. Since this number may be difficult to measure, you may want to round it to the nearest measuring spoon you have (1.5 or 1.25)

  Example 3:
  If you want to change portion sizes, you first have to find the total original yield and then adjust your recipe. If your original recipe yields 75 -¾ cup servings and you want 125 – ½ cup servings, you would multiply 75x3/4. The old yield is 56.25 cups. Your new yield, 125x ½ cup is 62.50. Following the same principle you would divide 62.50 by 56.25 and your adjustment factor is 1.11.

- Although mathematical calculations are necessary as a starting place, the recipe should be tested at its new volume because flavors and textures change as ingredient ratios vary.

b. Ingredient control

- Use the following steps to determine the quantity of food ingredients to purchase:

  - Determine the portion size of each food to be served.
  - Multiply by the number to be served. This number can be determined using forecasting or previous meal censuses.
  - Convert to the number of pounds necessary to yield the **REQUIRED EDIBLE PORTION** (EP). Edible portion is the consumable product after preparation.
  - Divide the EP by percentage yield (amount provided by one pound of commodity). Yield books or standardized recipes can be a source for determining purchase amount.
  - Convert to the appropriate purchase unit (pounds, cases, cartons, roasts, crates) of each ingredient or prepared food. Round upward to nearest whole unit if a partial case or crate is needed.

- Do not confuse volume equivalents with weight equivalents. Some ingredients are measured in volume, others by weight. For example, 1 c. water is 8 oz. in weight and also 8 oz. in a measuring cup. But a one-cup measure of flour weighs only 4 oz. Standardized recipes for baked products require weighing of ingredients.

c. Portion control and yield analysis

- **PORTION CONTROL** is essential to managing food service operations. Employees must be trained to weigh, measure or portion foods correctly to help maintain quantity control, costs, nutritional adequacy and customer satisfaction. Also, many special diets require specific portions of foods.

- Using the equipment specified by a standardized recipe helps ensure yield. Stainless steel pans for most standardized recipes are 12 x 20 inches in 2-to 8inch depths, with half-, quarter-, and third-size pans to accommodate smaller quantities. The 18 x 26-inch pan is standard for baking. The correct utensils should be used for portioning and serving.

- Food portions must be appropriate for the dishes, bowls and serving containers. The size of plates, bowls and glasses used has increased over the past twenty years, making "standard" servings appear quite small. Choose dishes that are appropriate for desirable serving sizes.

YIELD FROM SCOOPS and LADLES		
Sizes of Scoops	**Use**	**Equivalents**
No. 6	Entrée salads	2/3 cup
No. 8	Entrée, mashed vegetables	1/2 cup
No. 10	Cereals, meat patties, desserts	3/8 cup
No. 12	Salads, vegetables, desserts, muffins	1/3 cup
No. 16	Small muffins, small desserts, croquettes	1/4 cup
No. 20	Sandwich fillings, cupcakes, sauces	3-1/5 tablespoons
Sizes of Ladles		-
1 ounce	Relishes, sauces	1/8 cup
2 ounces	Gravy	1/4 cup
4 ounces	Vegetables	1/2 cup
6 ounces	Chili, soup	3/4 cup
9 ounces	Stew, chili, soup	1 cup
Ladles also come in 12, 24, and 32-ounce sizes.		

- **YIELD ANALYSIS** tests determine how much is obtained of an item (typically meat) from its as-purchased state to either its edible portion or as-served state. A yield test requires knowledge of actual yield in volume and weight of the finished recipe to determine how many 1 cup or 3 oz. portions will be obtained. Yield cannot be obtained by adding weights of the raw ingredients. A yield test should be run under actual serving conditions, measuring and weighing the finished recipe. If the cost is not within desired limits, the serving size must be modified, a different product purchased or the item removed from the menu.

$$\text{Yield Analysis Factor (YAF)} = \frac{\textbf{As Purchased Weight}}{\textbf{As Served Weight}}$$

For some products, a considerable amount of waste is removed. Peels of citrus, cores of sweet peppers, etc., which are trimmed before cooking or eating can have significant yield percentages.

COMMON CAN AND JAR SIZES

Size	Volume	Cans/Case	Products
6 oz.	6 fl. oz. (~3/4 cup)	48-72	Frozen concentrated juices and individual servings of single strength juices
8 oz.	7¾ fl. oz. (~1 cup)	48-72	Used mainly in metropolitan areas for fruits, vegetables and specialty items
No. 1 (Picnic)	9½ fl. oz. (~ 1 ¼ cup)	48	Condensed soups, some fruits, vegetables, meat and fish products
No. 300	14-15 oz. (~1 ¾ cup)	24	For specialty items, such as beans with pork, spaghetti, macaroni, chili-con-carne, date and nut bread, fruit and meat products
No. 303	16-17 fl. oz. (~2 cups)	24 or 36	Some ready-to-serve soups, meat and poultry products
No. 2	20 fl. oz. (~2 ½ cups)	24	Vegetable, fruits, juices, soups
No. 2 ½	26–29 fl. oz. (~2 ½ cups)	24	Fruits, vegetables, such as tomatoes, sauerkraut and pumpkin
No. 5	46 oz. 1 qt. 14 fl. oz. (~5 ¾ cups)	12	Juices, whole chicken, condensed soups
No. 10	6–7 lb. 5 oz. (~12 – 13 cups)	6	"Institutional" or "restaurant"-size container for most fruits and vegetables. Stocked by some retail stores

```
┌─────────────────────────────────────────────────────────────────────┐
│                       VOLUME EQUIVALENTS                              │
│                                                                       │
│   1 tablespoon  = 3 teaspoons          7/8 cup  = 14 tablespoons      │
│        1/8 cup  = 2 tablespoons          1 cup  = 16 tablespoons      │
│        1/8 cup  = 1 fluid ounce         ½ pint  = 1 cup               │
│         ¼ cup   = 4 tablespoons         ½ pint  = 8 fluid ounces      │
│        1/3 cup  = 5 1/3 tablespoons     1 pint  = 2 cups              │
│        3/8 cup  = 6 tablespoons        1 quart  = 2 pints             │
│         ½ cup   = 8 tablespoons       1 gallon  = 4 quarts            │
│        5/8 cup  = 10 tablespoons        1 peck  = 8 quarts (dry)      │
│        2/3 cup  = 10 2/3 tablespoons  1 bushel  = 4 pecks             │
│         ¾ cup   = 12 tablespoons                                      │
└─────────────────────────────────────────────────────────────────────┘
```

d. Forecasting production

- **FORECASTING** includes predicting trends and planning production for the immediate and distant future and balancing studies of the past and present. Forecasting is a prediction of food needs over a stated period using data of previous patterns and knowledge of scheduled special events, holidays, weather, etc.

- Considerations in forecasting production needs are historical data, internal and external factors.
  - ➢ Historical data include records of meals served, daily census, food left over, records on individual menu items. Records may show that only three out of five toppings for baked potato are used enough to keep them on the menu.
  - ➢ Internal factors include the size of plant, productivity of personnel and type of equipment. For example, customers want stir-fry items. This might require changes in equipment and training of personnel.
  - ➢ External factors include social, economic, political and environmental conditions. A switch, for example, to biodegradable containers for carry-out food service may be desirable based on consumer demand or environmental considerations.

- The production manager must know the estimated number of customers or the number of servings of each menu item in time to order from the procurement unit. Good forecasts are essential in planning smooth transitions from current to future output, regardless of the size or type of the food service (i.e., schools, hospitals and restaurants).

- Forecasts are based on past sales records and anticipated popularity of new menu items when offered with existing menu items. Good forecasting is important because preparing enough, but not too much of menu items, reduces waste while providing enough choices to patrons.

e. Production scheduling

- A **FOOD PRODUCTION SCHEDULE** is a control mechanism that specifies where, when and who will prepare menu items. Scheduling ensures efficient use of labor and equipment and minimizes production problems. Food production schedules should be developed at the same time menus are planned to prevent an imbalance of workloads, to allow adequate time for food preparation and to determine necessary equipment.

- Scheduling requires knowledge of dry and low-temperature storage capacity, preparation needs (assembly of ingredients, pre-preparation, cooking), workspace allocation, finishing (setting up salads, portioning desserts, slicing meats), storage prior to serving and staff capabilities.

- A production schedule will specify the following:
  - ➢ Name of each menu item.
  - ➢ Name of the employee assigned to a particular task.
  - ➢ Time preparation is to begin and is to be completed.
  - ➢ Details regarding ingredients and portion control.

- Management is responsible for developing the production schedule, for procedures to be followed and for supervision. Regular staff meetings can provide feedback.

4. Production systems

a. Conventional

- In the **CONVENTIONAL COOK-AND-SERVE** system, menu items are prepared from basic ingredients, and are held hot or cold until they are served. Production may take place in a kitchen on-site or in a separate kitchen that supplies several institutions or units. The cook-and-serve system allows control over menu, recipes and quality, but it is labor intensive. It is difficult to schedule a balanced workload that covers peak periods and minimizes employees on duty during slow periods.

b. Commissary

- In a **COMMISSARY,** a centralized production facility transports food (in bulk or proportioned) to satellite areas for service and possible final production (i.e., congregate feeding for seniors). Special considerations of this system include costs and logistics of transportation and maintaining culinary quality, food safety and sanitation of food products as they are held and transported.

c. Ready-prepared

- In a **READY-PREPARED** system, menu items are purchased already cooked and chilled or cooked and frozen on-site in preparation for reheating prior to service.

  - ➢ Foods may be purchased in any form, from basic recipe ingredients to fully prepared tems.
  - ➢ The system is efficient because the preparation is spread over the entire work period rather than occurring shortly before service, as in the cook-and-serve system.
  - ➢ It requires chilling and/or freezing equipment and adequate low-temperature storage space, as well as meticulous attention to food handling techniques to prevent bacterial growth.
  - ➢ The cook-and-freeze system maintains the quality of food because rapid freezing promotes smaller ice crystals.

d. Assembly serve

- In an **ASSEMBLY SERVE** (i.e., all convenience) system, most or all foods are procured in a ready-to-serve form (i.e., washed, chopped, preformed). Items may be fresh, frozen, dehydrated, canned and proportioned. This system has lower space needs and does not require a full kitchen. Lower labor costs and less skilled labor is needed, but food costs are higher. Schools, senior feeding sites and small volume feeders can attain cost savings by using assembly serve systems. Many fast food and sandwich restaurants are assembly-serve. Competitive bidding can reduce meal costs when large volumes of assembly serve meals are purchased.

e. Cook-chill

- In a **COOK-CHILL** system, food is prepared in advance and chilled in blast chillers, often for transport to other facilities. When it is time to serve the food, it is reheated to serving temperature.

f. Display cooking

- Open kitchens, or chef stations, are now popular where patrons can observe food preparation and plating. Examples include chefs preparing sushi, making pizza, plating desserts or stir-frying at tabletop ranges. This method uses food as entertainment and promotes interaction between the chef and patron.

5. Distribution and service

- Food may be delivered in bulk, individually portioned on trays or in a variety of other ways. In healthcare, senior feeding and school feeding settings, bulk foods may be transported in refrigerated and/or heated carts or insulated containers to sites where meals are served or trays assembled either on or off the premises. Time lapses between preparation and service and the safety and sanitation of transport vessels and vehicles and receiving temperatures must be monitored.

a. Type of service systems

(1) Centralized

- **PELLET SYSTEM** uses heated pellets in bases inserted under hot food plates.

Advantages
➤ Support equipment and system operation are conventional and uncomplicated.
➤ There is no requirement for a special plate; uses any standard-sized china. No special insulated delivery cart is required.

Disadvantages
➤ Provision for maintenance of cold items; such as milk, salads, ice cream, etc., is not made.
➤ Hot food cannot be held for long periods of time (maximum 45 minutes).
➤ Additional service pieces need to be inventoried, stored, transported, washed and sanitized.
➤ Potential for burns.

- **INSULATED COMPONENTS**

  Advantages
  - Only the dinner plate and food are heated; there are no pellet bases to heat.
  - No burn hazard to the attendant or patient because there is no hot pellet base or pellet disk.
  - No special delivery cart is required.

  Disadvantages
  - Patients often take attractive insulated components home, raising inventory costs.

- **HEAT SUPPORT CART**

  Advantages
  - Thermal energy can be controlled to plate and/or bowl as required.
  - Cart remains heated until tray is removed for service to the patient.
  - Each cart has an insulated drawer for ice cream and other frozen desserts.
  - Heat energy continues to be supplied to food during transportation.

  Disadvantages
  - Special motorized carts and trays with heaters are required.
  - The potential for maintenance/repair problems is high.
  - The cart and trays are dependent on the use of disposable dishes that can be uneconomical and aesthetically unacceptable.
  - No provisions are made for maintaining cold food temperatures except for ice cream.

- **CONTACT PLATE HEATER CART**

  Advantages
  - Reduced pantry labor due to reheating and refrigerating trays in the delivery carts.
  - Pantry can be smaller in size, and equipment costs for reheating ovens are eliminated.
  - Minimum intervention by employees after assembled tray leaves main tray assembly location.

  Disadvantages
  - Cart maintenance may be high due to complex electrical components.
  - Requirements for special dishes, usually disposables, can increase operating costs.
  - Inflexible presentation and rigid placement of food items.
  - Reheated only from chilled, not frozen, state.

- **PELLET AND SUBLIMATION REFRIGERATION**

  Advantages
  - A synergistic heat maintenance effect is achieved.
  - Simplicity of cart construction and ease of sanitation. The lightweight cart facilitates easy moving.

  Disadvantages
  - The operational cost and complexity of the required carbon dioxide cooling system is a consideration.
  - Patient trays are not completely assembled at central assembly point.
  - Final assembly is in patient areas requiring more staff time.

- **SPLIT TRAY**

  Advantages
  - ➤ Centralized supervision and control of the entire assembly process possible.
  - ➤ No reassembly in patient areas required.
  - ➤ Good hot and cold temperature retention.
  - ➤ Late trays easily accommodated within a reasonable period.

  Disadvantages
  - ➤ The cart is heavy, bulky and difficult to sanitize.
  - ➤ Initial costs and maintenance costs of carts are high.

- **MATCH-A-TRAY**

  Advantages
  - ➤ Same as described for split tray, except consolidation is required at the patient level.

  Disadvantages
  - ➤ Same as described for split tray. Additional labor must be supplied in patient areas to reassemble complete patient meals.

- **INSULATED TRAY**

  Advantages
  - ➤ Maintains hot and cold zones well without external heat or refrigeration sources.
  - ➤ Simplicity of transport is achieved.
  - ➤ Heavy carts are not required.
  - ➤ Less load on dishwashing facilities due to use of disposables.
  - ➤ No complex components to replace or repair.

  Disadvantages
  - ➤ Purchase of disposable dishes increases operational costs.
  - ➤ Food-holding time limited to 45 minutes.
  - ➤ Hot foods may take on a steamed appearance.
  - ➤ Trays can be difficult to sanitize due to deep wells.
  - ➤ Top and bottom tray compartments do not nest, increasing needs for storage space.
  - ➤ Presentation and placement of dishes is limited by tray construction.
  - ➤ Unattractive, institutional appearance.

- **COVERED TRAY**

  Advantages
  - ➤ Tray is a simple standard unit.
  - ➤ Equipment costs are low.

  Disadvantages
  - ➤ Requires an immediate and responsive transportation system.
  - ➤ High labor requirement for transport.
  - ➤ No thermal support, hot foods do not stay hot.

- **INTEGRAL HEAT OVENS AND CARTS**

  Advantages
  - ➤ Minimum intervention by employees is required.
  - ➤ Efficiency and speed of service is enhanced due to multiple meals reheated at the same time.
  - ➤ Integrally-heated dish acts as pellet system to continue to keep food hot longer.

Disadvantages
➢ Soups and cereals are difficult to reheat.
➢ Dishwasher time is increased, especially for breakfast service, because of food that sticks to dishes.
➢ On-going operation costs are high due to replacement and lease costs.
➢ An inflexible presentation of the tray and rigid placement of items may be a problem.

(2) Decentralized

- In **DECENTRALIZED SERVICE** bulk quantities of prepared food are sent hot and/or cold to serving pantries where food is portioned, assembled and reheated. Decentralized systems are suitable for large or spread-out facilities to minimize time between preparation and service. For example, a university with dining areas in several buildings or multiple senior feeding centers. Decentralized service reduces need for kitchen space, equipment and food production staff at multiple locations, but does require serving staff at each service location.

b. Equipment/packaging

- Equipment required depends on the food distribution system. In general:

  ➢ Counters should be kept clean and sanitized and should have attractive, easy-to-clean surfaces with insulation for hot and cold foods.
  ➢ Sneeze guards and shields should be provided for open food displays, and there should be adequate space to reach food and for service personnel.
  ➢ Serving utensils needed include a variety of ladles, long-handled spoons (perforated, slotted, solid) and assorted sized scoops and ice cream dippers. Each item must have its own serving utensil that is stored in a sanitary manner when not in use.
  ➢ Beverage dispensers, dish dispensers and temperature-controlled units for self-service are also required. Calibration on temperature-controlled units must be checked periodically.
  ➢ Tableware should be suitable for the type of service and menu. China quality, pattern and color should enhance the appearance of food as well as reflect the quality, price and ambiance of the food service organization.
  ➢ There should be enough dishes, flatware and trays to accommodate what is offered at any time. For example, there should be enough small dishes for cottage cheese served with an entrée and for ice cream served for dessert.
  ➢ Dishes and flatware chosen should be durable and easy to clean and stored in a sanitary manner. Plated silverware should be reinforced at points of greatest wear. Older individuals and those with arthritis find it hard to grasp flatware with slim handles.
  ➢ China, flatware and recyclable paper products may be more environmentally desirable than non-biodegradable plastic products. Costs, labor, sanitation and environmental concerns must be balanced in choosing such equipment.
  ➢ Equipment connected to waterlines must have a vacuum breaker installed to prevent backflow.

- All foods and utensils should be appropriately packaged and sealed so as to prevent or minimize contamination. Attention should be paid to excess or unnecessary packaging that can be difficult for customers to open and/or may contribute to excess waste or costs.

TOPIC C - SANITATION and SAFETY

1. Sanitation and food safety

- For complete information on food sanitation, refer to *ServSafe Coursebook*. NRA Educational Foundation, Chicago.

a. Principles

- Policies and procedures must be established for receiving, storage, preparation, display, service and transport of food and equipment, for the return of soiled dishes and for dishwashing designed to protect food from external contamination and the rapid growth of microorganisms. States may have rules that are stricter than national standards. The *FDA Model Food Code*, which serves as the standard, can be found by visiting **www.fda.gov/html.**

(1) Contamination and spoilage

- **CONTAMINATION** is the presence of unintended substances (i.e., biological, chemical, physical) in food. The following measures can be used to prevent contamination:

  - ➤ Purchase meat, poultry, dairy products and shellfish from officially inspected sources and reputable suppliers. Ask to see inspection reports and check date codes.
  - ➤ Purchase canned goods from approved commercial sources. Avoid home-canned foods. Discard canned foods if the cans or lids are dented, swollen, leaking, bulging or show signs of rust. Check date codes.
  - ➤ Dispense food packaged in small individual serving portions (i.e., milk, juice, crackers) in their original wrappers or containers.
  - ➤ Store foods at proper temperatures. Check refrigerator and freezer temperatures.
  - ➤ Cover food during transport and storage.
  - ➤ Use separate cutting boards for meat, poultry, fish, raw fruits and vegetables and raw and cooked foods.
  - ➤ Clean and sanitize cutting boards, utensils and work surfaces thoroughly after each use.
  - ➤ Keep cold foods at 40°F or colder and hot foods at 140°F or hotter. (Many states require 150°F or hotter.)
  - ➤ Thaw frozen foods in the refrigerator.
  - ➤ Store and process cooked and raw foods with separate equipment. Clean and sanitize containers and equipment between uses.
  - ➤ Use fresh eggs only if they are thoroughly cooked. Do not use eggs with dirty or cracked shells. Use pasteurized egg products for dishes that will receive little or no further cooking.
  - ➤ Wash fruits and vegetables immediately before using.
  - ➤ Cook foods to recommended temperatures.
  - ➤ Use one-stage and two-stage cooling methods for storing hot foods. Refrigerate cooked foods immediately in uncovered shallow containers and cover food after cooling.
  - ➤ Use plastic or metal tongs or scoops or automatic dispensers for ice.
  - ➤ Protect salad bar items with transparent shields or sneeze guards.
  - ➤ Control lighting, ventilation and humidity to prevent bacterial growth.
  - ➤ Store high-acid foods in stainless steel containers.

➢ Clean vents, fans and filters regularly.

➢ Discard chipped or cracked service ware. Do not touch service ware or tableware on surfaces that will come in contact with foods.

➢ Handle garbage properly. Store garbage in clean, covered, leak-proof containers.

➢ Instruct employees about proper hand washing methods, use of disposable gloves, hand sanitizers and hair restraints such as nets and caps.

- Food spoilage encompasses more than decomposition. Spoiled foods are: past the desired stage of development (i.e., ripeness); contaminated during production or handling; contaminated by microbes, insects or rodents; damaged by freezing, heating, drying or other processes; or may contain microorganisms and parasites that cause food-borne illnesses. Foods that are not fit to eat are spoiled and should be discarded.

- **CROSS-CONTAMINATION** is the movement of chemicals or microorganisms from one place to another. Food handlers can transfer chemical or bacterial organisms or substances while preparing food by not washing hands often, working while having a cold, cough, infection or communicable disease, or neglect of sanitation practices.

- A current contamination concern is contaminations by allergens or substances which can make a particular diner very ill. For some with food allergies, the presence of microscopic bits of flour (gluten) or nuts can cause a dangerous or even fatal reaction. Using a scoop for ice vanilla ice cream that was used for scooping butter pecan ice cream or residue from croutons on tongs assembling a salad, all cross-contaminate without the known presence of an allergen. Food service workers and servers must be trained and understand the ways of avoiding cross-contamination.

(2) Factors affecting bacterial growth

- When bacteria are present, they multiply readily when provided appropriate temperatures and growth medium, usually a warm, moist environment.

- Although any food can become contaminated, those considered **POTENTIALLY HAZARDOUS FOODS** provide a more favorable medium for the rapid growth of microorganisms and are often implicated in outbreaks of food-borne diseases.

- The acronym **FAT-TOM** is used to remember conditions favorable to the rapid growth of most food-borne organisms:

F = **Food source:** Protein-rich and some heat-treated carbohydrate foods provide a **food source** for microbial growth.

A = **Acid:** Slightly **acidic** (pH > 4.6) or neutral media favor bacterial growth. Molds, yeast and some bacteria can grow at pH levels less than 4.6.

T = **Time:** Foods kept at unfavorable temperatures for longer than 4 hours can provide sufficient **time** for bacteria to multiply to levels high enough to cause illness.

T = **Temperature:** The **temperature** danger zone between 41°F and 135°F favors rapid multiplication of organisms and production of bacterial toxins.

O = **Oxygen:** Most microorganisms grow when **oxygen** is present.

M = **Moisture:** Microorganisms grow and multiply best in foods with a water activity of 0.85 to 0.97.

(3) Signs and symptoms of food-borne illness

FOOD-BORNE ILLNESS

Causative Agent	Symptoms	Implicated Foods	Control Measures
Anisakiasis (parasite)	Tingling in the throat, abdominal pain, vomiting, coughing up small worms	Fish, raw seafood	Avoid raw seafood
Bacillus cereus diarrheal and/or emetic (bacteria)	Diarrhea, cramps, nausea, vomiting; onset 1-15 hrs	Rice, starchy foods; cooked ready-to-eat foods, meat products, soups, sauces, rice, pasta, vegetables	Cook foods thoroughly with careful time and temperature control; eat immediately after cooking; chill quickly
Campylobacter jejuni	Diarrhea, nausea, vomiting, cramps, fever; onset 1-10 days	Unpasteurized milk, raw poultry, and meat; shellfish; contaminated water	Use pasteurized milk; prevent cross-contamination with raw products, cook meat, poultry, and fish thoroughly
Clostridium botulinum (bacteria)	Diarrhea, vertigo, severe nervous system damage, respiratory failure, paralysis; infant botulism; onset 4-36 hrs	Improperly canned low acid foods (vegetables, meat, poultry, fish, vegetables, fruit); honey; garlic-in-oil mixtures, temperature-abused vacuum-packed foods	Use correct canning methods for low-acid foods, careful time and temperature controls for vacuum-packed foods; do not feed honey or garlic to infants
Clostridium perfrigens (bacteria)	Diarrhea, severe abdominal pain; onset 8-22 hrs	Cooked meat, poultry; reheated foods; improperly cooled foods	Careful time and temperature controls; cook food thoroughly; use quick-chill methods
Escherichia coli Enterohemorrhagic (EHEC); (0157:H7) is the most common strain in the US) Enterotoxigenic (ETEC) Enteroinvasive (EIEC) (bacteria)	Cramps, diarrhea, fever; may be dysenteric; may cause kidney failure, particularly in children; onset 2-6 days	Raw or under-cooked ground beef; raw milk; chicken; contaminated water; bean sprouts, unpasteurized juices, melons	Thoroughly cook ground meat to 155°F for 15 seconds; practice good personal hygiene; prevent cross-contamination; use caution when drinking water from unknown sources
Giardia (parasite)	Fatigue, cramps, nausea, weight loss, intestinal gas	Water, ice, salads	Use sanitary water source. Wash fresh produce

FOOD-BORNE ILLNESS

Causative Agent	Symptoms	Implicated Foods	Control Measures
Hepatitis A (virus)	Fever, fatigue, nausea, jaundice; onset 10-50 days	Contaminated seafood, water, ice; fruit juice, any food not receiving heat treatment	Obtain shellfish from approved sources; practice good personal hygiene; prevent cross-contamination; use sanitary water source
Listeria monocytogenes (bacteria)	Headache, fever, diarrhea, meningitis; most often affects fetuses, infants or pregnant women; onset 1 day to several weeks	Prepared and chilled, ready-to-eat food; raw milk, cheese; ready-to-eat luncheon meats; ice cream, frozen yogurt	Use pasteurized milk and dairy products; prevent cross-contamination, cook foods properly; some advise heating lunch meats
Norwalk Virus	Cramps, nausea, headache, fever, vomiting	Water, raw vegetables, fresh fruit, salads, shellfish	Obtain shellfish from approved sources; practice good personal hygiene; prevent cross-contamination; use sanitary water source
Rotavirus	Abdominal pain, diarrhea, vomiting, fever	Water, ice, some hors d'oeuvres	Use sanitary water source. Avoid cross-contamination
Salmonella (bacteria)	Fever, diarrhea, cramps, chills, vomiting, systemic infection, dehydration; onset 648 hrs; onset 3-4 weeks for delayed arthritic symptoms	Raw or undercooked eggs, poultry products; fish, protein foods and some fresh produce	Use proper food handling methods; avoid cross-contamination; cook egg and poultry dishes thoroughly to 165°F for at least 15 seconds, refrigerate quickly; good personal hygiene
Shigella (bacteria)	Fever; diarrhea; may be dysenteric; nausea; occasional vomiting and cramps; onset 1-7 days	Protein-rich salads; moist, mixed food; some raw produce, shrimp, milk products	Avoid cross-contamination; use good personal hygeine; cool foods rapidly
Staphylococcus aureus (bacteria)	Nausea, vomiting, diarrhea, cramps; onset 1-7 hrs	Meat, poultry, ham, egg products; tuna, potato and pasta salad; cream-filled pastry; cheese	Avoid direct hand contact with food; rapidly cool prepared foods; exclude employees with skin infections from handling food

FOOD-BORNE ILLNESS

Causative Agent	Symptoms	Implicated Foods	Control Measures
Streptococcus pyogenes (bacteria)	Fever, tonsillitis, scarlet fever, rheumatic fever; onset 2-60 hrs	Raw milk; devilled eggs	Use proper food handling tequniquesl use pasteurized milk; refrigerate food quickly
Trichinella spirallis (parasite)	Nausea, diarrhea, fever; thirst, sweating, chills, fatigue; onset 2-28 days depending on number of larvae ingested	Undercooked pork or wild game; ground meats	Cook pork and game meats to minimum internal cooking temperatures; rinse and sanitize equipment used in preparation or grinding of raw pork or meat products
Vibrio parahaemolyticus Vibrio cholerae Vibrio vulnificus (bacteria)	Diarrhea, cramps, fever, headache, vomiting; onset 4-96 hrs	Raw fish, shellfish (oysters, clams, mussels, scallops, crab, etc.)	Thoroughly cook fish and shellfish; refrigerate quickly; do not eat raw seafood; prevent cross-contamination
Yersinia enterocolitica (bacteria)	Various symptoms of gastroenteritis; may mimic appendicitis; onset 2-7 days	Meats; raw milk; poultry; tofu; non-chlorinated water	Thoroughly cook foods to minimum safe temperatures; wash vegetables carefully; purchase tofu that is fresh; use caution when drinking water from unknown sources

b. Sanitation practices and infection control

(1) Personal hygiene

- All employees should wash hands often, and always after handling food or using the rest room, using soap and warm water. They should use a paper towel to dry hands and turn off water. Proper hand washing includes scrubbing hands with soap for at least 20 seconds before rinsing. Rest rooms should be set up so that it is not necessary to touch door handles after hands are washed. This precaution avoids contaminating clean hands.

- Some facilities have automatic water turn-offs and wall-mounted hand dryers. Hands should be washed:

  - ➤ After every instance of contamination.
  - ➤ After visiting the restroom, coughing or sneezing.
  - ➤ Before starting to work; after handling raw food, especially of animal origin; and after handling any article (knife, cutting board, etc.) that has been in contact with raw food of animal origin.

> ➢ After smoking, eating, drinking or chewing gum.
> ➢ After handling garbage or trash.
> ➢ After cleaning tables or busing dirty dishes.
> ➢ After using any cleaning, polishing or sanitizing chemicals.

- Employees should be healthy and should observe safe food-handling practices.

- Employees who handle food should have a physical exam, including a tuberculin test, before being hired and at intervals thereafter.

- Employees with open cuts should not handle food. Cuts should be cleaned and bandaged, then covered with disposable gloves. Plastic gloves should be worn over bandages or any minor abrasions.

- Employees with contagious diseases of bacterial or viral origin, including colds and coughs, should not work in the food area. These diseases may spread to other workers and will increase the likelihood of contaminating food. Also, every effort must be made to protect clients/patients from illness transmitted by employees.

- Following an infectious illness, such as salmonellosis, workers may be free of symptoms but still able to transmit or transfer living organisms if personal hygiene rules are not followed.

- Carriers and those recovering from hepatitis may not handle food. Procedures for patients with transmittable diseases should be followed.

(2) Food and equipment

- Work surfaces should be kept clean, sanitized and well-organized.

- Only clean, sanitized utensils may be used in preparing, cooking and serving food.

- Clean dishes should be air-dried.

- Employees should not touch eating surfaces of clean dishes or flatware.

- Rodent and insect-control programs include both on-site sanitation and correct garbage handling, disposal of cartons, etc.

(3) Food storage

- Areas that store dry goods are required to have shelving to keep all products off the floor. Wherever possible, it should be away from walls.

- Grains should be stored in insect/rodent-proof containers (not paper) or in sealed containers, such as covered bins.

- Storerooms should have good lighting and be properly ventilated and temperature controlled. They should also have humidity controls to prevent formation of mildew and mold or growth of certain organisms.

- Most health codes require that cleaning supplies, including bleach, pesticides, solvents, be stored in a separate room from food.

- Perishable foods should be moved into refrigerators/freezers that have correct temperature and humidity controls, as quickly as possible.

- Food should be marked with date of purchase and/or use.

(4) Temperature control

- Failure to cool and reheat food properly is a leading cause of food-borne illness.

  - Temperature of freshly prepared items and food held for service should be checked every two hours.
  - Hot foods that do not meet temperature guidelines should be rapidly reheated to 165°F for 15 seconds. Foods reheated in a microwave need to be held at 165°F for 2 minutes to be safe.
  - Safe methods to cool foods include use of blast chillers, ice water baths, ice paddles or transfer to shallow pans and containers for more rapid chilling.
  - Thicker or denser foods take longer to cool. To more quickly cool roasts and larger cuts of meat, cut them in pieces.
  - Quick-chill methods of cooling reduce the temperature of freshly prepared items from 140°F or above to 40°F or below within 90 minutes.
  - The *FDA Model Food Code* recommends a two-stage cooling process in which the cooked food item is brought from 135°F (57°C) or above to 70°F (21°C) within 2 hours, then below 41°F (5°C) in an additional 4 hours. Food that cannot be cooled below 70°F within 2 hours must be reheated above 165°F for 15 seconds, and cooled again below 70°F within 2 hours. Using this method, foods may be reheated more than once as long as food has been properly handled at each step.
  - The one-stage cooling method requires foods be cooled to below 40°F within 4 hours.

- For fresh eggs, the receiving temperature should be 45°F or lower and the storage temperature should be 40°F or lower. Temperatures are taken of the air in the delivery truck or cooler, as it is difficult to measure the temperature of eggs in shells.

(5) Food handling techniques

- Direct hand contact with food should be avoided whenever possible. If contact is necessary, hands should be washed or disposable gloves worn. Employees should also avoid handling rims of glasses and parts of eating utensils that will be touched by food.

- Gloves of several types are used in kitchens. Rubber gloves are worn to protect hands from chemicals and water. Rubber gloves should be washed with soap and sanitized after use. Disposable gloves should be used and discarded after each specific task. For example, disposable gloves used to touch raw chicken should be discarded after use before another food is handled.

- For tasting, use a clean spoon each time a food is tasted during cooking.

- Employees should be informed of food handling practices upon hiring. The following should be checked by managers:

  - Employees are dressed in clean, neat, specified uniforms, including apron and name badge.
  - Uniforms should be put on at work. Aprons should be removed before using restrooms.
  - Hair is covered with a net or hat; beards are netted.
  - Employees wear closed shoes with non-slip soles.
  - Food handlers have no infectious sores, breaks in skin or transmittable diseases.
  - Finger cots or disposable gloves are worn over all hand bandages, or injured

IV. FOODSERVICE SYSTEMS (17%)

employees should be restricted to non-food-contact activities.

- ➤ Jewelry is restricted to a plain wedding band.
- ➤ Fingernails are trimmed, clean and free of nail polish.
- ➤ Hand washing procedures are strictly followed.
- ➤ Restrict smoking, eating and gum chewing to non-food-preparation areas.
- ➤ Different employees handle food and money or hands are washed between handling of food and money.

c. Regulations (government and other agencies)

- Federal law requires that all food service establishments be licensed and must display a current valid inspection permit. After inspections, action should be taken to correct all identified sanitation problems, even if the total score indicates that the inspection has been passed.

- Local health departments have regulations on safe sources of food, food processing and serving establishments, licensing, inspections, floor plan and equipment approval and food handling permits.

- The National Restaurant Association and the U.S. Public Health Service have sample inspection sheets that can be used by local agencies to use in inspections.

- The **NATIONAL SANITATION FOUNDATION (NSF)** develops standards and criteria for products, food service equipment and services that affect public health. They also have sanitation training materials available.

- The **OCCUPATIONAL SAFETY AND HEALTH ACT OF 1970 (OSHA)** uses standards contained in Part 1910, Volume 39, Number 125 of the *Federal Register*, dated June 27, 1974. Under OSHA, inspections are made and violations cited. Corrections must be made within a reasonable time or penalties will be levied.

d. Food safety

(1) Time and temperature control

MINIMUM SAFE INTERNAL COOKING TEMPERATURES	
Food product	**Standard time and hold**
Poultry, stuffing, stuffed pasta, casseroles, field-dressed game	165°F (74°C) for 15 seconds
Ground or flaked meats including hamburger, ground pork, flaked fish, ground game animals, sausage, gyros	155°F (69°C) for 15 seconds
Beef and pork roasts (rare)	145°F (63°C) for 4 minutes
Pork, ham, bacon, injected meats; beef steaks, veal, lamb, commercially raised game animals; fish; shellfish; shell eggs for immediate service	145°F (63°C) for 15 seconds
Any potentially hazardous food cooked in a microwave oven	165°F (74°C); let food stand for 2 minutes after cooking
Commercially prepared ready-to-eat food hot held for service	135 °F (57° C)

Source: *FDA Model Food Code*, revised 2005

- Water of dish machines should be clean and at proper temperatures:
Prewash	110°-140°F
Wash	140°-160°F
Power rinse	165°-175°F
Final rinse	165°-180°F

- Accuracy of gauges should be verified each meal by use of a maximum temperature thermometer and/or temperature sensitive strips.

- Temperatures should be documented as part of ongoing sanitation procedures and temperature logs maintained as records.

- Use properly calibrated thermometers, accurate within 2°F or 1°C, to measure temperatures. Measure internal temperatures at several locations in the thickest part of the food item. Clean and sanitize the thermometer after each use.

(2) Additives

- The FDA defines a **FOOD ADDITIVE** as "any substance used in the production, processing, treatment, packaging, transportation or storage of food , the intended use of which results or may reasonably be expected to result -- directly or indirectly -- in its becoming a component or otherwise affecting the characteristics of any food."

- Additives are substances added to foods that generally:
  - ➢ improve their flavor, smell, texture or color
  - ➢ extend storage life
  - ➢ maximize performance and/or
  - ➢ protect nutrient value

- Food additives are overseen by the FDA but the burden-of-proof for safety falls on the manufacturer.

- Additives that are on the **GRAS (GENERALLY RECOGNIZED AS SAFE)** list are exempt from the requirement of proving safety as they are seen as having "a reasonable safety of no harm from a product under the intended conditions of use."

- Pesticides were once considered food additives but the Food Quality Protection Act of 1996 re-defined food additives to exclude pesticide residues. While the FDA does monitor some pesticide residues in foods, they do not screen for all types of pesticides and residues of these chemicals can end up in the food supply.

- See Domain I for a discussion of specific food additives and their uses in food.

(3) Documentation and record keeping

- Proper procedures should be followed when receiving any shipment of goods (food or otherwise) to ensure the safety of food and minimize contamination. (Refer to Topic B Procurement, Production, Distribution and Service in Domain IV for procedures.)

- All food service establishments should keep records of the date of routine maintenance of all equipment and records of warrantees and repairs.

- Regular schedules of complete cleaning of equipment and storage areas must be followed and documented. Service manuals should be available for use in a language understandable to the equipment user.

- All in-service education regarding employee hygiene, handling of food, storage of food and use of equipment should also be documented.

- Maintain records of purchase and use of any hazardous materials.

(4) HACCP

- Procedures should be initiated and maintained in order to assure food quality and safety. **HAZARD ANALYSIS CRITICAL CONTROL POINTS (HACCP)** is a system that combines proper food handling procedures, monitoring techniques and record keeping, ensuring safe food handling throughout a food service operation. The goal of the HACCP system is to prevent, eliminate or reduce the risk of contamination or growth of microorganisms at every step in the food production process through effective control procedures.

- HACCP is based on seven principles:
  1. **Perform a Hazard Analysis:** Analyze your menu for potentially hazardous foods; consider your clients or population served and determine where food safety hazards (biological, chemical, physical) can occur.
  2. **Determine the Critical Control Points (CCPs):** Determine which steps in the operation are critical to a safe outcome and the last step at which you can intervene to prevent, control or eliminate a hazard from occurring. Usually this involves the cooking, chilling and holding processes or the receiving process for foods that will have no further cooking.
  3. **Establish Critical Limits:** For each CCP, determine the procedures the food handler must follow and the minimum and maximum criteria that must be met for hazards to be prevented, eliminated, or reduced to safe levels. Critical limits are often numerical (i.e., final cooking temperature of 165°F).
  4. **Monitor Critical Control Points:** To assure food safety, determine who will monitor CCPs, how CCPs will be monitored, frequency of monitoring and resources required for monitoring. The monitoring process should beongoing and employees should be properly trained.
  5. **Take Corrective Actions:** Whenever a food does not meet a critical limit, corrective action must be taken. Examples of corrective actions include cooking the item to the recommended temperature, reheating a food to 165°F for 15 seconds or discarding a food item after a specified time in the temperature danger zone.
  6. **Verify that the System Works:** Confirm the HACCP program is being followed according to your established procedures, monitoring actions and corrective steps. Periodically reevaluate each step in the process.
  7. **Record Keeping and Documentation:** Once a system is in place, maintain records to document compliance. Examples of records to keep include time-temperature logs, training sessions, corrective actions, complaints and calibration records.

(5) Recalls

- When manufacturers of equipment recall an item, it is usually for safety reasons, and should be addressed immediately. At times, it may cause problems with production, but since such recalls can cause serious problems, such as fires, the items must be repaired or replaced by the manufacturer.

- The same is true for food items that may be recalled by the distributor. The food items may be fresh, canned or frozen and must be discarded carefully. The area where the food was stored must be sanitized. In addition, any work space or receiving or loading dock that may have come into contact with the food must be carefully sanitized as well.

(6) Operational emergencies

- Operational emergencies, such as power outages, flooding, extreme weather conditions, fire, gas leaks, loss of communication systems, etc. can severely impact organizations and institutions.

- After emergency plans are employed, such as evacuation and putting out fires, the food service will be called upon to continue feeding the population served.

- Crisis management plans that include provision of emergency water, food and supplies will need to be implemented, depending on the nature of the emergency.

- A system identifying crisis coordinator and staff roles during an emergency, should be in place with all staff trained to respond in emergency situations.

(7) Bioterrorism

- Threats of bioterrorism that can cause anxiety about the safety of our food and water are a major concern, especially since September 11, 2001.

- The FDA and CDC urge monitoring of the safety of food from farm to table, including water supplies and imported foods.

- Agents likely to be bioterrorist weapons include anthrax, botulism, plague, smallpox, tularemia, salmonella and shigella.

- Food surveillance has increased since 2001. *FoodNet*, the Food-Borne Disease Active Surveillance Network which is part of CDC's Emerging Infections Program, a collaborative effort among CDC, USDA, and states has been formed. Also *Pulse Net*, developed by CDC is a system for public health agencies to track bacteria electronically and detect food-borne-illness outbreaks earlier.

- Governmental organizations charged with monitoring bioterrorism include USDA, Homeland Security Agency, Food Safety and Inspection Service (FSIS), Center for Disease Control (CDC) Center for Public Health Preparedness and the Food and Drug Administration (FDA).

2. Safety

a. Employee safety

- Employee safety is a legal, financial and ethical responsibility of management. Safety instructions including use of proper fire procedures and use of fire extinguishers should be given to all employees. In the workplace, some employees should receive training in first aid (including the Heimlich maneuver) and cardiopulmonary resuscitation (CPR). All employees should know building evacuation procedures. Emergency plans and exits should be clearly marked.

(1) Universal precautions

- The food service supervisor/employer has responsibility for (a) training employees regarding employee safety issues upon initial hire,0 as well as on a regularly scheduled basis, (b) following Occupational Safety and Health Act (OSHA) requirements and maintaining OSHA records and (c) providing as safe a workplace as possible. The food service director must know and act upon the organization's written safety regulations and hazard communication program.

- Employees must understand that food service operations can be dangerous places, with potential for falls, lifting injuries, burns and cuts, among other hazards. Employees must take responsibility for their own safety and for that of their co-workers once they have been taught correct procedures.

- Specific employee safety practices that should be addressed include:
  - ➤ Prevention of falls, both by providing slip-free floor surfaces and training personnel to keep floors dry and clean and to wipe up immediately after spills, and wearing appropriate shoes.
  - ➤ Appropriate employee hygiene, including maintaining clean uniforms, limiting

excessive jewelry and clothing (scarves, etc.) that could cause a safety hazard to the employee and or others.

➢ Correct methods of lifting and carrying heavy items; provision of and training in use of aids to prevent strains and back problems. This may include physical-fitness classes.

➢ First-aid equipment available and procedures to follow with cuts or burns.

➢ Rules for moving materials/food/equipment.

➢ Development of procedures to prevent both burns and fires and to ensure proper use of fire extinguishers.

➢ Proper use, cleaning, sharpening and storage of knives and slicers.

➢ Safe use of other equipment, including equipment with moving parts and their safety shields, electrical equipment, ladders and pressure equipment.

➢ Conditions under which accidents frequently occur (when employees are in a hurry, tired, stressed) and how to recognize those conditions in order to avoid accidents.

➢ Chemicals and other toxic materials used in food service for sanitizing and other purposes, their correct use, storage and abuse avoidance.

➢ Interactions that are dangerous, such as water and electricity.

(2) Equipment use and maintenance

- The vendor of chemicals/cleaning supplies must provide a **MATERIAL SAFETY DATA SHEET (MSDS)** for each product. The MSDS must be kept on site and must be available to employees and inspectors at all times. Review the MSDS prior to purchasing products to determine potential hazards, side effects or required protective devices (goggles, face shields, special composition gloves or aprons). Evaluate hazards, difficulty of use and skill level of the workers expected to use the products in relation to the expected benefit of using the product.

- Employers are responsible for providing a clean workplace including the following:
  ➢ A safe workplace, including asbestos control, fire deterrents and bio-safety regulation.
  ➢ Proper lighting.
  ➢ Sinks for hand washing.
  ➢ Adequate heating, cooling, ventilation and other air emission issues such as avoiding restricted refrigerants and other stratospheric, ozone-depleting agents.
  ➢ Noise control.
  ➢ Identifying, labeling, storing and disposing of toxic materials safely and substituting less dangerous materials, if possible.
  ➢ Complying with medical waste regulations.
  ➢ Keeping the number of employees exposed to dangerous situations at a minimum.
  ➢ Providing and encouraging use of personal protective clothing and equipment, such as eye goggles, disposable and mesh gloves.
  ➢ Providing alarm and monitoring systems.
  ➢ Designing work processes to minimize hazards.
  ➢ Planning, completing and acting upon regularly scheduled hazard inspections.
  ➢ Providing grounds, street and sidewalk safety.
  ➢ Complying with the Safe Drinking Water Act.

- Establishing a practice for emergency procedures.
- Investigating and reporting all accidents.
- Providing a good example in safe practice and habits.

- OSHA recommends employers establish workplace safety and health committees with membership including executives, supervisors and employees. Committees should meet at least monthly. Duties of the committee can include:
  - Developing procedures to handle safety suggestions.
  - Physically inspecting workplaces, one area at a time.
  - Conducting meetings to address accident prevention and other safety practices.
  - Investigating accidents and making recommendations to avoid future recurrences.
  - Providing workplace information on safe habits and practices (i.e., hand-washing signs and hand-washing sinks and soaps.)
  - Developing and revising safety rules and an emergency plan.
  - Recommending equipment, physical workplace changes to improve safety.
  - Promoting safety and first aid training and health and safety programming.
  - Maintaining records.

- Desirable safety features for equipment include the following:
  - Smooth, rounded corners on work surfaces; smooth, polished, welded seams, rounded corners and knee-lever drain controls on sinks; and table drawers with stops and recessed pulls.
  - Temperature controls; automatic steam shut-off when cooker doors open; side lift handles and condensation control devices for steam kettles; safety catches for steamer doors so that opening is not possible without first releasing steam.
  - Guards on slicers and chopping machines; brakes on mixers; recessed control knobs on ranges and ovens.
  - Wheel locks for mobile equipment.
  - All electrical equipment grounded; wiring not open or vulnerable to wear and tear.
  - Gooseneck venting on coffee urns so hot water overflows will not burn employees or customers.
  - Safety pilot lights and adequate venting for gas equipment.
  - Walk-in refrigerators and freezers that open from the inside.
  - Safe and adequate lighting.
  - Electrical cords that are intact, secure, and do not extend across work areas, traffic patterns or floors.
  - Sprinklers or water system over equipment that have open flames.

- General **LIGHTING REQUIREMENTS**: 70 foot-candles in areas for inspecting, checking and pricing; 50 foot-candles for dishwashing area; 30 foot-candles for general lighting. A **FOOT-CANDLE** is a measure of incandescent light.

(3) Personal work habits

- Employees must wear clean, safe clothing, with minimal jewelry, and closed, cushioned or rubber-soled shoes to avoid accidents (i.e., no apron ties or scarves that could get caught in equipment or necklaces that could dangle into a pot of soup.)

- In-service training should address work habits, including orientation of new employees, safety, sanitation, toxic chemical handling, and proper use and cleaning of equipment.

- Physical fitness of employees should be reviewed to ensure that they can perform assigned duties. New employees should be tested for tuberculosis before working with food. Some institutions require stool cultures for ova and parasites.

- Operational procedures and personal practices of employees should be observed to ensure compliance with safety standards.

- Disease transmission should be explained and safe work and food-handling practices, especially proper hand-washing technique, emphasized.

- Employees with colds, flu or other communicable diseases should not be allowed to work.

b. Safety practices

(1) Environmental conditions

- Equipment and physical facilities must be regularly inspected for safety.

- Permits, regulations and reports must be in compliance with regulations.

- Adequate hot-pads, long-handled spoons and so forth must be provided to avoid burns and scalding when preparing or serving foods.

- First-aid supplies and working fire extinguishers must be available and accessible.

(2) Regulations

- Assuring safety is the employer's responsibility.
  - Walk-in refrigerators can be opened from the inside.
  - Hot/cold water units and pipes, compressors, condensers and heat-producing units are insulated.
  - All sink drains must be indirectly connected to waste water mains.
  - Food and non-food items are properly labeled and stored separately.
  - Traffic through food preparation and service areas is controlled.
  - Pertinent safety practices are implemented.

- The **OCCUPATIONAL SAFETY AND HEALTH ACT (OSHA)** is also called the William-Steiger Safety and Health Act of 1970. The objective is to "assure safe and healthful working conditions for working men and women." Each employer must comply with safety and health standards, rules and regulations applicable to his or her operation. Inspections are conducted to check compliance under the following conditions:
  - There has been a catastrophe or fatality at the facility.
  - An employee complains of a hazard to safety or health.
  - The establishment is a "target industry." OSHA has identified bakery equipment as a special industry with particular rules.
  - The establishment is chosen as part of a random check.

- All establishments should have a current OSHA compliance manual.

(3) Fire safety

- Flammable or combustible materials should be stored away from heat sources.

- Fire exits should be well marked and unlocked at all times.

- Store oily rags in covered metal containers.

- Newer kitchens are required to have overhead sprinkler systems. Older kitchens should be evaluated to update present systems.

- Facilities must have accessible, up-to-date fire extinguishers approved by the **NATIONAL FIRE PROTECTION ASSOCIATION (NFPA)**, clearly marked as to type and proper usage. Check smoke alarms monthly.

- Employers should hold fire drills and employees should be trained to use fire extinguishers.

- All fire extinguishers should be checked annually by the local fire department. Fire extinguishers should be inspected and re-charged after every use.

- Clean range, oven hoods, and filters regularly.

- All electrical equipment and outlets should be in good repair.

FIRES AND EXTINGUISHERS

Combustible Material	Class of Fire	Type of Extinguisher	Markings
Wood, paper, cloth, cardboard, dry chemicals, plastic	Class A	Foam, soda acid, pump, gas cartridge, multipurpose	Triangle with capital letter A
Flammable liquids (cleaning supplies, grease, liquid shortening, oil)	Class B	Foam, carbon dioxide, multipurpose or ordinary dry chemical	Square with capital letter B
Electrical equipment (motors, switches, wires, frayed cords appliances)	Class C	Carbon dioxide, multipurpose or ordinary dry chemical	Circle with capital letter C
Combustible metals	Class D	Special extinguishing agents approved by recognized testing laboratories	Star with capital letter D

Note: There are also some multi-purpose extinguishers that carry multiple symbols.

IV. FOODSERVICE SYSTEMS (17%)

- Fire extinguishers are to be used different ways depending on what is to put out the fire.
  - ➢ Foam – Spray over fire.
  - ➢ Carbon dioxide – Spray at edge of fire first, then move toward the center.
  - ➢ Soda acid, gas cartridge, dry chemical – Direct at base of fire.

(4) Accident prevention

- The responsibilities of employer and employee delineated under universal precautions will help prevent accidents. All accidents must be reported according to OSHA rules.

c. Safety documentation and record keeping

- OSHA directives include the following:
  - ➢ Report all work-related accidents and illnesses and maintain records for five years.
  - ➢ Information must be kept current and posted annually.
  - ➢ Advise employees of their rights under OSHA.
  - ➢ Document the safety self-inspection program in writing.

TOPIC D - EQUIPMENT and FACILITY PLANNING

1. Facility layout

a. Equipment and layout planning

(1) Menu

- A facility should be planned and equipment selected after the basic menu determinations are made. If the menu determines the design and equipment, the results will be lower operating costs, greater productivity, more efficient service and higher quality products.

- Menu items should be selected to ensure a workload that is evenly distributed at work stations, resulting in an orderly and timely flow of production. A well-organized flow between processes minimizes steps, time and transport between work areas.

(2) Service system

- Food must be delivered quickly and in peak condition to the customer. The serving area may be in the kitchen itself, at various preparation centers where servers pick up orders for table service or assemble trays, or in a pantry or serving unit adjacent to or removed from the kitchen. In a cafeteria, the length and number of counters, the number of people served, the type of menu and the speed of service must be considered.

- Location is a major factor in marketing and sales potential of a facility. Whether the food service facility is within a building that houses other operations, is freestanding, is an existing building, or is being built to specifications, location must be considered. Location also influences sign design and appearance, road access and parking which, in turn, influences volume of business.

(3) Safety and sanitation

- Work areas should be designed to encourage optimal safety and sanitation.
  - ➤ Main traffic aisles should be a minimum of 5 feet wide or wide enough for carts and hand trucks to pass without interfering with workers in the area.
  - ➤ Aisles between equipment and worktables should have a clearance of at least 3 feet.
  - ➤ The area in front of ovens or kettles where contents are emptied should be 3½ to 4 feet across and deep.
  - ➤ Work aisles should be perpendicular to or parallel with main traffic aisles but separated from them.
  - ➤ Worktable heights are 36-41 inches for standing tasks and 28-30 for sitting tasks.
  - ➤ A minimum of 4 linear feet of workspace is recommended for each employees work area; 6 feet is preferable.
  - ➤ Maximum table reach for equipment should be 20 inches.
  - ➤ The highest shelf should be no more than 6 feet high.
  - ➤ Have non-skid step stools available.

- It should be arranged logically to allow specific areas for basic functions - with receiving away from the dining area; storage near receiving and kitchen; kitchen near dining; bar adjacent to dining; and clean-up area near kitchen, but away from food preparation area. The design should also allow for an office and an employee lounge or locker room. The flow of work and traffic patterns in serving and dining areas is crucial. The amount of room allocated to various areas depends on the type of facility.

- Special needs of physically-challenged persons should be considered. Handicapped access and restroom facilities may be a part of mandated codes.

(4) Privacy/accessibility

- A security system should be designed to meet specific needs (i.e., to protect fine wine, valuable art, china) as well as to guard cash and equipment and maximize food security and minimize the threat of deliberate contamination.

- Both outdoor and interior areas should be well lit.

- Metal or hard-core external doors and windows with metal frames are more secure than hollow-core doors and wooden windows. Exterior doors should have dead bolt locks.

- An alarm system should contact police, a security firm or the company headquarters if security is breached. Security cameras can monitor exterior doors and doors to store rooms and equipment rooms to avoid theft. Provisions should be made so storerooms (including refrigerators, liquor storage, etc.) can be kept locked.

- Most operations have internal security systems, such as a safe, for storing valuables.

- Prisons and facilities for the mentally ill have unique security needs and regulations' particularly concerning knives, sharp objects, hazardous equipment and locked doors.

(5) Codes and standards

- Construction should comply with federal, state and local building codes.

- The JCAHO standard reads, "The dietetic department/service is designed and equipped to facilitate the safe, sanitary and timely provision of food service to meet the nutritional needs of patients. The facilities and equipment of the dietetic department/service are in compliance with applicable sanitation and safety law and regulation."

- Facility requirements include:
  - Participation by all personnel in relevant in-service education and training programs.
  - Storage of food and non-food supplies under sanitary and secure conditions.
  - Food and non-food items stored separately.
  - Dishes and utensils cleaned in an area apart from food preparation.
  - Adequate space and equipment for preparation and food distribution, including modified diets.

- If federally funded, a facility must accommodate and offer employment to physically challenged individuals according to the Americans with Disabilities Act of 1990. Floor plans, access routes, doorways and aisles, tables, sinks and water fountains, etc. should be sized and placed to allow those in wheelchairs to use the facility.

(6) Fiscal aspects

- Economic factors play a large role in planning for equipment and layout because these factors influence selection of not only the design but the type of service as well.
  - Employee wages should be compared with costs of automation and convenience food to choose the type of service that will be best for the facility.
  - Costs of energy should be considered.

- Efficient use of labor is important for work flow.

- Good traffic flow allows more people to be served in a given period of time.

- Space should be made adaptable to varied uses in the event that needs change.

b. Planning team

(1) Composition

- The facility planning team generally includes an owner or representative of the institution, an architect, food facilities consultant, builder, food service operator and/or dietitian.

(2) Roles

- The architect/engineer interprets ideas of management and translates them into a physical plan. The architect provides knowledge of architectural and engineering principles, guides selection of designs and materials, prepares plans and specifications and guides construction. The architect is aware of codes and designs the facility to plan for compliance.

- The food facilities consultant guides preliminary goal-setting policies and procedures. This specialist can assist in developing an efficient operation, choosing equipment, meeting standards of safety and sanitation and providing an appropriate environment.

- The dietitian/food service operator must be experienced in operating a facility and be well informed in food management. The dietitian provides input as to functions, type of service and organization of work that influence the design.

- The owner/representative assesses need and arranges financing, reviews essential data in order to make decisions and has the final authority on plans and expenditures.

- The builder or contractor provides input regarding materials, construction features and contractual arrangements, including building permits; often subcontracts specific portions of building to electrical, plumbing, heating or other contractors; and supervises the actual construction.

(3) Responsibilities

- See roles and responsibilities described above.

2. Equipment specifications and selection

- Factors to be considered in selection of equipment include:
  - Needs of particular organization's menu plan.
  - Number and type of clients served.
  - Form in which food is purchased.
  - Style of service, length of serving period.
  - Number of labor hours.
  - Employee skills.
  - Accessibility and cost of utilities.
  - Budget.
  - Floor plan and space.
  - Adherence to codes and standards.
  - Type and amount of energy available.
  - Most food service equipment requires replacement after 9-14 years with dish machines, fryers, ovens, ranges and refrigerators expected to last 10 years.
  - Compliance with federal, state and local regulations and industry standards including National Sanitation Foundation (NSF), Underwriter's Laboratory (UL) or others.

- The CAPITAL VALUE of a piece of equipment is spread over a given number of years for accounting and planning purposes, estimating less value as the condition of the equipment declines. The accepted durability of equipment for accounting purposes is ten years, at a depreciation rate of 10% per year. Budgeting for replacement of equipment is based on projected years of life, depreciation, costs of maintenance and repair and the availability of new equipment with additional features such as added speed or added functions that reduce labor costs.

- A RANGE is a set of burners for heating food. Controls should be reached easily and should be located away from the heat. Handles should be made of nonheat-conducting material. Doors should be heavy-duty and balanced to prevent slamming. Hot tops use more energy to heat the heating plate, but offer more surface area for pots. Open burners are less costly, but each burner holds only one pot. All surfaces, including grease traps and vents, should be accessible for easy cleaning.

- **CONVECTION OVENS** cook faster and more evenly than traditional ovens, because a motor-driven fan circulates hot air within the oven. Stainless steel front and exterior are common, and doors may be glass or solid. Ovens are available with various sizes of fan motors. To prevent scalds, fans automatically turn off when doors open.

- **MICROWAVE OVENS** have been used in commercial food service for over 30 years. They are versatile, flexible, fast and an economical method for reheating frozen or prepared foods.
  - ➤ The oven operates through an electronic device known as a **MAGNETRON,** which produces high-frequency energy waves similar to radio or television transmission waves. A propeller produces an even wave pattern stirring the microwaves. Liquids in food absorb the wave energy; the electrons bounce around creating friction and heat.
  - ➤ Unevenness in the wave pattern results in hot and cold spots. Turning dishes and stirring food intermittantly help heat the entire food.
  - ➤ A microwave oven requires minimum floor space, less ventilation and less energy than conventional ovens. Reheating in a microwave can result in a 40-50% savings in energy costs over a range or oven. The amount of cooking power is controlled by wattage.
  - ➤ Microwave energy does not brown or caramelize food, but some ovens contain a heating element that will brown foods. A browning effect can be achieved on some foods with a commercial glazing preparation.
  - ➤ Ventilation is required for microwave cooking of many items. For example, baked potatoes must be pierced, and foods in plastic bags must be vented to release built-up steam.
  - ➤ Microwave cooking results are affected by quantity (small quantities cook faster than large quantities), temperature (warm foods cook faster than cold foods), shape (regular-shaped foods cook faster than irregular-shaped food) and density (porous foods cook faster than dense foods). In addition, salt, sugar, fat and water attract microwaves and speed cooking.

- **REFRIGERATION** is available in reach-in, walk-in, roll-in, pass-through, counter-top and display refrigerator configurations.

  - ➤ Good insulation helps conserve energy. Polyurethane is the most energy-efficient insulation. The thicker the insulation, the longer temperatures will be maintained. Energy is conserved because the compressor will run less.
  - ➤ Large compressors will maintain temperature better in hot and humid weather. A top-mounted compressor on a reach-in refrigerator permits relocation of the cabinet and makes it easier to clean and maintain.
  - ➤ Handles should be durable and have a safety grip. Vertical handles are easier to use because of the natural grip, but horizontal handles may be more durable with heavy kitchen traffic. Recessed handles are recommended in areas where handles may be damaged by moving equipment or supplies or where employees may bump into them.
  - ➤ Airflow is essential for maintaining uniform humidity and temperature levels in refrigeration units. Multiple air outlets provide maximum air circulation. Care should be taken not to block air outlets with refrigerator contents and not to line shelves with foil or pans that block circulation. This would cause the compressor to run more frequently to maintain temperature, thus increasing energy usage and potential compressor burnout.

- **WALK-IN REFRIGERATION** (includes refrigerators and freezers) uses poured-foam insulation, rather than frothed-in-place polyurethane, to assure an even temperature distribution.

  ➢ Doors should have cam-lift, self-closing hinges so they close and seal with a gentle nudge. Magnetic door gaskets ensure a tight seal. Inside safety releases should be checked for ease of operation. Heater wires in doors prevent accumulation of frost, ice or condensation.
  ➢ Shelving may be built-in or placed in separately. Stainless steel, louvered shelving is good for cleaning and air circulation. Shelving on casters facilitates cleaning.
  ➢ The amount of storage space needed is calculated by dividing the total amount of food to be stored (in pounds) by 15 (the pounds of food that can be stored in a cubic foot of storage):

  Total pounds food stored ÷ 15 = Space required in cubic feet

  ➢ One cubic foot can store up to 30 lb. of food, but 15 lb./cu. ft. is used in this formula to allow for wasted space for aisles, air circulation and unused space between containers and shelving.
  ➢ Walk-in units should have a door release from the inside and an emergency bell so that a person does not become trapped in a refrigerator or freezer.

- A **BLAST CHILLER** is designed to rapidly cool almost any type of food. This piece of equipment uses forced cold air to bring products from above 140°F to below 40°F in 90 minutes or less.

  ➢ It is typically used in cook-chill food service operations, but is increasingly seen in many kinds of food service operations because it helps meet important HACCP standards.
  ➢ The capacity of a blast chiller per load equals the number of persons the chiller can serve for 3 meals a day.

- The **ICE MACHINE** uses water and electricity to make ice.

  ➢ Ice is considered a food and must be handled like a food. The ice machine should be emptied, cleaned and sanitized regularly.
  ➢ A total system has 3 major components, ice production, storage and dispensing. Ice production may be as flakes or cubes. Ice storage, generally capacities from 400-500 pounds that refill automatically or manually. Stand or floor models must be insulaed and have a drain. Counter dispensers move ice from storage to glass (gravity feed is common.)
  ➢ Ice machines are rated according to the amount of ice the machine produces within a 24-hour period.

  Total ice available = Storage bin + the amount the ice machine can produce during peak periods

  ➢ Placement considerations for the ice machine include water source and drain , proximity to point of use, a cool, dry area, and adequate ventilation for the compressor.

- The selection of the size and type of **DISH MACHINE** depends on institutional needs, energy costs, space, supplies and labor. Low-temperature machines sanitize dishes through chemicals rather than heat. Blowers are used for air-drying dishes. Wiping dishes or utensils with cloths or towels destroys the sanitation of the dishwashing process. Booster heaters may be required if the hot water source is greater than 5 feet from the dish machine.

- Some operations use only a manual system for dishwashing, and some pieces of equipment (pots, pans and some utensils) require manual washing. In these instances, the equipment and utensils should be washed in a three-compartment sink using the following steps:
  1. Scrape or rinse any food or other debris from the equipment/utensil. Soak as needed to complete this process.
  2. Wash in warm soapy water (110°F or 42°C) in the first compartment using a sponge, scrubber or other appropriate tool.
  3. Rinse (dip in or spray with water) in the second compartment to remove all soap and food residues.
  4. Sanitize in the third compartment using either hot water or an appropriate sanitizer. If water is to be used, it should be 171°F (77°C), for at least 30 seconds. Chemical sanitizers such as chlorine (often in the form of bleach), iodine or quaternary ammonium compounds (quats) may also be used. The use of chemical sanitizers is dependent on water temperature, pH, water hardness, sanitizer concentration and contact time.
  5. Air dry all items.

- **FRYERS** should be chosen with production needs and safety in mind. Fryers may be gas fired or electric, freestanding counter models or built-in units. Capacities range from 15-130 lb. The type of fat used will vary. Accurate thermostats and fast heat-recovery features help ensure product quality and prevent fat deterioration. The **COLD ZONE** is the area in which crumbs and sediment fall. An accessible drain for removing and filtering fat and cleaning the fryer is an important feature.

- **PRESSURE FRYERS** cook more rapidly than conventional fryers because food cooks more quickly under pressure. The moisture given off by food or steam is retained during the cooking process, thus reducing the cooking time. The fat in a pressure fryer is not exposed to air, so heat is not lost. Tightly sealed lids are required to maintain pressure during operation.

- A **TILTING BRAISING PAN** is used to boil, stew, braise, grill or moist-heat roast. It has many other uses, such as grilling hamburgers, roasting turkeys and boiling eggs. Open-leg models are generally easy to clean and provide maximum access to operating parts. Counter and cabinet models are also available. Manual and power tilt models facilitate pouring off liquids and/or draining the pan. The distance between the gas or electric burners and the cooking surface determines energy efficiency. A condensate vent in the lid allows steam to be released without raising the cover.

- The **STEAM-JACKETED KETTLE** has a shell of stainless steel enclosing chemically pure water and rust inhibitors. The principle is the same as a double boiler -- controlled heat with little chance of burning the food. Steam-jacketed kettles are available in many sizes. A reliable thermostat and a pressure gauge are essential for the steam kettle. Tilting kettles provide a safe, easy method for removing heavy food items from the bowl. Many kettles have a tangent draw-off option that allows foods, like soup, to be released through a faucet at the bottom of the kettle.

- A **GRIDDLE** transfers heat from a burner to the griddle surface and then to the food. Griddles may be gas or electric, flat or sloped, grooved or smooth. Splash guards and a surface sloped toward the grease drawer protect the operator from splatters and prevent grease build-up.

- **PRESSURE STEAMERS** are available with one, two or three compartments that usually operate with three to five pounds of pressure. Safety valves release pressure if it reaches eight pounds. Automatic timers are used to prevent overcooking.

- **CONVECTION STEAMERS** supply steam continuously to an enclosed compartment, thereby creating a uniform flow and a consistently cooked product. The steamers provide a uniform temperature (212°F) directly across food at a high velocity. The steam blows condensation off cooking food instantly, vents out the cooled steam and replaces it with freshly heated steam. This process prevents a layer of cool air from forming above the cooking product. Since there is no pressure build-up, the door of a convection steamer can be opened at any time during a cooking cycle.

- A **COMBINATION OVEN/STEAMER** offers a single cooking chamber with the ability to cook in three cooking modes: hot air mode (convection oven); steam mode (convection pressure-less steamer); or a combination of both modes (circulating hot air with superheated steam.) The "combi-oven", as it is often called, may cook in all three modes independently, or in sequence, moving from one mode to another depending on the menu item. It is available in both gas and electric models.

- **SLICERS** usually have bases made of anodized aluminum, which is durable under normal operating conditions. Stainless steel blades or knives must be durable and maintain their sharpness. Blade width is determined by needs. Most are available with automatic and manual feed. Employee training about proper operating techniques, blade guard removal and cleaning and sanitizing procedures are necessary and will enhance safety. Slicers, when used continuously, should be cleaned and sanitized every four hours.

- **MIXERS** are essential equipment for production of entrées, mashed vegetables, desserts and baked goods. They come in sizes ranging from 5-to 20-quart bowls in bench models to 140-quart bowls in floor models. Capacity should be based on volume needs, space available and handling convenience.
  - ➤ Attachments for chopping, slicing and grinding increase versatility and are especially useful in smaller facilities that do not have separate pieces of equipment.
  - ➤ Bowls are raised or lowered by hand lifts on small machines and by power lifts on large machines. Transmissions allow speed changes while the mixer is operating.
  - ➤ Standard equipment on most mixers is one open-rim bowl (either heavily tinned or stainless steel), which facilitates easy cleaning and sanitizing. Tinned bowls are less expensive but not as durable.

- **VENT HOODS** are designed to exhaust 100% of the air above cooking equipment through exhaust ducts that lead outside of the food service area.
  - ➤ The size of hood is determined by the size of the equipment covered and by health and fire laws.
  - ➤ Clearance between the equipment and the hood should be enough to allow for

employee safety and efficient exhaust. Generally, a minimum of 6-ft 3- inches and a maximum of 7- ft are recommended as the distance between floor and lower edges of hoods.

➤ Large amounts of broiling and frying require calibrated exhaust hoods.

➤ Underwriters Laboratories (UL) rates apply to exhaust ratios. Failure to keep vents clean is a common sanitation violation and a potential fire hazard due to accumulation of grease.

- The capacity and motor size of a **WASTE DISPOSER** must be planned to meet the type and volume of food waste generated.

- **SOFT-SERVE ICE CREAM FREEZERS** are popular in many types of food service operations, especially schools and cafeterias. Care must be taken to select models that can be cleaned and sanitized correctly.

- The **COFFEE URN** heats water that is sprayed over coffee grounds and then allowed to drip through a paper, cloth or fine aluminum screen filter. Liners should be durable and removable for easy cleaning. Energy requirements should be evaluated. Lower amp and BTU requirements mean lower energy usage.

- Commercial **TOASTERS** efficiently provide high-quality toast with minimal energy usage. Production needs will determine the type of toaster to use. Pop-up toasters are less expensive, but conveyor toasters provide twice the volume of toast.

Preventive maintenance

- Information related to the purchase, recommended maintainence, warranty and repair of all equipment should be in a permanent record that is accessible.

- A maintenance and inspection schedule should be developed for all pieces of equipment, along with a mechanism for documenting these procedures. Records should be reviewed regularly to ensure compliance with the schedule and monitor for recurring issues with equipment maintenance. Frequent repairs may indicate need for replacement of equipment.

- To maximize usefulness, minimize repair and prolong the life of major equipment, use the following measures:

➤ Show a video or demonstrate equipment use and care to each employee who will handle the equipment, following the manufacturer's instructions.

➤ Appoint a single person to be responsible for maintenance (inspections, lubrication) of major equipment.

➤ Post special instructions or warnings related to the equipment, especially on equipment that gets hot or has sharp surfaces.

➤ Provide instruction manuals on the operation and care of equipment.

➤ Post simple instructions about the operation and cleaning of equipment. Use visuals demonstrating steps if literacy is an issue.

➤ Provide employees training on the proper operation, cleaning and sanitizing of equipment. Training in the language appropriate to the learner is desirable.

➤ Consider using **MAINTENANCE AGREEMENTS** (service agreements), which may save the facility the cost of employing skilled maintenance personnel and an inventory of spare parts. These agreements should specify what both parties entering into the agreement (i.e., response time, cost, convenience) should expect.

- A **WARRANTY** is a written statement provided by the manufacturer that guarantees a standard of performance for a given period of time and protects the purchaser from equipment defects. A warranty does not guarantee protection from wear occurring due to normal use during the warranty period. A warranty is a written guarantee of labor and parts, duration and conditions. The definition of parts may be limited. Some warranties cover replacement of defective parts only, not the labor to replace them.

- A **SERVICE CONTRACT** extends the coverage of a warranty after an initial phase for an additional cost. A service contract provides preventive maintenance and all repairs, including labor, for the duration of the contract.

- An easily accessible **REPAIR RECORD** should be available for each piece of equipment. It should specify type of equipment; trade name; manufacturer; model, serial and motor number; energy source; capacity; attachments; supplier; purchase price; new or used at purchase; guarantee or warranty; service agreement or free service period; and dates, cost and description of repairs.

Cleaning and care

- Equipment surfaces should be smooth and free of breaks, open seams, cracks, chips, pits and other imperfections. They should be free of difficult-to-clean internal corners and crevices.

- Food-contact surfaces of equipment should be accessible for cleaning and inspection without being disassembled (i.e., meat slicers). If equipment must be disassembled, simple tools should be kept near the equipment. Manuals for equipment should be available and employees should be trained to maintain equipment. Ease of assembly and cleaning should be a consideration when purchasing equipment.

- Equipment designed for in-place cleaning should allow cleaning and sanitizing solutions to be circulated throughout a fixed system to reach all interior food-contact surfaces. Equipment should have sealed electrical connections when pressure spray cleaning is used. Removing soil efficiently, effectively and safely must be balanced with environmental concerns. Price should not be the major determinant.

- Basic phases in determining cleaning efficacy are:
  1. Penetration of soil is established by wetting agents: water, soaps or detergents.
  2. Suspension loosens soil and flushes it away without being re-deposited. Fat requires an emulsifier; protein requires peptizing action that prevents "rings" or spots, as on glassware; sugars and salts are easily removed because they are water-soluble.
  3. Rinsing must remove soil and all traces of cleaning agents. This is usually effectively done with hot water and drying agents that eliminate film and streaks.

- Considerations regarding cleaning solutions include:
  - Care must be taken to use appropriate cleaners in correct amounts of dilutions. Some cleaners come in dispensers that release the right amounts for a single use.
  - Polyphosphate detergents are highly acceptable and provide a wide variety of options; some are non-toxic germicidals. Selection is determined largely by the hardness of the water.
  - Basic alkalis, such as caustic soda and soda ash, have poor water softening and rinsing qualities and high corrosive properties. Trisodium phosphate (TSP) is a good cleaning agent but leaves film and is harsh on hands and the environment.

- ➤ Abrasives and solvents may be necessary to remove some substances.
- ➤ Cleaning solutions should never be kept in the same containers or storage areas as food items. Cleaning solutions should be kept in the original labeled containers, in a locked cabinet distant from food handling areas.
- ➤ A utility sink should be provided for cleaning needs. Food preparation or hand washing sinks should never be used for cleaning chores.
- ➤ Many companies (i.e., Ecolab) that sell institutional cleaning supplies offer consultation as to appropriate products for specific facilities and provide training for employees.

Energy requirements

- Specifications should require equipment to meet exact voltages. There should be a separate electric plan for equipment, in addition to basic electrical needs,such as lighting. Equipment performance will be affected if electrical cycles are not accurate. The equipment should not cause failure of lights, refrigeration or cause other power outages.

- Charts are available from manufacturers to show output- per-hour for each size of machine. For example, the number of dishes that can be washed in an hour measures capacity of a dishwasher; the size of a mixer to be purchased is determined by volume per batch, mixing time and total quantity that can be produced in one hour. Most equipment comes in standard sizes and shapes that are adaptable to kitchen design and replacement.

Equipment selection

- The **JOINT COMMITTEE OF FOOD EQUIPMENT STANDARDS** states that equipment must be designed and constructed to exclude vermin, dust, dirt and splash or spillage from food that cannot under normal-use conditions be easily cleaned, maintained and serviced. Sanitation is encouraged by use of proper materials and construction (i.e., if on legs,equipment must be 6-8 inches off the floor). Proper spacing of equipment encourages safety. Local building, plumbing, electrical and sanitation codes apply to contractors installing equipment. Water, gas, waste-pipe lines, steam and electrical conduits must be planned for each piece of equipment to avoid interference with cleaning or placement of other equipment.

- Portable equipment, such as blenders, should be small and light enough to be moved easily by one person. It should have no utility connection, a utility connection that easily disconnects, or a flexible utility connection line of sufficient length to permit the equipment to be moved easily.

- Stationary equipment should be sealed to the table or counter or elevated on legs, with clearance, to facilitate cleaning. It may be floor mounted (sealed to the floor), installed on a raised platform or elevated on legs. Clearances of 6 inches from the floor and 12-24 inches from the wall will allow room for cleaning. Equipment may be cantilevered, projecting from the wall with only one end supported.

- Food service equipment must be installed in compliance with codes and according to the design on the blueprint.

Materials

- Durability of frames and of functional parts of equipment should be equal over the life of the equipment. For materials, aluminum and stainless steel are preferred for food service equipment. The American Society of Testing Materials (ASTM) sets standards of materials that can withstand unusual loads or stress. The American Society of Mechanical Engineers (ASME) sets safety standards for equipment using steam. The American Gas Association (AGA) sets criteria for seals on equipment meeting their standards.

- GAUGE is the thickness of a metal. It should be considered when selecting equipment. Thicker metal is tmore expensive, equipment and the gauge number is lower. Numbers 10 and 14 are most commonly used for food service equipment.

- GRIT refers to sandpaper used to polish stainless steel; No. 100 grit (polish) is comparable to a No. 4 finish.

- Finishes for stainless steel are:
  - No. 1: dull and rough
  - No. 2b: full finish, bright
  - No. 2d: full finish, dull
  - No. 4: Standard finish for food service equipment
  - No. 6: soft, velvety finish
  - No. 7: high glossy polish

- INCOLOY is a heat-conducting metal alloy that coats most heating element tubes and promotes efficient energy transfer. Quartz-sheathed tubes produce instantaneous heat, but the tubes are breakable and have a shorter life span.

- Other materials used for food service equipment include:
  - BRASS is a mixture of copper and steel.
  - MONEL is a mixture of nickel and copper.
  - ACRYLIC, LUCITE and PLEXIGLASS are usually clear; they are often used for covers, shields and sneeze guards.
  - MELAMINE is a form of plastic used for dishes and trays; it is durable, easily cleaned and lightweight.
  - FIBERGLASS is a combination of resin with glass for a durable substance.
  - POLYETHYLENE is the thermoplastic used for storage containers.
  - POLYPROPYLENE is a thermoplastic that can withstand high temperature; it is often used for dishwasher racks and cutting boards.
  - POLYSTYRENE cannot withstand high temperatures, it melts at 160°F; it is used for disposable cups (Styrofoam). There are environmental concerns about the lack of biodegradability and toxic chemicals released when polystyrene is burned.

COMPARISON OF MATERIALS USED FOR FOODSERVICE EQUIPMENT

Material	Advantages	Disadvantages
Wood	Cuts noise, attractive	Absorbs moisture and odors; hard to clean; encourages micro-organism growth
Copper	Conducts heat well and rapidly; attractive when clean	Needs polishing after use; very heavy, therefore makes equipment heavy; reacts with some food causing color changes
Aluminum	Easily fabricated; can be finished, etched or engraved; lightweight; withstands high temperatures and pressures; is hard and durable; does not corrode easily; has high thermal and electrical conductivity	Reacts with high-acid or alkaline foods and can discolor foods; if lightweight can dent or bow
Cast iron	Retains heat, cooks evenly; may impart some iron to food cooked in it.	Heavy; requires seasoning to avoid rusting; must be hand washed
Galvanized steel (combination of steel, chromium,	Steel and iron coated with zinc so it is less likely to corrode; common material for waste containers	Hard to clean; coating subject to wear
Stainless steel (combination of steel, chromium, nickel, carbon)	Quality material for foodservice; does not stain; cooks and cleans Well; durable if heavy enough well; durable if heavy enough	Expensive

TOPIC E – SUSTAINABILITY

- **SUSTAINABILITY** is based on the principle of meeting needs of the present without compromising the needs of the future and preserving natural ecology. A **SUSTAINABLE FOOD AND AGRICULTURE SYSTEM** helps to improve the health of the community by working together to have a locally-based and self-reliant system.

- The conservation of natural resources has become an important consideration for food and nutrition professionals. In healthcare, food service and community settings food and nutrition professionals are in a unique position to address conservation and sustainability issues.

- In many communities there is a degree of food insecurity because many to not have access to wholesome food because it is not affordable or because it is unavailable. These are often in low income areas and poor urban communities.

1. Food and water

- Conventional (industrial) agriculture practices, while capable of producing large quantities of food, can also negatively impact the natural environment in a variety of ways:
  - ➢ Excessive tilling, irrigation, heavy machinery and overgrazing of livestock can result in the depletion of topsoil, which limits the land's fertility and capacity for food production.
  - ➢ Excessive pesticides, fertilizers and livestock waste, used or generated through conventional farming, can deplete and/or contaminate waterways, impacting human water supplies (aquifers and reservoirs) as well as damaging wildlife ecosystems contained in lakes, streams and oceans and their potential food sources
  - ➢ Excess agricultural chemicals can also disrupt other natural ecosystems and impact natural processes in the food system (i.e., pollination from birds, bees).
  - ➢ Modern industrial agriculture methods, that favor genetically uniform plants, can limit crop biodiversity. This can result in less resistance to pests, pathogens, disease and cause climate/environmental changes.

- Organic agricultural methods can decrease some of these impacts, as they employ method,s such as crop rotation, cover cropping, and the use of organic materials rather than chemical fertilizers and pesticides.

- Genetically-modified crops may have some increased resistance to diseases, pests and environmental changes but such biotechnology may also result in negative impacts on other natural ecosystems

- Consumers' food choices can have a direct impact on the sustainability of a food system. The production of vegetable protein sources has been shown to be significantly more conservation-oriented and sustainable than animal-based proteins in both the energy used and the land needed to produce equal amounts. Also, livestock that is pasture-fed has been shown to use half as much energy to raise than grain-fed counterparts.

- Dietitians who work in local communities have to assess the local resources so they can educate the population about where they might access the most healthful food for the least amount of money. Nutrition professionals can encourage clients to make sustainable food choices including:

  - ➢ Eating a wide variety of whole foods.
  - ➢ Shopping at farmers' markets and other local locations that offer sustainably-produced foods, including heirloom varieties of crops. Many farmers' markets are accepting a SNAP card for payment.
  - ➢ Supporting food policies (at work and in the community) that encourage and maintain sustainable and locally based agriculture and food production systems including Community Supported Agriculture (CSA), farm to school, farm to college and/or farm to work programs, establish community gardens and cooperative buying programs.
  - ➢ Eating locally-grown foods reduces transportation costs and use of fuel.

- The conservation and protection of water supplies is vital, as water is essential to life and supplies are finite. Water supplies should be conserved to minimize the amount of polluted run-off generated, decrease impacts on wildlife habitats and ensure adequate supplies for the future. An added benefit of water conservation is decreased facility operating costs.

- Foodservice operations can decrease water usage through water efficient equipment (dish washers, etc.); spray nozzles and faucets with aerators and flow restrictors; and scraping foods from utensils, plates and equipment before rinsing or washing.

- Selecting food and beverages that require minimal packaging reduces waste. Filtered local water rather than bottled water is a sustainable option.

2. Non-food

a. Supplies

- Supplies should be purchased with sustainability in mind. This includes considering re-usable options (as opposed to disposable) when appropriate. Cost analyses should examine the feasibility of this, for example, reusable flatware and/or linens may cost more up front but reduce the cost of continuous purchasing down the road. Cost of maintenance should also be considered, such as labor and water use for washing flatware and/or linens.

b. Equipment

- A major consideration for sustainability of equipment purchase and use is energy consumption. Food service operations use considerably more energy than other operations within a given facility. Further, as energy costs increase food service operations incur a larger percentage of such costs, as their primary input (food) will also increase in cost due to increased costs associated with production, processing and transport. This will be in addition to direct increases in utility and energy usage costs.

- Considerations for sustainable practices related to equipment in food service facilities include:
  - ➢ Purchasing energy efficient equipment such as those that meet the federal Energy Star standards.
  - ➢ Using energy efficient cooking methods such as microwave, induction cooking and "supercookers", that combine methods for efficient cooking.
  - ➢ Energy audits can evaluate how a particular facility uses energy and pinpoint areas for more efficient usage.
  - ➢ Use insulation. Insulation is measured as a **K FACTOR THAT** reflects thermal conductivity. Higher K numbers mean proportionately better insulation, or less energy usage.
  - ➢ Evaluate lighting. Use energy-efficient fluorescent lights where suitable, clean lights regularly, paint walls and ceilings in light colors to reflect light, turn off lights in inactive areas.

- Facilities can more efficiently use energy for existing equipment by:
  - ➢ Minimizing preheating time.
  - ➢ Using timers for cooking.
  - ➢ Maintaining equipment in good working order (replacing seals on ovens and

refrigeration units; calibrating thermometers and thermostats).
- ➤ Using appropriate type and size of cookware for each piece of equipment.
- ➤ Running equipment at full capacity.
- ➤ Turning equipment off when not in use
- ➤ Making sure all equipment is in working order. A slow drip from a hot water faucet can use 40KWH of electricity a month.
- ➤ Opening refrigerator, freezer and oven doors only when necessary. Magnetic gaskets ensure tight closure. Install external thermometers in refrigerators/freezers to allow temperature checks. Glass windows in ovens permit a visual check of oven contents.
- ➤ Consolidating food in refrigerators and freezers and disconnect units when not in use.
- ➤ Saving refrigerator energy by pre-cooling hot leftovers, placing the pan of hot food on ice water and stirring the food until cool. Energy savings are offset by some labor costs.
- ➤ Scheduling energy-intensive cooking, such as baking and roasting, during non-peak hours when energy costs per unit are lower.
- ➤ Loading and unloading ovens quickly.
- ➤ Placing kettles and pots close together on range tops to decrease heat loss.
- ➤ Using the smallest piece of cooking equipment possible.
- ➤ Installing low water cut-off devices in dishwashing machines.
- ➤ Replacing outdated equipment with newer, more efficient models.

- Planners must know which type of available energy (electric, gas) is best suited for a particular need (fast-food grill differs from prepare-to-order or cafeteria); how much is needed to achieve desired results (centralized kitchen with large volume versus small restaurant); alternative ways to achieve the same results (electric grill versus charcoal); cost (incandescent versus fluorescent lighting); insulation techniques; and when proper standards for energy use are met.

Measures of energy

- **AMPERE** is a measurement of cycles per second of the current (flow).

- **CURRENT** is the amount of energy flowing. In equations, "I" is used to indicate current.

- One **KILOWATT-HOUR (KWH)** is 1,000 watts of power consumed in one hour.

- Energy costs are based on KWH.

- One **OHM** is a measure of electrical resistance.

- **VOLT** is a measure of electrical potential equal to one ampere of current passing through one ohm of resistance.

- **WATT-HOUR** is a rate of power consumption.

- **WATT** is a unit of power in electricity. One watt is one ampere of current overcoming one volt of electrical potential.

- **AC**, or **ALTERNATING CURRENT**, flows in two directions and each reversal is one cycle. AC is produced in a generator called an alternator.

- **DC**, or **DIRECT CURRENT**, flows in one direction and is produced in batteries.

- **FREQUENCY** is the number of cycles per second of alternating current.

    60 cycles/second = 60 Hertz (HZ)

- **HORSEPOWER** is a unit for computing the power of an engine. 1 HP = 746 watts of power.

- **PSI** stands for pounds per square inch, a measurement of gas pressure and water pressure in dish machines.

- **BRITISH THERMAL UNIT (BTU)** is a measure of a quantity of heat. It takes one **BTU** of heat to raise the temperature of 1 lb of water by 1° F. 4 **BTU** = 1 calorie 1 **BTU** = 0.252 calories 1 kcal = 3,968 **BTU**

- One **CALORIE** is the amount of heat required to raise the temperature of 1g of water by 1° celsius. It takes one kilocalorie of heat to raise one kilogram of water by 1° Celsius. Food calories are kilocalories.

- **CELSIUS (C)** is a method of measuring temperature. One degree Celsius is 1/100 of the temperature range between the temperature water freezes (0°C) and the temperature water boils (100°C). Normal body temperature is 37°C. Celsius temperatures may also be referred to as degrees **CENTIGRADE**.

- **FAHRENHEIT (F)** identifies 32°F as the freezing point of water and 212°F as boiling point. There are 180 degrees Fahrenheit in between. Normal body temperature is 98.6°F, although an individual's normal body temperature may be slightly higher or lower.

Sources of energy

- A kilowatt of electricity produces 3,413 BTU. It takes 30,000 BTU (about 7,500 calories) for an electric range to bring a 10-gallon pot of water at 50°F (10°C) to boiling (212°F). About 13,500 BTU perform the heating; the rest is lost from the range top. This process uses nearly 9 kilowatts (30,717) BTU of energy.

- A gas range must produce more actual heat than electricity to do the same job. Electricity is said to be 100% efficient, while gas is 70-75% efficient.

- Gas is measured in cubic feet and **THERMS**.

    100 cubic feet of gas = 1 Therm = 1,052,000 BTU

- Steam equipment has higher usable heat efficiency than gas or electric equipment. Steam is measured in 1,000-pound lots or horsepower. One horsepower steam equals 34,000 BTU. To be competitive, the cost to generate steam must be about the same as a therm of gas or about 290 times more than a kilowatt of electricity. The energy cost is a factor when purchasing steam equipment.

Energy requirements

- To compare energy sources, all energy can be converted to BTUs:

Electricity (kWh)	=	**3,413 BTU**
Natural Gas (cubic ft)	=	**1,000 BTU**
Oil (gal)	=	**140,000 BTU**
Steam (lb)	=	**1,000 BTU**

- To estimate energy needs, one must conduct an energy survey. Estimating facility energy requirements is not generally the responsibility of an entry-level dietitian.

- To estimate energy requirements one must list all equipment using energy, and determine how long the equipment will use energy. For example, the nameplate might say 100,000 BTU per hour. Extrapolate to hours per day, days per week and kwh per week; then compute cubic feet per hour from BTU to arrive at cubic feet of gas used per hour. The number of cubic feet of gas needed per day and per week can be computed by multiplying cubic feet per hour times hours per day times days operated per week.

- Employees should be given specific instructions on energy-saving procedures, and their adherence must be tracked. A chart showing monthly British Thermal Unit (BTU) use, plus in-service training and incentive programs, will help keep employees interested and motivated in conserving energy.

Energy conservation

- Energy conservation can yield as much as 20% savings in food service operations. Choice of equipment, layout, insulation, maintenance and other factors are all variables in cost of energy used.

- Management must originate, plan and implement energy-saving programs, beginning with programs that show the greatest potential savings: heating, air-conditioning, cooking food and heating water. The ease of making changes should also be considered (i.e., changing lights to lower watt bulbs or energy-efficient bulbs). Management should consult with utility companies and/or engineers to conduct an energy audit with the goal of reducing costs.

3. **Waste management**

   a. **Storage**

- Storage of hazardous wastes that could have environmental impact should always be done in accordance with local, state and federal regulations. MSDS (Material Safety Data Sheets) should be maintained on-site for all hazardous waste.

- Waste should be stored in tightly covered containers and removed regularly. Sanitation procedures are necessary to avoid insects and rodents.

   b. **Reduction**

- Creation of less waste overall (source reduction) is the most desirable strategy for dealing with waste. This can be achieved by purchasing products with minimal packaging , using both sides of a page for printing, using less "disposable" products and other strategies.

- There are some excellent systems for pulverizing all products, except metals, in a slurry and then extracting the water to drastically reduce the amount of waste, however these systems are expensive to purchase at this time.

c. Disposal

- When waste generation is unavoidable, recycling or composting is the best option for dealing with it. Many types of materials can be recycled into other products and food waste can be composted or used as animal feed. Institutions have varied procedures for recycling waste materials.

- As a last and least desirable/sustainable option, waste can be land-filled or incinerated.

- Opportunities to decrease waste are dependent upon the specific facility and the type of waste that is usually generated. However it is done, it is usually cost efficient/effective, as there will be less money (and other forms of energy) spent overall on waste removal.

This page intentionally left blank.

PROBLEM-BASED LEARNING, 141
PROBLEM-ORIENTED MEDICAL RECORD, 339
PROBLEM-SOLVING, 362
PROCESS CHARTS, 403
PROCESS EVALUATION, 158
PROCESS-ORIENTED EVALUATION, 159
PROCUREMENT DECISIONS, 433
PRODUCTION SCHEDULING, 453
PRODUCTION SYSTEMS, 454
PRODUCTIVITY, 345, 349, 350, 384, 403
PROFESSIONAL STANDARDS OF PRACTICE, 364
PROFIT MARGIN, 384
PROFITABILITY, 388
PROFITABILITY RATIOS, 384
PROFIT-AND-LOSS STATEMENT, 389
PROGRAM PROMOTION, 145
PROPRIETORSHIP, 387
PROPYL GALLATE, 43
PROSPECTIVE PAYMENT SYSTEM, 386
PROSPECTIVE STUDIES, 167
PROTEIN CALORIE MALNUTRITION, 256
PROTEIN DEFICIENCY ANEMIA, 281
PROTEIN DIGESTIBILITY CORRECTED AMINO ACID SCORES, 68
PROTEIN EFFICIENCY RATIO, 69
PROTEIN ENERGY MALNUTRITION, 256
PROTEIN-BOUND IODINE, 199
PROTEINS, 10, 67
PSI, 491
PSYLLIUM, 104
PTEROYLGLUTAMIC ACID, 74
PUBLIC HEALTH PROGRAMS, 234
PULMONARY, 125
PULMONARY CAPACITY, 126
PULMONARY VOLUME, 126
PULSES, 19
PURGING, 250
QUALIFIED HEALTH CLAIMS, 61
QUALITATIVE EVALUATIONS, 158
QUALITATIVE RESEARCH, 168
QUALITATIVE STANDARDS, 360
QUALITY CIRCLES, 355
QUALITY PRACTICE, 327
QUANTITATIVE EVALUATIONS, 158
QUANTITATIVE STANDARDS, 360
QUANTITATIVE STUDIES, 166
QUASI-EXPERIMENTAL RESEARCH, 167
QUETELET INDEX, 203
QUICK METHOD, 32
QUINOA, 30
QUINONES, 79
RADIATION, 441
RADURA, 448
RANDOM, 166
RANDOM BLOOD GLUCOSE TEST, 264
RANDOM RATIO DELAY SAMPLING, 403
RANDOM SAMPLE, 169

RANDOMIZED CLINICAL TRIAL, 167
RANGE, 176, 478
RANKING, 53, 444
RAPPORT, 156
RATING SCALE METHOD, 380
RATIO SCALES, 177
RAW FOOD COST, 393
RAW MILK, 25
RAW SUGAR, 50
RDA, 72
READY-PREPARED, 454
READY-TO-EAT MEAL, 412
RECALLS, 469
RECEIVING AND STORAGE, 433
RECEIVING CLERK, 437
RECOMMENDED DIETARY ALLOWANCES, 72
RECORDS, 162, 437
RECRUITING, 365
RECTUM, 121
RED CELL DISTRIBUTION WIDTH, 208
REDUCED, 60
REDUCTION, 492
REFEEDING SYNDROME, 320
REFERRAL SYSTEM, 237
REFLECTIVE LISTENING, 151
REFLEXOLOGY, 325
REFLUX ESOPHAGITIS, 109
REFRAMING, 151
REFRIGERATED EXTENDED SHELF LIFE, 447
REFRIGERATION, 479
REGIONAL ENTERITIS, 283
REGIONAL ILEITIS, 283
REGRESSION, 177
REGULAR DIET, 301
REIKI, 326
REMOVED PLANNING, 347
RENAL, 122
RENAL CALCULI, 294
RENAL RICKETS, 257
RENNIN, 27
REPAIR RECORD, 484
REPEATED-MEASURE DESIGNS, 166
REPLICATION, 174
REPRODUCTIVE, 133
REQUISITION FORM, 440
RESEARCH, 164
RESIDUE, 65
RESOURCES ALLOCATION, 385
RESPIRATORY, 296
RESPIRATORY ACIDOSIS, 296
RESPIRATORY ALKALOSIS, 297
RESPIRATORY QUOTIENT, 119, 296
RESTAURANT MENUS, 410
RESTING ENERGY EXPENDITURE, 200
RESTING METABOLIC RATE, 200
RETAIL CUTS, 11
RETENTION STRATEGIES, 380
RETINOL, 78